INTENSIVE CARE NURSING

Current Clinical Nursing
Series

INTENSIVE CARE NURSING

Current Clinical Nursing
════════════════════ Series

BARBARA J. DALY, R.N., M.S.N.
Assistant Director
Medical-Surgical Nursing
University Hospitals of Cleveland;
Assistant Clinical Professor
Frances Payne Bolton School of Nursing
Case Western Reserve University
Cleveland, Ohio

 Medical Examination Publishing Co., Inc.
an Excerpta Medica company

969 Stewart Avenue • Garden City, New York 11530

Copyright © 1980 by
MEDICAL EXAMINATION
PUBLISHING CO., INC.
an **Excerpta Medica** company

Library of Congress Card Number
78-78019

ISBN 0-87488-575-2

January, 1980

Printed in the United States of America

SIMULTANEOUSLY PUBLISHED IN:

United Kingdom : HENRY KIMPTON PUBLISHERS
London, England

Contents

10 : SPECIAL PROBLEMS IN CRITICAL CARE: DIC
by Barbara J. Daly, R.N., M.S.N.

Preface

Intensive care nursing in today's world provides the practitioner with unique challenges and responsibilities. Unlike other intensive care texts, this book is *not* premised on a conviction that intensive care nurses must have abilities more profound or skills of a higher level than those required of other nurses. However, it is our belief that nursing has advanced beyond the state of "a nurse is a nurse." Consequently, intensive care nursing does require abilities and skills that *differ* in direction and emphasis from other areas of clinical nursing.

The new graduate, the practitioner who desires to update his or her knowledge, and the practitioner new to the intensive care unit often share a common need to focus and supplement their learning in those areas relevant to critical care. This book is designed to provide the knowledge base necessary for data collection, interpretation and decision making in the ICU. It is not designed to provide an in-depth explanation of any one disease entity, but rather, to provide a broader overview of most of the conditions commonly encountered by the intensive care nurse.

The purpose of this book arose from working with intensive care nurses, orienting new graduates and providing workshops for the continuing education of nurses in practice. The motivation and eagerness to learn that has been displayed by those individuals has been, in turn, the motivating force behind this endeavor.

Contributors

MARTHA L. ALLEN, R.N., M.S.N., *Administrative Nurse Clinician,* Medical Intensive Care Unit, University Hospitals of Cleveland, Cleveland, Ohio; *Clinical Instructor,* Frances Payne Bolton School of Nursing, Case Western Reserve University, Cleveland, Ohio.

SHARON HUDEC CONWAY, R.N., M.S.N., *Administrative Nurse Clinician,* University Hospitals of Cleveland, Cleveland, Ohio; *Clinical Instructor,* Frances Payne Bolton School of Nursing, Case Western Reserve University, Cleveland, Ohio.

BARBARA J. DALY, R.N., M.S.N., *Assistant Director,* Medical-Surgical Nursing, University Hospitals of Cleveland, Cleveland, Ohio; *Assistant Clinical Professor,* Frances Payne Bolton School of Nursing, Case Western Reserve University, Cleveland, Ohio.

SUSAN M. DAUM, R.N., B.S.N., *Clinical Nurse I,* University Hospitals of Cleveland, Surgical Intensive Care Unit, Cleveland, Ohio.

VIRGINIA BURKE KARB, R.N., M.S.N., *Assistant Professor,* Medical-Surgical Nursing, University of Virginia School of Nursing, Charlottesville, Virginia.

BENITA C. MARTOCCHIO, R.N., Ph.D., *Associate Professor,* Medical-Surgical Nursing, Frances Payne Bolton School of Nursing, Case Western Reserve University, Cleveland, Ohio; *Clinical Associate,* University Hospitals of Cleveland, Cleveland, Ohio.

MARY T. REYNOLDS, R.N., M.S., *Nurse Practitioner,* V.A. Medical Center, Cleveland, Ohio; *Assistant Clinical Professor,* Frances Payne Bolton School of Nursing, Case Western Reserve University, Cleveland, Ohio.

HELEN SCHAAG, R.N., M.S.N., *Nurse Clinician,* V.A. Medical Center, Cleveland, Ohio.

WINIFRED J. WALTER, R.N., M.S.N., *Assistant Clinical Professor,* Public Health Nursing, Frances Payne Bolton School of Nursing, Case Western Reserve University, Cleveland, Ohio.

MARY ALEXANDRA (Sandy) WYPER, R.N., M.S.N., *Instructor,* Medical-Surgical Nursing, Frances Payne Bolton School of Nursing, Case Western Reserve University, Cleveland, Ohio; *Clinical Associate,* University Hospitals of Cleveland, Cleveland, Ohio.

Acknowledgments

As has been attested to by numerous others, the time and effort of many people is necessary in order to achieve the completion of any book. The authors and editor would like to express their appreciation to their friends and colleagues who have helped by providing assistance with proofreading, consultation on clinical material, and, most importantly, support and encouragement. Special thanks is also given to Elizabeth Lyons, who spent many long hours typing, retyping and assembling the manuscript.

For

my parents

The editor(s) and/or author(s) and the publisher of this book have made every effort to ensure that all therapeutic modalities that are recommended are in accordance with accepted standards at the time of publication.

The drugs specified within this book may not have specific approval by the Food and Drug Administration in regard to the indications and dosages that are recommended by the editor(s) and/or author(s). The manufacturer's package insert is the best source of current prescribing information.

CHAPTER 1

Physical Assessment of the Critically Ill

by Mary T. Reynolds, RN, MS, and
Winifred J. Walter, RN, MSN

INTRODUCTION

During the past ten years there has been a marked proliferation of knowledge in all areas of health care. These advances include vast increases in biochemical, physiological, and technological knowledge, as well as advances in the psychological and sociological aspects of health care.

During this same period, members of the nursing profession have realized the importance of and need to define nursing within a changing society. Nursing has undergone a significant role realignment in order to clarify independent and interdependent functions of nurses and to provide for a more apparent manifestation of nursing as an independent profession. Nurses have always been committed to work collaboratively with other professionals. In keeping with this commitment and in maintaining our own professional integrity, nurses in various settings have attempted to incorporate physical assessment skills and the Problem-Oriented System within the framework of the nursing process.

The nursing process is an intellectual and behavioral activity which nurses have been taught in their basic educational programs. The concept of the nursing process now incorporates more comprehensive patient assessment. The assessment focuses on the discriminative process through which the nurse uses particular skills and thought processes to identify patient needs.

In the Intensive Care Unit, the data gathered by the nurse depends upon the patient situation as well as the nurse's knowledge base, past experience, and creativity. For the critically ill person, the potential for life-threatening emergencies involving multiple organ systems requires that the nurse is prepared to make quick and accurate assessments.

This chapter will serve as a basis to assist the nurse in the Intensive Care Unit in the development and/or refinement of assessment skills that pertain to the care of the critically ill person. If the nurse in the Intensive Care Unit is equipped with a wide range of assessment skills, the nurse will develop a greater sensitivity in detecting subtle change in patient status that could be premonitory indications of impending organ collapse.

The nurse must have command of considerable subjective and objective data to accurately document changes in patient status. These data will provide sensitive parameters to assist in the assessment of patient status and upon which to base critical nursing interventions. For example, by auscultation of the lungs, coarse rales can be detected before secretions are visible around the endotracheal tube in a patient on a respirator; by auscultation of the heart, an increase in heart rate and an S_3 (one of the first indications of congestive heart failure) can be detected before the patient goes into frank failure; by observation of the patient's mental status, the nurse may detect aberrations which are often, especially in aged persons, the first signs of critical changes in physical status. In each of these instances, the nurse's assessment expertise can facilitate appropriate and accurate intervention, thereby averting total organ collapse and ultimate death of the patient.

How does the nurse in the Intensive Care Unit acquire additional assessment skills? First, it is important to remember that nurses have acquired a substantial knowledge base through basic nursing education programs. This knowledge base is used in making patient assessments. The new dimension which will be discussed in this and subsequent chapters is the use of tools and methods previously used only by physicians. These tools and methods have, in the past, been viewed as "magical" but in contemporary nursing practice, are nothing more than an addition to the nurses' extensive repertoire of knowledge and skills. These are already being incorporated into the basic curriculum of baccalaureate and master's degree nursing programs throughout the country.

Second, it is important that assessment skills be acquired

through systematic process. If there is a continuing education offering or hospital inservice program in the geographical area, it would be advisable to take advantage of one or the other. If neither of these routes is available, it is possible for the nurse to obtain this knowledge and skill independently. Independent learning requires a review of basic anatomy and physiology, interviewing techniques, and physical assessment techniques in the following systems: cardiovascular, respiratory, neurological, and renal. Because the acquisition of physical assessment skills includes the gaining of both knowledge and psychomotor skills, it is essential that the skills be obtained and refined through repeated use in clinical situations. In learning physical assessment skills, it is important to concentrate on normal findings and on normal variations before focusing on abnormal findings.

There are many articles and books available to assist the nurse in learning physical assessment skills. It is important to note, however, that even independent learning does not mean learning without the help of others. Two ways in which the nurse in the Intensive Care Unit can acquire the skills without a formal course are: by validation of the nurse's physical findings through comparison with the findings of the physical examination and by contracting with a competent practitioner in the work setting to give feedback on findings. Repeated feedback and experience are the keys to feeling secure in the identification of all physical findings, be they normal, abnormal, or normal variations.

Finally, it is important to remember that the key to any assessment is a systematic methodological approach. Only with a systematic approach, which is the most important but sometimes the most difficult aspect to learn, can accuracy be achieved.

Before beginning any assessment, the nurse needs the proper equipment. Table 1-1 is a list of essential equipment, important characteristics of the equipment, and the uses of the equipment to assess the physical status of individuals.

THE ORGANIZATION OF DATA: THE PROBLEM-ORIENTED SYSTEM

The Problem-Oriented System incorporates scientific methodology, and is an accepted method of recording patient data in many health care facilities. The Problem-Oriented System does away with

TABLE 1-1

Physical Assessment Equipment

Equipment	Characteristics	Uses
Stethoscope	Double barrel rubber tubing a) no longer than 12 inches b) internal diameter of ⅛ inch	Auscultation of: a) breath sounds b) heart sounds c) bowel sounds d) vessel sounds
	A diaphragm chest piece	The diaphragm: a) accentuates high frequency sounds b) should be placed firmly against the skin
	A bell chest piece approximately one inch in diameter	The bell: a) accentuates low frequency sounds b) should be placed lightly on the skin N.B. firm pressure will convert a bell to a diaphragm
Tape measure	Centimeter and inch	Measurement of difference in extremity circumference and abdominal girth
		Measurement of organ borders
Penlight	A concentrated and bright light source	Assessment of pupillary size and reaction
Safety pin		Detection of alteration in sensation
Q-tip		Assessment of corneal reflex
Reflex hammer	Wide edge and tapered edge	Assessment of deep tendon reflexes and plantar reflex

professional jargon and thus is an instrument of communication between all providers on the health care team. It is a uniform approach of recording patient care data. Because the Problem-Oriented System is uniform, it provides a scientific basis for both patient and clinician evaluation. The nursing process is also based on scientific methodology and the component parts of the nursing process reflect the component parts of the Problem-Oriented System, as shown in Table 1-2.

The Problem-Oriented System is based on the principle that the patient is the pivotal determinant of his care. What is the patient telling you (subjective data)? What are you observing about the patient (objective data)? What do the subjective and objective data mean in relation to present and/or potential problems for this patient (assessment)? What can you and the patient do to alleviate and/or prevent the problem (plan)? How has the plan worked in meeting the objective of prevention and/or alleviation (progress notes)?

TABLE 1-2

**The Relationship of the Nursing Process and
Problem-Oriented Charting to Scientific Methodology**
(University of Pittsburgh School of Nursing. Used with permission.)

Nursing Process	Scientific Method	Problem Oriented Charting System
	A. PROBLEM FINDING	
ASSESSMENT	1. Gathering Information	
	2. Examining Information	DATA BASE
	3. Interpreting Information	
	4. Identifying The Problem	PROBLEM LIST
	5. Stating The Problem	
	B. PROBLEM SOLVING	
PLAN	1. Developing Alternatives	
	2. Making A Decision	PLAN
	3. Deciding On A Plan Of Action	
INTERVENTION	4. Executing The Plan	PROGRESS
EVALUATION	5. Evaluating The Results	NOTES
REVISION	6. Re-defining Change	

Subjective data include all information obtained from the patient and/or significant others. These data consist of all historical as well as ongoing information obtained by the nurse in regard to the patient's physical, psychological, and social disturbances.

Objective data include all factual information about the patient. These data consist of all physical findings, diagnostic tests, and observations.

The assessment is an interpretation of the subjective and objective data collectively. The initial assessment is a simple statement of the patient's problems in terms of a diagnosis or need. The patient's problems are the basis for nursing interventions which include goals and plans for:

1. diagnostic information
2. treatment
3. patient education

The progress notes include subjective and objective data related to the patient's identified and/or new problems, an assessment of the patient's progress, and continuation or revision of the plans. In the Intensive Care Unit, where patients' actual or potential problems are complex and rapidly changing, flow sheets are an essential and integral part of the patients' progress notes. Flow sheets are only used to record objective data that are obtained at frequent intervals (i.e., lab data, I&O, BP, P, and levels of consciousness).

Figure 1-1 provides a schematic representation of the problem-oriented record.

THE COMPREHENSIVE HEALTH ASSESSMENT OF THE CRITICALLY ILL PERSON

Overview

The proficiencies involved in a comprehensive assessment of the critically ill person are interviewing, history-taking, and the physical assessment skills of observation, palpation, percussion, and auscultation.

Interviewing and the gathering of historical data are inseparable. Proficiency in these interdependent processes is the most important determinant of nursing intervention since 80-90% of the evidence leading to the patient's potential and/or actual problems is

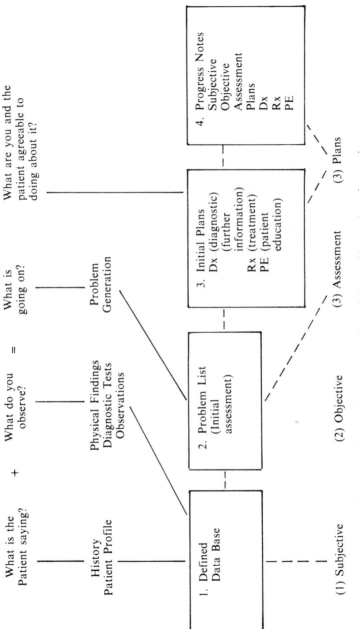

Figure 1-1. Schematic representation of the problem-oriented record.

obtained through historical statements and is thus dependent upon the skill of the interviewer in eliciting data that are as accurate and complete as possible.

Unfortunately, critically ill persons often are unable to communicate verbally for various reasons. Under these circumstances, the nurse must elicit the information from family members or significant others. Regardless of the circumstances, it is always important to include family members during the assessment of the critically ill person not only for the purpose of accurate assessment, but also as a means of providing emotional support to both the family and the patient.

Two crucial historical items to obtain at the onset are the manner in which the critically ill person usually copes with physical and emotional stress, and his usual response to confinement and the unfamiliar. This information is vital to the recovery of the critically ill person. It provides data which will enable the nurse to anticipate potential anxiety producing situations and assist the nurse in alleviating or preventing the patient's anxiety.

As mentioned previously, the physical assessment skills include observation, percussion, palpation, and auscultation. During the initial phase of learning and applying these skills, the nurse frequently experiences some degree of sensory deficit. This deficit is rarely a true sensory disability but rather a result of lack of experience in use of these techniques. Observation is a vital physical assessment skill to the nurse who cares for the critically ill person; minute changes in a patient's emotional, mental, and/or physical status are often the first premonitory signs of a life-threatening situation: restlessness often precedes overt signs of internal hemorrhage; confusion often precedes overt signs of dehydration in the elderly; changes in depth and rate of respiration often precede overt signs of acid-base disturbances. The remainder of the physical assessment skills (palpation, percussion, and auscultation) verify the historical and observational assessment and assist the nurse in localizing the problem.

Equally important as the skills for gathering a patient data base is the nurse's ability to make clinical judgments upon which to provide nursing interventions. The critically ill person is dependent upon both medical and nursing interventions. The emotional and social recovery of the critically ill person, however, is basically a function of nursing intervention. The emotional and social aspects of a critical illness are often overlooked, and the critically ill person may recover physiologically only to become emotionally and socially disabled.

This section will provide the nurse with the goals of and the steps in gathering a comprehensive data base upon which to assess the physical and psychosocial needs of the patient. The goals of the comprehensive health assessment are to:

1. Provide the nursing staff with a defined baseline for assessment of physiologic and psychosocial needs of the critically ill person.
2. To plan for and provide appropriate nursing interventions to meet the identified needs of the patient.
3. To evaluate the outcome of the nursing care.

The comprehensive health assessment provides the nursing staff with an understanding of the patient's current illness. It also provides an awareness of the psychosocial response of the patient and family to the illness. It is begun in the form of an initial immediate assessment, the purpose of which is to assess life-threatening processes, and is completed once the admission crisis is over.

STEPS IN GATHERING
A COMPREHENSIVE HEALTH ASSESSMENT

The Immediate Assessment

The purposes of the immediate assessment are twofold: first, to establish the baseline physical and emotional status of the patient upon which to measure his improvement or deterioration; second, to initiate appropriate intervention which will stabilize the patient's condition.

As the patient arrives in the unit, the nurse has to determine what information should be obtained in order to reach the goal of physiological stability. The data required in the performance of the initial immediate assessment include a brief history of the current physiologic deficit and a rapid physical assessment of the four major systems (cardiovascular, respiratory, neurological, and renal) vital to the regulation and maintenance of life. The following is a list of objective and subjective assessment parameters in the priority of performance. The methods for assessment will be discussed later in this chapter.

Objective Assessment Parameters

1. Determine the adequacy of respiratory status: observe for symmetrical chest movement; note rate, regularity, and depth of respiration; auscultate the lung bases for the presence of breath sounds (especially important if the patient is on a respirator), rales, and wheezing.
2. Determine the adequacy of cardiovascular status: auscultate for the heart rate and rhythm, note if the heart sounds are distant, obtain the blood pressure, determine the presence of major arterial pulses, inspect neck veins for distention, inspect the patient for gross hemorrhage, ascertain the color, temperature, and condition of the patient's skin, measure the CVP.
3. Determine the adequacy of neurological status: ascertain the patient's level of consciousness; establish orientation to time, place and person; observe pupillary size, equality, and reaction to light. Observe for movement of all extremities: if the patient is unable to move his extremities: 1) determine the reason for lack of movement from the conscious patient, i.e., pain, trauma, fracture to extremity; 2) if the patient is unconscious and there are no signs of trauma, apply painful stimuli, noting movement and whether it is purposeful.
4. Determine the adequacy of renal status: measure urine volume and specific gravity; test urine for presence of blood, glucose, ketones, and protein.
5. Inspect the extremities for equality in size, presence of edema, cyanosis, or ulcerations.
6. Obtain the patient's temperature and weight.

Subjective Assessment Parameters

While gathering the objective parameters, the nurse will elicit the following historical data from the patient or significant other (if patient is unable to talk):

1. What symptom is troubling the patient most at the time of arrival to the unit?
2. What were the precipitating factors that resulted in hospital admission?
3. Does the patient have any other concurrent illnesses?
4. Is the patient taking any medication?

5. Does the patient have any allergies to medication? If so, describe the type of reaction.
6. Does the patient have a bleeding tendency?
7. When did the patient last void, and color of urine?
8. When did the patient last have a bowel movement? (Color and consistency of stool.)
9. Who are the patient's significant others, their names and phone numbers?
10. Did patient receive a tetanus shot if there was a history of trauma?
11. When was patient's last meal?
12. If patient is female, is she pregnant?

As the nurse is establishing the historical and physical parameters, the patient should be in a position of comfort. In addition, all intravenous catheters and flow rates should be regulated and drainage tubes should be connected to the proper equipment. If the patient has a Foley catheter, the nurse should note the color, amount, and specific gravity of the urine; if the patient has no catheter, ask the patient to void. If the patient has a nasogastric tube, the color, amount, and hematest of drainage should be noted. The nurse should be able to complete this initial assessment within ten to fifteen minutes after the patient's arrival in the unit, although obtaining information from the family may require more time.

The Patient's History

The patient's history is usually obtained by the admitting physician. The nurse should review this history and be prepared to supplement it with historical data by which to make patient assessments and provide nursing interventions.

The purposes for reviewing the patient's history are to provide the nurse with baseline information about the patient, to conserve the nurse's time and the patient's energy by not obtaining redundant data, to provide the nurse with a starting point to begin data collection, and to determine data upon which to initiate nursing interventions. The patient's history is divided into six parts: the chief complaint, the history of current illness, the psychological, sociological, and cultural patient profile, the family history, the past health history, and the review of systems. The amount of historical data obtained depends upon the crisis situation. In fact, it is an essential nursing judgment to determine assessment priorities in the initial ICU period.

The Chief Complaint

This is the primary reason that the patient sought care, plus the duration of symptoms. This is recorded in the person's own words.

The History of Current Illness

This is a narrative of the critically ill person's chief complaint from the time of onset until his admission to the hospital. This portion of the history will tell the nurse the severity and rapidity of the illness, the rate at which complications arose, and the specific organ systems involved. This information will assist the nurse in the evaluation of the patient's physiological and psychological status. The nurse usually does not gather the history of current illness when the physician is present; however, when patients develop symptoms or signs in the ICU, the nurse should be able to use this model in order to systematically assess the symptom. Precise reconstruction of a symptom and events leading to it provide an accurate understanding of the underlying physiological or psychological processes.

As has been stated earlier, the method of interviewing is extremely important in eliciting valid data. A patient's symptoms should always be elicited by the use of nondirective questions to allow patients the opportunity to respond freely and spontaneously.

Table 1-3 describes the parameters which should be elicited for all symptoms reported by the critically ill person. Subjective information will be listed next to each parameter. Objective information gathered by the nurse will be listed in the last column.

The Family History

This refers to the summary of the age and state of health or cause of death of patient's parents and siblings with particular attention to the genetic, familial, environmental and communicable determinants of disease.

The Past Health History

This is the overall appraisal of the patient's general health and/or illness prior to the current illness. The past health history includes the following components:

TABLE 1-3

Model for Historic Description of Symptoms
(History of Current Illness)

Parameters for Analysis of Symptoms[10]	Subjective Data	Objective Data
1. Onset	When was the symptom first noticed?	Did nurse observe symptom at the time of onset?
2. Manner of onset	Did the symptom start suddenly or gradually?	Did the nurse observe a gradual or sudden onset?
3. Duration	How long did the symptom last?	Did the nurse observe the duration?
4. Precipitating factors	Did the patient recall anything previous to onset, e.g., ingestion of food, medicine, emotional factors, physical exertion, etc.	What was going on in the patient's environment previous to onset? Was the family visit disturbing? Was there a death or sudden emergency in the unit? Were there warning signals alarming on life support systems or ECG monitors?
		What was going on with the patient's physical status? Were there changes in mental status, vital signs, urinary output, breath sounds, central venous pressure, pulmonary artery pressure, drainage tubes? Was there a position change? Were there any treatment changes?
5. If the presenting symptom is pain, also include the following parameters in the analysis:		
a) Location	Ask the patient to point to the area. Does the pain radiate?	Observe where patient points to the pain. (N.B. Always record data using anatomical landmarks.)
b) Quality	Ask patient to describe the pain (e.g., sharp, dull, needlelike, aching, crushing, piercing, crampy, burning).	*(Continued)*

TABLE 1-3 (Continued)

Model for Historic Description of Symptoms
(History of Current Illness)

Parameters for Analysis of Symptoms[10]	Subjective Data	Objective Data
c) Intensity	Ask patient to describe severity of pain (e.g., mild, moderate or severe). Does the pain interfere with the patient's activities of daily living?	Observe facial expressions. Are there changes in vital signs? Is the patient breathless, perspiring? Observe position of patient.
6. Quantitative	Ask patient to describe frequency of symptom. If the symptom is excretory, elicit from patient the volume, color, and consistency of the substance.	Observe color, consistency, and frequency. Measure exact volumes.
7. Course	Ask patient if symptoms have persisted or changed in character.	Note changes in physical parameters since onset of symptomatology (e.g., vital signs, output, ECG monitor).
8. Associated symptoms	Ask the patient if there are any other signs or symptoms at the same time as the present one. If new symptoms have appeared, elicit the precise order of their appearance.	Observe for physical parameters described in *precipitating factors.*
9. Aggravating	Ask patient what makes the symptoms worse (e.g., positions, deep breathing, or coughing).	Observe for environmental and physical factors that affect the symptoms.
10. Relieving	Ask the patient what makes the symptoms less intense (e.g., sleep, medication, nursing measures, position).	Observe patient for signs of relief. Record relief measures in the nursing care plan.

1. A general statement of the patient's previous mental and physical health
2. Significant illnesses
3. Past hospitalizations
4. Accidents or injuries
5. Allergic reactions
6. Immunizations
7. Current medications

Information about the previous health status will assist the nurse to assess the present problems, predict responses, and plan for immediate and future care. The important parts of the *past health history* of which the nurse in the ICU should be aware are the following:

1. Significant Illnesses: Is there a past history of diabetes mellitus, cancer, heart disease, stroke, bleeding disorders, gastrointestinal or renal hemorrhage, hypertension, renal disease, mental/emotional problems, seizure disorders, or respiratory disease? What was the treatment? What were the effects of the treatment? What is the present treatment?
2. Current Medications (both patent and prescription): The rationale for these data is that concurrent chronic disease may require adjustment of present medications. Any acute illness superimposed on a chronic illness will necessitate a re-evaluation of the medication used to control the chronic illness. Certain medications such as steroids would need to be increased during the time of crisis. Medications such as aspirin may need to be discontinued since they could significantly affect bleeding time. Other medications can cause untoward drug interactions.
3. Allergic Reactions: Past allergic reactions to drugs and/or food must be established. Once established, the allergy must be recorded in a fashion easily visible to all staff in the Unit. If the nurse is gathering these data, she should have the patient (or significant other) describe the allergic reaction to the specific allergen since often what the patient has experienced is a side effect rather than an allergic response.
4. Immunizations: If the patient presents with trauma, it is imperative that the date of the last tetanus toxoid be ascertained.

The Review of Systems (ROS)

A systematic head-to-toe method for screening and uncovering symptoms in other body systems that may relate to the history of current illness or concurrent illnesses which were omitted in previous parts of the history is referred to as the Review of Systems. The system review includes previous and present symptoms related to the patient's physiologic and mental status.

The Psycho-socio-cultural Patient Profile

This is a collection of pertinent historical facts regarding the critically ill person's age and sex, relationship with his family/significant others and community, cultural background, religious background, occupation, education, pattern of daily living, including habits, recreational interests, and usual coping patterns. The patient's psycho-socio-cultural self significantly influences his response to illness, impending death, confinement, and ultimately, his psychosocial and physiologic recovery.

Although the nurse in the health care setting has traditionally collected these data, one often finds only limited attention given to this area in the ICU because the nurses are so busy with the continuous monitoring of changes and interventions concerned with maintaining vital systems. Because of this, little time is left to thoroughly assess the critically ill person's psycho-socio-cultural status. Careful attention to assessment of this area by asking salient questions of the patient or significant others will yield a more complete understanding of:

1. The patient's response in time of crisis.
2. Which therapeutic approaches can best be used to assist the critically ill person and significant others to cope with the sick role.
3. The basis upon which to provide meaningful person-centered nursing interventions with the goal of physiologic and psychosocial recovery.

Psycho-socio-cultural parameters to be assessed in gathering the patient profile are as follows:

1. Age
2. Sex
3. Ethnic background; primary language

4. Religious background (ascertain significance of #3 and #4 for patient at present time)
5. Marital status:
   a) children
   b) relationship with spouse and children
   c) relationship with significant others
   d) health status of family
6. Education
7. Occupation:
   a) job history
   b) How will hospitalization and subsequent recovery affect patient's job?
   c) What are the responsibilities?
   d) How does the person relate to others on the job?
8. Sources and adequacy of income while hospitalized and during recovery
9. Potential problems—secondary to hospitalization and recovery:
   a) financial
   b) care of family
   c) job
10. Expectations of treatment
11. Knowledge of and fears about illness
12. Living conditions:
    a) stairs to climb
    b) responsibility for running household
    c) number of people living in household
13. Personality:
    a) coping patterns with past illnesses or confinement
    b) description of self
14. Recreational interests:
    a) sedentary
    b) active
15. Pattern of daily living:
    a) usual sleep pattern
    b) food pattern, likes and dislikes, liquid intake
    c) exercise
    d) alcohol intake
    e) tobacco
    f) coffee intake

The information that a nurse in the ICU can use from the historical data provided by the critically ill person or significant other is unlimited. The nurse can use these data to plan for and carry out appropriate nursing interventions in order to achieve the goal of physiologic and psychosocial recovery. Table 1-4 lists possible historically significant data, potential complications superimposed on the acute health problem, and nursing interventions.

The remainder of this chapter is divided into critical subjective and objective data parameters for each of the four major vital systems: the respiratory system, the cardiovascular system, the neurological system, and the renal system. The sections on the respiratory, cardiovascular, and neurological systems include: (1) assessment parameters; (2) method of assessment; (3) deviations from normal; and (4) interpretation of findings. In addition, the section on the respiratory system provides an outline of basic anatomy and physiology which will assist the nurse in the interpretation and recording of physical findings. The section on the renal system includes subjective and objective data comparisons of dehydration, overhydration, and acute renal failure.

The subjective parameters for the respiratory and cardiovascular systems will be considered as a unit since many of the same symptoms occur as a result of either cardiovascular or respiratory pathology. The subjective parameters for these systems will follow the respiratory system and precede the cardiovascular system.

THE RESPIRATORY SYSTEM

The purpose of the respiratory system is to "promote the transfer of oxygen from the atmosphere into the lungs and the removal of carbon dioxide from the lungs."[16] The purpose of the assessment of the respiratory system is to determine subtle changes in the integrity of the system which would indicate decreasing efficiency. Recognition of these changes and prompt intervention by the nurse will increase the chances of survival for the critically ill person.

Basic Anatomy and Physiology of the Respiratory System:

The respiratory system consists of the nose, nasopharynx, larynx, trachea, main stem, lobar, and segmental bronchi, bronchioles, alveoli, and pleura. Anything that interferes with the ana-

TABLE 1-4

Historically Significant Data

Historical Data	Potential Complications	Nursing Interventions
Hypertension	Normotensive BP's could signify a shock state depending upon the severity of the hypertension	Report deviations of + or − 20 mm Hg from baseline BP
G.I. Ulcer	The patient is more prone to develop GI bleeding, especially if an NG tube is in place	1. Hematest GI drainage periodically. 2. From data obtained under patient profile develop a plan of care attuned to individual needs with the goal of decreasing stress
Diabetes Mellitus	Insulin requirements may be increased or decreased depending on the situation	1. Report deviations from usual pattern of control (determine usual pattern of control, e.g., dosage of insulin, what urine sugars run, etc.) 2. Test urine AC & HS for sugar and acetone. (2 gtt method with clini-test preferred) 3. Observe daily blood glucose level for deviations 4. Observe the patient for signs of hypo- or hyperglycemia 5. Know medications which produce false positives for urine glucose, e.g., Keflin
Seizure Disorders	Physiologic and/or psychologic stress may cause a decrease in the convulsive threshold	1. Report seizure activity (determine usual type and pattern of seizure activity, aura, and control measures) 2. Provide protection of the patient from the environment 3. From data obtained under the patient profile develop plan of care attuned to individual needs with the goal of decreasing stress
Coronary Artery Disease	These patients are prone to myocardial infarction and ischemia	Observe for chest pain, arrhythmias, and ventricular failure (determine previous angina pattern) *(Continued)*

TABLE 1-4 (Continued)

Historically Significant Data

Historical Data	Potential Complications	Nursing Interventions
Peripheral Neuropathy/ Arterial In- sufficiency of extremities/ edema/venous stasis	These patients are prone to decubiti and cellulitis	1. Change position of patient frequently 2. Provide skin care 3. Provide padding to prevent pressure of necessary equipment which must be next to the patient's skin
Heavy Alcohol Intake	These patients are prone to alcohol withdrawal and/or delirium tremens, which usually occur from 8 to 72 hours after alcohol withdrawal	1. Observe patient for trem- ulousness and hallucinations during the critical period 2. Make sure medication order is available in order to intervene quickly 3. Ask about vitamin B administration
Smoking	1. These patients are prone to respiratory complications 2. Possible loss of coping mechanism due to withdrawal 3. Often have thick, tenacious secretions	1. Vigorous pulmonary toilet 2. Develop plan for assisting patient to draw upon other coping mechanism (use data from patient profile)
Food Intolerance	1. Physiological stress superimposed on an already physically compromised system 2. There may be con- fusion of symptoms (e.g., epigastric distress may present as chest pain)	1. Prevent patient from receiving these particular foods (determine food intolerances and subsequent symptoms)
Anxiety over potential problems secondary to hospitalization	The anxiety may inter- fere with physiologic recovery	1. Talk with patient and family about problems, and plan with them for use of available community resources 2. Talk with patient and assure of ongoing planning throughout his hospital stay

tomical integrity of the respiratory system or with its surrounding structures such as the diaphragm, thoracic cage, muscles, abdominal viscera, and mediastinal structures, will produce a deficit in the efficient functioning of the system. Any deficit will in turn produce changes which the nurse will be able to detect on physical examination.

The right lung is shorter and wider than the left lung and has three lobes, whereas the left lung has two lobes. Because of the shape of the lungs, the left hemidiaphragm is lower than the right hemidiaphragm. Anteriorly, the apices of the lungs lie above the clavicles medially, while the inferior borders of the lungs lie at the sixth rib medially and at the eighth to ninth rib laterally. Posteriorly, the apices of the lungs lie above the scapula medially and the inferior borders of the lungs lie at the eleventh rib and may descend to the twelfth rib during inspiration. The right main stem bronchus is wider and shorter than the left and is at a 25 degree angle to the trachea; the left is at a 40-60 degree angle to the trachea. The trachea bifurcates into the main stem bronchi at the sternal angle. Figure 1-2 shows the anatomical landmarks of the thorax and lungs.

The *diaphragm* is the major muscle of ventilation and separates the abdominal and thoracic cavities. The excursion (i.e., movement) of the diaphragm is normally 3-5 cms with each respiration. The *intercostal muscles* are composed of the external intercostal muscles which increase the anterior-posterior diameter of the thorax and the internal intercostal muscles which play a role in forceful expiration.

The *accessory muscles* (scalene, sternocleidomastoid, trapezius, and pectoralis) are not active during resting ventilation, but their purpose is to increase the efficiency of movement of the diaphragm.[14] Since expiration is normally passive, the *expiratory muscles* (i.e., abdominal muscles) only come into play during active expiration. Like the accessory muscles, the expiratory muscles increase the efficiency of the movement of the diaphragm.

When describing physical findings of the thorax and lungs, it is important for the nurse to describe the findings in relation to anatomical landmarks. These include the sternal angle, the costal angle, and lines of reference.

The *sternal angle* (manubriosternal junction or Angle of Louis) is an important anatomical landmark of the thorax. It is formed by

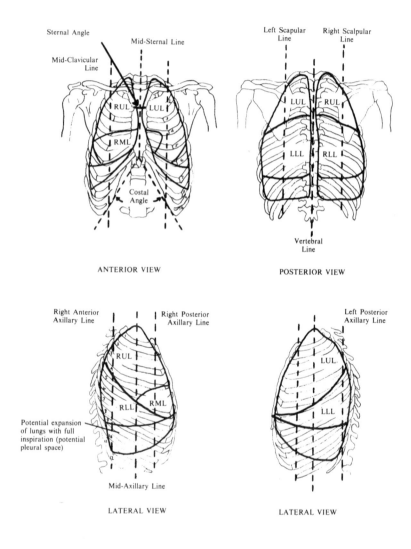

Figure 1-2. Anterior, posterior, and lateral views of lungs showing lobes and anatomical landmarks. (Adapted from: Hochstein E, Rubin AL: *Physical Diagnosis*. McGraw-Hill, New York, 1964, p. 105. Used with permission.)

the junction of the manubrium and the body of the sternum. It is located medially to the second right and left ribs. The *costal angle* is made up of the left and right costal margins as they join the sternum at the xyphoid process. This angle is normally less than 90 degrees but increases with chronic lung pathology, e.g., emphysema. As the angle increases, lung expansion decreases.

Lines of reference on the thorax include the midsternal line, the left and right midclavicular lines, the anterior, mid- and posterior axillary lines, the vertebral line, and the right and left scapular lines. The ribs and spinous processes of the thoracic vertebra are also important landmarks.

Auscultation of Breath Sounds

Breath sounds are the result of air passing through the tracheobronchioalveolar system during the respiratory cycle. They are loudest over the areas where the air flow is turbulent, i.e., major bronchi, and softest over the areas where air flow is more laminar, i.e., the alveoli, which comprise the major portion of the lung.

Breath sounds are divided into three categories: (1) vesicular; (2) bronchovesicular; and (3) bronchial. Vesicular breath sounds are normal and are heard over the major portions of the lung fields. Bronchovesicular breath sounds are normal when heard over the first and second intercostal spaces anteriorly and between the scapula posteriorly. Bronchovesicular breath sounds may also be heard over the lung apices anteriorly and posteriorly. When bronchovesicular breath sounds are heard anywhere else over the lung fields, they are abnormal and indicate a pathological process. Bronchial breath sounds are always abnormal when heard anywhere over the lung fields. Table 1-5 depicts the three categories of breath sounds and their characteristics, and Figure 1-3 is a schematic representation of these sounds.

Several principles of physics assist in the understanding of lung sounds. The first principle is that fluid and dense solids are better conductors of sound than air. This means that a patient who has a consolidation or mass in the lung tissue will have breath sounds that are accentuated or increased over that area in comparison to a symmetrical area. The second principle is that anything which interferes with the transmission of sound through the respiratory passages (i.e., lumens of the trachea, bronchi, or bronchioles) to the

TABLE 1-5

Breath Sounds

VESICULAR BREATH SOUNDS

1. Occur as a result of air movement in the bronchioles and alveoli.
2. Heard over all lung fields except the second intercostal spaces anteriorly, and between the scapulae posteriorly.

	Inspiration	Expiration
Pitch	Low	Lower
Volume	Soft and clearly audible	Softer and poorly audible
Duration	Longer	Shorter

BRONCHOVESICULAR BREATH SOUNDS

1. Occur as a result of a mixture of air movement in the trachea, bronchi, bronchioles, and alveoli.
2. Heard over the second intercostal spaces anteriorly, between the scapulae posteriorly, and may be heard over the apices.
3. A brief pause may be noted between inspiration and expiration.

	Inspiration	Expiration
Pitch	Medium	Higher
Volume	Louder than vesicular	Same as inspiration
Duration	Long and equal to expiration	Long and equal to inspiration

BRONCHIAL BREATH SOUNDS

1. Occur as a result of air passing through fluid or a dense solid.
2. Are *never* heard over the normal lung.
3. Can be simulated by listening to breathing over the trachea.
4. A pause can be heard between inspiration and expiration.

	Inspiration	Expiration
Pitch	High, blowing and hollow	Higher than inspiration
Volume	Loud	Louder than inspiration
Duration	Short	Longer than inspiration

stethoscope will diminish or completely obliterate the sound. These principles can be better understood by the following illustrations:

1. If a patient who has a consolidation in the lung takes a breath and you are listening over that area of the lung, the breath sounds will be more accentuated over that area in comparison

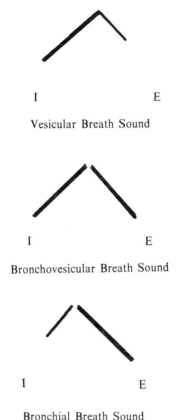

I   E

Vesicular Breath Sound

I   E

Bronchovesicular Breath Sound

I   E

Bronchial Breath Sound

Figure 1-3. Schematic representation of breath sounds.

to the same area in the opposite lung (fluid conducts sound better than air).

2. If the same patient with the same consolidation also had a bronchial plug completely obliterating the lumen of the bronchus leading to that area of the lung, the breath sounds would be absent (fluid conducts sound better than air, *but* the bronchial plug interferes with the transmission of sound).

3. If a patient had a pleural effusion, the breath sounds would be diminished or absent over that area (fluid conducts sounds bet-

ter than air, *but* the pleura are outside the lungs and the fluid is interfering with the transmission of sound).

Adventitious Sounds

Adventitious sounds are abnormal sounds which are superimposed on breath sounds and may indicate: secretions in the respiratory system, narrowing of the lumens of the trachea, bronchi, or bronchioles, or interference with movement of the pleura. Adventitious sounds are divided into three categories: rales, rhonchi, and pleural friction rub.

Rales are crackling or bubbling sounds which are produced by air flow through secretions. There are three types of rales:

1. *Fine Rales* originate in the alveoli, and are heard at the end of inspiration and rarely clear with coughing.
2. *Medium Rales* originate in the bronchioles, are heard midway through inspiration, and rarely clear with coughing.
3. *Coarse Rales* originate in the trachea and bronchi, are heard at the *beginning* of inspiration, and will clear at least in part with coughing.

Rhonchi are sounds produced as air passes through the trachea, bronchi, or bronchioles whose lumens have been narrowed, regardless of the cause of narrowing. There are two types of rhonchi:

1. *Sibilant Rhonchi* originate in the small bronchi and the bronchioles and produce a high-pitched wheezing sound.
2. *Sonorous Rhonchi* originate in the larger bronchi and the trachea and produce a low-pitched snoring sound.

Rhonchi are generally more audible on expiration because the lumen of the tracheobronchial tree is more narrow on expiration than on inspiration. Rhonchi may be heard during inspiration as well as expiration when there is greater obstruction. Rhonchi vary from respiration to respiration and may clear completely or partially to cough.

A *pleural friction rub* is a grating sound, like two pieces of leather being rubbed together, which originates in the pleura. A pleural friction rub is usually heard during the entire respiratory phase but may be heard only during inspiration and often is more audible during inspiration. Pleural friction rubs are heard best over the anterolateral chest wall, the area of greatest excursion, and are not affected by cough.

As can be seen in the previous description of adventitious sounds, it is important to have a patient cough and then to re-auscultate before making a judgment as to which adventitious sounds are present. When heard, adventitious sounds are recorded as to the anatomical site of auscultation and whether or not they clear to cough, as well as their occurrence in the respiratory cycle.

Techniques of Palpation, Percussion, and Auscultation:

Palpation for respiratory excursion, i.e., movement or expansion of the thorax (Figure 1-4), is done by placing the fingers of each hand over the lateral lower chest with the palms over the lower anterolateral chest. Place the thumbs along the costal margins with the thumbs pointing toward the xyphoid process. Squeeze the skin of the chest gently between your thumbs and ask the patient to breathe normally, then to breathe deeply. Allow the patient's thoracic movement to move your thumbs and hands. Note the movement of thumbs upward and outward, and symmetry of movements on inspiration. The same technique can be repeated posteriorly to determine thoracic expansion.

The technique of percussion is similar to the movement of the fingers when playing the piano. When tapping various organs of the body, different sounds are produced (i.e., over a hollow organ, such as the stomach, a tympanic sound can be heard; over an air-filled organ such as the lungs, a resonant sound can be heard, and over a compact organ such as the diaphragm, a dull sound can be heard).

Percussion is performed by placing the distal joint of the middle finger (the pleximeter) of the left hand (if you are right-handed) firmly over the area to be percussed. The whole middle finger must be lying flat or the sound will be distorted. In addition, make sure the remainder of the fingers, if resting on the patient's thorax, are five centimeters, i.e., spread as far as possible from the middle finger so as not to distort sounds. Flex the proximal and distal joints of the third finger (the percussing finger) of the right hand. With the tip of the percussing finger strike the distal joint of the pleximeter with a short vertical blow. Note the percussion sound; that is, note whether it is tympanic, resonant or dull (Figure 1-5).

When auscultating the lungs, it is important to do so in a systematic manner, comparing one area of one lung with the same area of the other lung (Figure 1-6). Place the diaphragm of the stethoscope firmly against the chest wall. Compare inspiration to expiration in

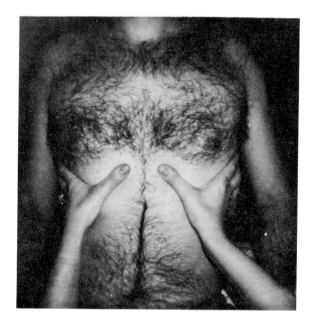

Figure 1-4. Palpation for respiratory excursion.

each area. Also compare breath sounds in each area to the symmetrical opposite area. Note the character of the breath sounds as well as presence of adventitious sounds.

Table 1-6 describes the parameters and methods of assessment utilized in the examination of the respiratory system.

Critical Subjective Data Parameters for the Respiratory and Cardiovascular Systems

The following symptoms are considered subjective when the patient reports them. They are considered signs or objective when the nurse observes them.

Dyspnea

This refers to difficult, troubled, or uncomfortable breathing. Dyspnea is caused by any pathological process that increases pulmonary venous pressure and produces pulmonary vascular congestion, e.g., congestive heart failure, pulmonary embolism, or

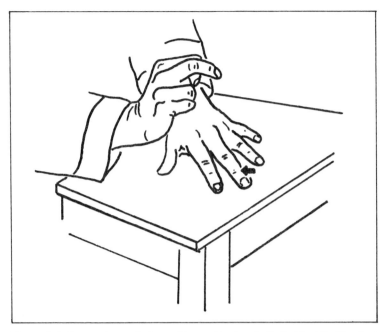

Figure 1-5. Percussion technique. (From: Hochstein E, Rubin AL: *Physical Diagnosis.* McGraw-Hill, New York, 1964, p. 143. Used with permission.)

shock lung. The pulmonary vascular congestion decreases lung expansibility, thus increasing the work of breathing. Dyspnea can also result from oxygen deficiency subsequent to failure of mechanical respiration or obstruction in the airway, or from compression of alveoli associated with pneumothorax or abdominal distention. The nurse should note if wheezing accompanies the dyspnea in order to determine whether or not the cause may be due to bronchospasm. The patient should also be observed for dyspnea on exertion, i.e., dyspnea which occurs when the patient changes position or ambulates. Dyspnea may also occur with postoperative pain or accumulation of secretions in the major airways.

Orthopnea

Dyspnea which occurs in a recumbent position is termed orthopnea. A patient may require two to three pillows to sleep comfortably, or the nurse may observe that the patient develops dyspnea when lying flat, but breathes easily when in a more upward posi-

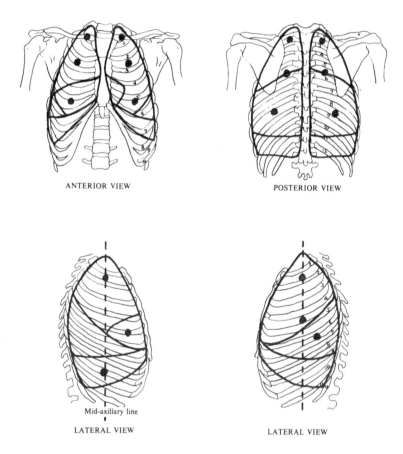

ANTERIOR VIEW

POSTERIOR VIEW

Mid-axillary line

LATERAL VIEW

LATERAL VIEW

Figure 1-6. Auscultatory sites (black circles represent stethoscope placement). Adapted with permission from: Hochstein E, Rubin AL: *Physical Diagnosis*. McGraw-Hill, New York, 1964, p. 6.

TABLE 1-6

Physical Assessment of the Respiratory System

Assessment Parameter	Method of Assessment	Deviations From Normal	Interpretation
I: Inspection and Palpation:			
Palpate the:			
A. Bony thorax and spine	Observe and palpate the sternum and spine for shape	1. Funnel chest 2. Pigeon chest 3. Lordosis 4. Scoliosis 5. Kyphosis	All of these deviations will interfere with normal respiratory capacity Patients with these deviations must be watched closely for signs of respiratory distress
B. Anterior-posterior (AP) diameter	Observe the AP (lateral) diameter of the chest and compare it with the transverse diameter	A ratio greater than 1:2	Normally the ratio of the AP diameter to the transverse diameter is 1:2 or less. The ratio may be increased in patients with emphysema
C. Slope of the ribs	Observe and palpate ribs in relation to the spine and sternum to determine their slope	A slope greater than 45°	This may indicate a chronic lung problem (e.g., emphysema)
D. Costal angle	Observe and palpate the costal angle to determine the angle (see previous description, p. 23)	A costal angle greater than 90°	This may indicate a chronic obstructive lung problem

(Continued)

TABLE 1-6 (Continued)

Physical Assessment of the Respiratory System

Assessment Parameter	Method of Assessment	Deviations From Normal	Interpretation
E. Movement of the intercostal spaces	Observe patient during both quiet and deep respiration for movement of the intercostal spaces	Retraction of intercostal spaces	Retraction occurs on inspiration and may indicate obstruction of the respiratory tract
		Bulging of intercostal spaces	Bulging occurs on expiration and may indicate a tension pneumothorax or a large pleural effusion
			Both retraction and bulging of intercostal spaces occur with severe emphysema and with severe asthma
F. Muscular development	Observe muscles of the chest for size and symmetry		Muscular development is usually more pronounced on one side depending on handedness
			Muscle mass will decrease the loudness, *but not* the characteristics of breath sounds. If minute differences in volume of sound occur with auscultation and one side has an increased

G. Trachea	Have the patient flex his neck. Palpate the trachea to determine its position (normally midline) by placing the little finger of the examining hand on either side of the trachea in the suprasternal notch	Decreased space on one side indicates tracheal deviation to that side	muscle mass, these differences can be accounted for and determined to be normal

Tracheal deviation may occur with a large pleural effusion, with an open pneumothorax, in obstructive atelectasis, or fibrosis of the lung or pleura |
| H. Respiratory excursions (i.e., movement or expansion of the thorax) | Observe the movement of the chest during quiet and deep respiration

Palpate the anterolateral rib cage bilaterally during quiet and deep respirations. (Use method described on p. 27) | Asymmetry of chest movements | A decrease in thoracic expansion indicates pathology on the side which lags. It may occur with acute pleurisy, chest pain, fractured ribs, pneumothorax or consolidation |
| **II: Respiratory rate, depth, and rhythm** | Observe patient and count respirations for a full minute without the patient's awareness

Always assess depth of respirations by palpation | A. Hyperventilation (increased rate and depth)

1. Tachypnea (increased rate) | Hyperventilation may occur with a pulmonary embolus, in peritonitis, severe hemorrhage, pneumonia, diabetic acidosis, fever and pain, hyperventilation with mechanical respirator |

(Continued)

TABLE 1-6 (Continued)

Physical Assessment of the Respiratory System

Assessment Parameter	Method of Assessment	Deviations From Normal	Interpretation
II: Respiratory rate, depth, and rhythm (Cont'd.)	of respiratory movements during quiet and deep respiration	2. Hyperpnea (increased depth)	Hyperpnea is a *critical sign* and indicates respiratory distress. If intervention is not immediate, the patient will develop acute respiratory alkalosis
		B. Hypoventilation (decreased rate and depth):	Hypoventilation may occur in any disease which affects the muscles of ventilation, e.g., Guillain-Barré syndrome; in any injury, deformity, or pathology of the bony thorax or lung which prevents normal movement of the chest, such as fractured ribs, severe scoliosis, or emphysema. Hypoventilation may occur with use of a mechanical respirator
		1. Bradypnea (decreased rate)	
			Hypoventilation also occurs with increased intracranial pressure and as a result of excessive alcohol or opiates
		2. Hypopnea (decreased depth)	Hypopnea is a *critical sign* and indicates respiratory distress. If intervention is not immediate, the patient will develop acute respiratory acidosis

III: Percussion:

A. Lung fields

Percuss lung fields (previously described on p. 27) over the intercostal spaces in a systematic symmetrical fashion. Begin at the apices and work down toward the bases, anteriorly, laterally, and posteriorly. Compare sounds from one area of the lung field to the same area of the opposite lung field. DO NOT percuss over bone as this dulls the percussion sound

Hyperresonance

A hyperresonance percussion tone may occur in emphysema and with a pneumothorax

Dullness

A dull percussion tone may occur in atelectasis, consolidation, or pleural effusion

Areas of dullness may occur due to the patient's position in bed (Figure 1-7)

Tympany

A tympanic percussion tone may occur with a large pneumothorax

B. Level of diaphragm

Percuss down posterior thorax on the right beginning at the 5th ICS until you reach an area of dullness. Mark the level

Increased levels of the diaphragm

Increased diaphragmatic levels may occur with increased intra-abdominal pressure

Remember that the dome of the hemidiaphragm is higher on the right than on the left. Also remember that

(Continued)

TABLE 1-6 (Continued)

Physical Assessment of the Respiratory System

Assessment Parameter	Method of Assessment	Deviations From Normal	Interpretation
	bed position distorts percussion sounds		
IV: Auscultation	Listen over lung fields in a systematic manner comparing breath sounds over symmetrical lung fields as previously described	Bronchovesicular breath sounds in lung fields other than over the apices, the 2nd right and left intercostal spaces, and the intrascapular areas	Bronchovesicular breath sounds occur with a small consolidation
	Breath sounds over the anterior and lateral chest wall are best heard with the patient in a supine position. If the patient is unable to sit up, listen to the posterior breath sounds with the patient first on his right side and then on his left side. These positions will prevent compression of lung tissue and misinterpretation of sounds	Bronchial breath sounds	Bronchial breath sounds occur as consolidation increases
		Diminished or absent breath sounds	Diminished or absent breath sounds occur with a large pleural effusion, in pulmonary emphysema, pneumothorax, and in obstructive atelectasis

Rhonchi occurs with bronchospasm, inflammation and secretions

Rhonchi

If the patient has a naso-gastric tube, clamp off the tube: the sounds from the suction will interfere with auscultation

If the patient is on a respirator and can be taken off, do so before auscultation. Respirators change the characteristics of breath sounds i.e., volume and duration

If the patient cannot be taken off the respirator, describe characteristics of the breath sounds carefully. The respirator does not cause adventitious sounds but will make adventitious sounds more difficult to hear

Chest tubes may produce a pleural friction rub in areas adjacent to the insertion of the tube

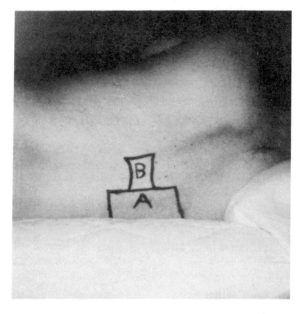

Figure 1-7. Effect of lateral recumbant position on percussion sound: (A) dullness next to bed; (B) dullness caused by pressure of viscera.

tion. Orthopnea is a sign of left ventricular failure. It is also seen in patients with emphysema or abdominal distention.

Cough

Cough is defined as "a sudden, forceful, noisy expulsion of air from the lungs."[3] It is a result of congestion of the bronchial mucosa which may occur with exudate, inflammation, or obstruction. The timing of the cough, i.e., early morning or at night, and absence or presence of sputum production are important observations. A cough that occurs in a recumbent position is often an early sign of congestive heart failure.

Sputum production

This also represents important subjective information. Sputum production is characterized by the amount, color, consistency, and odor of the sputum. Green or yellow sputum indicates an infectious process and a culture of the sputum should be obtained. Frothy pink or white sputum indicates acute pulmonary edema. Bloody sputum may indicate pulmonary infarction, coagulation disorder, cancer of lung, etc.

Chest pain

This is an extremely common symptom and can arise from any structure within the thoracic cage, i.e., the heart, lungs, pleura, the thoracic cage itself (ribs or sternum), or from extra-thoracic structures, such as muscles of chest, neck, shoulders, or upper abdominal viscera. The nurse should assess the chest pain using the model outlined for the history of current illness on p. 12.

Color

Changes in color of the skin and mucous membranes may indicate cardiac, pulmonary, renal or liver malfunction. Three color changes that the nurse in the ICU needs to assess are the presence of jaundice, pallor or cyanosis. Skin color is more accurately assessed in natural rather than fluorescent light. It is more important to note a change in color rather than to describe an absolute shade. Skin changes can be a sign of early shock because a decrease in cardiac output will stimulate the carotid baroreceptors to effect constriction of the arterioles and stimulation of sweat glands, producing the characteristic cold, pale, clammy skin.[1] The three color changes are:

1. *Jaundice:* Jaundice refers to skin which is yellow in color; it is most easily detected in the scleral tissue because bilirubin has a particular affinity for scleral tissue. Jaundice can occur as a result of increased destruction of red blood cells or impairment of the liver. It is difficult to detect true jaundice in artificial light because people with normal coloring look yellow under artificial light. Biliary obstruction and drug toxicity are also causes of jaundice. Regardless of the etiology, if jaundice is present, the color of the patient's stool and urine should be noted.

2. *Pallor:* This refers to a lack of red tones normally imparted to the skin and mucous membranes by the hemoglobin in the superficial blood vessels. Pallor is best evaluated by observing the conjunctiva, oral mucosa, and nailbeds. When looking at nailbeds for pallor, a reliable index is comparison of the patient's nailbeds to those of the examiner. Pallor may be a sign of pain, blood loss, or may be the patient's normal color.

3. *Cyanosis:* A bluish discoloration of the skin is termed cyanosis. It is dependent upon the presence of an absolute amount of unoxygenated hemoglobin, not on a ratio of oxygenated to unoxygenated hemoglobin. Because of the difficulty in quantifying cyanosis, every critically ill patient should have an arterial blood gas analysis. Cyanosis is most readily seen by examination of the ear lobes, oral mucosa at the base of the tongue, and the nailbeds. There are two types of cyanosis:

a) Central cyanosis, which is due to low arterial oxygen saturation and is seen in pulmonary diseases that interfere with ventilation and/or diffusion and in some congenital heart defects when there is a left to right shunt. The tongue is characteristically cyanotic.

b) Peripheral cyanosis, which results from low cardiac output due to congestive heart failure or peripheral vascular obstruction. Peripheral cyanosis is accompanied by a decrease in skin temperature and by mottling. In contrast to central cyanosis, the tongue is normal in color.

Peripheral edema

This is the gradual swelling of the lower extremities. Common causes of symmetrical peripheral edema are right ventricular failure, which is accompanied by an elevated central venous pressure, and peripheral vascular disease. Asymmetrical edema suggests a local obstruction as noted with a deep venous thrombosis, or a lymphatic obstruction. Noncardiovascular causes of edema may be due to liver or renal dysfunction. Fluid from the extremities shifts to the sacral areas when the patient is confined to bed.

THE CARDIOVASCULAR SYSTEM

The purpose of the cardiovascular system is to distribute, transport, and collect blood from diffusion sites (capillaries) within the body and to provide adequate perfusion to organs and tissues.[4] Assessment of the cardiovascular system is for the purpose of determining subtle changes in the integrity of the heart, veins, and arteries which would indicate decreasing efficiency of the cardiovascular system. Recognition of these changes and prompt intervention by the nurse increases the chances of survival for the critically ill person. It is necessary for the nurse to have a firm grasp of the following background information before she can begin cardiac auscultation.

Normal Heart Sounds

The first heart sound (S_1) results from sudden changes in the blood flow associated with closure of the mitral and tricuspid valves. The components of S_1, therefore, are sounds created by closure of the mitral valve (M_1) and the tricuspid valve (T_1). Recent investigations have shown that the beginning of ventricular contraction is a contributory factor in the creation of S_1.[5]

The second heart sound (S_2) results from sudden changes in the blood flow associated with the closure of the aortic and pulmonic valves at the end of systolic ejection. The aortic valve closes slightly before the pulmonic valve. The components of S_2, therefore, are sounds created by the closure of the aortic valve (A_2) and pulmonic valve (P_2).

Figure 1-8 is a pictorial description of the heart sounds in relation to the cardiac cycle. The dotted lines represent one cardiac cycle. The time interval between S_1 and S_2 is called *systole*; the time interval between S_2 and S_1 is called *diastole*.

Auscultatory Characteristics of Heart Sounds

S_1 is usually loudest at the apex of the heart. S_1 is a longer, lower pitched sound than S_2 and corresponds with the pulsation of the carotid artery. S_2 is usually loudest at the base of the heart and is a shorter, higher pitched sound than S_1. S_2, however, can be louder than S_1 at the apex in the younger or hypertensive patient. Figure 1-9 shows the relationship of the heart sounds to the electrocardiogram.

It should be noted that S_1 begins with the R wave and the S_2 occurs after the T wave. From the diagram, it can also be noted that the electrical impulse slightly precedes the resultant myocardial contraction.

Anatomical Location of the Transmission of Heart Sounds

The sound associated with closure of the tricuspid valve (T_1) is transmitted to the left lower sternal border (LLSB) at approximately the fourth or fifth intercostal space (ICS). The sound associated with closure of the mitral valve (M_1) is transmitted to the

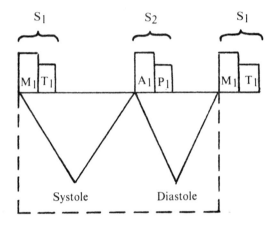

Figure 1-8. Heart sounds in relation to cardiac cycle.

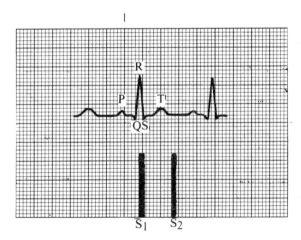

Figure 1-9. Relationship of heart sounds to the electrocardiogram.

fifth intercostal space (ICS) just medial to the midclavicular line approximately 7-9 cms from the midsternal line (MSL). The sites for transmission of valve sounds should not be confused with the anatomical location of the valves themselves.

The sound associated with aortic valve closure (A_2) is transmitted to the second intercostal space (ICS) immediately to the right of the sternal margin. It is also transmitted to the third intercostal space (ICS) immediately to the left of the sternal margin; this is known as Erb's point. The sound associated with the pulmonic valve closure sound (P_2) is transmitted to the second intercostal space (ICS) immediately to the left of the left sternal margin.

Techniques of Auscultation

A systematic method of listening to heart sounds is essential in order to avoid missing abnormal auscultatory findings. The examiner begins auscultation using the diaphragm of the stethoscope at the apex (Point of Maximal Impulse) and moves to the left lower sternal border, ascending gradually to the pulmonic area and across the sternum to the aortic area (Figure 1-10). Next, the order is reversed with the examiner moving from the aortic area to the apex, using the bell of the stethoscope. The bell accentuates low-pitched sounds and the diaphragm accentuates high-pitched sounds.

An excellent method to employ for auscultation of heart sounds is "inching," which is movement of the stethoscope small distances from one auscultatory area to another. Inching facilitates detection of all auscultatory sounds whereas data may be missed by only auscultating over the four major areas.

For a complete examination of the heart, the nurse should listen to the heart with the patient in both the supine and the sitting positions. For the critically ill person, however, the supine position alone is appropriate. When the heart sounds are "soft" or "distant," other positions may help to accentuate heart sounds. For example, with a patient who is obese or who has a barrel chest, the nurse is able to hear heart sounds more distinctly by listening over the xyphoid area with the patient sitting and leaning forward. Auscultation with the bell in the left lateral position will accentuate extra-heart sounds such as gallops or murmurs at the apex and the left lower sternal border.

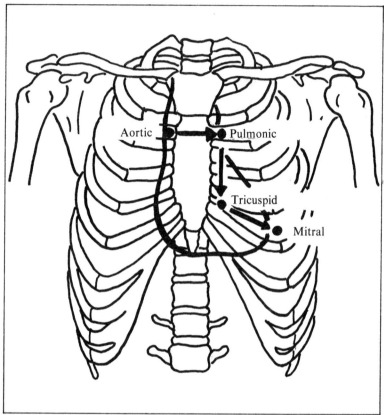

Figure 1-10. Auscultation of heart sounds. (From: Hochstein E, Rubin AL: *Physical Diagnosis*. McGraw-Hill, New York, 1964, p. 183. Used with permission.)

Inspection and Palpation for the Point of Maximal Impulse

Inspection and palpation of the anterior chest is best done when the patient is lying either flat on his back or with his head elevated no more than 45 degrees. In this position, the nurse observes for pulsations resulting from movement of the heart and great vessels by observing the chest wall tangentially. Any pulsation below the third intercostal space on the left precordium is known as the PMI, the area of the chest where the apex of the heart slaps against the chest wall; any pulsation above the 3rd ICS is not related to the heart but rather to the great vessels.[5] The PMI is normally located in the fifth

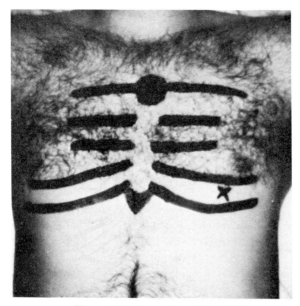

Figure 1-11. Location of the PMI.

intercostal space approximately 7-9 cms. from the midsternal line and medial to the midclavicular line (Figure 1-11). In a woman, this area lies over the distal one-third of the breast. The PMI is not always visible, but is usually palpable.

If the PMI is not palpable with the patient lying in the supine position, ask the patient to turn to the left lateral side. In this position, the heart moves closer to the chest wall and is thus more easily palpated. The examiner does not use the PMI palpated in this position as a reference point from which to measure, however, because placing the patient in the left lateral position displaces the heart laterally. However, one may use the PMI palpated in the left lateral position as a reference point for location of the PMI with the patient in a supine position.

The landmarks for measuring the PMI are the midsternal line horizontally and the midclavicular line vertically, according to the intercostal space where the PMI is palpated. The PMI is recorded thus: _ _ _ cms. from the midsternal line in the _ _ _ ICS, (at, medial to, or lateral to) the midclavicular line. The PMI is normally no larger than two cms. or the size of a nickel. The amplitude can be normally obliterated by too much pressure from the finger-tips.

Abnormal Cardiac Sounds

Split Second Heart Sounds (Table 1-7)

Under normal circumstances, the aortic valve closes slightly before the pulmonic valve. This phenomenon is due to the fact that left ventricular contraction slightly precedes right ventricular contraction. On expiration, however, closure of the aortic and pulmonic valves occurs almost simultaneously and thus is heard as a single sound. On inspiration, due to the decrease in intrathoracic pressure, there is an increase in venous blood to the right side of the heart which delays the closure of the pulmonic valve and results in a split sound. On expiration, the disparity in right atrial blood volume is not present, thus closure of the aortic and pulmonic valves is nearly simultaneous and results in a single sound. The splitting of S_2 into the two components (A_2 and P_2) on inspiration is *normal* and is referred to as a *physiologic split*. The physiologic split is best heard over the pulmonic auscultatory area at the *end of inspiration*. A physiologic split is heard easily in children, young adults, and thin persons.

A *paradoxical split* is abnormal and occurs when the second component (P_2) of the second heart sound is heard before the first component (A_2) due to reverse order of valve closure. This phenomenon may occur when closure of the aortic valve is delayed due to volume overload and increased pressure of the left ventricle a noted in aortic stenosis. On inspiration, the pulmonic valve (normally delayed) closes at the same time as the aortic valve with the result of a single sound. On expiration, however, the pulmonic valve closes earlier than the aortic valve, resulting in a *split sound on expiration*. This is an *abnormal* split sound and represents pathology as noted with any condition associated with volume overload of the left ventricle, or with left bundle branch block.

A *fixed split* is abnormal and occurs when there is a volume overload of the right ventricle. The closure of the aortic and pulmonic valves are in the normal sequence, but both components (A_2 and P_2) are distinctly heard with every second heart sound and do not change to become one sound during either inspiration or expiration. A fixed split is *abnormal* and may occur in right bundle

TABLE 1-7

Characteristics of Split Second Heart Sound

Respiratory Phase	Physiologic Split (Normal)	Paradoxical Split (Abnormal)	Fixed Split (Abnormal)
Inspiration	S_2 presents as two sounds $A_2 - P_2$	S_2 presents as one sound P_2A_2	S_2 presents as two sounds $A_2 - P_2$
Expiration	S_2 presents as one sound A_2P_2	S_2 presents as two sounds $P_2 - A_2$	S_2 presents as two sounds $A_2 - P_2$

branch block, pulmonary hypertension, and right ventricular failure secondary to either atrial or ventricular septal defect.

Murmurs

Murmurs are a result of turbulent blood flow. The turbulence in blood flow is due to structural changes or hemodynamic events occurring in the heart or great vessels. Murmurs are produced as a result of the following mechanisms:

1. Obstruction to forward flow, e.g., a stenotic valve or artery.
2. Backward flow across an incompetent valve, e.g., insufficiency of a valve.
3. Excessive flow or increased velocity of flow across normal structures, e.g., in pregnancy, hyperthyroidism, cardiac failure or anemia.
4. Turbulent flow in a dilated chamber, e.g., an aneurysm in a ventricle or aorta.
5. Shunting of blood through an abnormal passageway, e.g., a septal defect, patent ductus, or A-V fistula.

Murmurs are classified and recorded according to the following characteristics:

1. *Timing:* Murmurs are described as systolic or diastolic depending on where they occur in the cardiac cycle. Murmurs beginning with or after S_1 and ending before or at S_2 are termed *systolic*. Murmurs beginning with or after S_2 and

ending before or at S_1 are termed *diastolic*. Murmurs are further described in terms of specific occurrence in systole or diastole: early, mid, or late. A murmur that begins with one heart sound and is continuous to the other heart sound is referred to as a "holo" or "pan" systolic or diastolic murmur.

2. *Location:* Murmurs are described and recorded in relation to the anatomical landmarks or valve areas over which the murmur is heard loudest.

3. *Transmission:* Murmurs are described according to radiation from the area where the murmurs are heard the loudest. Murmurs may radiate from the area of loudest auscultation to other areas on the precordium and/or to the neck or axilla. Not all murmurs radiate, but recording the transmission of a murmur provides useful information about the origin of a murmur.

4. *Pitch:* Murmurs are described according to pitch. Pitch is related to the velocity of the blood flow. An increase in velocity of blood flow produces highest pitched sounds whereas a decrease in velocity produces lowest pitched sounds.[12]

5. *Quality:* Murmurs are described in terms of their quality, e.g., blowing, harsh, rumbling, or musical.

6. *Intensity:** Murmurs are described in terms of their loudness according to the following system:

   a) Grade I: Very faint; the examiner must strain to hear.

   b) Grade II: Faint, but readily heard.

   c) Grade III: Moderate, or the same loudness as the normal heart sounds.

   d) Grade IV: Louder than normal heart sounds and associated with a thrill (palpable murmur).

   e) Grade V: Extremely loud and associated with a thrill.

*Systolic murmurs are graded on a scale of I-VI, whereas diastolic murmurs, because they are less intense, are graded on a scale of I-IV.

f) Grade VI: Audible with the ear on or near the chest wall without the use of a stethoscope.

7. *Configuration:* Murmurs are described and may be diagrammed according to shape and intensity:

a) Crescendo: Intensity increases from onset of murmur.

b) Decrescendo: Intensity decreases from onset of murmur.

c) Crescendo-
   Decrescendo: Intensity increases and then decreases.

d) Sustained
   (plateau): Intensity remains the same throughout.

Murmurs commonly heard in the adult are the systolic ejection murmur, the holosystolic murmur, and the diastolic murmur. The *systolic ejection murmur* occurs most frequently. This murmur is short in duration and begins and ends early in systole. The majority of these murmurs heard near the apex or left lower sternal border are innocent or functional. Any systolic ejection murmur of Grade III or above usually denotes pathology. The two most common pathological systolic ejection murmurs are the murmurs of pulmonic and aortic stenosis. These murmurs are usually best heard at the base of the heart.

Holosystolic murmurs always represent heart pathology. They begin with S_1 and continue to the beginning of S_2, and may obscure the normal heart sounds. These murmurs are usually best heard at the apex. Holosystolic murmurs are associated with mitral insufficiency (most common cause), tricuspid insufficiency or ventricular septal defects.

Similarly, *diastolic murmurs* almost always represent pathology and are divided into two types, those caused by stenosis and those caused by incompetent heart valves. The murmurs caused by mitral or tricuspid stenosis are low-pitched and occur late in diastole; in contrast, regurgitant murmurs caused by aortic insufficiency are high-pitched and begin immediately after the second heart sound, ending before the first sound. Regurgitant murmurs caused by pulmonic insufficiency are usually high-pitched, but may also be low-pitched.[2]

Pericardial Friction Rub

Pericardial friction rubs originate in the pericardial sac and result from inflammation, infiltration, or infarction. Diseases commonly associated with rubs are pericarditis, acute myocardial infarction, trauma, uremia, neoplasms of breast and lung and postradiation therapy states. Pericardial friction rubs are high-pitched scratching or grating sounds that are heard best with the diaphragm of the stethoscope between the apex and the left sternal border. Pericardial friction rubs may be quite transient in nature and may be audible for only a few minutes to hours. They usually have two or three components and are often heard throughout the cardiac cycle.

Extra Heart Sounds

Extra heart sounds include the opening snap, the ejection click, S_3, and S_4. The two sounds which most commonly occur and which will be discussed here are the third heart sound, S_3, and the fourth heart sound, S_4. S_3, or ventricular gallop, and S_4, or atrial gallop, are both diastolic sounds and may occur independently or may both be present. An S3 represents an increase in mid-diastolic pressure, whereas an S4 represents an increase in end diastolic pressure.[2]

An S3 results from the rapid filling of the ventricle when the volume of early filling is increased or when there is decreased ventricular compliance. The third heart sound is heard at the left lower sternal border or apex and is often heard best in the left lateral position. S3 occurs early in diastole, is low-pitched, and is heard best with the bell of the stethoscope.

S3 can be differentiated from S2 by its lower pitch and its auscultatory site. In young children and adolescents an S3 is normal and results from transition of rapid to slow filling in a compliant ventricle. In adults, an S3 is usually abnormal and occurs secondary to right or left ventricular failure. If it is due to right ventricular failure, the best auscultatory site is at the left lower sternal border. If an S3 is due to left ventricular failure, the best auscultatory site is at the apex. An S3 is usually accompanied by an increased heart rate and is an *early* sign of ventricular failure.

The S4 is a sound created when the atrium contracts and ejects blood into a noncompliant ventricle. The fourth heart sound is heard best over the left lower sternal border or apex. An S4 sound occurs late in diastole, is low-pitched, and is heard best with the bell of the stethoscope. This sound can be differentiated from S1 because the S4 is a lower pitched sound. An S4 is commonly heard in patients during the acute phase of a myocardial infarction, in patients with hypertension, or in patients with aortic stenosis. It is not considered abnormal in patients after the age of 60 due to the normal aging process of the ventricle. Figure 1-12 represents the occurrence of heart sounds within the cardiac cycle.

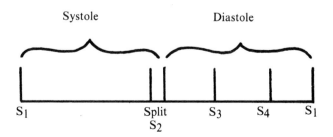

Figure 1-12. Occurrence of normal, split, and extra heart sounds in the cardiac cycle as heard at the apex of the heart.

Assessment of the Vascular System

The venous return of the vascular system is assessed by observation and/or palpation of the jugular veins and the extremities. The arterial flow of the vascular system is assessed by observation and palpation of the extremities and the peripheral pulses. The peripheral pulses are evaluated on the basis of presence or absence and the equality of amplitude in symmetrical areas. The contour of the normal pulse curve is a brisk upstroke and a downstroke which is more gradual. The force of the peripheral pulses correlates with the pulse pressure. All pulses except the carotids are palpated simultaneously to determine symmetrical characteristics. The characteristics of the peripheral pulses should be noted and documented preadmission or presurgery as baseline data. Generally, the peripheral pulses to be assessed include the carotid, radial, femoral, and pedal pulses. Figure 1-13 illustrates the location of the peripheral pulses. Pulses should be palpated routinely and frequently on all patients with a history of trauma or vascular surgery of any type.

It will be necessary in certain instances to assess other peripheral pulses, e.g., the popliteal pulse if the pedal pulses are absent or abnormal. Popliteal pulses are often difficult to palpate and require practice with a patient who has normal pulse volumes. The dorsalis pedis is not palpable in approximately 13% of the population.[3] When edema interferes with palpation of the pedal pulses, the nurse should elevate the extremity for a brief time and then re-palpate for the presence of a pulse.

In palpating pulses, only the middle and ring fingers should be used. The thumb and index finger should not have contact with the patient because both of these fingers have very strong pulses and the examiner may mistake his/her own pulsation for that of the patient.

If any pulse is absent or not equal to the contralateral pulse, the nurse should check the pulses proximal to that pulse to determine at what site the pulses begin to diminish. For example, if the radial pulse is absent, the nurse should then palpate the brachial pulse. If the radial and pedal pulses are full and equal, and the carotid and femoral pulses are full and equal, the nurse can assume that the midway pulses are functional because blood flow to the distal and proximal sites of the extremities is normal.

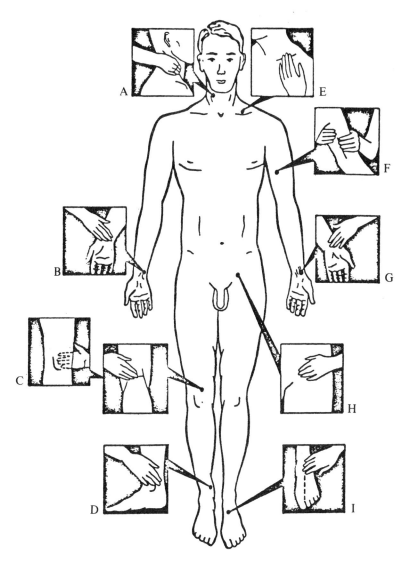

Figure 1-13. Location of pulses: A = carotid; B = ulnar; C = popliteal; D = posterior tibial; E = subclavian; F = high brachial; G = radial; H = femoral; I = dorsalis pedis. (From: Steedman RA: Postoperative Care of the Adult Cardiac Surgical Patient. In Zschoche DA, Ed.: *Mosby's Comprehensive Review of Critical Care*. C.V. Mosby Company, St. Louis, Mo., 1976, p. 239. Used with permission.)

Peripheral pulses are graded on a scale of 0-4 by the following system:

0	=	absent pulse
+	=	diminished (barely palpable)
++	=	average
+++	=	full and brisk
++++	=	bounding pulse

Pulses are easily recorded in the following manner:

	Carotid	Radial	Femoral	Dorsalis pedis	Posterior tibial
Right	++	++	++	++	++
Left	++	++	++	++	++

Table 1-8 describes the parameters and methods of assessment utilized in the examination of the cardiovascular system.

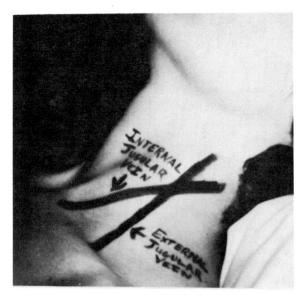

Figure 1-14. Location of the jugular veins.
(Refer to p. 61 of Table 1-8
for a more extensive description.)

TABLE 1-8

Physical Assessment of the Cardiovascular System

Assessment Parameter	Method of Assessment	Deviations From Normal	Interpretations
I: Heart:			
A. Heart and pulse rate and rhythm	Auscultate apical pulse and palpate radial pulse simultaneously for one full minute. ECG and arrhythmias will be discussed in the cardiovascular chapter	Pulse deficit	Occurs with various arrhythmias
		Pulse rate above 100	Tachycardia could be due to sepsis, ventricular irritability, hypovolemia, fever, congestive heart failure, pain, apprehension, or a chronotropic drug (e.g., Isuprel)
		Pulse rate below 60	Bradycardia could result from incomplete or complete heart block, or medications such as digitalis, or other antiarrhythmic agents
			A pulse increase or decrease of 20 beats from a baseline pulse is significant
B. Blood pressure	Take the blood pressure either by intra-arterial monitoring or sphygmomanometer at regular intervals, with the frequency of intervals determined by the patient's condition	Any elevation of 20-30 mm Hg systolic	The cause of an elevated **BP** may be peripheral vaso-constriction, hypercapnea, inotropic drugs, and/or increased intracranial pressure

(Continued)

TABLE 1-8 (Continued)

Physical Assessment of the Cardiovascular System

Assessment Parameter	Method of Assessment	Deviations From Normal	Interpretations
B. Blood Pressure (Cont'd)	Periodically, the nurse should check the BP by sphygmomanometer to compare it with the accuracy of the intra-arterial monitor	Any systolic pressure below 90 mm Hg, or any systolic drop of more than 20-30 mm Hg	Causes of lowered BP may be hypovolemia, shock, arrhythmias, poor myocardial contractility, or drugs such as antihypertensive agents, large doses of analgesics, and antiarrhythmics
	The arterial line is flushed intermittently with a heparinized solution to prevent clot formation		
	Observe for changes in the pulse pressure. Normally, the difference between the systolic and diastolic pressure is 30-50 mm Hg	Narrowed pulse pressure	Indicates a low stroke volume which may be caused by cardiac tamponade. If the cause is cardiac tamponade, there will also be a sudden rise in CVP and distant heart sounds
			Other causes are cardiogenic shock, heart failure, severe aortic or mitral stenosis[12]
		Widened pulse pressure	Occurs in aortic regurgitation, atherosclerosis, fever,[12] and increasing intracranial pressure

C. **The PMI**

With the patient in a supine position:

1. Inspect the chest wall for visible pulsations at eye level with the chest wall

2. If a pulsation is visible, place the examining fingers over the area and find the area of greatest amplitude

3. Measure the location of the PMI as previously described on p. 44

4. If a pulsation is not visible, place the examining hand over the left chest wall with the fingers resting over the lateral chest wall between the fifth and ninth ribs

Pulsation above the 3rd ICS

Displaced PMI

When the nurse detects changes in the pulse or the **BP**, she should report the **BP**, **P**, present ECG pattern, **CVP**, urine output, and the status of the breath sounds to the physician

May indicate an aneurysm of the ascending aorta

This may indicate either systolic overloading of the left ventricle or ventricular hypertrophy

N.B. Other factors influence the location of the PMI, such as shape of the chest wall, height of the diaphragm, and deformities of the thoracic spine or chest, including mediastinal shifts. A chest x-ray is, therefore, necessary to best determine cardiac size

(Continued)

TABLE 1-8 (Continued)

Physical Assessment of the Cardiovascular System

Assessment Parameter	Method of Assessment	Deviations From Normal	Interpretations
C. The PMI (Cont'd)	5. When examining a female patient, displace the breast upward with the palpating hand		
	6. Palpate for the PMI with the fingers. Begin laterally and move medially toward the sternum until the PMI is palpated		
	7. Determine the anatomical location of the PMI as previously described on p. 44		
	8. If unable to palpate the PMI in a supine position, place the patient in the left lateral position and proceed as previously described in number 6		
	9. Note the size of the PMI	Diffuse or enlarged PMI	This is known as a *heave*. If a heave is present, the PMI cannot be obliterated by the

		pressure of the fingertips and may be felt in several ICS
		A heave represents either an overload of the left ventricle or ventricular hypertrophy
D. Heart sounds	At each auscultatory area:	
	1. Identify the first heart sound which corresponds to the pulsation of the carotid artery. Note its intensity and the presence or absence of splitting. Splitting occurs when the two components of S_1 (i.e., closure of M_1 and T_1) can be heard distinctly on auscultation. Split S_1 sounds are normal	Very loud S_1
		May be a sign of mitral stenosis especially if it is associated with a diastolic murmur. Other causes may be fever, anemia, or tachycardia. Another cause is a shortened A-V conduction time, (P-R interval less than .10 second)[5]
		Diminished or very soft S_1
		Causes may include mitral insufficiency, decreasing ventricular contraction, delayed A-V conduction time. A faint S_1 will be heard if the A-V conduction is delayed; P-R interval beyond 0.22 second[5]
	2. Identify the second heart sound, note its intensity and the presence or absence of splitting. Splitting occurs when the separate components of S_2	Very loud S_2
		Common in young persons. May occur in hypertension or aortic insufficiency (which would be associated with a diastolic murmur)

(Continued)

TABLE 1-8 (Continued)

Physical Assessment of the Cardiovascular System

Assessment Parameter	Method of Assessment	Deviations From Normal	Interpretations
D. Heart sounds (Cont'd)	(i.e., closure of A_2 and P_2) can be heard distinctly on auscultation	Diminished or soft S_2	May occur in aortic stenosis, or pulmonary emphysema
	3. Compare the intensity of S_1 and S_2 at each auscultatory area	Distant or grossly diminished intensity of S_1 and S_2	If the heart sounds change in intensity and become barely audible, cardiac tamponade is probable
	4. Listen during the period between S_1 and S_2 in each auscultatory site for the presence of extra sounds and/or murmurs	Murmurs, extra sounds, paradoxical or fixed split second heart sounds	See pages 46-51 for interpretation of these sounds
	5. Listen during the period between S_2 and S_1 at each auscultatory site for the presence of extra sounds and/or murmurs. The key to successful auscultation is the ability to concentrate on and tune into, listening to one event at a time, and to selectively tune out the other events.		

II: Vascular system:

A. Jugular veins

The external jugular neck veins lie superficial to and cross the sternocleidomastoid muscles diagonally (see Figure 1-14, p. 54)

If the patient has a CVP line, use the CVP to assess the venous pressure; if not, do the following:

a) Place the patient in a 45° semi-recumbent position

b) Observe the external jugular vein for pulsation and distention

Jugular venous pulsations are not normally visible in the 45° semi-recumbent position. Jugular venous pulsations and distention may be visible in positions below this angle and are considered normal

Distention of the jugular veins

Distention of jugular veins above the level of the clavicle when the patient is in a sitting position indicates that the central venous pressure is over 15 centimeters of H_2O

An elevated central venous pressure occurs most commonly with right ventricular failure

If the nurse observes jugular venous distention she should assess the patient for other signs of failure, e.g., increased pulse rate, S_3, peripheral edema, and rales

Other causes of elevated central venous pressure are pericarditis, cardiac tamponade, superior vena cava obstruction, and pulmonary hypertension

(Continued)

TABLE 1-8 (Continued)

Physical Assessment of the Cardiovascular System

Assessment Parameter	Method of Assessment	Deviations From Normal	Interpretations
B. Major peripheral pulses		For All Peripheral Pulses:	
	1. Determine presence/absence	1. Inequality in pulse volumes and/or absence of pulse	May indicate an aneurysm, arteriosclerotic narrowing of the vessel, or external compression of the artery proximal to the point of palpation
	2. Determine amplitude		
	3. Determine equality in contralateral areas	2. Rapid, thready pulse with low amplitude	Rapid thready pulse is a sign of shock or severe ventricular failure
1. Carotid	The carotid pulse is located across from the thyroid cartilage and medial to the sternocleidomastoid muscle		
	1. Have the patient slightly extend his neck without turning his head	1. Absent bilateral pulses	Is the cardinal sign of cardiac arrest
	2. Place the examining fingers over one carotid until you determine the characteristics of the	2. Diminished pulse	May indicate an occlusion of the common carotid artery, a dissection of the aortic arch, or ineffective cardiac output

pulse. Repeat the maneuver with the other carotid

Only one carotid pulse is palpated at a time. Palpation of both carotids simultaneously results in a reduction of blood flow which could become critical in a patient who already has severe atherosclerosis

2. Radial		
The radial pulse is located on the flexor surface of the wrist medial to the distal portion of the radius	Unequal or absent pulse	May be due to previous arteriotomy or use of a monitoring catheter, or arteriosclerosis of the innominate artery
Place the patient's arm in a relaxed position and palpate the pulses simultaneously in contralateral extremities		
3. Femoral		
The femoral pulse lies just below the inguinal ligament midway between the superior iliac spine and the pubic tubercles	Diminished, unequal, or absent pulse	May indicate arterial obstruction of the iliac artery

(*Continued*)

TABLE 1-8 (Continued)

Physical Assessment of the Cardiovascular System

Assessment Parameter	Method of Assessment	Deviations From Normal	Interpretations
B. Major peripheral pulses (Cont'd)	Press deeply in the groin area and palpate pulses simultaneously in contra-lateral extremities		
4. Pedal pulses:			
a) **Posterior tibial**	The posterior tibial pulse is located just posterior to the medial malleolus		
b) **Dorsalis pedis**	The dorsalis pedis pulse is located on the dorsal aspect of the foot mid-way between the extensor hallucis tendon and the extensor digitorum longus tendon but may be lateral or medial to this area (see Figure 1-13, p. 53)		
	In some patients, the dorsalis pedis or posterior tibial may not be pal-pable in the same foot. If neither pulse is pres-	Diminished, unequal, or absent pulse	May indicate thrombus formation or narrowing of the lumen of the artery secondary to arteriosclerotic changes

ent in one extremity, then palpate the popliteal pulse

Dorsiflex the foot and begin to lightly palpate from the distalmost point

Palpate the pulses simultaneously in the contralateral extremities

C. Extremities

1. Size and symmetry:

a) With the legs in a flat position and midline, observe for symmetry and color of legs

b) Measure and record *daily*, the circumference of each calf and thigh with a tape measure:

(1) Measure to a point on the calf approximately 8" above the malleolus or 6" below the distal portion of the patella

c) Perform the same procedure with the arms if patient has IV catheter,

Red, tender, and/or edematous extremities

Indicates venous thrombosis, which is a continuous threat in bedfast patients because of a predisposition to pulmonary emboli. Venous thrombosis is an obstructive alteration of the vein which can be caused by mechanical, thermal, or chemical changes[6]

If the above signs are noted, check pulses proximal and distal to the site and the patient's body temperature

A difference of one inch in circumference without presenting symptoms is normal

(Continued)

TABLE 1-8 (Continued)

Physical Assessment of the Cardiovascular System

Assessment Parameter	Method of Assessment	Deviations From Normal	Interpretations
C. Extremities (Cont'd)	transvenous pacemaker, or CVP in the antecubital area		
	d) Palpate the legs for tenderness		
	2. Homans' sign: a) Place the patient's legs in a flat position and midline		
	b) Quickly and forcefully dorsiflex the foot while observing whether the patient experiences pain in the calf	Pain in the calf on dorsiflexion of the foot is a "positive" Homans' sign	A positive Homans' sign indicates a deep venous thrombosis
	3. Edema: a) Press the tip of the examining finger for approximately five seconds against	Bilateral edema except for sacrum	Indicates right ventricular failure, hepatic or renal failure, or a reduction in plasma albumin

an area of the patient's skin overlying a bony prominence, e.g., the medial malleus, tibia, or sacrum

b) Inspect the area for indentation

c) The extent of the edema is described in terms of the degree of indentation and its extension proximally

d) Compare findings with previous documentation

Unilateral edema of extremity

Indicates venous or lymph obstruction or an inflammatory process, e.g., thrombophlebitis.

If the patient has peripheral venous disease, he will have peripheral edema; therefore, the sacral area must be used to assess edema. In the adult, fluid must accumulate to approximately ten pounds before detected as pitting[3]

THE NEUROLOGICAL SYSTEM

The neurological system is the most vital organ system of control and regulation of body functions. "The nervous system is a complex array of specialized structures which serve to receive, store, and transmit information—thereby integrating the activities of spatially separated cells, tissues, and organs and making it possible for a multicellular organism to function as a coordinated unit in terms of growth, development, the ability to do work, and to adapt to changes in the environment."[13]

The purpose of the neurological system assessment is to determine initial changes in the integrity of the brain and spinal cord that could indicate physiologic deterioration of the critically ill person. The signs which the nurse continuously monitors to prevent deterioration are:

1. Mental status
2. Level of consciousness
3. Temperature
4. Blood pressure
5. Pulse rate and regularity
6. Respiratory rate, depth, and regularity
7. Cranial nerve function
8. Motor function
9. Deep tendon reflexes
10. Plantar reflex

Ongoing evaluation of the patient's mental status is often the earliest sign of neurological dysfunction. Therefore, the nurse needs to be continuously observant in documenting the patient's behavior.

Critical Subjective Data

Severe progressive headache

This may indicate increased intracranial pressure. The nurse should describe the headache using the parameters suggested in the history of current illness. *Vomiting and failing vision* along with protracted headache are definitive symptoms of increased intracranial pressure.

Visual changes

Changes such as blurring or clouding of vision, decreasing vision, partial or complete loss of vision, or scotomas all indicate damage to either the optic nerve or brain, secondary to injury, increased intracranial pressure, vascular or tumor lesions.

Critical Objective Data

Vital signs

Graphing of vital signs is an excellent assessment tool for the evaluation of increasing intracranial pressure. Changes in orientation, level of arousal, and muscular strength are the earliest signs of increased intracranial pressure. The classic changes in vital signs which occur are: elevation of systolic blood pressure with a decrease in diastolic pressure (widened pulse pressure); decreasing pulse rate which gradually becomes irregular; decreasing respiratory rate which gradually becomes irregular; and a gradual increase in body temperature.

Figure 1-15 depicts the changes in mental state, pupil size, blood pressure, pulse, respiration, and temperature before and after the onset of increased intracranial pressure.

Seizure

The nurse should note the starting point, progression, type of movement (clonic or tonic), and duration of the seizure. The level of consciousness preceding, during, and after the seizure, and any aura should also be noted. If the seizure is generalized, the nurse should determine whether it is followed by motor weakness or paralysis. If it is a localized seizure, the nurse should state the exact degree and part of the body involved as well as the length of time it takes the patient to recover.

The seizure should be described with minute accuracy in sequential order of the appearance of each component. Accurate observation and recording of seizures is essential in that it can assist the physician in determining the focal area of the brain that is irritated. Since seizures may also result from cardiovascular phenomena, it is also important to record the pulse.[2]

Changes in behavior

Signs of restlessness or confusion should be carefully noted by the nurse as these changes may result from increased intracranial pressure, hypoxia, pain, urinary retention, and/or deprivations

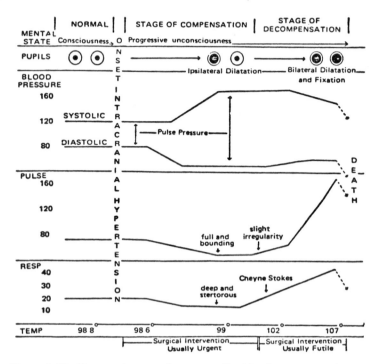

Figure 1-15. Changes in mental state, pupils, blood pressure, pulse rate, respiratory rate and temperature with increased intracranial pressure. (From: McCracken ML: Assessment Skills for the Nurse. In Hudak CM et al: *Critical Care Nursing*. J.B. Lippincott Company, Philadelphia, Pa., 1973, p. 290. Used with permission.)

which may lead to ICU psychosis. The nurse should also report any involuntary movement (e.g., picking at bedclothes with fingers, termed *carphology*). This sign occurs in the critically ill person and is a "grave prognostic sign."[3]

Pupillary abnormalities

Inability of the pupils to constrict briskly to a concentrated light source, unequal pupil size, or dilated fixed pupils are all progressive signs of increased intracranial pressure or cranial nerve damage. If the pupils are unequal on admission, the patient's previous records should be reviewed to document whether the unequal pupils may be a normal variation.

Weakness or paralysis of extremity(ies)

Weakness or paralysis may indicate spinal cord injury or cerebral vascular accident. Upper motor neuron lesions produce a spastic paralysis, whereas lower motor neuron lesions produce a flaccid paralysis. Grading of muscle strength, as described in many physical assessment books, will provide the nurse with a graphic representation of the patient's course.

Speech difficulties

Aphasia or dysarthria may be symptoms of a cerebral vascular accident or frontal lobe disease.

Nuchal or neck rigidity

When nuchal rigidity occurs, it is often accompanied by photophobia and is a sign of meningeal irritation.

Leakage of cerebrospinal fluid

In a patient with trauma, the nurse should observe for clear or serosanguinous fluid from the ears, nose, or head wound. This sign may indicate injuries from a basilar skull fracture, meningeal tear, or a depressed skull fracture. If the patient is alert, he may complain of drainage trickling in his throat.[9]

Incontinence of bowel or bladder

Incontinence may result from injury or disease processes related to the brain, spinal cord, or the local nerve supply to the bowel or bladder.

The development of any of these neurological signs or symptoms should be reported immediately to the physician along with the current status of the following parameters:

1. Vital signs
2. Mental status
3. Cranial nerve functioning
4. Gross motor movements
5. Deep tendon reflexes
6. Plantar reflex

With the exception of the vital signs, the succeeding section will describe the parameters and method of assessment utilized in the examination of the neurological system (Table 1-9).

The Deep Tendon Reflexes

Deep tendon reflexes are muscle stretch reflexes elicited by the tapping of a tendon which results in a rapid stretch of the muscle, thus producing the reflex. The basic mechanism of the simple reflex is as follows:

1. A receptor in the tendon sends impulses via afferent (sensory) fibers in the peripheral nerves to the posterior or dorsal root.
2. The impulse synapses in the spinal cord (anterior horn cells).
3. The impulse is sent via efferent (motor) fibers from the anterior horn to a muscle with resultant contraction.

The deep tendon reflex (DTR) depends on intact sensory nerve synapses in the spinal cord, motor neurons, neuromuscular junctions, as well as a competent muscle. DTRs do not depend on the motor function of the brain.

These reflexes are elicited most easily with a rubber percussion hammer. If a reflex hammer is unavailable, the nurse can use the ulnar aspect of her hand. A sudden brief blow is delivered over the site of muscle insertion. The limb must be positioned so that the muscle can be mildly stretched to evoke a muscular contraction (reflex). To deliver the blow, the examiner holds the reflex hammer loosely but firmly between the thumb and fingers so that it swings freely and strikes the tendon briskly.

When reflexes are not elicited by the usual procedure, which happens in very tense or muscular persons, they may be elicited by the use of reinforcement. Reinforcement is a phenomenon which lowers the threshold and increases the reflex response. Reinforcement is accomplished by asking the patient to perform a strong muscular effort in some part of the body away from that part being tested. When testing arm reflexes, ask the patient to clench his teeth or tighten his thigh muscles. When testing lower extremity reflexes, ask the patient to clench his fists or to pull against the sides of the bed. While the patient is distracted, strike the tendon. When eliciting reflexes while using reinforcement techniques, it should be recorded that reinforcement was used for the particular reflex since reinforcement may increase the reflex response.

TABLE 1-9

Physical Assessment of the Neurological System

Assessment Parameter	Method of Assessment	Deviations From Normal	Interpretation
I: **Mental Status:** (When assessing the patient's mental status, always let the patient know what you are doing; it may be particularly upsetting for the patient who is unable to comply)			
A. Orientation to time	1. Ask patient if it is morning, afternoon, or night 2. Ask patient what month it is 3. Ask patient what year it is	Inability to answer (2) and (3) correctly	In assessing orientation to time it is important to keep in mind that because of the ICU environment it is difficult for the critically ill person to keep track of time so that if the patient answers (2) and (3) correctly but misses (1), the patient may still be considered "oriented to time"
B. Orientation to place	1. Ask patient the name of the city in which he is	Inability to answer both questions correctly	Consider name of city and a hospital as correct answers. If patient was admitted in a critical state, the patient

(Continued)

TABLE 1-9 (Continued)
Physical Assessment of the Neurological System

Assessment Parameter	Method of Assessment	Deviations From Normal	Interpretation
B. Orientation to place (Cont'd.)	2. Ask patient where he is		may not know the proper name of the hospital, but if the patient knows that he is in a hospital, consider the patient "oriented to place"
C. Orientation to person	1. Ask patient who are the people walking around the unit	Inability to answer correctly	If the patient answers: "doctors" and "nurses" or equivalent, consider the patient "oriented to person" (The patient's inability to recognize place and person indicates a higher degree of cerebral impairment than does the disorientation of time)
D. Ability to calculate	1. Ask the patient to count backward by serial three's	Inability to answer correctly	The ability to calculate is dependent upon the patient's background and educational level and is difficult to evaluate. Ascertain these background factors and change questions accordingly (e.g., a person with a mathematical background should be given
	2. Ask the patient to do a series of sums (e.g., "what is the sum of $7 + 5 + 6$?")		

			more difficult calculations and a person with a deficient educational background should be given sums in terms of money)
E. Ability to abstract	1. Ask the patient to give you a list of things which belong to the same category, e.g., vegetables 2. Ask patient to interpret a familiar proverb, e.g., "What does it mean when you say that 'a stitch in time saves nine'?"	Inability to answer (1) and (2) correctly; repetition of question by the patient or a literal interpretation of (2) by the patient	A person with impaired judgment will either make literal interpretations or just rephrase the words. The earliest sign of cerebral impairment begins with the inability of the patient to make abstractions
F. Recent memory	1. Ask patient the details of why he came into the hospital 2. Ask patient what he had for his last meal	Inability to answer both questions correctly	The patient with diffuse organic cerebral impairment shows better retention of past events than of recent events[15]
G. Remote memory	Ask patient to name some capitals of certain states or when Pearl Harbor was bombed, or where the patient was born	Inability to answer correctly	(See F above)

(Continued)

TABLE 1-9 (Continued)

Physical Assessment of the Neurological System

Assessment Parameter	Method of Assessment	Deviations From Normal	Interpretation
H. Ability to follow simple commands	Ask patient to squeeze your finger, open his mouth, close his eyes, etc.	Inability to follow the command	This may indicate cerebral impairment. The patient will need further evaluation by physician to determine pathology
I. Affect and mood	Observe the patient for lability of affect and mood and changes from the patient's usual pattern	Lability, depression, euphoria, combativeness, inattentiveness, and restlessness	Changes in affect and mood are early warning signs of deficient organ function and should be reported immediately
II: Motor System:			
A. Movement of extremities	Ask the patient to move all extremities or observe patient's ability to move all extremities when he is changing positions	Inability to move all extremities	This may indicate beginning paralysis. (If patient is unconscious, he will be unable to move extremities spontaneously but application of a painful stimuli, e.g., pinching the soles of feet, should result in spontaneous withdrawal from painful stimuli)

B. Muscle strength	1. Upper extremities can be assessed by:	
	a) Instructing the patient to squeeze the examiner's index and middle fingers as hard as he can (to prevent pain to the examiner's fingers, cross the middle finger over the index finger before allowing the patient to grasp them)	Inability of the patient to prevent examiner from removing fingers from the patient's grasp	In the normal exam, the examiner should have difficulty removing his fingers from the patient's grasp
			Weakness of the grasp indicates weakness of the forearm
	b) Have patient extend his arms outstretched in front of him	Inability of the patient to maintain this position for five seconds	The weak arm will drift downward
	2. Lower extremities can be assessed by having the patient flex and extend his feet against the resistance of the examiner's hand	Inequality in strength	Muscle weakness of the extremities indicates damage to the pyramidal tract, i.e., to the motor pathway, the peripheral nerve, the neuromuscular junction, and/or the muscle. Muscle weakness should be reported to the physician immediately
C. Muscle tone	1. Feel the bulk of the muscle when it is relaxed (muscles should	1. Soft or "flabby" muscles	Hypotonicity

(Continued)

TABLE 1-9 (Continued)

Physical Assessment of the Neurological System

Assessment Parameter	Method of Assessment	Deviations From Normal	Interpretation
C. Muscle tone (Cont'd.)	feel firm, but not contracted)	2. Hard or contracted muscles	Hypertonicity
		Decreased resistance to movement	Flaccidity or hypotonicity is characteristic of lower motor neuron lesions (N.B. the DTR's in that extremity are absent)
	2. Ask patient to move, flex, and extend his extremities. If the patient is unable to move extremities, the nurse should put the extremities through the full ROM. (If there is increased resistance, stop and proceed to extend or flex the extremity slowly; if there is any pain, stop and do not proceed to move the extremity)	Sudden passive movements that are met with resistance initially but, when the resistance is overcome, movement continues easily	Spasticity
		Steady contraction of flexor and extensor muscles which results in continued increased resistance throughout full range of joint movement	Rigidity
			Spasms and rigidity are associated with hypertonicity which is due to and characteristic of upper motor neuron lesions. (N.B. DTR's are very brisk and may exhibit clonus)

III: Cranial Nerves (I-XII)

A. Olfactory (I):

  Have patient close his eyes and occlude one nostril and ask the patient to identify familiar odors such as coffee or tobacco (The olfactory nerve is not usually tested in the ICU.)

1. Sensory nerve

2. Function: smell

  Inability to report odor correctly

  Many people have normally lost their ability to smell, so this may be difficult to interpret

B. Optic (II):

1. Sensory nerve

  Have patient read large print, covering one eye at a time

  Inability to read the print or identify letters

  May indicate injury to or pressure on cranial nerve II

2. Function: sight

  The funduscopic exam also is a part of the assessment of the optic nerve, but will not be discussed as a part of this chapter

  Find out from patient why he can't read, e.g., is his vision blurred, before making an interpretation

C. Oculomotor (III):

1. Motor nerve

  A. Assessment of pupil constriction:

  1. Observe pupillary size and equality

2. Functions:

  2. Pupillary reaction is tested by shining a bright source of light into the patient's eye. The examiner

  a) constricts pupil

  Inability of the pupils to constrict

  Pupils failing to constrict may be a sign of increased intracranial pressure

  b) elevates eyelids

  Inability of the pupils to constrict equally

(Continued)

TABLE 1-9 (Continued)

Physical Assessment of the Neurological System

Assessment Parameter	Method of Assessment	Deviations From Normal	Interpretation
c) controls uplateral, upmedial, inmedial, and downmedial movement of the eye (tested with cranial nerves IV and VI)	brings the light from the side of the head and shines the light directly on the pupil	Unequal pupil size; constricted pupils; dilated pupils	Dilatation of pupils usually occurs on the same side as the brain damage
B. Assessment of eye and eyelid movement		Ptosis of the eyelids	Indicates injury to or pressure on cranial nerve III
		Inability to follow the examiner's finger up and medial, down and medial, and/or medial	
D. Trochlear (IV):	The muscles of eye movement are controlled by cranial nerves III, IV, and VI, and are tested as a unit by having the patient raise his eyelids (III) and then asking the patient to follow the nurse's finger while keeping the patient's head motionless (III, IV, VI). The nurse moves her hand in a wheel-spoke pattern: ✱	Inability of the patient to follow the examiner's finger down and lateral	Indicates injury to or pressure on cranial nerve IV
1. Motor			
2. Function:			
a) controls downlateral movement of the eye			

E. Abducent (VI): 1. Motor 2. Function: a) controls outward movement of eye	An alternate method of testing cranial nerves III, IV, and VI, when the patient is unconscious is to take hold of the patient's head and quickly move it from side to side, while at the same time observing the direction of the eye movements (this is known as the Doll's Head or Doll's Eyes maneuver)	Inability of the patient to follow the examiner's finger laterally Movement of the eyes in the same direction as the turned head	Indicates injury to or pressure on cranial nerve VI The normal finding is that the eyes move together in the opposite direction of the turned head
F. Trigeminal (V): 1. Sensory and motor nerve 2. Functions: a) controls sensation from the anterior scalp to the chin including the cornea and the mucous membrane of the mouth	The corneal reflex is tested by asking the patient to look upward and approaching the patient from the side, touching the cornea lightly with a piece of cotton rolled into a fine strand. N.B. use tip of sterile applicator for this test	Inability to blink eye	The expected response is blinking the eye. (If cranial nerve is not intact, the nurse needs to provide measures to prevent dryness and ulceration of the cornea)
b) controls opening and closing of the jaw	Ask patient to clench teeth and to open his mouth against the resistance of the examiner's hand	Inability to perform request	Indicates injury to or pressure on the motor portion of cranial nerve V

(Continued)

TABLE 1-9 (Continued)

Physical Assessment of the Neurological System

Assessment Parameter	Method of Assessment	Deviations From Normal	Interpretation
G. Facial (VII):			
1. Sensory and motor nerve	Observe patient while talking; ask patient to wrinkle his forehead, frown, and smile. (The sensory portion is not usually tested in the ICU)	Asymmetry of movement	Indicates injury to or pressure on the motor portion of cranial nerve VII
2. Functions:			
a) controls movements of the muscles of the face			
b) controls sensations of taste to anterior 2/3 of tongue			
H. Acoustic (VIII):			
1. Sensory nerve	Test the hearing (cochlear) portion of cranial nerve VIII by occluding one ear and ask if the patient can hear the ticking of a watch held close to the opposite ear	Inability to hear watch ticking	This method only tests for gross hearing losses but may indicate damage to the acoustic nerve
2. Functions:			
a) controls hearing			
b) controls equilibrium	Due to the acuity of illness of the patients in the intensive care	Sensations of vertigo, tinnitus, or disturbances in balance	Vertigo, tinnitus or disturbances in balance may indicate a vestibular lesion

	unit, it is difficult to test the equilibrium (vestibular) portion of cranial nerve VIII because testing involves a number of balance maneuvers		
I. Glossopharyngeal (IX):			
1. Sensory and motor	Because of their close proximity, cranial nerves IX and X are tested together		
2. Functions:			
a) controls swallowing	Test to see if the gag reflex is intact by stimulating the posterior pharynx with a tongue blade	Absence of gag reflex	Absence of the gag reflex is a critical sign. The nurse should take precautionary measures to prevent the patient from aspiration (i.e., no food or fluids, frequent suctioning, and nasogastric drainage)
b) controls taste sensation of posterior 1/3 of tongue	Ask patient to swallow	Inability to swallow	Indicates injury to or pressure on cranial nerve IX and the motor portion of cranial nerve X
	Ask patient to speak	Hoarseness	
J. Vagus (X):			
1. Motor and autonomic nerve	The autonomic portion of the vagus nerve is not assessed as part of the neurological exam		
2. Functions:			
a) controls swallowing and speaking			

(Continued)

TABLE 1-9 (Continued)

Physical Assessment of the Neurological System

Assessment Parameter	Method of Assessment	Deviations From Normal	Interpretation
b) slows heart, constricts bronchial muscles, etc.			
K. Accessory (XI):			
1. Motor nerve	Ask the patient to move his head to the right and to the left against resistance from the examiner's hand	Inability to perform movements against resistance	Indicates injury to or pressure on cranial nerve XI
2. Function:			
a) controls movement of trapezius and sternocleidomastoid muscles	Ask the patient to shrug his shoulders against resistance from the examiner's hands		Intactness of this nerve is important in the use of assistance devices for quadriplegic patients
L. Hypoglossal (XII):			
1. Motor nerve	Ask the patient to stick out his tongue	Any deviation of the tongue from the midline position	The tongue deviates to the weak side and indicates injury to or pressure on cranial nerve XII
2. Function:			
a) controls movement of the tongue			

Evaluation of Deep Tendon Reflexes

Reflexes are evaluated by their presence or absence, symmetry, and briskness of response in all extremities. The following grading system (0-4) is generally used when recording deep tendon reflexes and the plantar reflex:

	0	absent reflex
+	1	barely visible or sluggish reflex
+ +	2	active or average reflex
+ + +	3	brisk reflex
+ + + +	4	hyperactive response with clonus

Clonus is a rhythmic oscillation between flexion and extension or a rapid repetitive contraction of a muscle and is characteristic of upper motor neuron lesions.

A stick figure is one of the simplest methods for recording reflexes. Figure 1-16 represents recording of the normal deep tendon and plantar reflexes:

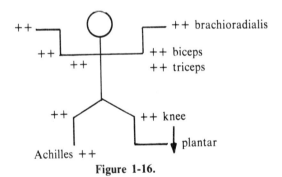

Figure 1-16.

Reflexes are reduced or absent with lower motor neuron disease, spinal shock, peripheral neuropathy, and severe myopathy. Reflexes are increased with upper motor neuron disease.

Table 1-10 summarizes the assessment of DTR and plantar reflexes, and includes:

1. the name of the reflex
2. the site of innervation
3. the site of stimulus
4. the method of assessment
5. the expected response

TABLE 1-10

Physical Assessment of the Deep Tendon and Plantar Reflexes

Reflex	Site of Innervation	Site of Stimulus	Method	Expected Response
Brachioradialis	C5, C6, Radial nerve	At the insertion of the brachioradialis tendon, which is immediately above the styloid process of the radius	Have the patient flex his elbow at a 90° angle with the forearm and palm between pronation and supination. Allow the forearm and hand to rest on the abdomen or thigh. Place the index finger against the distal end of the patient's radius approximately one to two inches above the styloid process of the radius. Strike the index finger (this compresses the tendon) with the tapered edge of the reflex hammer (see Fig. 1-17A, p. 91)	Flexion of the elbow and supination of the forearm
Biceps	C5, C6, Musculocutaneous	At the insertion of the biceps tendon, which is at the inner aspect of the elbow medially	Have the patient's arm semi-flexed at the elbow with the palm down. Place the index finger or thumb over the biceps tendon on	Flexion of the elbow with contraction of the bicep muscle

Triceps	C7, C8, Radial nerve	At the insertion of the triceps tendon, which is immediately above the olecranon process	the inner medial aspect of the elbow. Strike the finger or thumb which is compressing the tendon with the tapered edge of the reflex hammer (see Figure 1-17B, p. 91) Have the patient's arm flexed at the elbow with the palm of the hand toward the body of the forearm and hand resting on the upper abdomen. Strike the tendon just above the olecranon process with the tapered edge of the reflex hammer (see Figure 1-17C, p. 91)	Extension of the forearm with contraction of the triceps
Quadriceps (knee or patellar)	L2, L3, L4	At the insertion of the patellar tendon, which is immediately below the patella	Support the patient's knees from behind and lift them until they are flexed at approximately a 45° angle with the patient's heels resting on the bed. Strike the patellar tendon with the wide edge of the reflex hammer (see Figure 1-17D, p. 91)	Extension of the leg at the knee with contraction of the quadriceps muscle

(Continued)

TABLE 1-10 (Continued)
Physical Assessment of the Deep Tendon and Plantar Reflexes

Reflex	Site of Innervation	Site of Stimulus	Method	Expected Response
Achilles	L5, S1, S2	At the insertion of the Achilles tendon, which is the ankle	Flex patient's knee at a 75° angle. Place the lateral portion of the foot on the opposite leg while allowing the lateral portion of the leg to rest on the bed. Dorsiflex the foot slightly with your hand. Strike the Achilles tendon with the wide edge of the reflex hammer (see Figure 1-17E, p. 91)	Plantar flexion of the foot
Plantar Reflex	L4, L5, S1, S2	Sole of foot	Stroke the lateral aspect of the sole of the foot from the heel to the ball of the foot. When the examiner reaches the ball of the foot continue the motion medially across the entire ball of the foot.	Flexion of the toes
				The Babinski sign is an abnormal plantar reflex with the extension of the large toe and fanning of the other toes

Use a closed safety pin or the unnotched side of a key and apply firm pressure to evoke the response (see Figure 1-17F, p. 91)

The Babinski sign is often referred to as the single most important reflex in neurology. When this sign is present, it is pathognomonic of pyramidal tract or upper motor neuron disease. Nervous system defects will produce this abnormal response early in the disease. The Babinski sign frequently precedes other signs of organic disease of the neurological system. For these reasons, it is imperative to include the plantar reflex in the quick neurological assessment

Levels of Consciousness

In determining levels of consciousness, the nurse uses the previously described assessment parameters for mental status. "Impairment of consciousness occurs on a continuum. The descending order of the continuum is from spontaneous verbal and motor activity and attentive cooperation to complete absence of any motor or reflex responses."[17] Following are the levels of consciousness listed in decreasing order of cerebral functioning:

1. *Loss of ability to abstract:* The patient becomes inattentive, is unable to think at his customary speed and level and becomes increasingly difficult to arouse.
2. *Confusion:* The patient becomes disoriented to time, then to place, and finally to person (others and self). This is followed by the inability to follow simple commands.
3. *Stupor:* The patient responds to the spoken word either by moaning and groaning or does not respond at all. The deep tendon and plantar reflexes are intact at this level.
4. *Semi-comatose:* The patient loses the ability to cooperate and it therefore becomes necessary to use painful, rather than verbal, stimuli to elicit a response. Painful stimuli can be applied by pressing against the supraorbital bone, rubbing the sternum, pinching the Achilles tendon, or using a pin on the palm of the hand or the sole of the foot. Painful stimuli must be applied with great care to prevent injury to the patient. When the patient first becomes semi-comatose, the response to pain is purposeful, such as resistance or withdrawal. Later, the responses are decerebrate, such as chewing or hyperventilating. During the semi-comatose state, the corneal and cough reflexes may still be present and the deep tendon reflexes usually are present. Measures should be taken to guard against respiratory failure.
5. *Comatose:* The patient is unable to respond to any external stimuli. There is a loss of all basic reflex response.

When recording the patient's level of consciousness, it is advisable to describe the actual phenomenon observed and/or elicited from the patient rather than to use the above terms because the terms may be misinterpreted and lead to ambiguity. When monitoring a patient for signs of improvement or deterioration of consciousness, it is important that the nurse be aware of the patient's

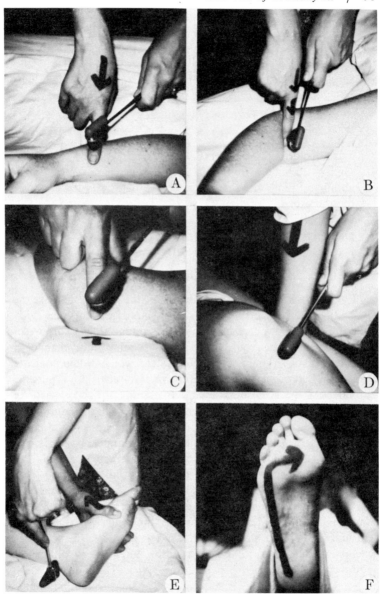

Figure 1-17. (A) Testing for the brachioradialis reflex; (B) testing for the biceps reflex; (C) testing for the triceps reflex; (D) testing for the quadriceps reflex; (E) testing for the Achilles reflex; (F) testing for the plantar reflex.

position on the continuum and the direction in which his condition is progressing.

The neurological parameters that need to be assessed when the critically ill person first is admitted to the ICU and monitored thereafter at regularly prescribed intervals are:

1. mental status
2. pupil size, shape, equality, reaction to light
3. extra-ocular eye movements
4. ability to swallow
5. ability to move all extremities or if patient is unconscious, motor response to stimuli
6. vital signs
7. plantar reflex

THE RENAL SYSTEM

The purposes and primary functions of the renal system are the regulation and concentration of solutes in the extracellular body fluid and the excretion of metabolic end products. The purpose of the assessment of the renal system is to determine initial changes in the integrity of or burden on the system which would indicate physiologic deterioration or improvement of the critically ill person.

Nurses in the ICU must be able to assess fluid and electrolyte balance and recognize warning signs and symptoms of kidney malfunction since patients whose conditions warrant observation in the ICU frequently manifest abnormalities in renal function. All assessments and interventions are directed toward recognition of premonitory signs and prevention of acute renal failure.

If the nurse in the ICU detects a decrease or increase in urinary output, he or she should immediately check the patient's urine specific gravity and systematically assess the above parameters to determine if there is a problem with fluid balance or if the patient is developing acute renal failure. In addition, the nurse should determine weight changes of the patient and review the intake and output for the past 48 hours. The following findings should be immediately reported to the physician: the status of each parameter, weight changes, intake and output for the past 48 hours, and the patient's current BUN, creatinine, hematocrit, and serum sodium, potassium chloride, and bicarbonate.

As can be noted, assessment of renal status, unlike cardiovascular, respiratory, or neurological, is dependent primarily upon observation of secondary signs and symptoms. There are few, if any, single findings which will definitively indicate changes in renal function. For this reason it is especially important that the nurse be particularly thorough in assessing all factors related to fluid and electrolyte balance.

Table 1-11 includes subjective and objective parameters for assessment of dehydration, overhydration and acute renal failure.

TABLE 1-11

Assessment Parameters of Dehydration,
Overhydration, and Acute Renal Failure

Parameters	Dehydration	Overhydration	Acute Renal Failure
General Symptoms	Thirst is the earliest symptom of water loss Dryness of mouth	Shortness of breath, salivation, lacrimation	Symptoms are minimal at first and include anorexia and tiredness[s]
Buccal Mucosa	Dry	Moist	*
Saliva	Thick and decreased	Excessive and frothy	*
Temperature	May be elevated	Not affected	*
Pulse	Rapid with postural changes (a rise of 20 beats or more per minute with position change, i.e., lying to standing)	Rapid, sometimes bounding, without postural changes	
Blood Pressure	Postural changes (a systolic drop of ten or more mm Hg with the position change) concomitant with pulse changes (the pulse increases and the BP decreases with the position change)	May be elevated or decreased but is not affected by postural changes	*

(Continued)

TABLE 1-11 (Continued)

Assessment Parameters of Dehydration,
Overhydration, and Acute Renal Failure

Parameters	Dehydration	Overhydration	Acute Renal Faure
Weight (5% change in body weight is considered significant)	Loss	Gain N.B. The patient who is NPO should lose weight; if his weight remains the same over time, he is becoming over-hydrated	*
Urinary Output	20-30 cc per hour	May be increased or decreased depending on the solute load	Less than 10 cc per hour
Specific Gravity	Usually greater than 1.020	May be increased or decreased depending on the solute load	Isotonic: 1.008-1.015; remains fixed and does not change with alterations in fluid therapy
HCT	Increased	No change (MCHC is decreased and MCV is increased[8]	*
CVP	Low	High	*
Pulmonary Wedge Pressure	Below 16 cm of H_2O	Above 16 cm H_2O	*
Neck Veins	Flat	Distended	*
Breath Sounds	Normal; secretions, if present, will be thick and tenacious	Rales; secretions will be thin and frothy	Normal or rales
Heart Sounds	Normal	Presence of S_3	*

*Indicates that these parameters may reflect dehydration or overhydration depending upon the fluid status of the patient.

REFERENCES

1. Ayres S: *Care of the Critically Ill*. 2nd Ed. Appleton-Century-Crofts, New York, 1974, p. 146.
2. Davies B, Director, Cardiac Catheterization Laboratory: Personal Communication. Veterans Hospital, Cleveland, Ohio, 1977.
3. DeGowin EL, DeGowin RL: *Bedside Diagnostic Examination*. 3rd Ed. Macmillan Publishing Co., New York, 1976, p. 270.
4. Detweiler D (Ed.): Circulation. In Brobeck JR (Ed.): *Best and Taylor's Physiological Basis of Medical Practice*. 9th Ed. Williams and Wilkins Company, Baltimore, Md., 1973, pp. 1-3.
5. Frank MJ, Alvarez-Mena SC: *Cardiovascular Physical Diagnosis*. Year Book Medical Publishers, Inc., Chicago, Ill., 1973, p. 73.
6. Gilbert C: Physical Appraisal of Circulatory Function. In Sana JM, Judge RD (Eds.): *Physical Appraisal Methods in Nursing Practice*. 1st Ed. Little, Brown, and Company, Boston, Mass., 1975, p. 189.
7. Ginsberg DJ, Chief, Renal Service: Personal Communication. Veterans Hospital, Cleveland, Ohio, 1977.
8. Goldberger E: *A Primer of Water, Electrolyte, and Acid-Base Syndromes*. 5th Ed. Lea and Febiger, Philadelphia, Pa., 1975, p. 304.
9. Hendee RW, Hudak CM: Pathophysiology of the Central Nervous System and Management Modalities. In Hudak CM (Ed.): *Critical Care Nursing*. J.B. Lippincott, Philadelphia, Pa., 1973, p. 274.
10. Hochstein E, Rubin AL: *Physical Diagnosis*. McGraw-Hill, New York, 1964, p. 6.
11. Hudak CM, et al.: *Critical Care Nursing*. J.B. Lippincott, Philadelphia, Pa., 1973.
12. Prior JA, Silberstein JS: *Physical Diagnosis*. 4th Ed. C.V. Mosby, St. Louis, Mo., 1973, p. 275.
13. Schwartz IL, Siegel GJ: Excitation, Conduction and Transmission of the Nerve Impulse. In Schwartz IL (Ed.): General Physiological Processes. In Brobeck JR (Ed.): *Best and Taylor's Physiological Basis of Medical Practice*. 9th Ed. Williams and Wilkins Company, Baltimore, Md., 1973, pp. 1-29.
14. Shapiro BA: *Clinical Application of Respiratory Care*. Year Book Medical Publishers, Inc., Chicago, Ill., 1975, pp. 18-19.
15. Steegmann AT: *Examination of the Nervous System*. 3rd Ed. Year Book Medical Publishers, Inc., Chicago, Ill., 1970, p. 186.
16. Stone WE: Uptake and Delivery of the Respiratory Gases. In Youmans WB, Siebens AA (Eds.): Respiration. In Brobeck JR (Ed.): *Best and Taylor's Physiological Basis of Medical Practice*. 9th Ed. Williams and Wilkins Company, Baltimore, Md., 1973, pp. 1-6.

17. VanMeter MJ, Diehl EA: Detection of Alterations in Neuromuscular Functioning. In Sana JM, Judge RD (Eds.): *Physical Appraisal Methods in Nursing Practice.* 1st Ed. Little, Brown, and Company, Boston, Mass., 1975, p. 189.
18. Zschoche DA, Ed.: *Mosby's Comprehensive Review of Critical Care.* C.V. Mosby, St. Louis, Mo., 1976.

CHAPTER 2

Care of the Patient With Cardiovascular Disease

by Mary Alexandra (Sandy) Wyper, RN, MSN, and
Barbara J. Daly, RN, MSN

INTRODUCTION

This chapter will discuss nursing care of the patient with a primary disorder of the cardiovascular system. There will be three major divisions. The first section will be devoted to a discussion of normal anatomy and physiology. This will be an overview, designed to review those aspects of the structure and function of the heart necessary for an understanding of the pathological features of cardiac disease, and the rationale underlying intervention.

Although many patients in Intensive Care Units have problems related to the cardiovascular system, or suffer interference with cardiac mechanisms secondary to another disease process, such as the patient who develops arrhythmias while hypoxic, this chapter will deal only with patients whose primary disorder is cardiac in nature. The second major section of this chapter will discuss care of the patient who has suffered a myocardial infarction, and the third section will deal with patients who have undergone cardiac surgery.

The framework utilized for these discussions will be the nursing process (assessment, analysis of the data, goal identification and intervention, and evaluation) applied to problems in meeting each of the basic needs. It is hoped that by structuring the chapter in this way, the reader will be able to choose appropriate intervention measures indicated in the care of any individual patient. By identifying the manner in which cardiac dysfunction interferes with other physiological and psychological processes, rather than presenting only a stereotype of common care measures utilized in caring for the "cardiac patient," the reader can then utilize specific relevant aspects of the chapter in caring for any patient, regardless of primary diagnosis.

ANATOMY AND PHYSIOLOGY

Structural Anatomy

The heart is a muscular organ, lying in the mediastinum, whose major function is to act as a pump in propelling blood. The heart is covered by a loose fibrous sack called the pericardium. The actual cardiac muscle tissue, the myocardium, is covered by the epicardium on the outside, and on the inside by the endocardium, which also covers the valves and papillary muscles.

Chambers and valves

The heart is conveniently thought of as two halves, the right and left side, divided by a fibrous septum. Each side consists of a collecting chamber, the atrium; and a pumping chamber, the ventricle (Figure 2-1). The right heart receives blood from the systemic circulation and pumps blood to the lungs where carbon dioxide is given off and oxygen picked up. The pulmonary circuit is considered to be a low pressure system; consequently, the myocardium of the right ventricle is much thinner than the left, reflecting the lesser degree of work involved in pumping blood through the pulmonary system.

The left atrium receives oxygenated blood from the lungs; the left ventricle delivers this oxygenated blood to the tissues. Although, for discussion purposes, the left and right sides of the heart are sometimes treated as distinct and separate chambers, it is important for the nurse to understand at the outset that pathology of any one part of the heart will eventually affect all components. That is, although the patient may initially have right-sided heart failure, eventually the alterations in muscle function and pressures generated will lead to left-sided failure.

The passage of blood into and out of each chamber is regulated

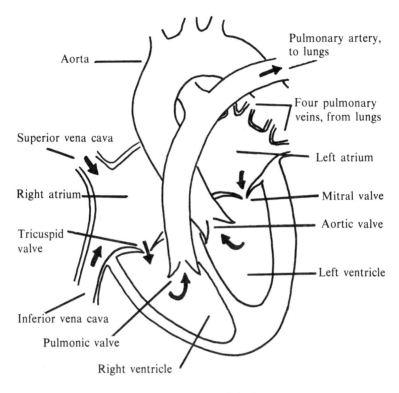

Figure 2-1. Structures of the heart.

by four valves. All of the valves consist of flaps, or cusps, which open to allow the passage of blood in one direction; and then snap closed, preventing the retrograde flow of blood. The mitral and tricuspid valves have an additional attachment to the muscle wall, which the pulmonic and aortic valves do not have. The leaflets of the valve are connected to chordae tendineae, which are inserted in the papillary muscles, anchored in the myocardium itself. The chordae tendineae prevent the leaflets from inverting and allowing this backward flow of blood.

The atrium and ventricle are separated by the tricuspid valve on the right, and the mitral valve on the left. The tricuspid valve has three leaflets, and the mitral, in corresponding position on the left, has two leaflets. These are also referred to as atrio-ventricular (A-V) valves. Each ventricle also has a valve at the outlet. Blood flows out from the right ventricle through the pulmonary valve and from the left ventricle through the aortic valve.

Blood vessels

The complete circuit of blood, then, is as follows. Venous blood returns from the tissues to the heart and empties into the right atrium via the superior and inferior vena cavae. It passes from the right atrium to the right ventricle (via the tricuspid valve), and is pumped out to the lungs via the pulmonary artery. Oxygenated blood returns to the heart via the pulmonary veins, enters the left atrium and passes through the mitral valve to the left ventricle. The left ventricle, which is the major pumping chamber, ejects the blood through the aortic valve into the aorta for passage to the tissues.

The blood supply for the myocardium is provided by two coronary arteries, which originate as ostia lying in the aorta, just behind the leaflets of the aortic valve. The left coronary artery immediately divides into two branches. The left anterior descending artery (LAD) lies on the apex of the heart and supplies the left ventricular myocardium, the anterior septum, and anterior papillary muscle, and has several diagonal branches. The other main branch, the circumflex coronary artery (CCA), descends posteriorly, supplies the lateral and posterior portions of the left heart, and has several smaller marginal branches (Figure 2-2). If the CCA extends as far as the interventricular groove on the posterior aspect, the circulation is considered to be "dominant left."[2] The right coronary artery (RCA) supplies the right side of the heart, a portion of the septum, and, most importantly, the sino-atrial node in more than half of all individuals, and the atrio-ventricular node in almost everyone. If the RCA provides the major blood supply for the posterior left ventricle, the circulation is considered to be "dominant right."

The coronary arteries are particularly susceptible to the development of atherosclerotic plaques. In addition, the coronaries are quite narrow and are subject to large compressive forces when the heart contracts during systole. Unlike all other arteries, flow through the coronaries is greatest during the diastolic phase of the cardiac cycle, when the heart is relaxed. Another significant difference in the arterial blood supply to the myocardium is the extent of oxygen extraction. The heart extracts 75% of the available oxygen in

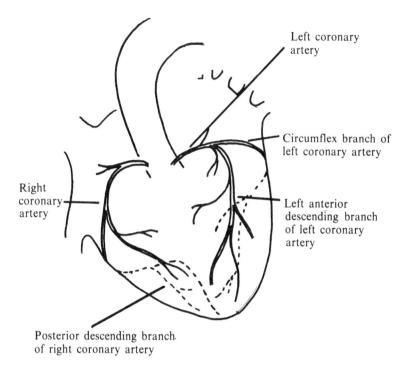

Left coronary artery

Circumflex branch of left coronary artery

Right coronary artery

Left anterior descending branch of left coronary artery

Posterior descending branch of right coronary artery

Figure 2-2. Coronary arteries.

the arteries, in contrast to other organs, which remove an average of 25%. This means that the muscle cannot increase oxygen extraction to any great degree, and increased oxygen needs, as with fever, stress, or exercise, must be met by increasing coronary blood flow. It has been documented that in the presence of 80% or greater obstruction of the artery by an atherosclerotic plaque, the myocardium will inevitably suffer ischemia.[11]

Cardiac muscle

Cardiac muscle cells have certain characteristics which make them particularly effective in ensuring that the heart is able to pump effectively. First, the cells, like other skeletal muscle cells, are composed of striated filaments of actin and myosin. Secondly, these cells, which are responsible for the contractility of cardiac tissue, are arranged in a tight meshwork fashion that facilitates the conduction of impulses from one cell to another.

Conducting tissue

By far the most unique aspect of cardiac tissue is the ability to automatically initiate electrical impulses which result in mechanical contraction. The sino-atrial (SA) node is a group of specialized pacemaker cells, located in the right atrium, just below the entrance of the superior vena cava. The SA node cells are capable of "automaticity"—that is, they are capable of spontaneously generating an electrical impulse, which is then conducted in a wave-like fashion across the atria. Then, providing all cells are intact and capable of responding normally, a contraction results.

The impulse originating in the SA node is thus conducted to the second locus of pacemaker tissue, the atrio-ventricular (AV) node. Some of the impulses will reach the AV node earlier than others, due to their conduction along internodal pathways, which are bundles of specialized conduction tissue able to speed this forward transmission. The AV nodal fibers delay the further transmission of impulses; this allows time for the atria to completely empty into the ventricles.

Beyond the AV node, the conduction system is composed of fibers arranged in a bundle (AV bundle of His) extending from the AV node through the interventricular septum, dividing into the right and left bundle branches, which lie to either side of the septum. The left bundle branch divides into a posteroinferior and anterosuperior aspect, and both right and left bundles separate into a profuse network of smaller branches, termed Purkinje fibers, at the apex of the heart and spread upward along the lateral aspects of each ventricle. The His-Purkinje system is able to transmit an impulse from the AV node through both ventricles in just 0.03 seconds due to the large number of junctions between cells.[10]

Physiology

In discussing cardiac physiology, it is convenient to focus upon the function of the heart as a pump, and upon the electrophysiological processes which are necessary to initiate the pumping action. However, it must be understood that this separation of mechanical and electrical function is an academic one only, and that many events take place simultaneously in the heart to bring about rhythmic coordinated contractions.

Pumping function

The mechanical aspects of the cardiac cycle begin with the filling of the atria with blood delivered through the venous system. This is a continuous flow of blood, and upon entry into the atrium, some of the blood will immediately also flow through the A-V valve into the ventricle. The contraction of the atrium, initiated by the SA node, is responsible for the delivery of most of the remaining blood in the atrium. When the ventricle begins to contract, higher pressures are generated and the A-V valves close. This is called the isovolumetric period, when there is a change in ventricular pressure but no change in volume. As this high pressure is generated, the pulmonic and aortic valves open and the ventricles eject about 70 ml. of blood. This is termed the stroke volume. When the ventricles begin to relax, the ventricular pressure immediately drops, and the pressure in the arterial system is then higher than in the ventricles. This higher pressure in the pulmonary artery and aorta closes the pulmonic and aortic valves.

The cardiac cycle is timed so that as the ventricles are in the phase of contraction, or systole, the atria are in diastole and are filling. Just after the aortic and pulmonic valves close, the A-V valves open and the ventricles refill.

Adequate oxygenation of the tissues depends in large measure upon an adequate cardiac output. Cardiac output, defined as the volume of blood ejected by the heart per minute, in turn is affected by several variables. The formula for determining cardiac output (C.O.) will immediately point out the first two determinants.

Cardiac Output = Stroke Volume x Heart Rate/Minute

As is obvious, if either stroke volume or heart rate falls, the cardiac output will decrease; if either stroke volume or heart rate increases, C.O. will increase. What is less obvious is the observation that with very high heart rates (greater than 150 beats per minute) there is inadequate time for the ventricles to fill completely between each contraction, and stroke volume falls as a result. In this case, the greater frequency of contraction results in a decrease, rather than an increase, in cardiac output.

Two other significant factors affecting stroke volume, and thus cardiac output, are preload and afterload. In discussing preload, one must review the mechanism of Starling's Law. This law states that stretching any skeletal muscle, including the heart, will result in an increased force of contraction. This stretching of the myocardium comes about by increasing the volume of the chambers. As was mentioned above, under normal conditions, the heart ejects a stroke volume of 70 ml. with each contraction; this is not the entire content of the ventricle, however. By the end of each filling phase or diastole, the ventricle contains about 120 ml. of blood; this is termed the *end-diastolic volume*. After the contraction phase or systole, about 50 ml. remain in the ventricle; this is termed the *end-systolic volume*.

Preload is equivalent to end-diastolic volume. If ventricular filling increases, there will be an eventual compensatory increase in cardiac output. This comes about through several steps. First, if, for example, there is an increased flow of blood from the veins into the heart, as with higher central venous pressures caused by administering intravenous fluids, there will be a rise in end-diastolic volume, or preload. The myocardium will initially eject its usual volume of 70 ml., thus leaving a greater proportion of the blood in the ventricle, or increasing end-systolic volume. When the ventricle then fills again with the next cycle, ventricular volume increases even more because both the incoming volume of blood is greater and the already present volume of blood is greater. The result of this increased volume is a stretching of the muscle fibers and increased force of contraction, which raises stroke volume. Thus, increasing the preload of the heart causes an increase in cardiac output.

It is essential to note at this point that this ability of the heart, referred to as Starling's Law, operates only within physiologic limits. That is, persistent over-distention of the ventricles will eventually lead to a decrease in cardiac output as the ventricular muscle hypertrophies and becomes less effective. Sudden, severe over-distention can also exceed the limits of myocardial expansibility and result in a less effective contraction.

Afterload is a factor which more often operates to cause a decrease in stroke volume. Afterload refers to the pressure which exists in the vascular system into which the ventricle must pump. Increases in pressure, as caused by vasoconstriction or hypertension, for example, represent an increased resistance to pumping, which will reduce the ability of the ventricle to eject its stroke volume, and cardiac output will fall. Under normal conditions the heart automatically compensates for increased afterload. The initial fall in stroke volume results in an increased end-systolic volume, and the sequence described earlier then begins. The increased end-systolic volume will add to the filling volume at the end of the next diastole to cause an increased preload. This, in turn, causes an increased force of contraction, which is then able to overcome the increased afterload and maintain a normal stroke volume. Again, however, persistent increases in afterload will eventually lead to myocardial hypertrophy.

The last significant factor which ordinarily regulates cardiac output is sympathetic control. Sympathetic stimulation causes innervation of all myocardial cells, including the SA node, through the action of the catecholamines, epinephrine and norepinephrine. It results both in an increased heart rate and an increased contractility, or a more forceful contraction without a change in muscle fiber length. Parasympathetic stimulation, mediated via the vagus nerve has no effect on contractility, but decreases SA node rate and A-V node excitability, through the action of acetylcholine.

Electrophysiology

As with other muscles, the process of contraction involves an initial stimulus, which causes the movement of ions across the cell membrane. This in turn causes a change in the electrical charge, generating a current which flows along the cell membrane, from one cell to another, causing contraction.

In its resting state, the cardiac cell membrane is relatively impermeable to sodium and potassium. The existence of high concentrations of sodium and low concentrations of potassium outside the cell, in comparison to low concentrations of sodium and high concentrations of potassium and of negative ions inside the cell, causes the outside to be positively charged and the inside to be negatively charged *in comparison to each other*. Impulse initiation results from an increased permeability to sodium ions, which diffuse quickly across the cell membrane into the cell. This reverses the electrical charge, and the outside of the cell becomes negative in comparison to the inside. Shortly after this, potassium begins to diffuse out. This process is termed *depolarization*; the existence of different electrical potentials at different cells causes current to flow (Figure 2-3).

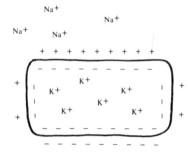

Cardiac cell in normal resting state. Extracellular fluid is high in sodium, and intracellular fluid is high in potassium. The presence of a high concentration of negative ions within the cell makes the inside of the cell negative in comparison to the outside.

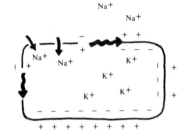

In depolarization, sodium diffuses into the cell and the electrical potential on either side of the cell membrane is reversed. This generates current, which then spreads along the cell membrane, depolarizing the other areas of that cell and neighboring cells.

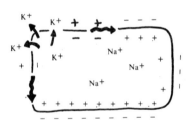

In repolarization, potassium has diffused out of the cell, reducing the number of positive ions in the intracellular fluid and restoring the relatively negative intracellular charge. Sodium and potassium pumps later restore the usual concentrations of the ions on either side of the membrane.

Figure 2-3. Cell depolarization and repolarization.

Before the next depolarization occurs, the concentrations of sodium and potassium will have been restored on both sides of the cell membrane. This process is termed *repolarization*.

With this understanding, the reader can see how essential normal serum potassium levels are for conduction to take place. Hypokalemia, or the existence of abnormally low concentrations of potassium outside the cell makes it more difficult for the restoration of electrical charge to occur, and enhances the ability of all cardiac cells to stimulate a contraction. This may result in conduction defects, and also allows stimuli to arise from areas other than the normal pacing cells of the SA node or A-V junctional region. An abnormally high concentration of potassium outside the cell reduces the difference in electrical charge across the membrane, making the cell relatively less negative. This, then, requires a stronger than normal stimulus to cause depolarization, and contraction becomes weaker and more irregular.

Adequate calcium levels are also required for effective myocardial contraction. The major action of calcium is a facilitation of the movement of the actin and myosin filaments, enabling a smooth, strong contraction. Calcium also appears to have some ability to lower the threshold of excitation of cardiac cells.[10]

MONITORING AND DIAGNOSTIC TECHNIQUES

Electrocardiogram

Of all the monitoring and diagnostic techniques available, the electrocardiogram is certainly the most common, and the one about which the nurse must be most knowledgeable. There are many excellent texts and programmed instruction manuals available which will provide the nurse with a sound foundation in ECG interpretation; this section is not intended to serve that function, but only to give the reader a brief review of the technique involved.

When depolarization and repolarization occur in the heart, the current generated diffuses throughout the body. This current can be detected by electrodes of opposite polarity placed on the skin and connected to a device similar to a galvanometer, which measures current. Addition of an amplifier and a recorder comprise the other major parts of the ECG apparatus. A cardiac monitor, of course, has the same components, in addition to an oscilloscope, for constant display of the tracing.

The deflection produced by the recorder will vary as to direction depending on the direction of current flow: an upward or positive deflection is produced by current flowing towards the positive electrode, a downward or negative deflection is produced by current flowing towards the negative electrode, and current that flows in a line perpendicular to the axis (imaginary line connecting the two electrodes) will produce either a straight, isoelectric line (no deflection) or a deflection that is equally positive and negative.

The placement of the leads then determines the appearance of the ECG recording for any given current flow. Various locations are utilized in order to obtain a comprehensive and exact recording of all impulses. The various leads are assigned numbers, and are defined as follows:

Lead   I: Left arm electrode positive, right arm negative
Lead   II: Left leg electrode positive, right arm negative
Lead III: Left leg electrode positive, left arm negative

In addition to these bipolar leads, nine unipolar leads are possible. In the unipolar lead, only one positive electrode is used, and the center of the heart provides the other pole. There are three unipolar limb leads: aVR, using the right arm electrode; aVL, using the left arm electrode, and aVF, using the left leg electrode. Six chest electrodes (V leads) make up the remainder of the twelve lead ECG.

The deflections produced, regardless of lead used, provide information about the heart's electrical activity. The tracing is made on a waxed graph paper by a heated stylus; the height of each deflection reflects voltage, and horizontal distance reflects time. The first deflection is produced by atrial depolarization and is termed the P wave. The atrial repolarization wave usually cannot be seen. The largest complex, the QRS, corresponds to depolarization of the ventricle. The T wave is the last complex normally seen and reflects ventricular repolarization. These are shown in Figure 2-4 as they would appear in a Lead II tracing.

Vectorcardiography

This is a further sophistication of the recording of the heart's electrical activity. A *vector* can be defined as a force which has both magnitude and direction. The objective of vectorcardiography is to determine the *mean vector* of a given electrical force, most importantly ventricular depolarization or the QRS wave. Although we commonly refer to ventricular depolarization as one event, it actually is a sequential process, occurring first across the ventricular septum, then through the endocardial aspect of the left ventricle, proceeding towards the epicardium. Thus, the size and thickness of the ventricular wall affect the resultant tracing. The average of all vectors obtained can be used to project the mean QRS axis, which can

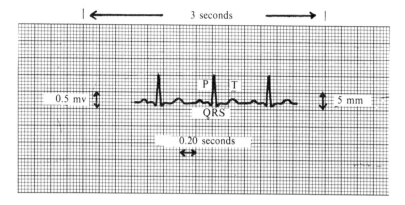

Figure 2-4. ECG complexes, Lead II.

be thought of as an angle on a plane and expressed in degrees. Right or left axis deviation occurs when the mean QRS axis is in an abnormal plane or when the actual position of the heart in the individual's chest is abnormal, as might be caused by tumors or pregnancy, or by hypertrophy due to valve disease.

Echocardiography

Echocardiography is one of the many diagnostic techniques made possible by the discovery that ultrasonic sound waves may be directed towards substances or structures, and the resultant reflection of the wave recorded to yield information about composition, size, and shape. Direction of the ultrasonic beam toward the heart and recording of the referred echoes are used to diagnose valvular disease, pericardial abnormalities, and specific structural abnormalities, such as tetralogy of Fallot.

Cardiac Catheterization

Cardiac catheterization and coronary angiography are probably the two most valuable diagnostic procedures available to the cardiologist and cardiac surgeon. By inserting a catheter through a peripheral vein and threading it up into the right heart, pressure readings and oxygen samples may be obtained, as well as visualization of the ventricle through fluoroscopy. Right heart catheterization also usually involves advancing the catheter into the pulmonary artery to obtain pressure readings.

Left heart catheterization is somewhat more difficult since it involves cannulation of an artery and passage of the catheter retrograde from ventricle to atria. Ventricular angiography is extremely valuable, however, in diagnosing valve disease, aneurysm formation, and determining hypokinetic areas which can be detected only by watching the ventricle as it actually contracts and fills.

Coronary angiography is performed by directing the catheter to the coronary ostia and injecting dye. The visualization of coronary arteries and localization of obstructive lesions have made the current coronary artery revascularization techniques possible.

Pulmonary Artery Catheterization

The development of the Swan-Ganz catheter and the technique of bedside pulmonary artery catheterization provided the first way to accurately and directly assess left ventricular function in the Intensive Care Unit. Formerly, left heart function was assessed indirectly by arterial and central venous pressure measurements. Changes in arterial pressure, however, can be caused by several factors, such as hypovolemia or peripheral vasoconstriction in the presence of normal ventricular function. The central venous pressure will vary with right ventricular function, which often, but not always correlates with left-sided function, and consequently, is not reliable. Consider the following situation:

Mr. A. has been admitted to the CCU from the emergency room with a diagnosis of transmural myocardial infarction. He has been persistently hypotensive; arterial pressures, obtained via an intra-arterial line, have remained in the range of 76/50. He is restless, diaphoretic, and has put out only 30 cc. of concentrated urine in the past three hours. An initial trial of volume replacement of 300 cc. has had no discernible effect.

To administer more fluid at this point would necessarily run the risk of fluid overloading an injured and failing left ventricle and producing pulmonary edema. On the other hand, use of potent vasopressors can be avoided if it can be determined that the patient is still hypovolemic and that the left ventricle would be able to generate an adequate cardiac output after additional volume is given.

By inserting the pulmonary artery catheter, the pressures in the pulmonary circuit were found to be somewhat low. An additional 750 cc. of D5W was administered to the patient in order to achieve a normal mean pulmonary artery pressure. At this point his arterial pressure rose to 110/74, and urine output increased to 40 cc./hour.

The Swan-Ganz pulmonary artery catheter is inserted via a peripheral vein (the brachial, subclavian, jugular, or femoral) and threaded up into the right atrium. It is advanced through the tricuspid valve, and out into a small segment of the pulmonary artery. Once in place, a balloon at the tip of the catheter can be inflated, thus occluding the pressure generated from the right side of the heart. The pressure then obtained, via transducer, is that which exists in the pulmonary capillary bed and reflects left-sided function. If the ventricle is failing, for example, and unable to maintain a normal cardiac output, fluid will accumulate in back of the ventricle, in the pulmonary system and left atrium, and the pressure in the capillaries will be elevated. If, on the other hand, high venous pressures exist, as the result of right heart failure secondary to chronic obstructive pulmonary disease, or cor pulmonale, and the left ventricle does not have impairment in function, the pulmonary capillary pressure, when the balloon is inflated, will be normal. Because the catheter must be wedged in a small segment of the arterial tree in order for the balloon to occlude the segment, the capillary pressure is often referred to as the *wedge pressure*. The usual appearance of the tracings as they appear on the oscilloscope and normal values are shown in Figure 2-5.

Once in place, the position of the catheter is continually monitored in order to detect movement. Two possible hazards are that the catheter may slip back into the ventricle, which can lead to ventricular irritability and arrhythmias, or that the catheter may advance itself far enough to be constantly wedged, even with the balloon deflated, thus occluding a portion of pulmonary blood supply and leading to pulmonary infarction. Both of these events require the immediate repositioning of the catheter.

Readings of pulmonary wedge pressure are ordinarily taken by the nurse by inflating the balloon for several seconds every few hours, or after any major change in treatment regime. A more recent addition to the original catheter now also makes it possible for cardiac output determinations to be done.

The pulmonary artery thermodilution catheter has two additional lumens added to the original Swan-Ganz design (Figure 2-6). In addition to the balloon lumen and tip or distal lumen, there is a proximal lumen which terminates in a portal about 13 cm. from the end of the catheter, which places it roughly at the entrance of vena

Average Pressures
(in mm Hg)

Pulmonary Artery:
20/8-35/15

Mean: 15-24

Right Ventricle:
20-35/5

Pulmonary Wedge:
5-15

Right Atrium:
1-6

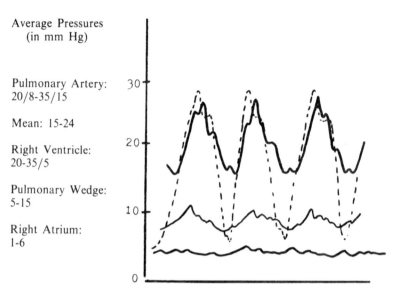

Figure 2-5. Pulmonary artery catheter readings.

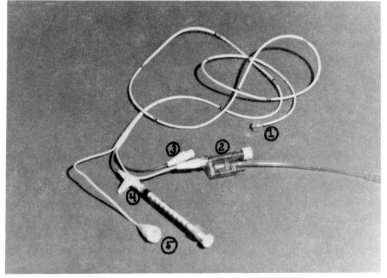

Figure 2-6. Thermodilution catheter: (1) inflated pulmonary artery balloon; (2) Sorenson Intraflo, a constant infusion device, connected to the distal lumen; (3) proximal lumen; (4) stopcock and TB syringe used to inflate the balloon; (5) thermistor lumen.

cava to the atrium. The fourth lumen terminates at the thermistor located near the end of the catheter. The basic technique involves the injection of a known volume of solution of a known temperature through the proximal lumen, and measurement of the change in temperature over time, as the solution passes the thermistor. The calculation is done by a bedside computer which attaches to the thermistor lumen. Determination of cardiac output provides an extremely accurate method by which to assess the effect of various treatment regimes, such as the use of vasodilators or inotropic agents.

MYOCARDIAL INFARCTION

Pathophysiology

Definitions

Acute myocardial infarction is the death or necrosis of a group of myocardial cells, and occurs when these cells sustain a period of irreversible anoxia. The anoxia is a result of an imbalance between myocardial oxygen supply and oxygen demand and is usually (90-95% of cases) a consequence of coronary atherosclerosis. Although the term "coronary thrombosis" has been used synonymously with "myocardial infarction" in the past, current evidence suggests that inadequate perfusion is only rarely due to a primary clot in a major coronary artery or in one of its branches.[24] Myocardial ischemia and injury are terms used to describe transient, reversible periods of moderate and severe anoxia which commonly precede infarction. Patients with any of these conditions are said to have coronary artery disease.

Predisposing Factors

Much has been written previously regarding the process of coronary atherosclerosis, and the reader is referred to a cardiac nursing text for an in-depth discussion. By way of a brief review, coronary artery disease typically starts with the proliferation and thickening of the inner arterial wall (intima) and progresses to the deposition of fatty materials, which often become calcified, between the intima and the medial layer of the wall. These deposits are called atheromas. As the disease continues, the lumen of the artery becomes narrowed, and decreased perfusion to cells served by the vessel results. Initially, the patient may be symptomatic only under circumstances of increased oxygen demand (i.e., physical or emotional stress); however, as the obstruction to blood flow increases, less stress is required to elicit symptoms of ischemia. Ultimately, a vessel becomes totally occluded (either as a result of progressive atheroma growth or because the roughened surface of the vessel wall predisposes to thrombus formation), and infarction ensues.

In spite of intensive research in the area, little progress has been made in identifying the exact cause of coronary atherosclerosis or in decreasing the mortality associated with this process. Various studies in the past decade have shown that over half of all the annual deaths in the United States are due to some form of cardiovascular disease, and that coronary artery disease is the principal cause of all the cardiovascular deaths. Certain diverse factors have been identified as rendering an individual "at risk" for the development of coronary atherosclerosis. These factors include a family history of coronary artery disease, cigarette smoking, elevated serum cholesterol levels, the absence of female hormones, and an intense, hard driving, achievement-oriented personality. This list is not all inclusive but intended to indicate some of the many areas where research is currently being directed in an attempt to prevent or slow the development of coronary atherosclerosis in our population.

The diagnosis of coronary artery disease is usually based on the patient's clinical presentation, coronary angiography and stress testing by electrocardiogram. Medical treatment is aimed at slowing the progression of the disease process and includes steps to reduce risk factors, steps to reduce myocardial oxygen demands, and relief of symptoms. In recent years myocardial revascularization procedures, commonly called coronary by-pass operations, have been employed with increasing frequency to prevent the ultimate consequences of coronary occlusion. Nursing care of the patient undergoing by-pass surgery is discussed in the surgical section of this chapter.

Alterations in Cellular Metabolism

The clinical consequences of a myocardial infarction are best understood in the light of the metabolic consequences of anoxia. A decrease in oxygen supply principally affects the aerobic or energy producing phase of cellular metabolism. However, glycolysis, or the anaerobic phase, is altered as well in that there is an increased production of lactic (rather than pyruvic) acid. It is thought that the pain associated with coronary artery disease results from the action of this increased lactic acid on pain receptors.

Cells which are not adequately perfused show altered ability to perform their normal functions. These functions include the special properties of cardiac cells. Cellular death occurs when the oxygen supply is decreased to the point that energy production ceases. One of the principal uses of cellular energy production is the maintenance of its membrane. With no energy available, the membrane collapses, and the intracellular contents are spewed into the interstitial compartment. The number of cells that die is related to the size of the area perfused by the occluded artery and to whether collateral circulation has previously been established. Whatever the extent of the actual zone of infarction, it is surrounded by cells that are injured (severely anoxic), and injured cells are surrounded by an area of ischemia. The complications that occur as a result of an infarction can be related to all three states of anoxia. The primary site of a myocardial infarction is, in the great majority of cases, the left ventricle. The infarction process may extend into the atria or into the right ventricle but rarely starts in these areas.

Diagnosis

The goals of diagnostic procedures are first to determine whether an infarction has, in fact, occurred and second to determine the location and extent of the infarction if possible. The patient's presenting symptoms, electrocardiogram, lab work, and clinical status must all be evaluated in order to achieve these goals.

The most common presenting symptom of myocardial infarction is substernal pain which often has a strong pressure component. The pain has been described as a crushing or heavy sensation—"like an elephant standing on my chest." The pain typically lasts for several minutes and is unrelieved by rest, nitroglycerin, or changes in body position. Radiation of the pain into the left arm, jaw, or groin is frequently noted, and on occasion the pain may occur *only* in one of these radiation sites. Accompanying the pain may be diaphoresis, nausea, vomiting, a strong urge to defecate, and a sense of impending doom. Although the above description may be "classic" for a myocardial infarction patient, it is important to remember that the infarction may be "silent" about 15% of the time. Silent MIs may occur in patients who have a decreased level of awareness (such as those under anesthesia, those in diabetic coma, or patients who are psychotic), or in patients who have an enormously high pain threshold or the ability to deny the pain experience. Infarctions in these patients are usually discovered in retrospect because of changes in their electrocardiograms, or because they seek medical assistance for some complication of the infarction process.

The electrocardiogram is usually considered to be the most definitive diagnostic tool for myocardial infarction and is certainly most helpful when the typical changes are present. It should be noted, however, that in the absence of typical changes, a probable diagnosis may still be made based on the patient's clinical history and his laboratory findings. The reader is referred to a text on electrocardiography for a specific discussion of the use of the 12 lead electrocardiogram in the diagnosis of myocardial infarction. Important points, however, include: (1) the nature of the changes indicate not only whether an infarction has occurred, but also, (2) the location of the infarction in the left ventricle (anterior, inferior, lateral, posterior or a combination of these sites), and (3) the extent of the infarction process relative to the thickness of the ventricular wall (i.e., transmural or nontransmural). These considerations are extremely valuable in predicting probable complications for a specific patient and in planning specific types of assessment and intervention.

Changes in certain laboratory values occur with myocardial infarction, and considerable progress has been made in the area of identifying changes that are specific for damage to the heart. An elevated WBC and ESR are to be expected because of the injury and inflammation which has occurred. More specific determinations can be made from elevations in serum enzyme levels since cardiac cellular death releases intracellular enzymes into the general circulation. Enzymes most frequently elevated are: SCPK, SGOT, SLDH, and SHBD. Since these enzymes are found in numerous other body tissues as well as in cardiac tissue, the exact pattern of elevation becomes important. The accompanying chart (Table 2-1) depicts the relative pattern of elevation found with myocardial infarction with respect to the usual upper limits of normal. Aside from the pattern of elevation, isoenzyme determinations have increased the specificity of this test. SLDH for example, is made up of 5 distinct components, only two of which are specific for cardiac muscle. While an increase in total SLDH might not indicate myocardial damage, an elevation in the cadiac isoenzymes definitely would. SHBD is similar in specificity to SLDH isoenzymes, in that the other conditions which produce elevations should be clearly differentiated from MI based on the clinical presentation.

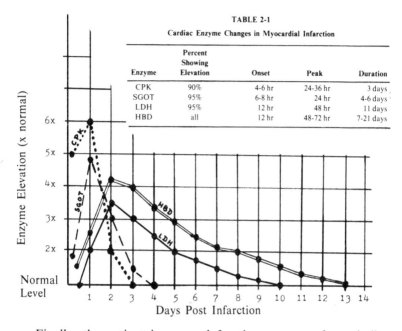

TABLE 2-1

Cardiac Enzyme Changes in Myocardial Infarction

Enzyme	Percent Showing Elevation	Onset	Peak	Duration
CPK	90%	4-6 hr	24-36 hr	3 days
SGOT	95%	6-8 hr	24 hr	4-6 days
LDH	95%	12 hr	48 hr	11 days
HBD	all	12 hr	48-72 hr	7-21 days

Finally, the patient is assessed for the presence of any indications of complications frequently associated with the infarction process. The location of the infarction is often a key to the type of complication that might be expected—for instance, inferior MIs are usually associated with an occlusion in the right coronary artery which subsequently may result in altered functioning of those portions of the heart's electrical system which are also perfused by the right coronary artery. Some alterations in electrical activity are not specific to the location of the infarction, such as the occurrence of premature ventricular contractions which arise from the zone of ischemia. Infarction may result in mechanical failure as well and also may give rise to thrombus formation on the surface of the injured ventricle. Patients may arrive in the emergency room or Intensive Care Unit with clinical signs of acute pulmonary edema or a cerebrovascular accident that, in retrospect, are traced to an acute myocardial infarction. Complications will be discussed in greater detail in the section following general nursing care.

Stages of Healing

Pathological findings indicate that necrosis of cells does not become evident until the infarction is approximately 5-6 hours old.

Hence, a person who dies "suddenly" following an MI (within one hour of the onset of symptoms) may not show evidence of this insult on post mortem examination. The phagocytic process, or invasion of the necrotic area with white cells, gets underway within the first 24 hours after the infarction. The first 4-5 days of the healing process are clinically crucial because enlargement of the collateral circulation is beginning to occur, and the zone of injured or severely anoxic cells is usually pushed in one direction or the other. Increased myocardial oxygen requirements related to activity, stress or some drugs such as digitalis may result in the ultimate infarction of this zone. Minimal oxygen requirements may allow adequate perfusion via collateral vessels and a decrease in the anoxia back to a state of ischemia. During the next 10 to 15 days, the collateral circulation continues to enlarge, fibroblasts produce connective tissue in the area of infarction, and the ischemic cells slowly regain their normal functional abilities. These phases of healing generally correlate with the period of hospitalization for the relatively uncomplicated infarction patient. Healing is not complete during this time, however, and for the next several months scar tissue replaces the previously necrotic muscle, and the surrounding functional myocardium hypertrophies to compensate for the loss of contractility in the area.

GENERAL NURSING CARE OF THE MI PATIENT

The activities of the nurse who is caring for a patient with an acute myocardial infarction should be directed toward (1) promotion of healing of the damaged area, (2) prevention of complications resulting from the infarction or from the patient's state of relative immobility, and (3) prompt detection of complications and initiation of measures to reverse those that do occur. A basic needs framework will be used to discuss data collection, analysis, and plans for intervention and evaluation.

Oxygen Needs

The patient's ability to meet his oxygen needs may be significantly altered by the infarction process, and it is in this area that the nurse must be the most astute in her understanding of the pathological process and in her ability to assess the patient. Assessment of this need area is somewhat complicated by the fact that alterations in either the circulatory system or the respiratory system, or both, can result in decreased cellular oxygenation.

Nine physiologic factors are involved in meeting oxygen needs. Circulatory components include blood volume, blood carrying capacity, blood vessels, and a pumping heart. Respiratory components include respiratory control, airway, thorax mobility and respiratory membrane. One additional factor, the ability of the cells to utilize O_2, is disturbed only in rare circumstances such as carbon monoxide or cyanide poisoning.

The factor most likely to be altered by the infarction process is the heart's ability to act as a pump. Structural damage to the myocardium may decrease the stroke volume component of the cardiac output equation, although an increase in heart rate may compensate for this alteration. Arrhythmias associated with the infarction process may also decrease pumping efficiency due to either very slow heart rates (for which an increase in stroke volume may not be possible) or very rapid heart rates which may lead to decreased ventricular filling time. It is clear that circulation to the heart itself is compromised by the presence of coronary atherosclerosis which decreases the patency of the blood vessels involved.

Other factors necessary for meeting oxygen needs may be secondarily affected by either treatment modalities or by other complications of the infarction process. Morphine sulfate, for instance, which is commonly used to control pain and apprehension may lead to depression of respiratory centers and may decrease heart rate as well. Bedrest may induce decreased thorax mobility, decreased available respiratory membrane due to atelectasis, and venous stasis which promotes thrombus formation. The development of left ventricular failure may lead to pulmonary congestion which also decreases the availability of an adequate respiratory membrane.

Assessment

Some of the parameters utilized in the assessment of oxygen status are clearly related to the circulatory system, some are clearly related to the respiratory system, and others may indicate that a problem is present without clearly identifying the source. If an alteration in the patient's ability to meet his oxygen needs is noted, knowledge of the source of the problem is certainly an immense aid to planning appropriate intervention.

The most commonly evaluated circulatory parameters are heart rate and rhythm, heart sounds, blood pressure, and the presence and quality of peripheral pulses. Venous distention, skin color and temperature, and capillary refill also represent types of data that may be considered to be directly related to circulatory status. Thorax shape and mobility, respiratory rate and rhythm, character of respirations (muscle groups used, subjective feelings of dyspnea, etc.), and breath sounds represent types of data that are usually considered to be directly related to the respiratory system.

Some overlap can be noted in the data categories of the previous outline. Alterations in skin color, for example, may be due to either respiratory or circulatory problems. Abnormal breath sounds may indicate secretions blocking a major airway or fluid accumulation in the alveoli as a result of left ventricular failure. General signs of hypoxia, such as decreased activity tolerance or changes in mental status also do not clearly identify the source of the problem nor do alterations in arterial blood gas levels. Decreased urinary output may be related to inadequate circulation or simply to a hypovolemic state. Invasive assessment parameters will be discussed in the section dealing with specific complicatons.

Analysis of data

Although the initial assessment of any patient admitted to an Intensive Care Unit would include all of the above parameters (see chapter on assessment), the ongoing assessment of the myocardial infarction patient should be specifically directed toward those parameters which would reflect alterations related to the infarction process or treatment modalities as outlined above. Any pre-existing alterations in the patient's ability to meet his oxygen needs would additionally need to be considered in the data analysis. Representative nursing diagnoses in this need area for a patient with a myocardial infarction would include: (1) actual or potential decreased capacity of the heart to act as a pump, related to structural damage; (2) decreased thorax mobility related to bedrest; (3) decreased capacity of the heart to act as a pump related to slow (or fast) rate arrhythmia; (4) potential respiratory depression related to morphine administration.

Goals, intervention, evaluation

General goals for all myocardial infarction patients relative to oxygen needs would include the following:

1. The patient's oxygen requirements will not exceed his ability to meet them as evidenced by lack of chest pain, maintenance of normal skin color and temperature, maintenance of acceptable heart rate with activity (see section on activity needs), absence of dyspnea with exertion.
2. The patient will not develop atelectasis as evidenced by lack of decreased or absent breath sounds.
3. The patient will not develop venous thrombosis as evidenced by absence of a positive Homans' sign, warmth, redness and pain.
4. The patient will not develop respiratory depression as evidenced by maintenance of normal respiratory rate.

Other goals would relate to specific nursing diagnoses and would probably evolve in relationship to a complication of the infarction process.

Interventions should be directed toward the "related to" segments of the nursing diagnosis (e.g., decreased pumping capacity *related to arrhythmia*), and may be of several types. Continuing assessment or data collection is needed to monitor changes in the patient's status and to recognize new alterations in physiologic factors related to oxygen needs. Other nursing actions may be directed toward maintaining the patient's present ability to meet the need, and yet others will be aimed at reversing an identified problem.

Oxygen therapy is frequently instituted for myocardial infarction patients, although the use of this therapy varies from institution to institution. In some institutions, all patients receive approximately 40% O_2 (usually via nasal prongs or face shields) for the first 24 to 48 hours of hospitalization. In other instances, oxygen therapy may be reserved for those patients who have episodes of chest pain, arrhythmias, or some other complication or who show clinical signs of hypoxemia. Valencia and Burgess (1969) state that some hypoxemia is usual following myocardial infarction even in the absence of specific complications, although the exact cause of the hypoxemia appeared to be variable.[23] Another study indicated that 40% O_2 was helpful in improving oxygen delivery and cardiac output only in cases of patients who were severely hypoxemic.[22] Further clinical research is needed to determine the effectiveness of low to moderate flow oxygen therapy as a general intervention for the MI patient.

The benefit of writing goals in specific behavioral terms is the ease with which evaluation can be carried out. The process of evaluation consists of the collection and analysis of data which would indicate goal attainment. When the evidence suggests that the goal has not been achieved, reassessment is required to determine whether or not the goal is stated in observable terms, is congruent with the patient's present and potential capabilities, is attainable with the available resources and within an identifiable period of time, and whether or not the interventions are appropriate.

Nutritional Needs (Food, Fluid, and Electrolytes)

An individual is generally considered to be meeting his nutrition needs when there is a balance between his intake of calories, carbohydrate, protein, fat, water, vitamins and minerals and his body's need for these substances. The infarction process, in and of itself, does not alter the body's ability to meet this need although it may result in some alterations in the usual requirements, and peripheral factors relative to the patient's clinical status or to treatment modalities may create a situation in which nursing assistance is needed. Limited mobility, for example, may result in a decreased requirement for calories, but an increased requirement for bulk and fluids. If the patient is on a selective diet, he may not display much interest in, or have enough energy for selecting foods that meet his nutritional requirements. Low cholesterol diets are frequently ordered for the MI patient. If this represents a change in his usual dietary pattern, explanation of the rationale for this order will certainly be required, and even though the explanation is provided in a careful, thoughtful manner, the diet may still seem dull and tasteless. This is especially true if a sodium restriction is required as well. The benefits of insistence on profound dietary modifications during the first phase of hospitalization are open to question, although it seems certain that such changes may be required ultimately.

Assessment

Parameters for assessment of nutrition needs include the patient's current height and weight; usual dietary patterns; history of weight gain or loss; laboratory studies such as FBS, hematocrit and hemoglobin, serum electrolytes, cholesterol, and triglycerides; general appearance and energy level; and intake of food and fluids since admission.

Analysis of data

The patient's nutritional status prior to hospitalization will be enormously significant in the evaluation of his current status. Areas for special concern would be: demonstrated hyperglycemia or hypercholesterolemia, obesity, electrolyte imbalances (particularly hyper- or hypokalemia), and inadequate or excessive fluid intake. Representative nursing diagnoses in this need area for a patient with a myocardial infarction would include (1) obesity related to excessive caloric intake, (2) hypercholesterolemia related to patient's previous dietary patterns, (3) hypokalemia related to diuretic therapy and inadequate intake, (4) fluid volume deficit related to inadequate intake, and (5) anorexia related to pain (or unfamiliar foods, or anxiety, etc.).

Goals, interventions, evaluation

A general patient goal in this need area as identified in the *A.N.A. Standards of Cardiovascular Nursing Practice* is "The individual maintains a dietary intake which is compatible with therapeutic and personal goals."[1] This goal can be adapted to correlate more specifically with identified nursing diagnoses and to facilitate evaluation. Appropriate goals for a patient with myocardial infarction relative to nutrition would include:

1. The patient has a fluid intake of at least 2,000 cc per 24 hours (or the limit of a fluid restriction if one exists).
2. The patient maintains an oral intake pattern that does not compromise his O_2 needs as evidenced by lack of chest pain or arrhythmias following meals.
3. The patient establishes or maintains an "ideal" body weight for his height and frame type.
4. The patient maintains a normal serum potassium level.
5. The patient explains the rationale for prescribed dietary modifications.
6. The patient selects foods that are compatible with his therapeutic regimen.
7. The patient expresses a willingness to modify his diet in accordance with therapeutic regimens.

Nursing interventions will again be of various types. Teaching, counseling, and motivating the patient and his family will be prime activities, as will collaboration with the dietary department regarding choices of foods, management of fluid restrictions and arrangement of frequency and size of feedings. In most Intensive Care Units, the patient is assisted with feeding only when there is evidence that this activity causes an excessive energy expenditure or results in arrhythmias, or when treatment modalities limit the patient's mobility. Most patients much prefer to feed themselves, and the boost to their morale that results from this type of self-care should be an important consideration.

The process of evaluation will be the same throughout and is contingent upon both establishing goals in terms which can be evaluated and carrying out goal-directed interventions.

Elimination Needs

Elimination needs are met through adequate functioning of the urinary and gastrointestinal systems and through the individual's ability to carry out toileting activities. As was the case with nutrition needs, the infarction process itself does not alter the body's ability to meet this need unless complications occur (i.e., decreased circulation to the kidneys), but the treatment regimen of rest and limited mobility may lead to alterations in normal functioning and alterations in the patient's ability to manage toileting activities.

Assessment

Factors to be assessed in this need category include fluid output relative to fluid intake; intake of solid foods; pattern of urination relative to normal; pattern of bowel elimination relative to normal; weight pattern (especially rapid gains or losses); presence of edema; serum electrolyte, creatinine, and blood urea nitrogen levels; urine chemistries, medications which affect gastrointestinal motility; and physical and environmental factors which may inhibit normal toileting activities.

Analysis of data

The importance of considering the patient's usual elimination patterns in the data analysis cannot be overemphasized. Not only is the patient often the first to notice an alteration in function, but he may also be knowledgeable about interventions which have been effective in the past.

Constipation is a well-known result of immobility and lack of bulk or fluid in the diet and is, therefore, a potential problem for the MI patient. Stool softeners are given on a wholesale basis in the intensive care unit because of the need to prevent the patient from straining during defecation. It has long been discussed that straining at stool may reflexively slow the heart because of parasympathetic stimulation. An equally serious potential problem is the great surge of venous return that occurs when straining ceases. If a venous thrombus has formed and is loosely attached to the vessel wall, this rush of fluid may easily lead to embolization.

Low urine output is a finding which must be analyzed in an especially careful manner. Questions to be considered are, first, is this urinary retention or decreased urine formation? Urinary retention may be the result of lack of privacy or inability to void in a recumbent or semi-recumbent position. If the bladder does not appear to be distended, the next question to ask is whether the decreased urine formation merely reflects low fluid intake or is possibly an indication of inadequate circulation to the kidneys.

Representative nursing diagnosis in this need area would include: (1) potential constipation related to bedrest, present diet, unfamiliar environment, morphine, etc., (2) decreased urinary output related to low fluid intake, and (3) diarrhea related to quinidine therapy.

Goals, interventions, evaluation

General patient goals for this need area are the following:

1. The patient maintains his normal pattern of bladder and bowel elimination as evidenced by . . . (a descriptive statement concerning the patient's normal bladder and bowel elimination— i.e., "a formed stool every other day").
2. The patient's toileting activities do not stress his O_2 needs, as evidenced by maintenance of baseline pulse and blood pressures, lack of pain, and lack of arrhythmias.

Nursing interventions are primarily directed toward ensuring adequate intake of fluid and solids, so that normal elimination patterns are maintained. In addition, the patient may require assistance in identifying food intolerances and in communicating these to the dietary department. When alterations in normal elimination patterns occur, the nurse is in the best position to inform the patient of, and discuss with him, alternative types of therapeutic interventions. Finally, the nurse takes steps to ensure maximum privacy for toileting activities and provides whatever assistance is needed to keep energy expenditure at a minimum during this time. The common practice with MI patients is to allow the use of the bedside commode and to assist males to a standing position if this facilitates voiding, as energy expenditure for these activities is less than that involved in moving on and off the bedpan.

Comfort, Rest, and Sleep Needs

The needs that comprise the next category are highly interrelated and are often grouped together under the heading of "rest." The component parts, however, represent a type of continuum since discomfort (physical or emotional) will certainly alter the patient's ability to obtain rest and, ultimately, sleep. These needs assume considerable importance in the care of the MI patient because the potential for discomfort is as great as the need for rest.

The amount of pain that an individual will have during or following a myocardial infarction is extremely variable. As noted earlier, the actual infarction event may be characterized by severe pain or by discomfort that is so minimal that the patient may not seek medical assistance. Following admission to the Intensive Care Unit, some patients experience no further episodes of pain while others may require frequent analgesia. Continuing episodes of pain may be related to the size of the infarction, the relative absence of collateral circulation, and increased myocardial oxygen requirements. Control of the pain is essential, not only to meet the patient's comfort needs, but also to relieve anxiety and reduce sympathetic stimulation (both of which may increase oxygen demands) and to promote rest and healing.

Sources of general discomfort for the MI patient are many and variable. IVs, monitoring electrodes, sensory overload associated with the ICU environment (in some units where the structure provides the equivalent of a private room, the problem may be more sensory deprivation), nausea, lack of mobility, and post MI fever are just a few of the potential etiologies.

Similarly, general discomfort, pain, stress, an unfamiliar environment, and interruptions in circadian rhythm may all contribute to insomnia. In summary, the myocardial infarction patient is a prime candidate for the development of alterations in his ability to meet comfort, rest, and sleep needs.

Assessment

Parameters for this need area include the patient's subjective reports of pain, discomfort, fatigue, or insomnia; objective evidence of same (listlessness, tense muscles, increased heart rate, fixed body position, irritability, pinched facial expression, etc.); usual sleep pattern; usual methods employed to promote comfort, relaxation and sleep; sleep pattern noted in the hospital; response of the patient to analgesia; environmental considerations; and laboratory values which would indicate malnutrition or altered ability to meet oxygen needs which would therefore result in decreased energy production.

Analysis of data

Pain, discomfort, fatigue and insomnia are the common nursing diagnoses that relate to the need category of comfort, rest, and sleep. All of these diagnoses are potentially valid for the MI patient; however, it is essential that the "related to" segment of the diagnosis be identified. Fatigue related to sensory overload is a much different problem from fatigue related to hypoxemia. This category is also one in which the diagnosis can and should be validated with the patient. The nurse may have misinterpreted some of the data, or may find that she and the patient do not have the same perception of the likely etiology of the problem. If the patient feels that his insomnia is related to noise on the unit, nursing measures to induce relaxation will probably be of little help without steps to decrease the auditory stimuli. Validation of the diagnosis will also facilitate establishment of goals and ultimately the evaluation of interventions.

Goals, intervention, evaluation

General goals for the MI patient in this need area include the following:

1. Patient maintains his normal sleep pattern as evidenced by . . .
2. Patient is well rested as evidenced by subjective statements regarding this, a relaxed appearance, mental alertness, willingness to participate in A.D.L. as permitted . . .
3. Patient states he is comfortable—or reports prompt relief of symptoms of discomfort.

The diffuse nature of the possible etiologies for alterations in the MI patient's ability to meet his needs for comfort, rest, and sleep, makes a specific discussion of nursing interventions impossible.

Control of pain related to myocardial ischemia is generally achieved with morphine sulfate given either subcutaneously, intramuscularly, or intravenously. Morphine has the advantage of reducing anxiety and decreasing the sympathetic response to pain. The disadvantages of this intervention are respiratory depression and slowing of the heart rate. The latter consequence is sometimes avoided by the simultaneous administration of Atropine, although this practice is by no means universal. Much has been written about nonpharmacologic measures to reduce pain and discomfort. The reader is referred to general nursing texts for an in-depth discussion.

Rest is legislated for the MI patient by the medical activity order, but this is not to say that the desired amount of rest is, therefore, achieved. Strict bed rest, for as long as 3 weeks, was the practice of the past. The emotional stress associated with forced dependency, particularly when the patient was asymptomatic, and the significant hazards of immobility for which these patients were at risk, seemed however to outweigh the benefits to be achieved by this regimen. Currently, the practice in most Intensive Care Units is to allow some liberalization in the activity order although a great deal of variability can still be noted. The nursing implications of this situation involve at least two different responsibilities. The first is assisting the patient to accept and cope with whatever activity restrictions are in force. If the patient understands the rationale for the order, he is more likely to cooperate and to deal openly with his feelings. This should facilitate the achievement of emotional, as well as physical rest. The second of the nursing responsibilities is assessment of the patient's physiologic responses to both physical activity and events which may be emotionally disturbing (i.e., emergencies within the unit, visits from family or friends, news relative to his diagnosis or prognosis, etc.) so that the nurse can intervene as needed to promote optimum rest. Daytime sedation, usually in the form of tranquilizers, is often used to facilitate "rest," and it is usually the nurse who is in the best position to assess whether this intervention is effective or is interfering with the patient's normal sleep pattern.

Clinical research regarding the nature of sleep has revealed many interesting phenomena which are beyond the scope of this discussion, but some general knowledge in this area is essential for the

ICU nurse. In brief, sleep patterns are of two different types: (1) nonrapid eye movement (NREM) sleep which has four distinct phases, and (2) rapid eye movement (REM) sleep, so named because of the coordinated rapid movement of the eyeballs that can be noted during this time. REM sleep is thought to be the phase in which most dreaming occurs and is characterized by slight increases in pulse, blood pressure, and oxygen consumption. Nocturnal angina and episodes of duodenal ulcer pain have been demonstrated to occur during the REM sleep stage. The amount of time an individual spends in the REM sleep state generally increases as the length of the sleep period increases (i.e., if an individual sleeps for several consecutive hours, he will spend more time in REM sleep during the later hours than during the early ones). REM sleep has been demonstrated to be decreased in a patient taking barbiturates and in a patient who sleeps for only short periods at any one time. When an individual is deprived of one of the normal sleep stages, the cessation of the situation responsible for the deprivation results in a rebound effect; that is, the body will attempt to make up the deprivation. It would clearly seem undesirable for the MI patient to be in a situation of making up lost REM sleep.

Nursing implications to be derived from these findings are (1) the importance of arranging medication schedules and assessment activities in such a way that the patient is able to obtain several hours of uninterrupted sleep during the night; (2) the benefits of using relaxation methods to promote sleep rather than relying on the effectiveness of barbiturate sleeping medications; and (3) the need for close observation of the patient who has been taken off barbiturate drugs for indications of increasing incidence of physiologic changes associated with REM sleep.

Activity Needs

Activity is necessary to maintain the integrity of the musculoskeletal system, to promote the optimal functioning of other body systems, and to promote a feeling of fitness and well-being in the individual. When a person has no internal restrictions on his mobility, can carry out his own activities of daily living, and gets sufficient exercise, he is usually considered to be meeting his activity needs.

The patient with a myocardial infarction presents a dilemma in this particular need category. The need to rest the myocardium has previously been established, yet the need to prevent the physical and psychological hazards of immobility must be considered. The on-going questions to be answered, therefore, are how much activity is "enough?" and "what data would indicate that the cardiovascular system has been excessively stressed?"

Assessment

Assessment in this area involves determining the patient's pre-illness activity status, his potential for activity, and his response to activity. Parameters include the patient's usual level of activity (active/sedentary), his usual approach to, and capability for carrying out activities of daily living, range of motion in the joints, muscle size and strength, activity order, actual activity in relation to the written order, and physiologic responses to activity such as pulse rate, blood pressure, character of respirations, and subjective feelings of well-being versus tiredness.

Analysis of data

Data analysis should revolve around several questions such as (1) does this patient's current activity level meet his needs for both activity and rest? (2) is he as active as his physical status permits? (3) how well does he tolerate those activities in which he does participate? (4) is this patient particularly prone to any hazards of immobility, and if so, which ones? The hazards of immobility are a common topic of discussion in every nursing course and will not be reviewed at length; however, the point must be emphasized that every patient is not equally at risk. A valid nursing diagnosis, even a potential one, must be based on specific data about the specific patient at hand. To illustrate, a generally healthy, well-nourished patient who is capable of turning himself in bed is not at risk for decubitus ulcers as a result of a few days on bed rest. The question of assessing activity tolerance is of special concern to the ICU nurse since "progressive ambulation" is often at her discretion. One set of guidelines for this assessment has been proposed as follows: the activity is too strenuous (1) if the pulse increases 20 beats or more per minute over the pre-activity pulse; (2) if the pulse exceeds 120 beats per minute during the activity; or (3) if upon completion of the activity, the pulse does not return to the pre-activity level within three minutes.[19] Other indications that an activity is compromising the body's ability to meet its oxygen needs are dyspnea and an increased incidence of abnormal cardiac electrical activity. Representative nursing diagnoses in this need area would include the following: (1) decreased mobility related to a "strict bed rest" activity order; (2) potential decreased R.O.M. in shoulder related to limited mobility and history of arthritis, (3) decreased activity tolerance related to low caloric intake (or anemia, or reduced pumping ability of the heart, etc.).

Goals, interventions, evaluation

The goal for this need area suggested by the *A.N.A. Standards for Cardiovascular Nursing* is: "The individual maintains an activity pattern which is compatible with therapeutic and personal goals."[1] The essence of this goal can again be adapted to correlate with specific nursing diagnoses. General goals for all patients would include:

1. The patient maintains an activity level which is sufficient to prevent hazards of immobility as evidenced by lack of atelectasis, or lack of skin breakdown, etc.
2. The patient's activity level does not exceed his activity tolerance as evidenced by lack of arrhythmias, pulse increase of less than 20 beats per minute, lack of chest pain or dyspnea during the activity.

Interventions will greatly depend on the patient's physical and emotional status. The nurse will need to determine which activities the patient is able to, and should be encouraged to carry out actively, and which activities should be passive. When the patient is able to carry out some activities independently, the nurse may need to teach him the most efficient, energy-saving procedure. For example, it has been found that patients who can turn themselves in bed frequently do a Valsalva maneuver in the process because they hold their breaths while pulling themselves over. The nurse can demonstrate the correct procedure for this activity as well as for other repositioning activities. Special challenges are presented by the patient who exhibits no interest in self-care activities and by the patient who will not accept any activity restriction. The first situation may indicate that the patient is experiencing grief related to his diagnosis or prognosis; the second situation is more characteristic of a patient who is undergoing denial. These reactions will be discussed more fully in the section on psychological needs, but both represent a threat to the patient's optimal activity status. The nurse may well need to collaborate with other members of the health team to determine the most appropriate interventions.

Sexual Needs

Sexual needs may seem like a low priority consideration for a patient in the Intensive Care Unit, but patient responses to opportunities to discuss concerns about sexual functioning have indicated that this is definitely not the case. The notion that a damaged heart may mean the end of normal sexual functioning is widespread in our society, and there is the potential for at least some concern on the parts of the patient and sexual partner, no matter what their age or marital status. In terms of physiology, the infarction process may alter the patient's ability to participate in the sex act only to the extent that such energy expenditure compromises his oxygen needs. In relation to emotional status, the patient may experience some degree of sexual disequilibrium because he (or his partner) fears that such activity may result in pain, another infarction, or even death.

Assessment of sexual needs

Data concerning the patient's current status, relative to this need area, may be obtained by observing the quantity and quality of his interactions with significant others and with the health care team, determining what activities he associates with his usual sexual role, and simply by asking whether he expects that there will be any change in his sexual functioning or relationships with significant others as a result of this illness.

Analysis of data

Indications of possible sexual disequilibrium include lack of warm interactions with significant others, preoccupation with personal appearance, aggressive sexual behavior, questions regarding long-term effects of the pathology, and simple verbalization of concerns about sexual functioning. A representative nursing diagnosis in this need category would be sexual disequilibrium related to inadequate knowledge about the potential for future sexual activity.

Goals, intervention, evaluation

A general goal relative to sexual needs would be that the patient maintains sexual integrity. Integrity, in this instance, should be interpreted broadly to include not only the ability to carry out the usual sexual role, but also an optimal concept of self as a sexual being.

Interventions will usually involve: (1) allowing the patient to express his feelings and concerns; and (2) providing factual information regarding sexual functioning to the patient and the sexual partner, (3) facilitating communication between the patient and the physician, (4) facilitating communication between the patient and significant others. The nurse must recognize her own feelings concerning sexuality and determine the extent to which these feelings will influence the ability to intervene effectively. The importance of assessing the patient's status relative to sexual needs cannot be ignored, and the nurse must be aware of situations in which the expertise of other members of the health team is required. Some intensive care units have prepared their own brochures concerning sexual activity following a myocardial infarction, and there are a variety of other publications available which the nurse can suggest if the patient's physician is in accord (see suggested reading list).

SECONDARY NEEDS

The remaining needs are called secondary needs, according to Maslow's hierarchy.[17] They are secondary in that they do not relate to the primary physiologic needs which must be satisfied to some degree before an individual can move upward and attempt to fulfill psychosocial needs. However, physical safety, which falls in this category, is far from a secondary consideration in the intensive care unit since failure of the health team to ensure that this need is met could threaten the patient's life. Emotional security, love and belonging, and self-esteem are not needs that tend to be primary motivating factors in the behavior of a critically ill patient, but the experience of unexpected hospitalization and the diagnosis of a myocardial infarction may certainly threaten the patient's ability to meet these needs. Consequently, nursing intervention in these areas may significantly reduce some of the emotional stress of the ICU patient.

Safety Needs

Safety needs encompass a variety of component parts such as sensory status, environmental considerations, mobility, maintenance of skin and mucous membrane integrity, and mental/emotional state. The emphasis of this discussion will be on those components most likely to be influenced by treatment in the intensive care setting.

Perhaps the most important potential source of threat to the safety status of the MI patient is the complex electrical equipment which is utilized in his care. Awareness of electrical safety has been greatly increased since the advent of intensive care units, and the reader is especially urged to review the report of the Inter-Society Commission on Heart Disease Resources.[9] The two primary considerations are grounding of the electrical equipment and the potential for these patients to have a "direct current pathway" to their hearts. The nature of the electrical hazard involved is the small amounts of current which may leak from equipment that is not properly grounded (i.e., has an intact ground wire which communicates with the internal body of the equipment and is connected to the ground wire in the power cord and to the hospital grounding system via a three-pronged plug). If a piece of electrical equipment is not properly grounded, leakage current will seek another pathway to "ground" (the lowest available level to which current may flow), and that pathway may involve the patient who is connected to ground by his monitoring or ECG electrodes.

A second hazard is called "ground current" and occurs when two pieces of electrical equipment are not grounded at the same voltage level. This may happen when the pieces of equipment are plugged into separate wall outlets and no provision has been made for a common ground level throughout the unit. If something provides a low resistance pathway between the pieces of equipment (the patient, for example), ground current will flow from the higher level outlet to the lower level outlet, through the patient. The nurse can form the same type of pathway by touching a piece of electrical equipment and the patient simultaneously. She may provide the missing link in the ground current circuit. The situations described thus far may result in the patient receiving painful shocks or burns, but are not likely to be death-producing if he has normal, dry, intact skin. A more serious problem arises when the patient has a "direct current pathway" to his heart—a pathway that penetrates the normally protective skin. Such a pathway may take the form of an intracardiac ECG electrode, a transvenous pacemaker, or even steel thoracotomy sutures. Microshocks, far below the threshold of sensation (.001 volt), may cause ventricular fibrillation if they are allowed to reach the heart via a direct current pathway.

The general goal for this aspect of safety needs is that the patient does not receive any shocks or burns nor does he develop any arrhythmias related to improper grounding or functioning of electrical equipment. Most modern units have electrical designs which provide common grounds and often include alarm systems which warn of electrical hazards. If a common ground has not been provided, the nurse will need to be diligent about limiting the number of pieces of electrical equipment connected to the patient to those which are absolutely essential; plugging all equipment in the same or closely adjacent wall outlets; insulating direct current pathways; prohibiting the use of *any* ungrounded equipment; and remaining alert for any indications of equipment malfunction. Routine inspection of unit grounding systems and equipment should be made by the maintenance department, and it may be necessary for the nurse to insist that this be done.

Other threats to the MI patient's safety status are altered mental functioning related to narcotic medications, sensory overstimulation or sensory deprivation, and infection related to intravenous catheters or pacemakers.

Psychological Needs (Security, Love and Belonging, and Self-esteem)

In order to effectively assist a patient to cope with the psychological reactions that accompany a myocardial infarction, the nurse will need to understand the impact of the diagnosis and course of treatment on his needs for security and self-esteem, and also the normal psychological reactions to loss.

Security is threatened by an unfamiliar environment, an unfamiliar patient role, and an often uncertain diagnosis and prognosis. From the time of admission onward, it is essential to assess the patient's *perception* of the reason for his confinement in an Intensive Care Unit, the nature of his illness, the cause of his illness and his expectations regarding the outcome of treatment. The nurse can build trust and relieve anxiety by providing simple, factual explanations, orienting the patient to his role and responsibilities and to his surroundings, structuring the environment, and establishing the reliability of the health care team. It will be helpful to recall that while a low level of anxiety may serve to facilitate learning, moderate and severe anxiety inhibit this activity so that instructions and explanations may have to be repeated frequently.

Many progressive ICU's allow a family member or significant other to remain in the patient's presence when this is judged to contribute positively to the maintenance or restoration of the patient's security. Observing the quality of interactions between the patient and his significant others will also provide data which will assist the nurse in assessing the patient's ability to meet love and belonging needs. In addition, it should be remembered that the stress of the illness and the hospitalization on family and friends may be such that they will require assistance with meeting their own security needs and with providing support to the patient.

The etiology of alterations in the MI patient's ability to meet his self-esteem needs is the body image change which may accompany this illness event; the patient often views himself as no longer "whole." Technically speaking, while the person might be much less "whole" following a surgical procedure which totally removes another body organ, our society places an enormous emotional significance on the functioning of the heart.

The MI patient can hardly ignore the threats to his body image that are posed by the symptoms which accompany the actual infarction event, the forced dependency created by the treatment regimen, and the actual or perceived need to significantly alter his life style. Depending upon the degree to which his psychomotor skills contributed to his self-image in the past, the unexpectedness of the illness, and the effectiveness of his coping skills, the patient may experience profound feelings of loss and undergo a series of emotional reactions which can be simply summarized as "grief and mourning."

The common first response to loss is denial, and this coping mechanism is utilized frequently by MI patients during the first few days of hospitalization. This is a mechanism which protects the ego and may manifest itself by inappropriate cheerfulness, unwillingness to comply with activity restrictions, or by statements of disbelief concerning the diagnosis. The nurse does not encourage the use of denial but neither is it necessary to actively break down this defense mechanism. Acceptance of the patient's feelings, explanation regarding the therapeutic regimen, and provision for the patient to maintain some control over his care are the most useful interventions. If the patient's level of denial is so extreme that his behavior threatens his life or well-being, firm controls will have to be established.

The second response to loss is the awareness and acknowledgment phase. This phase commonly occurs about 5 to 14 days following the loss event and may be characterized by considerable anger, irritability and attempts to fix blame. If the patient feels that his life style or some specific activity he undertook were in some way responsible for the infarction, this state may also be characterized by guilt. Anger is not a maladaptive response since it gives the patient an opportunity to move from a position of relative helplessness to one of relative power; however, the health team and the patient's significant others must be prepared for the possibility that they may be the targets of this emotion. Again, the staff will need to allow the patient to express his feelings without reacting in a retaliatory manner. The patient should not, of course, be permitted to be abusive, both for the sake of the staff and because, ultimately, this behavior will serve to increase his feelings of guilt.

Anger may be followed by depression, which is characterized by sadness, crying, dependency, lack of interest in his progress or care, and preoccupation with dying. During this phase, the nurse needs to saturate the patient's dependency need before she can assist him back to a state of self-care within the limits imposed by the treatment regimen. She matches his mood and conveys an understanding and acceptance of not only his feelings but also of his right to have these feelings. It is not a simple matter to distinguish a normal depressive reaction to loss from a situation of clinical depression, but the nurse is often in the best position to begin to question whether the patient is clinically depressed. Some Intensive Care Units have built-in procedures for psychiatric evaluation. The nurse should not hesitate to initiate whatever referral mechanisms are available when the patient's response seems to extend beyond "normal."

In summary, the diagnosis of myocardial infarction and the resultant treatment regimen pose significant threats to the patient's ability to meet his self-esteem needs. The nurse must understand the nature of the threats, be able to assess each patient's psychological responses to the diagnosis, and intervene in ways that will restore or maintain the specific individual's feelings of value and worth.

COMPLICATIONS OF MYOCARDIAL INFARCTION

Attention will now be directed toward specific complications associated with the infarction process. The aims of this discussion are: (1) to establish the physiologic basis for each complication, (2) to correlate the complication with a specific type of infarction (by location or extent) when possible, (3) to place the complication in the proper prognostic perspective, (4) to identify the consequences of the complication on the previously discussed basic needs and thus provide the means for assessment, and (5) to identify current treatment modalities. In short, the nurse must know what she is looking for, how to recognize it when she sees it, and what her responsibilities are for setting the intervention machinery into motion.

COMPLICATIONS RELATED TO ALTERATIONS IN THE HEART'S ELECTRICAL ACTIVITY

Arrhythmias of the Sinus Node

Sinus bradycardia

The inherent ability of the SA (sino-atrial) node to initiate the heart's electrical activity can be depressed by an inadequate supply of blood and oxygen. Coronary occlusions high in the right coronary artery, which commonly result in inferior infarctions, may compromise circulation to the sinus node via the SA nodal artery. The result is a decrease in heart rate, or sinus bradycardia (see ECG criteria in Table 2-2). Another etiology of sinus bradycardia is increased activity of the parasympathetic nervous system. This event occurs naturally at night or during periods of rest and as a response to activities such as vomiting or straining to defecate.

Sinus bradycardia is not generally considered to be a serious complication of myocardial infarction, although the potential for two undesirable consequences exists. A decrease in heart rate may lead to decreased cardiac output if stroke volume cannot compensate accordingly. In this instance, the patient will show clinical evidence of a failure to meet O_2 needs, manifested by chest pain,

TABLE 2-2

Electrocardiographic Characteristics of Cardiac Arrhythmias Associated with Acute Myocardial Infarction

Interpretation	ECG Characteristics
Sinus Rhythm	P waves present and regular (i.e., P-P intervals do not vary by more than .16 seconds) Atrial rate 60-100 Each P wave is followed by a "QRS" (verifies conduction into the ventricles)
Arrhythmias of the Sinus Node:	
A. Sinus Bradycardia	P waves present and regular Atrial rate less than 60 (rarely less than 45 without some ectopic activity) Each P wave followed by a "QRS"
B. Sinus Tachycardia	P waves present and regular Atrial rate above 100 but not often greater than 150 Each P wave followed by a "QRS"
Ventricular Arrhythmias:	
A. Premature Ventricular Contractions	Use atrial rate to identify basic cardiac mechanism *PVCs:* "QRS" complex premature in time Not associated with a P wave "QRS" wide and bizarre with T wave usually sloping in the opposite direction from major "QRS" deflection Usually followed by a pause

	Special types:
	1. *End-diastolic*
	    PVC is *barely* premature
	    Next regular sinus P wave is superimposed on front of PVC
	2. *Interpolated*
	    PVC is "sandwiched" in between two consecutive sinus beats
	    No pause following PVC
	    This PVC is an "extrasystole"
	    results in a heart rate which is faster than the atrial rate
	3. *Multifocal*
	    PVCs of varying "QRS" configurations in the same lead. Indicates increased ventricular irritability

(Continued)

TABLE 2-2 (Continued)

**Electrocardiographic Characteristics of Cardiac Arrhythmias
Associated with Acute Myocardial Infarction**

Interpretation	ECG Characteristics
A. Premature Ventricular Contractions (Cont'd)	4. *"R on T"* PVC is *very* premature—begins during the previous T wave Likely to hit the "vulnerable" period which may result in V. Tach. or V. Fibrillation
B. Ventricular Tachycardia	More than 3 consecutive PVCs As an established rhythm, heart rate is rapid (120-250) Ventricular rhythm generally regular except for occasional "capture beats" Sinus P waves may be seen unrelated to the "QRS" complexes May be considered relatively benign if ventricular rate is less than 120
C. Ventricular Fibrillation	No recognizable "QRS" complex Bizarre, erratic electrical activity—a lethal arrhythmia ECG absolutely necessary for diagnosis
Conduction Defects:	
A. Bundle Branch Blocks	P waves present and followed by "QRS" complex Use atrial rate to identify basic cardiac mechanism "QRS" complex prolonged ($>$.10 seconds)
1. Right Bundle Branch Block	"QRS" wider than .10 seconds *Lead QRS configuration* V-1 rSR′ or notched R V-6 qRs — s wave wide

2. Left Bundle Branch Block	"QRS" wider than .12 seconds
	Lead QRS configuration
	V-1 qrS, rS, or "QS"
	      s wave wide
	V-6 *no* initial q
	      wide, notched R

(Continued)

TABLE 2-2 (Continued)

**Electrocardiographic Characteristics of Cardiac Arrhythmias
Associated with Acute Myocardial Infarction**

Interpretation	ECG Characteristics
B. First Degree A-V Block	"Misnomer"—no impulses are blocked P waves present and followed by "QRS" Use atrial rate to identify basic cardiac mechanism P-R interval prolonged beyond .20 seconds
C. Second Degree A-V Block	P waves present and regular Use atrial rate to identify basic cardiac mechanism Each P is *not* followed by a "QRS"
1. Mobitz I (Wenckebach)	Periodic nonconducted P wave Cyclic prolongation of P-R interval until one sinus impulse (P wave) is not conducted P-R interval before nonconducted P wave longest; P-R interval after nonconducted P is shortest
2. Mobitz II	Periodic nonconducted P wave P-R interval remains constant for conducted beats Conducted "QRS" complexes are prolonged
3. Advanced	Frequent nonconducted P waves (at least every other P is not conducted; i.e., 2:1 block or worse) P-R intervals constant
D. Complete Heart Block (Third Degree)	P waves present but unrelated to "QRS" complexes Interpretation made from changing P-R interval (i.e., P waves appear at varying places relative to "QRS" complexes—no *true* P-R interval) Ventricular rate and rhythm depend on site of subsidiary pacemaker 40-70, regular, "QRS" appears normal: probably junctional 20-40, less regular, "QRS" appears wide and bizarre: probably ventricular
E. Ventricular Standstill	P waves present No "QRS" complexes No heart rate or rhythm; a lethal arrhythmia

decreased blood pressure, decreased mental alertness, etc. The other consequence is electrical in nature. The slower the underlying sinus rate, the greater the potential for the initiation of electrical activity by sites other than the sinus node (ectopic foci). Hence, sinus brady-cardia may lead to an increased incidence of ventricular ectopic ac-tivity (usually in the form of PVCs), which, although probably not hemodynamically significant in and of themselves, must be taken seriously as a warning of impending trouble.

Sinus bradycardia is usually not treated unless the patient does develop either symptoms of decreased cardiac output or evidence of increased ectopic activity. Atropine, given either subcutaneously or intravenously, is a common form of treatment but has been used much more judiciously than in the past because of side-effects related to urinary retention and mental confusion in the elderly. If Atropine is contraindicated, or if the results are not satisfactory, a temporary pacemaker may be used.

Sinus tachycardia

The pathophysiology of the infarction process itself does not predispose to this arrhythmia, but several related sequelae do. If the patient develops left ventricular failure, for example, the rate of the sinus node will increase in a compensatory attempt to maintain car-diac output. Post MI fever, because of the increased metabolic de-mands placed on the body, would tend to increase the heart rate, as would physical exercise. In the above instances, sinus tachycardia (see ECG criteria in accompanying chart) may not be a mal-adaptive response. However, in situations in which the sinus node is simply responding to an excitatory stimulus (such as norepi-nephrine, released from the sympathetic nervous system in response to emotional stress, or caffeine ingestion), the increase in heart rate again may compromise the patient's ability to meet his O_2 needs.

Increases in heart rate reduce both ventricular filling time and coronary artery perfusion time. The clinical consequences of these effects will be related to the status of myocardial functioning and the degree of coronary atherosclerosis present. In short, some patients may experience angina or show signs associated with decreased car-diac output.

Sinus tachycardia is also not considered to be a serious problem unless the patient is symptomatic. Every effort should be directed at identifying the predisposing factor(s), so that appropriate treat-ment can be aimed at the cause of this arrhythmia.

Arrhythmias from Ventricular Ectopic Foci

Ventricular arrhythmias

The MI patient is particularly prone to the development of ventricular arrhythmias because of the presence of an ischemic area surrounding the infarct which acts as an excitatory stimulus. These arrhythmias can be viewed on a continuum, starting with premature ventricular contractions (PVC), through ventricular tachycardia (VT), to ventricular fibrillation (VF).

PVCs are the result of a ventricular ectopic focus which has been made irritable by any of a number of stimuli. The reader is referred to a text on electrophysiology or electrocardiography for an indepth discussion of excitatory stimuli. Ischemia has been mentioned previously and is an important stimulus in the MI patient, but fever, hypoxemia, hypokalemia, and digitalis toxicity are also likely influencing factors.

PVCs (see chart) occur in the great majority of MI patients regardless of the location or extent of the infarcted area. They are generally considered to be a "warning arrhythmia"—that is, not hemodynamically significant unless they interfere with the patient's normal electrical activity at very frequent intervals. If this occurs, cardiac output may be diminished, and the patient will experience difficulty meeting his O_2 needs.

Most ICUs have specific criteria for instituting treatment for PVCs *in the MI patient*. It should be noted that these criteria may not apply to patients with other clinical conditions. Examples of some common treatment criteria include frequency (6 or more per minute), proximity to the previous normal cardiac complex ("R on T" type), number of apparent ectopic foci responsible (more than one), and number of consecutive PVCs (2 or more).

Treatment is aimed at suppressing the irritability of the ectopic focus in order to prevent the development of more catastrophic arrhythmias. Lidocaine given intravenously, first as a bolus (1 mg./kg. body weight) and then as a continuous infusion of 1-4 mg./minute, is currently the drug of choice for ventricular arrhythmias. Pronestyl may also be used, either alone or in combination with Lidocaine; Dilantin and Inderal are occasionally employed. Lack of a prompt response to antiarrhythmic drug therapy should signal the need to search out other potentially reversible predisposing factors (hypokalemia, hypoxemia, etc.).

Ventricular tachycardia represents increased irritability of a ventricular ectopic focus, and may appear as 3 or more consecutive PVCs interrupting a sinus rhythm, or as an established rhythm at a rate which is often in excess of 150 beats per minute. Ventricular tachycardia is an ominous sign for two reasons. Both the rapid heart rate and the lack of synchronization between atrial and ventricular mechanical activity associated with the arrhythmia, contribute to a distinct decrease in cardiac output. Secondly, the decreased C.O. of ventricular tachycardia will certainly compound the ischemic state already present in the ventricle of an MI patient, and ventricular fibrillation may follow closely if this arrhythmia cannot be reversed.

Treatment for ventricular tachycardia which persists as an established rhythm should be determined by the patient's clinical status. If the C.O. has decreased to the point where the patient has lost consciousness, immediate reversal is mandatory. Additional doses of Lidocaine may be given, although the manufacturer suggests that 200-300 mg. per hour is the maximum safe dose. Prompt reversal is often achieved at this point with cardioversion (synchronized precordial shock).

Cardioversion is similar to defibrillation in that DC current applied to the chest wall is transmitted to the heart in sufficient quantities to act as an excitatory stimulus which initiates concurrent depolarization of all cardiac cells. This event frequently disrupts the firing of the ectopic focus and allows the sinus node to regain control of the heart's electrical activity. The difference between cardioversion and defibrillation is simply that in the former procedure, the equipment is synchronized to fire at a specific point in the cardiac cycle (generally a QRS complex triggers the discharge of electrical energy), with the aim of preventing the development of ventricular fibrillation. This chaotic electrical activity can result from stimulation of the ventricles, either internally or externally, during the vulnerable period of repolarization (approximately the peak through the downstroke of the T wave). If synchronized cardioversion equipment is not immediately available and/or specific ICU policies allow the nurse only to defibrillate and not to cardiovert, then defibrillation must be employed for the unconscious patient with ventricular tachycardia.

When ventricular tachycardia renders the patient symptomatic (i.e., shows clinical evidence of decreased cardiac output) but still conscious, greater variety in treatment modalities exists. The aim remains to reverse the arrhythmia as quickly as possible, and cardioversion may still be employed. In this instance, however, some type of premedication is indicated before the shock is delivered. Valium is commonly used because of its muscle relaxant and amnesic properties.

Ventricular fibrillation is the result of such rapid chaotic firing of an ectopic focus, that the ventricles are neither electrically activated as a unit, nor do they mechanically contract as a unit. Instead, individual muscle fibers contract and relax with the result that the ventricles "twitch" rather than propel blood. Cardiac output drops to zero, and the patient appears clinically dead. Studies too numerous to cite indicate that this arrhythmia is responsible for the great majority of "sudden deaths" following myocardial infarction. Once the patient is admitted to an Intensive Care Unit, however, early recognition and prompt treatment of warning arrhythmias have dramatically reduced the incidence of primary ventricular fibrillation (occurring in patients without other complications which might explain the presence of the arrhythmia). In fact, in-hospital mortality associated with acute myocardial infarction has been demonstrated to be related to complications *other than* ventricular fibrillation.[14]

Treatment for ventricular fibrillation is without controversy, and consists of the immediate application of unsynchronized precordial shock at approximately 400 watt seconds (joules) of electrical energy. The exact energy level may vary slightly from unit to unit. If the first shock is not successful, the general policy is to recharge the defibrillator and administer a second shock immediately. If the procedure is still unsuccessful, cardiopulmonary resuscitation should be instituted promptly while additional therapeutic maneuvers are undertaken. Most commonly, the patient will be intubated so that a higher percent of oxygen than available in expired air can be delivered. A properly placed endotracheal tube will also maintain an open airway. Intravenous administration of sodium bicarbonate is essential to reverse the metabolic acidosis which is sure to accompany the clinical condition. Acidosis will hinder successful reversal of ventricular fibrillation. In addition, epinephrine is used to coarsen fine fibrillation (increase the voltage of the chaotic electrical activity seen on the monitor or ECG machine) and thus facilitate defibrillation. Epinephrine also stimulates the sinus node which must be capable of resuming control of normal electrical activity if this treatment is to be successful.

Other ectopic arrhythmias

Impulse initiation from ectopic foci in the atria or junctional areas is not a common occurrence in uncomplicated myocardial infarction.[14] Right coronary artery occlusion may cause enough ischemia in the region served by the A-V nodal artery (junctional area) to enhance the automaticity of pacemaking cells found in that area, sometimes to the extent that the sinus node is temporarily usurped by this lower pacemaker. This is not, however, a serious problem. The appearance of atrial arrhythmias is a good indication that other complications, such as pump failure or extension of the infarction into the atrium, have occurred.

Conduction Abnormalities

Conduction abnormalities which occur as a result of acute myocardial infarction can be divided into two categories: (1) those involving the A-V node, and (2) those involving the intraventricular conduction system. Although some variability exists, blocks involving the A-V node are more commonly associated with inferior myocardial infarction and those involving the intraventricular conduction system are associated with anterior infarctions. A review of the mechanism of blood supply to these portions of the cardiac conduction system should make the reason for the above correlations evident. As a group, A-V blocks are somewhat less serious than intraventricular blocks. However, all forms of second degree block and complete heart block, as well as most forms of bundle branch blocks, are associated with an increase in MI mortality rates.[14] Specific ECG criteria for the conduction abnormalities appear in the accompanying chart. The following discussion will be limited to cause, hemodynamic effects, and usual treatment.

1. *First degree A-V block:* First degree A-V block is not a "block" at all, but rather an abnormal delay of impulses as they are transmitted through the A-V node. It has no hemodynamic consequences, and the patient's heart rate is governed by the underlying sinus mechanism, not the conduction defect. It is considered to be a warning arrhythmia and is generally not treated.

2. *Bundle branch blocks (BBB):* A bundle branch block results in delayed electrical activation of the ventricles due to failure of *at*

least one of the divisions of the intraventricular conduction system to propagate supraventricular impulses. Bundle branch blocks also do not have any hemodynamic consequences as long as all impulses initiated by the sinus node are conducted into the ventricles (even if the route of conduction is abnormal). The bundle branch blocks are considered to be serious complications, however, because of the propensity for sinus rhythm with bundle branch block to deteriorate into second degree or even complete heart block, and because of the increased mortality noted to be associated with these conditions.

The bundle branch blocks are classified according to QRS duration and morphology as (a) Right bundle branch block, (b) Complete left bundle branch block, (c) Left anterior hemiblock, and (d) Left posterior hemiblock. The latter two classifications represent situations in which the pathology is localized to *one half* of the left bundle branch system. The potential seriousness of these conditions is shown in the following mortality statistics reported by Kleiger et al:[14]

Type of BBB	Mortality
RBBB + LAH	75%
LBBB	40%
RBBB + LPH	25%

Right bundle branch block or left anterior hemiblock (the most prevalent intraventricular conduction defect) were not associated with increased mortality when they occurred alone.

The bundle branch blocks are an example of a clinical situation in which treatment is preventative in nature. To reiterate the point, bundle branch blocks, in and of themselves, do not cause alterations in cardiac output. However, because of the possible sequela, it is the policy in many ICUs to place temporary transvenous pacemaker wires in patients who exhibit the more worrisome types (i.e., especially in RBBB with LAH and almost certainly if the patient exhibits any degree of A-V block).

3. *Second degree A-V blocks:* Second degree A-V blocks occur when some, but *not all* of the impulses initiated by the sinus node are conducted into the ventricles. There are three types of second degree A-V block and they vary in terms of cause and hemodynamic effects:

a) *Mobitz I (Wenckebach):* This arrhythmia is a result of malfunction in the A-V node, which conducts sinus impulses with increasing difficulty until one impulse is not conducted at all. At this point the cycle usually resumes again and continues until another sinus impulse is not conducted. This arrhythmia has the potential to decrease the heart rate and thus reduce cardiac output, but each case must be judged on its own merits. The actual heart rate will depend on both the number of impulses initiated by the sinus node and the number of nonconducted impulses (i.e., the faster the basic sinus rate, the greater the net heart rate will be at any given frequency of nonconduction).

In addition, whether the resultant heart rate will actually render the patient symptomatic is difficult to predict. Mobitz I is probably the least serious form of second degree A-V block, and may not be treated unless the patient shows clinical signs of decreased cardiac output, or the frequency of nonconducted impulses appears to be increasing. If treatment is indicated, a pacemaker is the most reliable approach.

b) *Mobitz II:* This arrhythmia is also characterized by periodic or occasional nonconduction of sinus impulses, but in contrast to Mobitz I, the site of pathology is in the intraventricular conduction system. The presence of a persistent intraventricular conduction defect is demonstrated by the prolonged QRS duration of the conducted sinus impulses. The nonconducted sinus impulses represent transient episodes of *bilateral* bundle branch block.

Mobitz II presents the same potential for decreasing cardiac output as does Mobitz I. The net heart rate depends on both the basic sinus rate and the frequency of nonconducted impulses. The effect of the net heart rate on the specific patient's cardiac output is again an individual matter. Because it indicates a severely diseased intraventricular conduction system, however, this arrhythmia is usually taken much more seriously than Mobitz I, and a temporary transvenous pacemaker may be placed, even though the patient is clinically asymptomatic. In this instance, the use of the pacemaker is precautionary—the goal being to have it in and capable of functioning before Mobitz II deteriorates into a more hemodynamically serious arrhythmia.

c) *Advanced second degree A-V block:* Advanced second degree block does not represent pathology which is different from Mobitz I or Mobitz II but is simply the progression of one of these arrhythmias to a point where at least half of the sinus impulses are not conducted into the ventricles. This condition is certain to cause a significant decrease in heart rate and usually in cardiac output as well. Even if the basic sinus rate were at the upper limits of normal (i.e., 100), the maximum heart rate for a patient with advanced second degree block would be only 50 beats per minute. Slower heart rates are not unusual, and on occasion electrical impulses initiated by subsidiary pacemakers in the junctional region or ventricular myocardium are present.

Treatment is aimed at increasing the heart rate and thus the cardiac output. Pacing is the only reliable method of treatment although in some situations a sympathomimetic drug, such as Isoproterenol, may be used to stimulate the junctional region until an artificial pacemaker can be placed. It must be noted that the treatment does not reverse the pathology, but merely prevents the patient's clinical condition from deteriorating.

Second degree A-V blocks which occur as a complication of the infarction process may be transient, particularly if the pathology involves the A-V node. Hence, normal electrical conduction may return following several days of maintenance therapy with an artificial pacemaker. The belief that conduction defects involving the A-V node may be due to inflammation or edema in that area has led to the use of steroids as an adjunctive treatment in some institutions.

4. *Complete Heart Block:* The failure of any impulses initiated by the sinus node (or any other supraventricular focus) to be transmitted into the ventricles is known as third degree or complete heart block. As a direct result of the infarction process, complete heart block represents the final progression of pathology involving the A-V node or the intraventricular conduction system. Hence, an arrhythmia that starts as either Mobitz I or Mobitz II can deteriorate into advanced second degree block and then to complete heart block. The progression can occur quickly, a fact which necessitates observation of the patient's monitor at frequent scheduled intervals once any form of second degree block is noted.

There are other etiologies of conduction abnormalities besides inadequate circulation to various portions of the cardiac conduction system. Although this is not intended to be an in-depth discussion of electrophysiology, it is important to recognize the role that various cardiac drugs may play in causing conduction abnormalities up to, and including, complete heart block. At toxic doses, digitalis preparations, Procainamide and Quinidine all have the potential for depressing the activity of the conduction system. Patients with cardiac arrhythmias or pathologies requiring these medications, even if the conditions are not related to acute myocardial infarction, are also "at risk" for conduction defects.

Complete heart block is a serious arrhythmia that has been demonstrated to be associated with a significantly increased mortality rate.[14] Heart rate in this arrhythmia depends on the ability of one of the heart's subsidiary pacemakers to initiate electrical activity which can be transmitted into the ventricles. If the block is at the level of the A-V node, the potential for a junctional pacemaker to take over (usually at a rate between 40-70 per minute) exists. In this instance, cardiac output may not be severely compromised. If the block is in the intraventricular conduction system, however, the only subsidiary pacemaker capable of stimulating the ventricles is within the ventricles themselves and normally operates at a rate between 20-40 per minute. Not only is this rate likely to be too slow to maintain an adequate cardiac output, but it will also predispose to ventricular irritability which may prove to be lethal. If neither of the subsidiary pacemakers takes over, ventricular standstill results, and the patient will exhibit signs of clinical death. Cardiopulmonary resuscitation should be instituted immediately.

As with the second degree blocks, the aim of treatment for complete heart block is to increase the heart rate to a point at which cardiac output is sufficient for the patient's metabolic needs. The patient is usually maintained with a temporary pacemaker until either the block subsides or it becomes apparent that the problem is persistent enough to warrant the installation of a permanent pacing system. Patients who have shown evidence of bifascicular block in the intraventricular conduction system and develop CHB may be candidates for permanent pacemakers even if the block subsides. Isoproterenol may again be utilized to stimulate the subsidiary pacemakers until a pacemaker catheter can be placed, but increased ventricular irritability is a side effect of this drug, and management of the patient becomes exceedingly complex at this point. Early recognition and treatment of arrhythmias which may predispose to complete heart block are obviously of great importance in the ICU.

In summary, arrhythmic complications of myocardial infarction primarily interfere with the patient's ability to meet his needs for oxygen *if* the specific arrhythmia significantly decreases cardiac output. In two instances, ventricular fibrillation and ventricular standstill, the arrhythmias are death-producing. Assessment of the patient must include continuous knowledge of his heart rate, understanding of the potential for his current heart rhythm to affect heart rate or to lead to a death-producing mechanism, and ability to detect clinical signs of insufficient oxygenation of vital organs.

CARDIAC PACING

The reader is referred to the references at the end of the chapter for detailed information regarding artificial cardiac pacemakers. A general overview of this treatment modality is presented here to acquaint the ICU nurse with some of the basic concepts involved.

Rationale

Cardiac pacing "works" because of one of the special properties of cardiac cells—"excitability." This property refers to the ability of the cell to initiate a wave of electrical activity in response to a stimulus. In the case of pacing, the stimulus is electricity. A wave of depolarization is initiated by the cardiac cells which come in contact with the pacing stimulus.

Purpose

The purpose of cardiac pacing is *control of heart rate*, at least in terms of establishing a minimum rate. Unfortunately, pacing technology has not yet devised a technique for increasing the paced rate as the patient's metabolic needs increase, or for inhibiting the onset of rapid rate arrhythmias. Control of heart rate is useful clinically to achieve one of two general results: (1) maintenance of an adequate cardiac output and (2) suppression of ectopic foci that are resistant to more conventional forms of treatment.

Components of the Pacing System

A pacing system has two principal components, the pulse generator (or "pacemaker") and the pacing catheter or electrode.

The pulse generator is powered by batteries of varying types and life expectancies. Batteries used in temporary systems have life expectancies that are commonly measured in hours. Those used in permanent systems have more variable capabilities ranging from 18 months to 10 years. Some types are now rechargeable. The pulse generator is adjustable in terms of both rate of stimulation and strength of stimulation. The latter is measured in milliampere units (MAs), and must be of sufficient strength to actually result in depolarization of cardiac cells. It should be noted that pacing affects *only* electrical activity—it cannot insure mechanical contraction of the cells.

The pacing catheter, or electrode, delivers the electrical stimulus from the pulse generator to the heart. If the catheter makes contact with the outer surface of the heart, such as would be the case if it were placed during a cardiac or thoracic surgical procedure, the pacing method is *epicardial*. If the catheter makes contact with the inner surface of the heart via the venous system, the pacing method is *endocardial*. The term *transvenous* is frequently used in place of endocardial. Depending on the nature of the specific arrhythmia which required the use of a pacemaker, the catheter may be placed in either the atrium or the ventricle. Although somewhat unphysiologic, ventricular pacing is by far the more common approach and *must* be employed when the underlying problem is a conduction abnormality. In the absence of conduction defects, atrial pacing is possible, and results in synchronization of atrial and ventricular mechanical activity. Atrial pacing is, however, technically difficult and not often undertaken. More complex systems allow for both atrial and ventricular pacing, and are currently reserved for patients who also have a significant element of mechanical, as well as electrical, failure.

Types of Pulse Generators

Two types of pulse generators have been used in the Intensive Care Unit. The oldest and simplest type is known as the "fixed-rate" pacemaker. This unit is designed to deliver a preset number of impulses per minute regardless of what the patient's natural heart rate might be at the time. The advantage of this type of pacemaker is its lack of vulnerability to malfunction. The disadvantage is that impulses from the pacemaker may compete with the heart's natural electrical activity and could arrive in the ventricles during the vulnerable period of the cardiac cycle—i.e., the time during which a stimulus may initiate ventricular fibrillation.

A more flexible type of pulse generator and one which is used more frequently is the "demand" pacemaker. This unit will also send impulses at a preset rate but only if the heart's natural electrical activity does not achieve this minimum rate. The unit contains a mechanism which is designed to sense "QRS" or ventricular depolarization complexes. In the most commonly used models, known as ventricular-inhibited demand pacemakers, a "QRS" complex occurring before the preset pacing interval will shut off the pacing component. As an example, if the pacemaker is set for a rate of 75 per minute, it will fire *only* when there has been no "QRS" complex (either paced or natural) for 0.8 seconds (60 sec. $\div$ 75 = 0.8 sec.). A properly functioning demand pacemaker should eliminate the threat of competition and is therefore the treatment of choice for virtually all arrhythmias.

Complications of Pacing

Complications of cardiac pacing are many and variable. Infection, rejection, and thrombus formation are related to the presence of a foreign body. Loss of ability to "capture" or cause depolarization may be related to displacement of the pacing electrode, breakage of the electrode, or changes in the patient's clinical condition which require higher energy output from the pulse generator. Lack of stimulation from the pulse generator can result from loss of battery power or electronic component failure. Loss of a special function such as "sensing" may also be due to component failure or improper electrode positioning. Stimulation of noncardiac sites can produce hiccoughs, muscle twitching and epileptic seizures.

Perhaps the most serious potential complication is accidental electrocution. This aspect was discussed under safety needs, but to reiterate the main point, patients with temporary pacing catheters of any type in place have a "direct current pathway" to their hearts and are extremely vulnerable to ventricular fibrillation initiated by "microshocks" or electrical currents which are far below the threshold of skin sensation.

Nursing Responsibilities Related To Cardiac Pacing

Nursing responsibilities related to cardiac pacing include assisting the patient to meet his needs for safety, comfort, and psychological security, and monitoring the function of the pacing system.

Safety

Several aspects of physical safety must be considered. First, the patient should be protected from electrical accidents. Interventions include: (1) ensuring proper grounding of all equipment with which the patient comes into contact; (2) ascertaining the presence of a common unit ground or plugging of all electrical equipment into the same or closely adjacent wall outlets; (3) enclosing the pulse generator (in temporary systems) in a semi-opaque surgical glove or other insulating material; (4) covering the tips of noninsulated pacing electrodes (transvenous) with a rubberized material such as short lengths of a tourniquet; (5) wrapping and insulating epicardial pacing catheters that are not connected to a pulse generator; and (6) ensuring that the pacing catheter is manipulated only by someone wearing insulating gloves.

Second, the patient should be protected from infection. The implantation procedure is done under sterile conditions, and it is frequently the policy to cover the catheter portal of entry with an antibacterial cream and a dry sterile dressing. Both the entry site and venous route to the heart require frequent inspection for signs of inflammation. If the patient has a permanent pulse generator, this incisional area would be included as well.

Third, temporary pacing systems should be protected from dislodgement. This is generally achieved by securing the pulse generator in such a way that it cannot be accidentally dropped or knocked from the patient's bed, pulling out the pacing electrode in the process. The pulse generator may be fastened to the patient, his gown, or a piece of close-by *stationary* equipment.

Comfort

Potential sources of discomfort for the patient with a pacemaker are incisional pain (from either the catheter insertion site or the pulse generator site in permanent systems), stiffness if the catheter is inserted by way of an arm vein, and hiccoughs or muscle twitching if the pacemaker stimulates noncardiac sites. Nursing interventions in this instance are directed toward relief of symptoms.

Psychological security

The fact that a pacemaker is necessary, on even a temporary basis, for the maintenance of normal cardiac function can hardly be less than frightening for the patient. The rationale for this treatment and an explanation of the steps of the insertion procedure, as well as the expectations that will be held of the patient during and after the procedure, should be given in the simplest possible terms. The actual insertion event is often a time of great stress for the staff, as well as for the patient. The resultant anxiety may be easily communicated and can impede any real learning on the patient's part; hence, explanations may need to be repeated frequently. The patient who has a permanent pacemaker has even greater learning needs. Patient teaching programs can be facilitated by the use of information booklets provided by pacemaker manufacturers and by the excellent materials available from the American Heart Association.

Monitoring function

Because of the wide variety of pacemaker types, it is essential that the ICU nurse understand exactly what performance is expected of each specific pulse generator used in her unit. Information booklets provided by the pacemaker manufacturers should aid in gaining this understanding, which is of paramount importance in monitoring the function of the system. In the case of a demand pacemaker, there are three specific assessments to be made on a continuing basis. First, does the pacemaker fire appropriately—i.e., does a pacemaker spike or artifact appear on the monitor every time that a natural QRS complex (or P wave if atrial pacing) does not occur in the preset time interval? Does the needle indicator on the face of the pulse generator deflect appropriately to signal that the pacemaker is firing? Second, does the pacemaker sense appropriately—i.e., does it recognize a natural QRS complex and withhold its stimulus accordingly? Lastly, does the pacing stimulus result in depolarization of the ventricles (or atrium in atrial pacing)? Does a QRS (or P wave) immediately follow each pacemaker artifact? This is referred to as "capture" and is essential if the pacemaker is to achieve the desired results.

Additionally, the monitor should be observed for evidence of arrhythmias, such as PVCs, which are related to the presence of a potential source of trauma in the heart (the pacing catheter). The patient should be assessed for data which indicate whether or not the paced rate is adequate to maintain cardiac output.

COMPLICATIONS RELATED TO ALTERATIONS IN THE HEART'S MECHANICAL FUNCTION

Pump Failure

In the broadest sense, there are several complications of myocardial infarction that can be grouped together as those relating to an inability of the heart to function as a pump. The discussion in this section will be confined to situations in which the myocardium is failing but still structurally intact. Subsequently, in the next section, complications related to loss of structural integrity, which also result in pump failure, will be considered. In more specific terms, left ventricular failure, pulmonary edema, and cardiogenic shock are "pump failure" complications and represent a continuum associated with significantly increased mortality.

The etiology of pump failure is the loss of contractile ability in the infarcted cells. The size of the infarcted area is certainly a factor which will weigh heavily on the potential for pump failure to develop, but infarct size cannot always be determined ante mortem, and other related factors have been demonstrated. Many studies have indicated that pump failure is significantly more likely to occur in patients who are over 60 years of age, who have a history of previous infarctions, or who have sustained an anterior infarction.[14,18] These complications are responsible for the great majority of in-hospital deaths related to myocardial infarction.

Left ventricular failure

A patient with mild left ventricular failure may not exhibit overt clinical symptoms; consequently, attention must be directed toward the early detection of subtle findings. Early detection and treatment may prevent progression of this pathology to the stages associated with high mortality.

The early consequences of pump failure are compensatory efforts by the heart to maintain cardiac output (i.e., persistent sinus tachycardia at rest), increased circulation time, and mild pulmonary congestion which may be detectable only on x-ray. The appearance of fine pulmonary rales or an abnormal third heart sound would tend to confirm the diagnosis of ventricular failure. The keys to early detection of this problem are aggressive assessment of those particularly susceptible patients and the development of a high index of suspicion at the first indication of difficulty.

At this point it would perhaps be useful to review the etiology of some additional signs of failure (often called congestive heart failure) because their presence indicates yet another problem. Peripheral edema, venous distention, and increased central venous pressure readings are all indicative of right ventricular failure and/or fluid volume overload. Because the infarction process almost always involves the *left* ventricle, the appearance of the above signs would indicate that primary left ventricular failure has been reflected backward through the pulmonary circulation to the right ventricle. Right ventricular failure may also develop as a consequence of a major pulmonary embolus.

The basic need most likely to be affected by the pump failure complication is, of course, the need for adequate cellular oxygenation. As long as the failure remains at the mild stage, treatment is primarily aimed at fluid and sodium restriction, so as not to overtax the tenuous myocardium, and diuresis. Oxygen may or may not be given. The use of digitalis preparations at this stage is also somewhat controversial due to the resultant increased myocardial oxygen consumption. Both the pathology and the treatment modalities may influence the patient's fluid, electrolyte, and nutritional status, but the main concern of the ICU nurse is to reduce the cardiac workload by keeping physical and emotional stress to a minimum.

Pulmonary edema

Pulmonary edema represents a more severe form of left ventricular failure, with signs and symptoms which primarily reflect effects behind, rather than beyond, the pump. Incomplete ventricular emptying causes increased end-diastolic volume and pressure which is quickly passed back to the left atrium and subsequently to the pulmonary circulation. The blood vessels of the pulmonary vasculature are extremely low resistance vessels, which means that a substantial increase in blood volume is necessary before the pressure in these vessels rises to the point of forcing fluid out into the interstitial spaces or into the alveoli themselves. The onset of pulmonary edema may be gradual in a patient who does not respond to treatment for mild left ventricular failure or may appear quite suddenly, especially if the patient has been inadvertently overloaded with fluids.

Pulmonary edema results in a double assault on the patient's ability to meet his oxygen needs. Not only is the left ventricle failing to pump blood efficiently to the systemic circulation, but oxygen exchange in the lungs is also hampered by the presence of the edema fluid. The patient will be dyspneic, pale, and apprehensive. His breath sounds will be moist, and he may expectorate frothy, sometimes pink-tinged sputum.

Interventions aimed at relieving discomfort and improving oxygenation include assisting the patient to a high Fowler's position with support from pillows or an over-bed table if possible and delivering O_2 in a manner that is the least frightening for the patient (i.e., a tight fitting face mask will probably not be tolerated well), and possibly utilizing positive pressure to force edema fluid out of the alveoli. Sedation is also helpful in relieving apprehension and reducing oxygen demands, and a bronchodilating agent such as Aminophylline may be utilized. In addition, venous return to the heart is decreased either by actual reduction of blood volume (phlebotomy or diuresis) or by sequestration of blood volume in the extremities through the use of rotating tourniquets. Rapid acting forms of digitalis are commonly employed to improve cardiac output.

A great potential exists for disturbances in fluid-electrolyte and acid-base balance due to poor tissue perfusion in the systemic circulation and the combined use of digitalis and diuretic agents. Serum electrolyte levels and arterial blood gases require frequent monitoring. It is clear that attention must also be directed toward promoting the psychological security of the patient and his family.

Cardiogenic shock

All episodes of left ventricular failure are associated with some decrease in cardiac output and may result in systemic hypotension. The point at which the patient becomes symptomatic (i.e., shows evidence of decreased perfusion of vital organs such as the kidneys and the brain) is commonly considered to be "shock," regardless of the actual arterial blood pressure. A patient who has a history of hypertension may become symptomatic at blood pressure levels that would be considered normal in a nonhypertensive individual. Kleiger *et al.* define cardiogenic shock as (1) systolic BP < 90 mm Hg; (2) signs of peripheral vasoconstriction such as cold, pale extremities; (3) urine output < 25 cc./hour; and (4) confused sensorum.[14]

The ICU nurse is in a position to see many examples of shock, such as hypovolemic, neurogenic, and septic shock; it is important to understand that the primary deficit in cardiogenic shock is the failing myocardium. Cardiogenic shock is a syndrome which may occur in association with frank pulmonary edema, although this is not always the case. Mortality associated with this complication of myocardial infarction is variously reported to be from 80 to 100%.

The pathophysiology of cardiogenic shock is complex; however, some of the essential features are as follows:

a) Initially, cardiac output and arterial pressure may be maintained by compensatory mechanisms such as increased heart rate and peripheral vasoconstriction. Significant vasoconstriction hinders indirect blood pressure measurement (i.e., auscultatory method), therefore direct arterial pressure catheters are often employed. This method allows continuous monitoring of systolic, diastolic, and mean arterial pressures which can be used to evaluate the results of treatment.

b) Inadequate perfusion of the coronary arteries serves to compromise an already decreased oxygen supply, leading to arrhythmias and further worsening of mechanical performance.

c) Inadequate perfusion of the kidneys initiates a cycle of sodium and water retention which compounds the overloading of the right ventricle and pulmonary circulation.

d) Inadequate perfusion of body cells initiates increased anaerobic metabolism and production of metabolic acids (particularly lactic).

e) Metabolic acidosis is often profound and will facilitate the development of cardiac arrhythmias and lead to peripheral vasodilation. The acid-base imbalance may be further compounded by respiratory acidosis resulting from inadequate pulmonary exchange of oxygen and carbon dioxide.

f) Inadequate perfusion of the pancreas is thought to result in the release of an enzyme, MDF or myocardial depressant factor, which further stresses the already failing myocardium.

In short, a vicious chain of events which is difficult, if not impossible to break is initiated. From the mortality figures it is clear that treatment is usually not successful. The primary goals are maintenance of a mean arterial pressure which will prevent irreversible damage to vital organs such as the brain and kidneys, improved oxygenation of the myocardium as well as all body tissues, and restoration of a normal acid-base balance. Reduction in pump failure mortality currently appears to be related to the refinement of medical or surgical procedures "which limit the size of the infarction and prevent the death of ischemic but still viable myocardium."[14]

Fluid balance is a particularly complex aspect of treatment since the use of diuretics may render the patient hypovolemic. The use of the Swan-Ganz catheter, which allows for measurement of pulmonary capillary pressure (a reflection of left atrial and thus left ventricular end-diastolic pressure), pulmonary artery pressure, and central venous pressure has greatly improved fluid management and also permits more immediate evaluation of other treatment modalities.

Vasopressor drugs are commonly employed, sometimes in combination with agents which increase myocardial contractility (have a positive inotropic effect) and also cause some vasodilation. This combination is an attempt to maintain arterial pressure and at the same time promote circulation to vital organs suffering from vasoconstriction, particularly the kidney. Dopamine is frequently used in low doses (1-5 mcg/kg./min.) to promote renal vasodilation. Other vasodilating agents, such as nitroglycerine and Nitroprusside, may also be used to reduce afterload and promote cardiac output.

Oxygen therapy is essential, although the exact mode of delivery is somewhat variable. Attention must be directed to maintenance of a clear airway and, when possible, body positioning that facilitates respiration and prevents pooling of secretions.

Constant monitoring of blood pressure, heart rate and rhythm, urinary output, arterial blood gases and pH, serum electrolytes, BUN and other determinations, and complex measurements such as CVP or pulmonary pressures make attention to the patient's comfort and emotional status seem like low priority items. In addition, control of pain may be difficult because of the hypotensive effect of many analgesic medications, yet this consideration is essential not only from the aspect of comfort but also because pain itself may compound hypotension. The probable outcome of this complication demands that the ICU nurse exert the maximum possible control over environmental and interpersonal factors which will promote the security and dignity of the patient and his family.

Loss of Structural Integrity

Three complications of myocardial infarction disrupt the structural integrity of the heart and have serious, if not lethal, consequences. They are (1) rupture of the intraventricular septum, (2) rupture of a papillary muscle, and (3) rupture of the free wall of the ventricle.

Ventricular septal rupture

This complication is most likely to occur in patients who have sustained an anteroseptal or massive anterior infarction. Its occurrence is indicated by the sudden onset of severe left ventricular failure, possibly including shock, and the physical finding of a loud pansystolic cardiac murmur. These same findings are also characteristic of mitral insufficiency resulting from papillary muscle rupture; consequently a definitive diagnosis must often be based on the results of emergency cardiac catheterization. In the case of a ruptured intraventricular septum, oxygen tension and diastolic pressure are increased in the right ventricle due to the shunting of blood across the septum.

Supportive treatment is the same as that discussed under pump failure. Surgical repair of the septal defect is attempted at some institutions as soon as possible, and at others, only if the patient is able to survive the acute period.

Papillary muscle rupture

Patients with both anterior and posterior infarctions may be predisposed to this complication which is a result of necrosis at the insertion site of one or more papillary muscles. The signs and symptoms are generally the same as those discussed above under septal rupture. The significant consequence of papillary muscle rupture is the resultant mitral insufficiency. Part of the left ventricular volume is shunted backwards into the atrium and pump failure again occurs. Death is almost a certainty without surgical repair of the valvular defect.

Ventricular rupture

Mortality associated with ventricular rupture approaches 100%. It occurs most often in females and in patients who remain hypertensive following an infarction. The latter finding associates cardiac strain with this complication.

Cardiac tamponade is the result of ventricular rupture, and a presumptive bedside diagnosis can be made from the combination of electrical mechanical dissociation (electrical activity as noted on the ECG machine or monitor does not correlate with evidence of mechanical contraction such as heart sounds or peripheral pulsation), and failure of external cardiac massage to produce palpable pulsations. The definitive diagnosis must, of course, be made at autopsy. Emergency attempts to repair the rupture surgically are unsuccessful, largely because necrotic tissue is difficult to suture. The further development of synthetic materials, such as those that are used to repair septal defects, may offer some hope to an occasional victim of this complication.

Other Complications

There are two final complications of the infarction process which may occur in the acute phase. They are pericarditis and thromboembolism.

Pericarditis

Inflammation of the pericardial sac is thought to be a response to the presence of necrotic tissue in the heart. The patient will exhibit clinical signs of an inflammatory reaction such as fever and malaise; he usually has chest pain which is substernal in location but pleuritic in nature (worse on inspiration and in a supine position). The major diagnostic clue related to pericarditis is the presence of a pericardial friction rub which is heard while doing auscultation of the chest. Treatment is generally supportive in nature, although in some instances steroids may be employed or, to reduce the possibility of cardiac tamponade, anticoagulation may be discontinued.

Thromboembolism

The major thromboembolic threat associated with myocardial infarction is the development of mural thrombi or clots on the endocardial surface of the injured ventricle. The consequences of embolization of these thrombi are serious and may take the form of a cerebrovascular accident or an arterial embolus of an extremity.

Although the use of anticoagulants following myocardial infarction remains controversial, prevention of mural thrombi in patients who have sustained a transmural infarction is the most clear-cut indication. Anticoagulants have not been demonstrated to improve coronary circulation or prevent the extension of a coronary thrombus if one, in fact, exists. Nursing management should be sufficient to prevent the development of peripheral venous thrombi.

CARDIAC SURGERY

Introduction

The third section of this chapter will discuss the nursing care of the patient who has undergone cardiac surgery. The framework of the nursing process, utilized in the previous section on the care of the myocardial infarction patient, will again be followed. It will be important for the reader to note that many of the considerations involved in meeting the basic needs of the MI patient apply equally to the surgical patient. For example, nursing responsibilities and the rationale underlying the maintenance of proper fluid balance in the patient with left ventricular failure are essentailly the same, regardless of whether the primary cause is large ischemic and hypokinetic areas secondary to infarcts, or hypertrophy secondary to valvular disease. Therefore, while mention will be made of the pathological consequences of disorders amenable to surgical correction, repetition of nursing intervention will be avoided. Instead, the focus will be upon consequences of the disease entity and surgical procedure itself which interfere with meeting the patient's basic needs in ways not discussed earlier, or which necessitate nursing interventions different than those appropriate for the nonsurgical patient.

Cardiac surgery has been perfected to the point where innumerable variations in technique and procedure are available. This chapter will not attempt to cover the field of congenital defects and pediatric cardiac surgery, which is an area where tremendous advancements have been and continue to be made. In the adult patient, the great majority of procedures are for the treatment of valvular disease or coronary ischemic disease. Exceptions are those patients who reach adulthood before undergoing correction of congenital disorders, patients with diseases of the pericardium secondary to another disease process, such as metastatic cancer, and patients with structural abnormalities, such as ventricular aneurysm or cardiac tumors (e.g., atrial myxomas). Only those conditions and procedures related to aortic valve disease, mitral valve disease, and coronary revascularization will be discussed, as representative of the most common problems.

Extracorporeal Bypass

The development that has probably had the greatest impact on cardiac surgery is the use of the extracorporeal circulatory device, or the cardiopulmonary bypass pump. The first successful use of the bypass pump was in 1953;[13] since then several refinements have been made. The essential requirements for safe, effective extracorporeal circulation include: (1) a pumping mechanism; (2) a gas exchange system; (3) temperature control; (4) filtration; and (5) suction. Although the specific pump models vary in the exact way these functions are accomplished, all are able to accomplish these five tasks.

The three most common types of pumps used today are the bubble oxygenator, the membrane oxygenator, and the disc oxygenator. The bubble oxygenator accomplishes gas exchange by bubbling oxygen through a column of blood, and has the disadvantage of producing a great deal of turbulence, which can damage blood cells. The disc oxygenator involves filming blood onto a series of discs, which then rotate through a gas-filled chamber, where exchange of O_2 and CO_2 occurs. This system is somewhat slower than the bubble oxygenator and also produces some trauma to cells. The membrane oxygenator does not expose the blood directly to gas but rather layers the blood across a thin, semipermeable membrane, and exchange occurs by osmosis. This type of pump probably causes the least damage to cells because it involves the least manipulation of blood. Disposable plastic pumps are used in most institutions today.

The technique of bypass is similar for all types of equipment and surgical procedures. Before beginning, the patient must be heparinized to prevent clotting. The blood is removed from the venous system by means of cannulas placed in the superior and inferior venae cava or the femoral vein. Oxygenated blood is returned, after circuit through the pump, via cannulas in the aorta, the femoral, iliac or subclavian arteries. Bypass is usually begun and discontinued gradually.

The pump itself must be primed with fluid before bypass is started in order to avoid removing a large amount of vascular volume from the patient. A variety of priming solutions may be used, including dextrose and water, albumin, and Ringer's lactate; blood is not usually used because of both the expense and the dangers associated with transfusion (approximately 5 units of blood would be needed).

Some surgeons prefer to use hypothermia while operating, particularly with pediatric procedures. This is done by cooling the blood in the pump. Most often, only mild hypothermia is employed (28°-30°C). The advantages of this are to reduce metabolic rate and thus oxygen need and to reduce bleeding.

Filtering of the blood from the pump is necessary for several reasons. First, gas bubbles must be removed before returning the blood to the arterial circulation. Second, blood products (fragmented cells and clots) must be removed. Third, blood and tissue debris, fed into the pump by the "scavenger" or auxiliary suction lines to maintain a bloodless field in the heart and chest must be cleared.

As can be seen, several dangers are inherent in the use of extracorporeal circulatory devices. The cannulation itself, particularly if peripheral vessels are used, may result in damage to the vessel intima and eventual thrombus formation. The use of nonblood priming solutions causes hemodilution, which may be severe enough to produce hypoxia and hypotension. Thrombocytopenia may transiently occur with pumps which traumatize the blood; with cell destruction, fibrinolysin activity also increases, and fibrinogen levels may fall. These two effects both contribute to bleeding, which may be further aggravated by inadequate heparin reversal with Protamine sulfate.

The changes in all blood components, including protein, are thought to cause a variety of postoperative symptoms, collectively termed postperfusion or postpump syndrome. The symptoms vary considerably, and may include fever, splenomegaly, atypical lymphocytes, headache, confusion, blurred vision, tremors, and rash. Most of these resolve spontaneously within a few days, but the fever may persist for several weeks.

SURGICAL PROCEDURES

Aortic Valve Disease

Diseases of the aortic valve may produce stenosis, insufficiency, or both. The most common causes are (1) rheumatic scarring; (2) calcification; and (3) congenital malformation.

Aortic stenosis

Stenosis refers to the narrowing or restriction in valve opening. Regardless of the cause, the result is that the left ventricle must generate a higher than normal pressure during systole in order to eject the stroke volume. As described in the anatomy and physiology section, it is able to do this by stretching and generating a more forceful contraction; however, ventricular hypertrophy is an inevitable consequence.

The three classic symptoms of aortic stenosis are angina pectoris, dizziness or "fainting spells," and clinical congestive heart failure. Angina is probably secondary to an inability to perfuse the hypertrophied myocardium. Syncope reflects the left ventricle's inability to increase cardiac output when necessary, as with exercise, or even to maintain an output sufficient to compensate for changes in posture. With the inevitable failure of the ventricle, pulmonary edema, hypotension and shock may occur.

On x-ray, the left ventricle is obviously enlarged. The second heart sound is abnormal, split or absent. The systolic pressure is usually low, and the pulse pressure decreased. Aortic stenosis is not usually associated with arrhythmias, except in very severe cases. Diagnosis is based on cardiac catheterization.

Aortic insufficiency

Insufficiency, or incompetence, refers to the incomplete closing of the valve, allowing regurgitation, or the retrograde flow of blood. Aortic insufficiency may have many causes, such as endocarditis, which destroys the valve cups, rheumatic disease, severe hypertension, Marfan's syndrome (a connective tissue disease), and aortic aneurysm with upward dissection. Stenosis may also progress to the point where the valve leaflets are unable to close completely.

The consequences of this disorder are related to the regurgitation of blood from the aorta back into the left ventricle during diastole. This additional load results in an increased end-diastolic volume when the ventricle receives its normal load of blood from the atrium. The persistent increase in end-diastolic volume will eventually lead to left ventricular hypertrophy.

Signs and symptoms include those associated with congestive heart failure, in the presence of a bounding pulse. The increased stroke volume, caused by the end-diastolic volume, and flow of blood back into the heart during diastole, result in an increase in pulse pressure (increased systolic, decreased diastolic). The diastolic pressure is often heard down to zero, reflecting the persistent turbulence of the blood. Carotid pulsation is frequently visible, and a diastolic murmur can be heard. As with stenosis, ventricular hypertrophy is evident on x-ray, and cardiac catheterization confirms the cause.

Surgical intervention

Correction of aortic stenosis or insufficiency by repairing the valve (valvuloplasty) is only rarely possible in the adult. Replacement of the valve is the treatment of choice. Prosthetic valves may be of synthetic or artificial material, or of organic material. The Starr-Edwards (Figure 2-7A) consists of a ball in a cage, as does the Smeloff-Cutter. The ball rests in the ring base, occluding blood flow during diastole; during systole the ball is pushed upward, to the top of the cage, allowing blood flow through the ring. The Bjork-Shiley design involves a disc which remains seated in the ring base and flips sideways with systolic flow (Figure 2-7B).

All artificial valves produce some turbulence to blood and damage to cells, requiring postoperative anticoagulation. The biologic prosthetics more closely simulate normal flow characteristics and do not require long-term anticoagulation. Although autografts (the patient's own tissue, such as pericardium) and homografts (from cadaver donors) have been attempted, only heterografts (from another species, usually porcine) have proven to be very successful, and these are gaining more popularity.

A midline sternotomy is the incision used for aortic valve replacement. Extracorporeal bypass is always necessary. The diseased valve is excised and the prosthesis sewn in place; the entire procedure, without complicating factors, requires three to four hours.

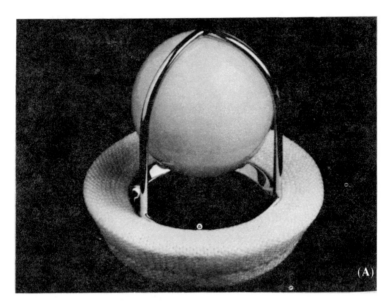

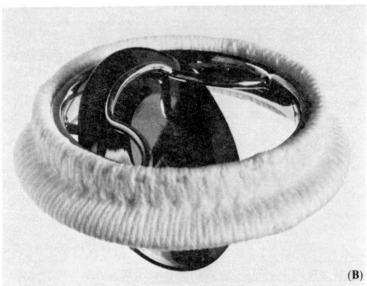

Figure 2-7. (A) Starr-Edwards valve, manufactured by Edwards Laboratories, Division of American Hospital Supply Corporation, California; (B) Bjork-Shiley valve, manufactured by Shiley Laboratories, California.

Mitral Valve Disease

Mitral disease, like aortic disease, is most often the result of rheumatic fever, and is the most common rheumatic disorder.[13] Unlike aortic disease, mitral stenosis and mitral insufficiency affect cardiac dynamics in sharply different ways. Stenosis is much more common in females than males (4:1) than it is in insufficiency (2:1).[20]

Mitral stenosis

The inability of the mitral valve to open normally may be primarily related to fusion of the commissures, thickening and calcification of the cusps, or thickening and shortening of the chordae which normally prevent inversion of the cusps but allow opening. The specific cause of the stenosis is significant in the surgeon's choice of corrective procedure, as will be discussed later.

The consequence of stenosis of the mitral valve is an increase in the systolic pressure in the left atrium, as the myocardium attempts to overcome the increased resistance to flow. Atrial hypertrophy develops, and the higher pressures may be reflected back into the pulmonary circuit, producing pulmonary hypertension, and even right ventricular failure, in severe cases.

The most frequently occurring signs and symptoms include dyspnea, exertional and nocturnal, which is the result of the changes in the pulmonary vasculature, and hemoptysis, caused by increased bronchial vein pressure, again secondary to pulmonary hypertension. Atrial fibrillation, common in the distended left atrium, is often associated with the development of mural thrombi, which then become systemic emboli. Echocardiogram and/or cardiac catheterization are diagnostic.

Mitral insufficiency

Insufficiency may also be caused by rheumatic disease, or may result from papillary muscle dysfunction, such as might result from myocardial infarction. As described on page 101, the papillary muscles and chordae serve to anchor the valve leaflets and prevent inversion when high pressures are generated in the chamber.

As with mitral stenosis, insufficiency produces atrial hypertrophy. The etiologic factor, however, is not an increased systolic pressure, but rather an increase in diastolic volume, as the incompetent valve allows the regurgitation of blood back into the atrium during ventricular systole. This enlargement is more severe than in mitral stenosis, sometimes producing what is termed "giant left atrium." Left ventricular hypertrophy may also ensue as a consequence of increased atrial volume.

The clinical manifestations of insufficiency are similar to those seen in stenosis—angina, hemoptysis, and dyspnea—but are generally less severe. Electrocardiograph reveals atrial fibrillation, but also indicates left ventricular hypertrophy, in contrast to mitral stenosis. Cardiac catheterization and ventricular angiography confirm the diagnosis.

Surgical intervention

Repair, rather than replacement, of a diseased mitral valve, in contrast to aortic valves, is often possible. It is always preferable to preserve the natural valvular apparatus and avoid the problems associated with the use of a prosthesis if it is possible to adequately repair or correct the defect. Although pure mitral regurgitation can sometimes be corrected by repair and suturing of the valve, valvulotomy is more often performed for mitral stenosis. Mitral valve procedures may be performed through a right or left thoracotomy incision, or through a median sternotomy.

Commissurotomy refers to the reopening of a stenotic valve; this may be done as an "open" procedure, utilizing cardiopulmonary bypass, or as a "closed" procedure, without bypass. The closed procedure is performed by making a small incision in the left atrium, and using a finger or dilator to widen the opening of the valve and free the leaflets. The opening in the atrial wall is held closed around the surgeon's finger or the dilator by a purse-string suture while the repair is taking place. While closed commissurotomy has the advantages of being a simpler procedure, less time consuming, and avoids the complications associated with the pump, many believe that adequate repair cannot be achieved if the surgeon cannot visualize the valve and that either the stenosis will persist, or insufficiency will be caused. Consequently, open commissurotomy is preferred by many, particularly when the extent of the disease is uncertain.

The same considerations relevant to the choice of aortic prosthesis apply to decisions regarding mitral prostheses. The most commonly used mechanical devices include the Kay-Shiley, Starr-Edwards, Cutter, and Beall valves. Use of porcine grafts for mitral valve replacement is becoming more common, although the long-range success of these valves has yet to be demonstrated.

Morbidity and mortality, as with aortic valve replacements, seem to be primarily related to two variables—the effectiveness of the prosthetic valve, and the degree to which advanced, intractable disease is present. Effectiveness of the valve refers to the frequency of associated complications, such as embolization, dislodgement, and hemolysis. As valve disease progresses, irreversible damage to the myocardium also progresses. Surgery is generally indicated when the symptoms of the disease cause limitations in the life style or indicate the possibility of sudden death, as is the case with the angina and syncope of aortic stenosis.[3] Past this point, the effectiveness of valve replacement in reversing or preventing further cardiac decompensation and the ability of the heart to withstand surgery decrease, and mortality increases.

Coronary Artery Revascularization

Coronary artery disease is, as was described earlier, one of the most frequent sequelae to atherosclerosis and a leading cause of death in this country. The first attempts to revascularize the myocardium were made as early as 1935; in a procedure developed by Dr. Claude Beck, the pericardium and epicardium were abraded and muscle or other tissue was grafted to the myocardium in an effort to increase the blood supply to the myocardial cells.[5] The use of vein and artery grafts, sutured to the aorta and implanted in the coronary sinus (Beck II), or in a tunnel created in the myocardium (Vineberg), was the next development in revascularization procedures. Several variations were made in the technique used, but it was not until selective coronary arteriography was developed that direct bypass procedures were possible. By determining the exact percent of obstruction and location of the lesion, it became possible for the surgeon to use vein grafts anastomosed at the aorta to "jump" or bypass the diseased segment by implanting the vein distal to the atherosclerotic plaque (Figure 2-8). Various methods of endarterectomy are also used in conjunction with the bypass operation.

There still exists some controversy concerning patient selection for this procedure. As with valve replacement, the basic principle is to operate when the mortality associated with only medical treatment of the disease exceeds the mortality associated with surgical

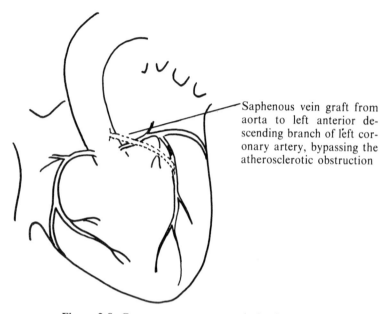

Saphenous vein graft from aorta to left anterior descending branch of left coronary artery, bypassing the atherosclerotic obstruction

Figure 2-8. Coronary artery revascularization.

intervention, and when there is good likelihood that the graft will remain patent. The factors which affect mortality and patency rates, however, are numerous. Among the more obvious of these are age and general state of health; the older individual who has major noncardiac disease, such as COPD, is a poor surgical candidate. The overall mortality for coronary artery disease without revascularization is 5%;[8] surgical mortality in the patient with chronic pulmonary disease or advanced liver disease is much higher.

Other considerations relate to technical factors. As outlined by Diethrich, the likelihood of vein graft patency decreases under the following conditions: diseased aorta, arterial anastomoses of less than 1.5 mm., long vein grafts, diseased vein segment, severe atherosclerosis and diabetes.[6] He reports a patency rate of 83% although the rate varies considerably from institution to institution, depending on the criteria used to select patients.

Another approach is choosing patients for surgery according to the disease process itself. Patients with intractable angina are prime candidates, as medical therapy has already been proven unsuccessful. More recently, even patients who have very unstable angina have been shown to tolerate the bypass procedure with greater relief of symptoms and lower rate of infarction and death than when treated only medically.[4] Patients who have documented coronary artery disease, but are asymptomatic, are perhaps the most controversial group; the trend is more and more towards early elective operation if the patient is otherwise healthy, in order to prevent myocardial ischemia. The last consideration involves an assessment of left ventricular function. The patient who already has a severely damaged ventricular myocardium will not tolerate surgery well, and will experience little benefit from revascularization.

GENERAL NURSING CARE
OF THE CARDIAC SURGERY PATIENT

The overall objectives of the nurse caring for the patient who has undergone cardiac surgery are quite similar to those applicable to the care of the myocardial infarction patient. They are: (1) promotion of healing of the areas subjected to surgical intervention; (2) prevention of complications resulting from either the surgical procedure itself or the related disease entity; and (3) prompt detection of complication and initiation of measures to reverse those that do occur. As with the previous section on nursing care of the M.I. patient, a basic needs framework will be utilized; the reader is encouraged to review that section before proceeding further.

Oxygen Needs

All surgical patients have some interference in their ability to meet oxygen needs. This interference may be caused by any or all of the following factors: use of cardiopulmonary bypass, the administration of general anesthesia, the presence of the thoracotomy incision, pain, and subsequent use of analgesics, and blood loss.

Use of extracorporeal circulatory devices has been associated with a postoperative syndrome referred to as "pump lung."[21] Pathological changes noted include a decrease in lung distensibility, impaired oxygen diffusion, interstitial edema and inflammation. Although the exact etiologic mechanism is not known, this syndrome is thought to be related either to the loss of surfactant or the deposition of microemboli in the pulmonary capillary system, both secondary to cardiopulmonary bypass.

The effects of general anesthesia on pulmonary function are well known. These are further aggravated by the necessity, for most procedures, to collapse the lungs.

Postoperative activity orders vary a great deal, but some period of bedrest is, of course, required. Often, because of either an initial period of hemodynamic instability or a focus on complicated, intricate monitoring devices, the patient is also permitted to remain supine, rather than having his position changed.

As with all thoracic procedures, the presence of the incision itself restricts breathing to some extent, partially because of pain and partially because of fear on the part of the patient of tearing the incision or generating more pain. Thoracotomy incisions are generally less painful than abdominal incisions and are not associated with as great a change in $AaDO_2$ (see Chapter 3), but even the patient with a median sternotomy, which causes less pain than lateral incisions, requires analgesic. Morphine sulphate is the usual drug of choice, and this, in turn, can produce respiratory depression.

The last factor that may interfere with the meeting of oxygen needs is blood loss. As mentioned, use of cardiopulmonary bypass results in a certain degree of hemodilution. Whole blood transfusions are usually given intraoperatively to restore hemoglobin levels, but some further blood loss is inevitable. A mediastinal chest tube is inserted in surgery and left in place for 24-48 hours in order to facilitate drainage and provide a means by which to estimate blood loss. Excessive volume loss, in addition to the reduction in hemoglobin, may lead to a reduction in cardiac output and subsequent interference in oxygen delivery to the tissues. Another factor which may contribute to bleeding is the use of large amounts of stored blood, to which acid-citrate dextrose (ACD) has been added. ACD inactivates calcium, which is an essential component of the clotting process. A third potential cause of postoperative bleeding is, of course, small vessels that were not ligated during surgery.

Left ventricular failure and cardiac arrhythmias may also occur. The ways in which they interfere with oxygen delivery are the same as with the MI patient.

Assessment

Methods of assessment of pulmonary status and postoperative ventilation are not unique to cardiac surgery patients. Rate and quality of respirations, quality of breath sounds, presence, quantity and nature of secretions are all observations that must be made at least hourly during the first 24 hours. Arterial blood gases should be drawn in the immediate postanesthetic period and then every twelve hours during the first 24-48 hours.

In addition to the usual circulatory parameters, blood loss must be carefully monitored. Drainage from the chest tube should be measured hourly until the tube is removed. In many ICUs, it is standard procedure to calculate the blood balance; that is, blood administered is recorded, blood lost is recorded, and the difference between the two calculated as 'x' number of ccs. positive or negative balance.

Analysis of data

The analysis of data obtained must have, as an essential component, the integration of all observations and evaluation as to relative significance and true causative factor. For example, if the patient's nailbeds are cyanotic, but his arterial oxygen saturation level is adequate (90% or greater), the causative factor is probably circulatory rather than primarily respiratory in nature. The patient may be experiencing a decreased cardiac output and/or peripheral vasoconstriction which is producing the peripheral cyanosis. On the other hand, if the patient is restless and disoriented, but blood pressure, heart rate and rhythm, and all other neurological signs are normal, a respiratory cause should be sought. The most important part of the nursing diagnosis is the careful evaluation of all elements in order to construct a diagnosis which will appropriately direct intervention.

Goals, interventions, evaluation

Although there may be many goals, depending on the analysis of the cause of interference with this need, two of the primary goals that should direct intervention with every cardiac surgery patient are:

1. The patient does not suffer interference with meeting oxygen needs due to postoperative respiratory insufficiency of any

nature (e.g., respiratory infection, atelectasis, or inadequate pulmonary function).

2. The patient does not experience inadequate oxygen delivery due to diminished blood volume.

The first intervention measure designed to assure reaching the first goal is thorough preoperative teaching. This may be the responsibility of the general division nurses, the respiratory or physical therapist, or the ICU nurse, depending on institutional practice. Having the ICU nurse visit the patient preoperatively has many advantages, which will be discussed later; because the ICU nurse is the practitioner primarily responsible for assuring adequate respiratory function postoperatively, it seems most practical for her to be involved in preoperative preparation. This preparation includes explanation of coughing and deep breathing exercises, demonstration and practice by the patient.

Coughing and deep breathing should begin as soon as the patient is out of surgery and should be performed at least every hour for the first eight hours, then every two hours, then every four, with the progression depending on the patient's progress. Supplemental oxygen is usually administered for the first few days, and it may be necessary to gradually wean the patient from this. In some Critical Care Units, patients are kept intubated on the respirator until the first postoperative morning, in order to reduce the likelihood of inadequate oxygenation and to reduce the work of breathing; however, this has the disadvantage of discomfort for the patient, increasing risk of infection, and further delay in the resumption of normal respiratory function. Although devices such as blow bottles may be ordered, there is no substitute for frequent coughing and deep breathing.

A second essential intervention is the appropriate administration of pain medication. The patient will not be able to generate an effective cough if he is in severe pain or afraid of aggravating pain. It is not sufficient for the nurse to wait for the patient to request pain medication; assessment of the need for analgesia is part of the nurse's role, not the patient's. Administration of too much narcotic can also further interfere with adequate respiration, and part of the nurse's assessment of the patient's pain should be the judgment of how much analgesia is required. She should have the option of reducing the dosage if she has observed that the ordered dose produces respiratory depression.

The third essential component of respiratory intervention is that of mobilizing the patient. While on bedrest, the patient should be turned at least every two hours. Even severe hypotension does not contraindicate turning the patient side-to-side slightly. Most patients will also breathe more easily in the initial postoperative period if the head of the bed is kept slightly elevated 10°-20°.

Adequate blood volume and hemoglobin levels are assured by careful monitoring of blood loss and appropriate blood replacement. Chest tube patency and proper functioning of the suction apparatus are both the responsibility of the nurse. A common practice is to replace the patient's blood loss cc. for cc.; that is, if 200 cc. are lost, 200 cc. of whole blood are given. The advantage of such a practice is that it makes it possible for the nurse to maintain the patient's intravascular volume without over-transfusing the patient or letting the patient become hypovolemic. The nurse is usually able to use her judgment as to when to begin blood replacement. Because it is somewhat difficult to exactly assess the patient's blood volume postpump during the initial eight postoperative hours, monitoring of the patient's CVP, blood pressure, pulse, and urine output will provide the most reliable indicators of the need for transfusion. Losses that might be expected postoperatively are: up to 200 cc. in the first two hours, 50 cc. per hour in the next four, and 10-30 cc. thereafter, with blood loss stopping after 12-24 hours.

Nutritional Needs (Food, Fluid, and Electrolytes)

Because of the patient's inability to meet any of his own nutritional needs in the immediate postoperative period, this area is clearly within the province of the Intensive Care staff.

Fluid and electrolyte balance, as with blood balance, are subject to major abnormalities secondary to the use of the pump. In addition, the cardiac surgery patient is also subject to the same effects of anesthesia and stress to which any surgical patient is subject. This includes an initial sodium and water retention in response to inappropriate ADH secretion. Cardiac patients are also frequently diuresed preoperatively, which may result in dehydration and potassium deficits. On the other hand, hemolysis of RBCs will release large amounts of potassium into the serum, as will the use of large amounts of bank blood, which contains many hemolyzed cells.

The patient may be started on oral intake as soon as he is awake. Most often these patients are quite thirsty, reflecting their "dry" state. A problem that is sometimes encountered in trying to advance the patient's diet is postoperative ileus and gastic distention. This does not occur frequently enough to warrant routine use of nasogastric tubes, but it is a possibility.

Assessment

The most common postoperative situation in respect to the need for adequate nutrition and fluid and electrolyte balance is one in which the patient is oliguric for the first 8-12 hours, with hypokalemia and mild hypernatremia. This should be assessed through the routine practice of obtaining serum electrolytes immediately after surgery and each subsequent morning, and by hourly measurements of urine output, with specific gravity every two to four hours. Daily weights should also be a standard practice with cardiac patients.

Analysis of data

As with each need, however, the simple observation of the existence of the problem is not sufficient; the nursing diagnosis must propose a causative factor. Intervention with the patient who is oliguric because of low cardiac output secondary to a failing left ventricle will be quite different than intervention when oliguria is caused by a decreased cardiac output secondary to dehydration. Use of the pulmonary wedge pressure in determining the ventricle's need for or ability to tolerate an increased vascular volume is invaluable. If the pulmonary artery catheter has not been placed, the nurse must rely upon more traditional assessment tools: CVP, blood pressure, urine specific gravity.

Goals, interventions, evaluation

The myocardium that has been subjected to a surgical procedure cannot tolerate the stress of an overloaded vascular system. Consequently, the goal is to maintain a fluid balance that is sufficient for metabolic processes and organ perfusion, but does not cause decompensation in cardiac status. The daily weight is the single most reliable tool in evaluating this; some weight gain is to be expected as the patient becomes rehydrated, but this should not exceed 0.5 kg./day.

In addition to preventing fluid overload, the urine output must be maintained in order to prevent accumulation and deposition of cell and tissue break-down products, related to use of the bypass device, in the renal tubules. Output is usually maintained by the administration of diuretics, most commonly Lasix. The physician must be notified if the output remains below 20 cc./hour for two consecutive hours.

Potassium supplements are administered intravenously until the patient can tolerate an oral intake. For severely hypokalemic patients, 40 mEq. of KCl can be diluted in 100 cc. of D_5W and administered over four hours. The usual potassium requirement is 65-125 mEq. of potassium per day, and it is not usually necessary to supplement with more than 40 mEq. The nurse, in this case, has the responsibility of safeguarding the infusion to prevent too rapid administration, which could produce arrhythmias.

Oral intake is progressed as the patient tolerates, usually beginning with ice chips or sips of water as soon as the patient is awake. Bowel sounds should be assessed every four hours to insure that an ileus has not developed. Some postoperative nausea and vomiting, requiring a return to NPO status, is not uncommon. The intravenous intake should be titrated with the oral intake; that is, as the patient begins to take fluids by mouth, his IV rate should be immediately decreased. If the patient can tolerate an oral intake, it is preferable that he receive fluids, electrolytes, and vitamins through this route, both for his own comfort and to avoid causing sudden imbalances.

Elimination

There is not usually any major interference with the meeting of elimination needs related to cardiac surgical procedures. There may, however, be some minor disturbances or alterations in normal patterns of elimination secondary to the postoperative regimen of NPO status, bed rest, and use of bladder catheters.

Assessment

The most valuable source of data in respect to this area is a thorough preoperative assessment of the normal bladder and bowel patterns of the individual. It will be especially helpful to know if the patient has had problems in the past following previous surgeries. Depending upon the length of stay in ICU and the practice in regard to leaving catheters in place, the definitive identification of problems may not be possible until the patient has returned to the general division.

Analysis of data

As the use of indwelling bladder catheters declines with more knowledge about how these catheters lead to urinary tract infections, difficulty voiding becomes a more common problem in postoperative care. The problem assumes importance in that the nurse cannot assess renal function without knowledge of urinary output, and the dilemma is the question: Is the patient not voiding because he is truly oliguric, or is there adequate urine production but interference in micturition?

Goals, interventions, evaluation

Prostate enlargement and difficulty voiding is a common problem with the older male patient, and both male and female patients often have difficulty with voiding in bed. The nurse should not hesitate to get the patient out of bed to void, providing hemodynamic parameters are stable. If the patient has not voided within the first eight postoperative hours, a catheter must be inserted in order to rule out or determine oliguria.

Comfort, Rest, and Sleep Needs

The cardiac surgery patient is virtually guaranteed of interference in meeting these needs. There are three major causative factors: incisional pain, frequent medical and nursing intervention, and environmental factors.

Assessment

In assessing the degree of disturbance, it is essential that the nurse not lose sight of the fact that these disturbances, while very predictable, still present difficulties to the patient in terms of meeting his physiological and psychological needs. It is not difficult for the clinician to become so accustomed to the presence of postoperative pain in the cardiac patient that she no longer perceives this as a problem, but rather as simply requiring a routine kind of intervention. This kind of framework will prevent her from making a comprehensive assessment of the many factors which should be examined.

The extent of interference with comfort, rest, and sleep should be gauged by a comparison with the individual's "normal state," an assessment of how he is coping with the disturbance, and observation of precipitating and relieving factors. Although some incisional pain is inevitable, it is helpful for the nurse to note when it is at its worst, to what extent it is interfering with coughing, deep breathing, and other activity, and to what extent it is preventing rest and sleep. It is also reasonable to ask to what extent is anxiety a contributing factor in the patient's perception of pain.

In assessing sleep needs, the nurse should keep in mind that although the patient appears to be sleeping for one- to two-hour periods throughout the entire day, he is probably not achieving normal REM sleep. Consequently, although his total sleep may add up to 12 hours, he can be expected to have relative sleep deprivation.

Analysis of data

In synthesizing observations, the nurse should first attempt to construct a nursing diagnosis which will specify the most significant causes of the interference. For example, the diagnosis might be: interference with comfort needs due to severe incisional pain, not relieved by moderate doses of analgesia. This diagnosis would direct her intervention towards the administration of higher doses of medication. On the other hand, a diagnosis of severe incisional pain related to a high anxiety level, manifested by muscle tension and a state of hyper-alertness, will direct intervention perhaps towards the use of a tranquilizer-muscle relaxant such as diazepam.

The second aspect of the analysis should be an examination of how each separate need—comfort, rest, and sleep—is exaggerating or influencing the other needs. It is to be expected, for example, that the patient who is suffering severe pain will not be able to meet his sleep needs; the appropriate intervention, however, should be focused on relieving pain, not on using sedatives to insure sleep. Likewise, the patient who is sleep deprived will often perceive more pain.

Goals, interventions, evaluation

Because some interference in meeting these needs is inevitable, the related goals are directed towards limiting the extent of interference or the consequences of the interference. Some usual goals would include:

1. The patient does not experience interference in other need areas

because of limitations imposed by severe pain (e.g., he is not unable to participate in necessary coughing and deep breathing exercises because of pain; he is not unable to eat because of pain, etc.).

2. The patient suffers no untoward psychological complications because of lack of rest and/or sleep. (This complication will be discussed more fully later in the chapter.)

Interventions, of course, depend upon the identification of the cause of the interference. Morphine sulfate is the drug of choice for incisional pain and should be given fairly frequently during the first 48-72 hours. The patient is then often switched to an oral analgesic such as acetaminophen or codeine.

If the care activities of the ICU staff are determined to be a significant factor in preventing rest or sleep, much can be done to reschedule care and prevent unnecessary interruptions. All too frequently the prevailing belief is that the patient is in the ICU for physical care and it is just not possible, nor appropriate, to allow him 3-4 hours of uninterrupted rest. There are very real constraints imposed by physiological needs that dictate frequent vital signs, turning, ambulating, etc., but there is no reason that these activities cannot be grouped so as to prevent days of constant, every half-hour, interruptions of rest. It is also well within the nurse's province to prevent other medical and paramedical personnel from nonessential interventions during a designated rest period; for example, if patient has just gone to sleep, and his condition is stable, chest x-rays, blood drawing, and ECG can probably all be rescheduled for later.

The environment of the Intensive Care Unit has been found to be generally detrimental in that it is often noisy, disturbing, and presents to the patient many abnormal stimuli. If the patient seems to be reacting adversely to these influences, transfer out of the ICU as soon as possible should be given priority. In the meantime, an effort should be made to minimize those factors which are most disturbing, such as noise, lights, etc.

Activity Needs

As with rest needs, the activity needs of the cardiac surgery patient are not usually different than any other surgery patient.

Unless the patient has suffered an infarct during surgery, or already has left ventricular failure, he should have the same activity and rest needs and tolerance for activity as any other patient. The surgical intervention itself, however, imposes some restrictions.

Assessment

Parameters for assessment are the same as those with the MI patient. The presence of a sternal incision adds a significant limitation to initial ambulation, but should not interfere with ability to carry out range of motion exercises in bed. Interestingly, many patients say that the groin incision, made for the insertion of the bypass pump or for obtaining a segment of the saphenous vein for grafting, presents as much of a restriction to activity as does the chest incision. Lateral thoracotomy may be expected to restrict arm motion more than midline sternotomy incisions, and the nurse should assess to what extent the patient is avoiding the use of, or having difficulty using, that arm.

The use of the bypass pump and presence of heart disease should also alert the nurse to the increased potential for activity limitation due to myocardial ischemia. Although the patient should be able to quickly achieve the preoperative level of activity, the development of chest pain of a different quality than incisional pain dictates a return to bedrest and an immediate ECG, particularly in the coronary revascularization patient.

Analysis of data

The reader is encouraged to review the section of data analysis relative to activity needs in the MI patient, if this has not yet been done, as the same four questions are applicable to the surgery patient as are the guidelines for judging activity tolerance.

Of special importance in the surgery patient is the risk of thrombus formation and embolization from the operative leg. Leg exercises can cause some degree of discomfort in the surgery patient, unlike the MI patient, and the nurse must sometimes be especially diligent in assisting the patient to do these. The medical patient is also more likely to quickly resume normal activities after hospital discharge, assuming no psychic overlay, than is the surgical patient, who will still be experiencing some physical discomfort. Consequently, early intervention and teaching of the need for gradual but consistently increasing activity is necessary.

Goals, interventions, evaluation

Most patients should be assisted to sit on the side of the bed within the first 12-24 hours after surgery. If this is tolerated, the patient can then sit in a chair at the bedside for 10-15 minutes on the first postoperative day, and again, for a longer period later in the day, and should be assisted to ambulate in the hall by the fourth day.

As with all needs of the cardiac patient, if the specific intervention does not seem effective, it is helpful for the nurse to re-evaluate the extent to which anxiety is a contributing factor. It is not uncommon for the patient to be fearful of moving too much or too fast, or be so concerned with the sound of the cardiac monitor or presence of intravenous and drainage tubing that he is unable to move about freely.

Sexual Needs

Interference with the meeting of sexual needs is not ordinarily a concern in the immediate postoperative period. However, as the patient begins to perceive himself as progressing and moving away from the critical, life-threatening period, he often will have questions regarding the resumption of normal sexual activity. Usually this point is not reached until after the patient has been transferred out of the ICU, but some patients can benefit from the opportunity to discuss their concerns early in the postoperative period.

Assessment, analysis, goal identification, and intervention are essentially those previously mentioned. Probably of utmost importance, and thus well worth mentioning again, is the nurse's own attitude toward the individual's sexual needs, sexual behavior, and her own role in intervention in this area. Overt sexual behavior on the part of the patient is sometimes observed, and in order to intervene therapeutically, the nurse must be comfortable with or at least aware of her own feelings and any difficulty she might have in dealing with this area.

Psychological Needs
(Security, Love and Belonging, and Self-Esteem)

The earlier discussion of the individual's response to loss, and threat to body image is equally applicable to the surgical patient. This patient is often under a double threat, in a sense, in that he may have already suffered a myocardial infarction or period of critical illness and been hospitalized in an acute care area, with all of the attendant difficulties in adjusting to the sick role and threat to life. The surgical experience then presents another insult to the patient's emotional stability.

Fears commonly associated with cardiac surgery include death, loss of function, disfigurement, financial worries, pain or intolerable sensations, and loss of role relationships. A great deal of research has been done in an attempt to determine how best to assist the patient in dealing with these fears and eliminate complications such as severe anxiety and delirium.

The preoperative visit is the most valuable single method by which to both assess the patient's status and initiate intervention. It was well established by Janis that the degree of anxiety manifested preoperatively is a reliable indicator of the amount of stress experienced in the postoperative period.[12] Patients who exhibit a moderate anxiety level generally have less difficulty following surgery than do patients who exhibit a very low level or a very high level. The individual who is very actively and strongly denying any concerns about the forthcoming surgery is not able to receive the support and assistance he requires and remains unprepared for the experience. The individual who manifests extreme anxiety probably has unrealistic fears, often grounded in past unresolved conflicts or fantasies, and thus cannot gain reassurance from reality oriented information. Both of these individuals, then, are at high risk for serious interference with the meeting of psychological needs.

For patients who are able to express moderate anxiety, a factual, information-giving, and supportive approach seems most effective. Patients benefit from a brief, but realistic description of the *sensations* they can expect; for example, the existence or working of the monitor is irrelevant in and of itself, but the patient should be told to expect to hear the beeping noise, to feel the adhesive gel pads on his chest, not to be surprised by the sounds of the various alarms in the unit, etc. The significant part of having an intravenous line or chest tube is what it feels like to the patient. Less than factual information prevents the patient from anticipatory preparation and will result in feelings of anger and resentment. Even unpleasant sensations, such as the pulling of the chest tube or the need to ambulate, should be briefly explained, with reassurances about the availability of analgesia.

The preoperative visit also provides an opportunity for the ICU nurse to assess the emotional status of the patient's family and the quality of the interaction between the patient and spouse, children, parents, or siblings. Often the patient receives ample opportunity to discuss his feelings and ask questions of nurses, physicians, social worker, etc., but the family remains ignored. It is usually helpful for significant others to remain in the room, while the ICU nurse is explaining the postoperative routine to the patient, but then for the nurse to also talk with the patient and family separately.

Figure 2-9 is an example of a method of recording the preoperative visit, topics discussed, and pertinent observations. It can be easily filled out in duplicate so that the staff of the general division can have access to the information and the staff in the Intensive Care Unit can also review it.

The preoperative visit, although sometimes time consuming if many patients have to be seen, is well worth the effort. Even if the patient is already well prepared in terms of information, it reinforces to him and his family the concern of the staff with all aspects of his illness and recovery. It also eliminates some of the strangeness and unfamiliarity of the environment of the ICU if the patient is able to recognize a familiar nurse. Some institutions have solved the problem of many patients to visit each day by doing group teaching; this is a less individualized approach, but does make it possible for each patient to at least receive some preparatory teaching and explanation.

COMPLICATIONS

This section will provide a brief review of those complications which are potential occurrences in the postoperative period following cardiac surgery. Again, complications which were discussed under the earlier section on the myocardial infarction patient will not be repeated, except insofar as there are specific factors which relate to the surgical intervention itself.

Complications Related to Alterations in the Heart's Electrical Activity

The surgical patient is prone to postoperative arrhythmias for several reasons. First, the manipulation involved in repair of valves

PREOPERATIVE TEACHING NOTE

NAME_____

ADDRESS _____

SURGERY AND DATE _____

BRIEF MEDICAL HISTORY (Include previous hospitalizations
and current medications)

How long have you had heart trouble?
When did you decide to have heart surgery?
What made you decide to have the surgery?

SOCIAL HISTORY
Occupation: What kind of work do you/your husband do?
If retired: How long have you been retired/unable to work?

Marital Status: Children: Religion:

QUESTIONS ASKED (Note if none asked or if asked by others
present, e.g., wife)

TEACHING (Check topics covered)

___ 1. Physical set up of ICU
___ 2. Monitor
___ 3. IV's
___ 4. Oxygen
___ 5. Catheter
___ 6. Chest tube
___ 7. Vital sign routine
___ 8. Activity (turning, OOB)

___ 9. Pulmonary care (explain that
       P.T. will visit; demonstrate
       coughing and deep breathing
       and have patient practice)
___ 10. Pain medication
___ 11. Diet
___ 12. Length of stay in ICU

GENERAL COMMENTS

General appearance (e.g., overweight, healthy);

Physical assessment — Color: Breath sounds:
                       Pulses: Apical:
                       Vital signs:

Behavior during interview: (e.g., lying quietly, pacing, smoking, sitting up)

Attitude: (e.g., disinterested attentive, seemed to want to end visit, very
talkative about history, disn't want to discuss surgery — *Include
patient's comments*)

Figure 2-9. *Preoperative visit record.*

or placement of bypass grafts produces a certain amount of inflammation and subsequent edema. The more extensive the work on the myocardium itself, the greater will be the resultant increase in irritability, leading to ectopic activity. This is evidenced by the very frequent occurrence of arrhythmias, both atrial and ventricular, in the first few postoperative hours.

Suture placement through or near pacing tissue or major conduction pathways may also lead to the various kinds of blocks. The block may be temporary, if it is the result of edema, or may be permanent if it is the result of actual disruption of pathways by sutures. Generally a temporary pacemaker will be used until the inflammatory process has had time to subside and the permanence of the conduction defect can be assessed.

A third and often significant factor leading to arrhythmias is hypoxia. Postoperative respiratory depression, atelectasis, and/or pneumonia may all result in a decreased pO_2, which again makes the myocardium more irritable and susceptible to the activity from ectopic foci.

Because all of these factors are of a potentially temporary basis, frequent titration of anti-arrhythmic dosage is necessary. The physician must rely upon the observations of the nurse of the monitor pattern and trend in arrhythmias in order to appropriately determine medication dosage. This includes not only the ECG pattern itself, but the relationship of ectopic activity to time of pronestyl administration, for example, or to ambulation, or to pulmonary treatments.

In general, the longer the time since surgery, the less likely it is that arrhythmias will occur. Although patients do sometimes develop new ectopic foci on the second or third day, it is unusual for this to happen if there have been no previous arrhythmias.

Complications Related to Alteration in the Heart's Mechanical Function

Decreases in cardiac output, pulmonary congestion, and frank cardiogenic shock may all occur in the surgical as well as the medical patient. The most significant factor is not the surgical procedure itself, but the extent of underlying disease. The patient with advanced valvular disease that has resulted in severe ventricular hypertrophy, and the patient who has already had ventricular damage secondary to infarct, comprise the group at greatest risk.

Excessive bleeding may temporarily lead to a reduction in cardiac output. Bleeding that is excessive in amount, or prolonged past the first 24 hours, indicates either a vessel that is not properly ligated or a coagulopathy. Usually the latter is ruled out first by laboratory data such as prothrombin time, clotting time, fibrinogen levels, etc., in order to avoid returning the patient to surgery unnecessarily. Unless the bleeding is profuse and hemodynamic collapse is a real danger, the patient will not be taken back to surgery for 24-48 hours, even if a clotting disorder has been ruled out, because small bleeders will sometimes clot off by themselves and obviate the need for re-operation.

Tamponade is a life-threatening condition that is possible following any cardiac procedure. It occurs when blood or fluid accumulates under the pericardium, thus compressing the heart and restricting filling and effective contraction. Signs and symptoms include restlessness and diaphoresis, hypotension, narrowed pulse pressure, rising CVP, neck vein distention, paradoxical pulse (peripheral pulses disappear on inspiration, and systolic pressure is heard 10-15 mm lower during inspiration than expiration), widened mediastinum, and distant heart sounds. This complication requires immediate recognition and should be the first possibility investigated when hypotension occurs. Initial treatment might be a pericardiocentesis in order to relieve the restriction to pumping, but often the patient is taken back to surgery without delay so that the pericardium can be drained and the site of bleeding repaired at the same time.

Complications Related to the Procedure

There are several complications which may result from the surgical technique or procedure and which, while not affecting the heart itself, are of a serious nature. Air embolization is always a threat in open heart procedures. The air may originate from the the pump, as mentioned earlier, or may be trapped in the heart after closure. The usual method to eliminate any air bubbles involves placement of ventricular or aortic vents—needles placed in the uppermost portion provide an escape route for the air bubbles, which will rise to the surface. The patient is also put in the head-down position in order to facilitate the venting. Unfortunately, despite these maneuvers, a very small percentage of patients do suffer varying degrees of cerebral damage due to air embolization, and this is part of the reason why the neurological assessment of the patient awakening from anesthesia is so significant.

Embolization of blood clots or tissue debris is also a possibility and occurs most commonly in patients who have undergone repair or replacement of the mitral valve. It is also more common when the femoral vein has been cannulated by bypass.

Wound dehiscence is another possible complication and occurs more often with a median sternotomy incision than a lateral thoracotomy. Unlike abdominal incisions, there is not a large muscle mass which can apply tension on a weak incision, nor are large amounts of adipose tissue usually a problem; however, the sternotomy incision involves the splitting and wiring of a bone, the sternum, and is a much slower healing process. Nonunion of the sternum is a possibility, as with any bone break, and some patients do have to return to surgery for re-wiring of the sternum. This may occur any time from a week to a month postoperatively.

A complication which has received a great deal of attention in the literature is postoperative psychosis. The psychological disturbances range from slight confusion or mood alteration to vivid hallucinations with paranoid ideation. The incidence of post-cardiotomy delirium has been variously reported as occurring in 20%-57% of patients.[15] Attempts to correlate the incidence with significant factors have not produced uniform results, although the incidence frequently seemed higher in older patients, in those whose preoperative condition was worse, and in patients who had a prolonged time on cardiopulmonary bypass.[7] The actual causative factors generally fall into three categories: 1) existence of an unidentified emotional disturbance preoperatively which is aggravated by the stress of surgery; 2) the uniqueness or abnormality of the ICU environment; and 3) a physiologic occurrence, such as microemboli or alteration in catecholamine level.[16]

Because the physical environment of the patient is the factor most subject to control by the health care team, efforts have been made to more specifically examine the exact mechanism by which the environment could cause a change in the patient's emotional state. Originally it was thought that this was a sensory deprivation experience, but it now seems that a more accurate description would be overload of sensory abnormalities. That is, the environment of the Critical Care Unit subjects the patient to sensations, sounds, and sights which are, compared to his field of previous experiences, totally abnormal; depending upon the adequacy of preoperative preparation, he has little or no ability to interpret these perceptions and judge their significance to himself.

This complication, while not life-threatening, is a major disturbance to the patient and can prolong the convalescent period and even necessitate continued psychiatric care. Consequently, it is well worth the effort of the ICU staff to minimize the chance of occurrence. This can be done in three ways: 1) identification of patients who might have serious unresolved emotional conflicts, preoperatively; 2) modification of the ICU environment to minimize "abnormal" disturbances and emphasize "normal" factors, such as turning lights off at night, allowing patients to have familiar objects such as family pictures around and allowing frequent family visits; and 3) transfer of the patient out of the Intensive Care setting back to a general division as soon as possible.

REFERENCES

1. American Nurses Association: *Standards of Cardiovascular Nursing Practice*. American Nurses Association, Kansas City, Mo., 1975, p. 8.

2. Andreoli K, et al.: *Comprehensive Cardiac Care*. 3rd Ed. C.V. Mosby, St. Louis, Mo., 1975, p. 4.

3. Behrendt DM, and Austen WG: *Patient Care in Cardiac Surgery*. Little, Brown, and Company, London, 1972, p. 1.

4. Bender HW, et al.: Unstable coronary artery disease. *Annals of Thoracic Surgery* 19:521-527, 1975.

5. Diethrich EB: A brief history of coronary arterial surgery. *Heart and Lung* 4:369-371, 1975.

6. Diethrich EB: Aortocoronary bypass—classification and results. *Heart and Lung* 4:381-389, 1975.

7. Elsberry NL: Psychological responses to open heart surgery. *Nursing Research* 21:220-227, 1972.

8. Erlich IB: Patient selection and preoperative evaluation. *Heart and Lung* 4:373-379, 1975.

9. Green HL, et al.: Electronic equipment in critical care areas: Status of devices currently in use. (Inter-Society Commission for Heart Disease Resources.) *Circulation* 43(1):A 101+, 1971.

10. Guyton AC: *Textbook of Medical Physiology*. 5th Ed. W.B. Saunders, Philadelphia, Pa., 1976, p. 173.

11. Herman MV, and Gorlin M: Pathophysiology of Ischemic Heart

Disease. In Levine HJ (Ed.): *Clinical Cardiovascular Physiology*. Grune and Stratton, New York, 1976, p. 472.

12. Janis IL: *Psychological Stress*. John Wiley and Sons, New York, 1958.
13. King OM: *Care of the Cardiac Surgical Patient*. C.V. Mosby, St. Louis, Mo., 1975.
14. Kleiger RE, et al.: Mortality of myocardial infarction treated in the coronary care unit. *Heart and Lung* **4**:215-225, 1975.
15. Kornfeld DS, et al.: Psychiatric complications of open heart surgery. *New England Journal of Medicine* **273**:287-292, 1965.
16. Lazarus HR and Hagens JH: Prevention of psychosis following open heart surgery. *American Journal of Psychiatry* **124**:76-87, 1968.
17. Maslow A: A theory of human motivation. *Psychological Review* **50**:370+, 1945.
18. Mulligan CD: Continuing evaluation of coronary care. *Heart and Lung* **4**:227-232, 1975.
19. Pitorak E and Wood J: Nursing the Patient Having A Problem with Some Aspect of Transporting Material To and From Cells. In Beland I and Passos J (Eds.): *Clinical Nursing: Pathophysiological and Psychosocial Approaches*. Macmillan Publishing Co., New York, 1975, p. 641.
20. Ryan TJ: Mitral Valve Disease. In Levine HJ (Ed.): *Clinical Cardiovascular Physiology*. Grune and Stratton, New York, 1976, p. 526.
21. Sanderson RG: *The Cardiac Patient*. W.B. Saunders, Philadelphia, Pa., 1972.
22. Sukumalchantra Y, et al.: Correcting arterial hypoxemia by oxygen therapy in patients with acute myocardial infarction: effect on ventilations and hemodynamics. *American Journal of Cardiology* **24**:838, 1969.
23. Valencia A and Burgess JH: Arterial hypoxemia following acute myocardial infarction. *Circulation* **40**:641, 1969.
24. Whipple GH, et al.: *Acute Coronary Care*. Little, Brown, and Company, Boston, Mass., 1972, p. 41.

SUGGESTED READING LIST

Pathophysiology

Grotto AM: Recognition and management of the hyperlipoproteinemias. *Heart and Lung*. 1:508, 1972.

Griffith G: The life cycle of coronary artery disease. *Heart and Lung* 1:63, 1972.

Oliver MF: The metabolic response to a heart attack. *Heart and Lung* 4:57-60, 1975.

Rosenman RH: Observations on the pathogenesis of coronary heart disease. *Heart and Lung* 1:68, 1972.

Smith A, et al.: Serum enzymes in myocardial infarction. *American Journal of Nursing* 73:277-279, 1973.

Westfall UE: Electrical and mechanical events in the cardiac cycle. *American Journal of Nursing* 76:231-235, 1976.

Electrocardiography, Arterial Monitoring, and Diagnosis

Bilitch M: *A Manual of Cardiac Arrhythmias*. Little, Brown, and Company, Boston, Mass., 1971.

Bologni V: The Swan-Ganz pulmonary artery catheter: implications for nursing. *Heart and Lung* 3:976-981, 1974.

Fisch C: Electrophysiologic basis of clinical arrhythmias. *Heart and Lung* 3:51-56, 1974.

Marriott HJL: *Practical Electrocardiography*. 5th Ed. Williams and Wilkins Company, Baltimore, Md., 1972.

Meltzer LE, Pinneo R, Kitchell JR: *Intensive Coronary Care*. 3rd Ed. Charles Press Publishers, Bowie, Md., 1977.

Phibbs B: *The Cardiac Arrhythmias*. C.V. Mosby, St. Louis, Mo., 1973.

General Nursing Care of the M.I. Patient

Gentry WD, Haney F: Emotional and behavioral reaction to acute MI. *Heart and Lung* 4:738-745, 1975.

Griffith GS: Sexuality and the cardiac patient. *Heart and Lung* 2:70-73, 1973.

Hackett TP, et al.: The coronary care unit: an appraisal of its psychological hazards. *New England Journal of Medicine* 279:1365-1370, 1968.

Hamilton WP, Lavin MA: *Decision-Making in the Coronary Care Unit*. C.V. Mosby, St. Louis, Mo., 1972.

Lawson B: Easing the sexual fears of the cardiac patient. *R.N.* 37(ICU):1-5, 1974.

Long B: Sleep. *American Journal of Nursing* 69:1896-1899, 1969.

Moskowitz L: Vasodilator therapy in acute myocardial infarction. *Heart and Lung* 4:939-945, 1975.

Scalzi C: Nursing management of behavioral responses following an acute myocardial infarction. *Heart and Lung* 2:62-69, 1973.

Strain JJ: Psychological reactions to acute medical illness and critical care. *Critical Care Medicine* 6:39-44, 1978.

Vinsant M, et al.: *A Common Sense Approach to Coronary Care: a Program*. C.V. Mosby, St. Louis, Mo., 1972.

Winslow EH: Visual inspection of the patient with cardiopulmonary disease. *Heart and Lung* 4:421-429, 1975.

Complications of Myocardial Infarction

Bjerkelund CJ: Anticoagulant therapy in acute M.I. *Heart and Lung* 4:61-67, 1975.

Cole JS, McIntosh HD: Electroshock hazards in the coronary care unit. *Heart and Lung* 1:481-484, 1972.

DeMaria AN: Atropine: Current concepts of its use in acute myocardial infarction. *Heart and Lung* 3:135-137, 1974.

Dorr KS: The intra-aortic balloon pump. *American Journal of Nursing* 75:52-55, 1975.

Kones R, Benninger G: Digitalis therapy after acute myocardial infarction. *Heart and Lung* 4:99-103, 1975.

Miller R, et al.: Procainamide: reappraisal of an old antiarrhythmic drug. *Heart and Lung* 2:277-283, 1973.

O'Rourke ME: Cardiogenic shock following myocardial infarction. *Heart and Lung* 3:252-257, 1974.

Selzer A: The use and abuse of quinidine. *Heart and Lung* 1:755-780, 1972.

Tanner G: Heart failure in the M.I. patient. *American Journal of Nursing* 77:230-234, 1977.

Vismara LA, et al.: Cardiocirculatory effects of morphine sulfate: mechanisms of action and therapeutic application. *Heart and Lung* 3:495-499, 1974.

Pacemakers

Furman S: Recent developments in cardiac pacing. *Heart and Lung* 7:813-826, 1978.

Manwaring M: What patients need to know about pacemakers. *American Journal of Nursing* 77:825-830, 1977.

Spence M, Lemberg L: Cardiac pacemakers I: modalities of pacing. *Heart and Lung* 3:820-827, 1974.

——: Cardiac pacemakers II: indications for pacing. *Heart and Lung* 3:989-995, 1974.

——: Cardiac pacemakers IV: complications of pacing. *Heart and Lung* 4:286-295, 1975.

Winslow EH, Marino LB: Temporary cardiac pacemakers. *American Journal of Nursing* 75:586-591, 1975.

Postoperative Nursing Care

Benzing G, Edwards L: Immediate postoperative care after cardiac surgery. *Heart and Lung* 3:415-422, 1974.

Futral JE: Postoperative management and complications of coronary artery bypass surgery. *Heart and Lung* 6:477-486, 1977.

Jillings CR: Phases of recovery from open heart surgery. *Heart and Lung* 7:987-994, 1978.

Lasater KL, Grisanti DJ: Postcardiotomy psychosis: indications and interventions. *Heart and Lung* 4:724-729, 1975.

Wilson WS: Aortocoronary bypass surgery II—an updated review. *Heart and Lung* 3:435-454, 1974.

CHAPTER 3

Care of the Patient With Respiratory Problems

by Barbara J. Daly, RN, MSN

ANATOMY

The respiratory system is composed of two major divisions: the upper airway and the lower airway. The upper airway consists of the nose and nasopharynx, the mouth and oropharynx, and the larynx. The nasal cavity, mouth, and pharynx have a mucosal lining which serves to heat inspired air to body temperature and humidify it to 65% or 75% humidity. The average adult loses about 300 cc. of water per day in this way. In addition to this heating and humidifying function, the nose and nasopharynx also act as a filter for inspired air. Large particles in the air (10 microns) are removed by hair follicles in the vestibule of the nose, and smaller particles are trapped by the sticky mucus lining of the air passageways. Once entrapped, this debris is removed either by sneezing, coughing, or by the slow, gradual movement of cilia. Cilia are thin filaments lining most of the respiratory tract down to the terminal bronchioles; they constantly move forward and backward in a wave-like fashion and propel the mucus layer and trapped particles up into the pharynx.

The larynx is considered the last portion of the upper airway. It is covered by the epiglottis, which closes reflexively during swallowing to prevent aspiration of food and fluids into the respiratory tract. The larynx is composed of several half rings of cartilage, and one complete ring; the cricoid cartilage. The vocal cords are located in the upper portion of the larynx, above the cricoid cartilage. The functions of the larynx are: (1) air passage, (2) further filtering, (3) speech, (4) protection from aspiration, (5) blockage of the airway by the epiglottis in order to generate positive pressure for a cough.

The lower airway is sometimes further divided into the large airway (trachea and bronchi) and the small airway (bronchioles and alveoli). The trachea is about 12 cm. long in the adult and, like the larynx, consists of half-ring or "D" shaped cartilages, with the flat fibrous membrane portion on the posterior side, lying next to the esophagus. The trachea divides at a point termed the carina into the right and left main stem bronchi (Figure 3-1).

The right bronchus is wider and shorter than the left and extends more vertically from the trachea. The left main stem bronchus is narrower, longer, and extends at a 45° angle from the trachea. The right bronchus then divides into three branches, one for each lobe, and the left divides into two. These lobar branches, also called secondary bronchi, further divide into segmental bronchi. The respiratory tree continues branching into progressively smaller units, termed bronchioles. The bronchi are partially supported by cartilage and individually have a much greater surface area; the bronchioles have no cartilaginous structure and because they are so numerous, have collectively a total surface area many times that of the larger airways. The last subdivision of the passageways is called the terminal bronchiole, and it has been estimated that there are about one million of these.[4] Each bronchiole leads to an alveolar duct, and finally alveoli (Figure 3-2).

The alveoli, numbering about 300 million, are blind pouches. It is in the alveolar sacs and alveolar ducts that gas exchange takes place. The alveolus has a fluid lining which is continuous with the mucus lining of the larger airways. This lining is composed partially of *surfactant,* a phospholipid responsible for reducing the surface tension in the alveoli. Below the fluid lining is the alveolar epithelium and then an epithelial basement membrane. This basement membrane is separated in some places from the capillary membrane by a very thin interstitial space and in some places is in direct apposition to the capillary endothelial basement membrane. These layers together are sometimes termed the *respiratory membrane.*

The blood supply for all of the respiratory tract, except the alveoli, is composed of bronchial arteries and veins. The bronchial

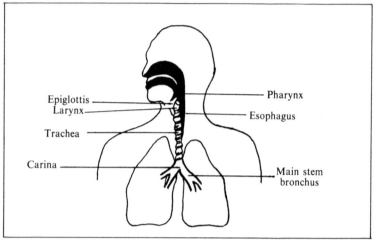

Figure 3-1. Large airways (From: AC Guyton: *Textbook of Medical Physiology.* 5th Ed. W.B. Saunders, Philadelphia, Pa., 1976, p. 526. Used with permission.)

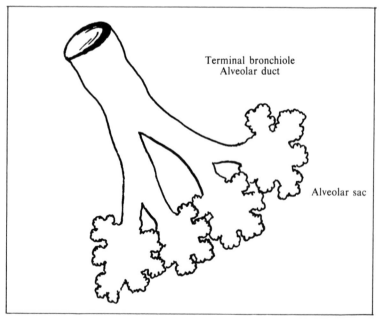

Figure 3-2. Schematic representation of bronchiole and alveoli.

artery arises from the aorta, and the bronchial veins empty back into the pulmonary veins. Lymphatic drainage is supplied through the peribronchial space at the hilum, and eventually joins the right lymphatic duct.

The lungs themselves are attached to the body only at the hilum, where the larger airways and blood vessels enter (Figure 3-3). They are covered, however, by the visceral pleura, a porous serous membrane, from which lymphatics drain. This visceral pleura lies next to and is contiguous with the parietal pleura, which lines the inside of the thoracic cage. In infancy and childhood, the thorax grows more rapidly than do the lungs; as the thorax expands, pulling the parietal pleura with it, away from the visceral pleura, a vacuum is created between the two pleural membranes. This negative pressure (in comparison to atmospheric pressure) is maintained, providing there is no disruption of the pleural membrane. As each breath is taken, the thorax moves out, pulling the parietal pleura further away, and negative pressure increases.

VENTILATION

Ventilation, or the process of moving air in and out of the body, is accomplished by the action of the intercostal muscles, the ribs, and the diaphragm. Contraction of the diaphragm causes it to lower and flatten, thus elongating the thoracic cavity; this contributes the major portion of the change in lung volume during inspiration. The remaining increase in volume is due to the movement of the ribs up and out, changing the anteroposterior diameter of the lungs. The scalene sternocleidomastoid, trapezius, and pectoralis muscles are termed accessory muscles because, while not normally active in respiration, they can be used to assist when deep breathing is necessary, as with exercise, or in respiratory distress.

When the thoracic cavity enlarges through the movement of the ribs and diaphragm, the lungs, held against the parietal pleura, also enlarge. With the change in volume, the intra-alveolar pressure becomes slightly negative in relationship to atmospheric pressure (1 to 3 mm. Hg). A vacuum is created, and air then rushes into the lung.

When inspiration stops, expiration passively occurs through elastic recoil of lung tissue and muscles. The surface tension in the alveoli also causes a tendency for the walls of the alveoli to collapse together. The abdominal muscles may be used to assist in pushing

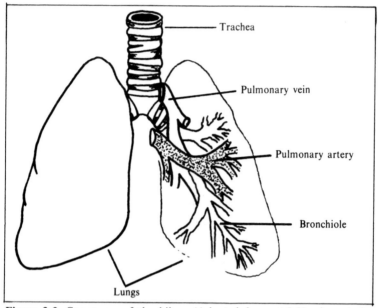

Figure 3-3. Structures of the hilum (Adapted from: AJ Vander, et al.: *Human Physiology: The Mechanics of Body Function.* 2nd Ed. McGraw-Hill, New York, 1975, p. 285. Used with permission.)

the diaphragm up by elevating the contents of the abdominal cavity. As pressure is thus exerted on the lungs by the recoiling structures, the intra-alveolar pressure becomes greater than atmospheric pressure and air is forced out.

GAS EXCHANGE

The underlying purpose of respiration is to supply oxygen for cellular metabolism and eliminate the carbon dioxide formed. In order for this to occur, both internal and external respiration is necessary. External respiration refers to the exchange of gases between blood and environment; internal respiration refers to the exchange between blood and tissues.

Diffusion

Before proceeding further with the discussion of gas transport, a brief review of the characteristics and laws governing gases is necessary. First, it must be recalled that gases are composed of discrete molecules in constant motion; the molecules will spread throughout any volume by diffusion. Oxygen, therefore, can move from the alveolus through the alveolar-capillary membrane into the blood by simply diffusing, providing the membrane is intact and there is no obstruction, as with fluid or secretions.

The rate of diffusion is dependent upon four factors. First, the thicker the membrane through which the gas must diffuse, the slower the diffusion. Second, the smaller the surface area, the slower the diffusion. These two principles explain why diseases that damage alveoli or cause fibrosis and thickening interfere with oxygen transport. Third, the more soluble the gas in the fluid of the membrane, the faster diffusion will occur. Carbon dioxide is 20 times as soluble in water as oxygen, and consequently, even when the interstitial pulmonary bed is congested as in pulmonary edema, the movement of CO_2 is not hampered, although the rate of oxygen diffusion is considerably slower. The fourth factor governing gas diffusion is that the greater the pressure difference on either side of the membrane, the faster the diffusion.

The amount of a specific gas in a mixture of gases may be described in two ways—percentage or partial pressure. Percentage refers to the number of molecules of that specific gas, compared to the total. Thus, air is comprised of 78.6% nitrogen, 20.8% oxygen, 0.04% CO_2, and 0.50% water vapor. Percentage figures provide information about the composition of a gas, but do not yield information about the diffusion power—for that, the partial pressure is much more useful.

The pressure of a gas is defined as the pressure which that gas exerts on the walls of its container. Thus, atmospheric pressure is the pressure which all of the gases in the atmosphere exert on any structure—the earth, buildings, individuals. Pressure is commonly measured in millimeters of mercury. (Recently, the term *torr* has been used to mean one mm.Hg, named after Torricelli, the inventor of the barometer).

Dalton's law states that the total pressure exerted by a gas mixture is the sum of all of the partial pressures of each individual gas. For example, atmospheric pressure, 760 mm.Hg, is the sum of the pressure exerted by nitrogen, the pressure exerted by oxygen, the pressure exerted by carbon dioxide, and the pressures exerted by all of the other gases.

The pressure that each specific gas in the mixture exerts is proportional to the concentration of its molecules in that mixture. Thus, knowing that the atmosphere is 21% oxygen, and that the total atmospheric pressure is 760 mm.Hg, we can calculate the partial pressure of oxygen in air as follows:

$$760 \text{ mm.} \times 21\% = 159.6 \text{ mm.Hg}$$

When air enters the respiratory passages it becomes humidified. The partial pressure of water in the air on an average day is 3.7 mm.Hg; by the time air reaches the alveoli, it has been humidified and exerts a pressure of 47 mm.Hg.

Because the diffusion of gas molecules is related to the amount of pressure exerted on the walls of their container, not just the concentration, partial pressure is used rather than percentages in discussing blood levels of various gases. Table 3-1 summarizes this information for the three commonly measured gases and water.

Note that alveolar air is comprised of a mixture whose composition is roughly the average of inspired and expired air. This is because, first, diffusion is constantly taking place, so that the oxygen inspired is being utilized while CO_2 is diffusing from the blood into the alveoli and accumulating. Second, as will be discussed in more detail later, the lungs do not completely fill and empty with each breath. Rather, each breath exchanges only about 1/8 of the total lung capacity. Thus the air inspired is mixed with the volume remaining in the lung, which contains more CO_2; each breath exhaled mixes with the atmospheric gas in the upper airway, which contains more O_2.

TABLE 3-1

Concentration of Gases in Inspired, Expired, and Alveolar Air

Gas	Inspired Air		Expired Air		Alveolar Air	
	partial pressure	%	partial pressure	%	partial pressure	%
N	563	74	566	74.5	569	74.9
O_2	149	20	120	16.0	104	13.6
CO_2	0.3	0.04	27	3.6	40	5.3
H_2O	47	6.2	47	6.2	47	6.2
Total	760	100	760	100	760	100

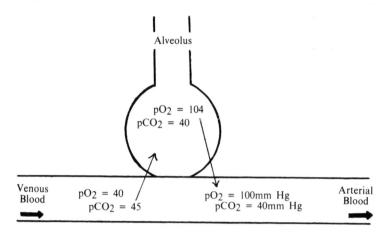

Figure 3-4. Gas diffusion across the alveolar-capillary membrane.

Venous blood flowing into the pulmonary capillaries has relatively little oxygen (pO_2 = 40), having returned from the systemic circuit where oxygen was utilized by the tissues. The difference between the capillary pO_2 level and the alveolar pO_2 (104 mm. Hg) establishes the pressure gradient which favors diffusion of oxygen from the area of high concentration (the alveolus), to the area of low concentration (the capillary) (Figure 3-4). The same situation exists to favor the movement of CO_2 in the opposite direction, from the capillaries into the alveoli.

Oxygen Transport

Once oxygen diffuses across the alveolar-capillary membrane into the blood, it has to be transported to the tissue cells for use in metabolism. This can occur in two ways. A very small amount dissolves in plasma, and a much greater amount (97%) combines with hemoglobin.

In the normal individual, each gram of hemoglobin can combine with 1.34 ml. of oxygen. This is a loose, easily reversible combination, effected by the concentration of oxygen, temperature, pH, and the concentration of CO_2. High pO_2 favors the binding of O_2 to the heme portion of the hemoglobin molecule and low pO_2 favors the release or dissociation of oxygen. Because of this, in the alveolar capillaries, where the pO_2 is the highest, O_2 binds most readily; in the tissues, where pO_2 is low, O_2 is released.

If the hemoglobin is carrying the maximum amount of oxygen, each 100 cc. of blood will carry 20 ml. of oxygen (15 Gm. Hgb/100 cc. x 1.34 ml. O_2/Gm. of Hgb = 20 ml. O_2/100 cc. blood). The term *saturation* refers to the degree to which oxygen molecules have combined with all of the available hemoglobin; i.e., hemoglobin that is 98% saturated is carrying almost all of the oxygen possible, while hemoglobin with a saturation of 50% has combined with only about half as much oxygen as it is capable of carrying. Hemoglobin that is completely saturated with oxygen is termed oxyhemoglobin, and hemoglobin that has released oxygen is called de-oxygenated or reduced hemoglobin.

The oxygen-hemoglobin dissociation curve is a graphic display of the extent to which saturation is affected by the concentration of oxygen in the blood (pO_2) (Figure 3-5). As can be seen, this relationship is not linear, but rather is represented by an S-curve, indicating that hemoglobin combines readily with oxygen and will be 80% or more saturated with pO_2s as low as 60. However, once the pO_2 drops below this, the curve shifts and saturation decreases sharply. Not only does this relationship favor the release of oxygen at tissue sites, as mentioned, but it also means that, in clinical practice, when caring for patients with pO_2s of 60 or above, we can be confident that most tissue oxygen needs are being met.

Figure 3-5 also demonstrates the effect of pH, pCO_2, and temperature. Increased hydrogen ion concentration (decreased pH), increased pCO_2, and increased temperature all cause the curve to shift to the right, indicating increased oxygen release, or lower saturations for a given level of pO_2. This is a beneficial adaptive mechanism in that many states of increased metabolism, such as exercise or fever, which increase oxygen needs of the tissues, tend to increase body temperature and lower pH, thereby providing a mechanism for meeting the larger oxygen demand. The effect of CO_2, which favors the release of oxygen at tissue sites, is called the *Bohr effect.*

The oxygen-hemoglobin dissociation curve is also helpful in understanding the effects of anemia. In the anemic patient, without pulmonary problems, the available hemoglobin will be completely (98%) saturated. However, the tissues will still be receiving a reduced oxygen supply. For example, if the patient's hemoglobin measures 7.5 Gm./100 ml. of blood, that 100 cc. of blood will carry only 10 cc. of oxygen, rather than the normal 20 cc. of oxygen.

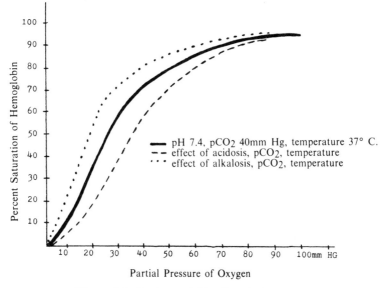

Figure 3-5. Oxyhemoglobin dissociation curve.

$$1 \text{ Gram of Hgb} = 1.34 \text{ cc. of } O_2$$
$$7.5 \text{ Gram} \times 1.34 = 9.95 \text{ cc. } O_2$$

Because the available hemoglobin is already fully saturated, attempts to administer oxygen and raise the pO_2 will not effect tissue oxygenation. Tachycardia and stimulation of the bone marrow to increase RBC production are compensatory mechanisms to meet the body's oxygen needs.

Carbon Dioxide Transport

Transportation of CO_2 in the blood also occurs in several ways, similar to oxygen. A small percentage dissolves in plasma and is transported as free CO_2. An additional small percentage combines with hemoglobin ($HbCO_2$). The majority of CO_2 is transported in the red blood cell, through the action of the enzyme carbonic anhydrase.

Within the RBC, CO_2 combines with water to form carbonic acid. Carbonic anhydrase facilitates this and accelerates the rate of reaction. Once carbonic acid is formed, it immediately dissociates into the bicarbonate ion and hydrogen ion, as shown on p. 206.

$$CO_2 + H_2O \underset{\text{anhydrase}}{\overset{\text{carbonic}}{\rightleftharpoons}} H_2CO_3 \rightleftharpoons HCO_3^- + H^+$$

These reactions take place almost immediately, creating a state of chemical equilibrium. Once dissociated, the bicarbonate ion is free to diffuse out of the cell. The hydrogen ion cannot penetrate the cell membrane and combine with hemoglobin; consequently, in order to keep the ionic charge of the cell constant, chloride ions diffuse into the cell in exchange for the bicarbonate. This is termed the "chloride shift" (Figure 3-6).

The ability of CO_2 to combine with hemoglobin is effected by pO_2 levels, just as oxygen saturation is effected by pCO_2 levels. As would be expected, low pO_2 levels, as exist at the tissue sites, favor the binding of CO_2 with Hgb, and high pO_2 levels, as exist in the al-

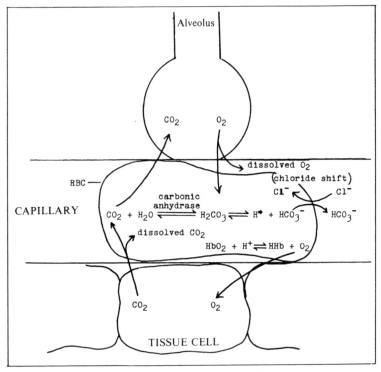

Figure 3-6. Oxygen and carbon dioxide transport.

veoli, favor the release of CO_2 from hemoglobin. This reaction, called the *Haldane effect,* causes twice as much CO_2 to be picked up from the tissue as would otherwise occur.

CONTROL OF RESPIRATION

Stimulation and control of respiration is a complex process involving several separate mechanisms. The major respiratory center is located in the medulla; this center, containing both inspiratory and expiratory neurons, is responsible for the involuntary control of respiration. Rhythmic, coordinated breathing is further insured by the action of the apneustic and pneumotaxic centers in the pons. The output of the respiratory center is transmitted to the diaphragm via the vagus nerve, and to the intercostals and abdominal muscles via nerve roots from the thoracic and lumbar portions of the spinal cord.

The inspiratory-expiratory cycle is aided by a feedback mechanism originating in the lungs. Stretch receptors in the bronchi and bronchioles are stimulated during lung inflation and send inhibitory impulses via the vagus through the brain stem to the respiratory center to stop inspiration.

At steady state, these mechanisms result in a regular, even pattern of breathing. In order for the body to respond to changing needs, they must also be able to stimulate varying respiratory patterns. This ability is based on a sensitivity to levels of CO_2, hydrogen ions, and oxygen.

The central chemoreceptors in the medulla, the major center, are responsive to changes in CO_2 and hydrogen ion concentration in the cerebrospinal fluid, which bathes the medulla. The CO_2 content of the CSF roughly approximates that of arterial blood; when CO_2 rises, the chemoreceptors stimulate an increase in both respiratory rate and volume. This increased alveolar ventilation results in the excess CO_2 being exhaled; the level of CO_2 in the CSF then falls back to normal, and the increased respiratory drive ceases. If the level of CO_2 continues to rise despite this compensatory mechanism, it will exert a depressing effect on the medulla and respiratory depression will result. However, if the level of CO_2 becomes progressively but slowly elevated over time, as in certain disease states, the central chemoreceptors become refractory and no longer respond to hypercarbia (elevated pCO_2).

In this case, respiratory drive is dependent on peripheral chemo-receptors, located in the bifurcation of the common carotid arteries and in the aortic arch. The aortic and carotid bodies, both receiving an extremely rich arterial supply, are sensitive primarily to O_2 levels, and, to a much lesser degree, to CO_2 levels. When the pO_2 of arterial blood falls, the medullary center is stimulated, via the vagus from aortic chemoreceptors and via the glossopharyngeal nerve from the carotid bodies, and alveolar ventilation is increased. Persons with chronically elevated CO_2 levels are said to function on this "oxygen drive."

The significance of a basic understanding of the central mechanisms of respiration lies in its application to clinical practice. First, knowledge of the way in which high levels of CO_2 can depress respirations will assist the nurse in identifying impending respiratory failure regardless of what pO_2 is achieved. Second, an understanding of the dependence of the patient with chronic hypercarbia on low oxygen levels to stimulate respiration will alert her to the danger of supplemental oxygen administration without close blood gas monitoring.

ASSESSMENT

Assessment of the individual with respiratory problems may be divided into four aspects: physical assessment, pulmonary function, arterial blood gases, and miscellaneous tests and procedures. It should be emphasized that no one tool or method is sufficient by itself; thus, blood gases, for example, are of no use when interpreted without taking into account clinical observation.

Of all methods, observation and physical assessment will provide the nurse with the greatest amount of and most valid information for decision-making in the Critical Care Unit. The first chapter introduced the reader to the skills of physical assessment. To review, there are four methods: inspection, palpation, percussion, and auscultation. Even without formal education in the physical assessment skills, the critical care nurse should be able to use each of these methods to some extent in gathering data concerning the respiratory status of her patient.

Physical Assessment

Inspection is the method most familiar to nurses and most easily utilized; in fact, it should be viewed not as an intermittent activity, but rather as a continual intellectual process. Each and every time the nurse approaches the patient, a series of observations should automatically be reviewed. These may be posed as the following questions:

What is the overall appearance of the individual? When first approached, is the patient lying comfortably and quietly, or does he appear disheveled and tired, indicating he has not been resting? Is his skin warm and dry, or cool and clammy? Does he have a great deal of equipment and paraphernalia surrounding him, or is his environment clean, restful, and therapeutic? Is he alone or does he have significant others with him? What medications has the patient received recently?

The first area of observation, as can be seen, is quite general. The purpose of asking these questions first is to establish a framework against which more specific data can be evaluated. Behaviorists term this the gestalt, or the "whole," which will be different than merely the sum of parts. Often, beginning practitioners tend to focus observations too quickly. Specific data are gathered which are both appropriate and valid; however, without first having established a gestalt, errors may result.

First, the specific observation may lead to an invalid conclusion. For example, the patient may appear restless and agitated. Knowing that the patient's most recent arterial blood gas indicated mild hypoxia, the nurse could easily conclude that the low pO_2 was causing the restlessness. However, if she first assesses all facets of the total situation, in addition to specific clinical observations, she may discover that the patient's wife is overdue to visit and he is concerned about why she is late, and this is, in fact, the basis for his agitation.

Second, the direction of inquiry may not be valid or most appropriate. When approaching the patient, the nurse comes with a certain predetermined focus; that is, she already has certain data which will specify the direction of inquiry, such as diagnosis, history of the patient and knowledge gained from previous contact, from the shift report, and from the care plan. This will direct her to focus on breath sounds, monitor pattern, or peripheral circulation, etc., and most often the direction will be appropriate. However, given that each patient is not a closed static entity, but rather an open active system in constant dynamic interaction with the environment, there is no limit to the amount or degree to which change will occur. Approaching the patient with a closed pre-set focus will inevitably lead the nurse into errors of omission.

Consider the following situation:

> The night nurse has learned from report that Mr. Smith is a 67-year-old patient with a history of mitral stenosis and COPD who underwent a mitral valve replacement two days ago. He has been in the Intensive Care Unit since surgery and has progressed fairly well. He has been in atrial fibrillation since surgery and has required continued monitoring for this; he has seemed quite anxious about his monitor pattern and heart rate and asks many questions of the nurses. It is reported that Mr. S. had had a great deal of difficulty in resting because of his anxiety and the noise in the ICU; he has not slept well the previous two nights. On assessment, the patient appears restless and somewhat diaphoretic, with a heart rate of 122. His breath sounds are moist in all lobes, but he states he is unable to cough because he is so tired; he is slightly disoriented as to date and time. The nurse, knowing the patient's history of anxiety, knowing that his major postoperative problem has been atrial fibrillation, concludes that the patient is fatigued, and that sleep deprivation and the anxiety frequently associated with cardiac surgery are the cause of the patient's confusion. She then administers 6 mg. morphine sulfate for pain and 100 mg. secobarbital for sleep. Within one hour the patient's respiratory rate decreases to 6 and he becomes unarousable. Arterial blood gases demonstrate severe hypoxia, elevated pCO_2, and acidosis.

Had the nurse not approached the patient with a pre-determined focus on cardiovascular problems and not viewed his primary diagnosis in isolation, she would have been able to make a more comprehensive assessment. Had her observations included an analysis of earlier blood gas results, and a more thorough investigation of his pulmonary status, including his history of COPD, she would probably have correctly identified the cause of his disorientation as hypoxia and would not have administered the narcotic and sedative which lead to respiratory depression.

The next question to be asked is: What is the patient's behavior? This question, while somewhat open-ended, is specific to the respiratory patient in that the first indication of inadequate oxygenation is a change in behavior. The question must be asked both prospectively and retrospectively—What is the patient's behavior right now and how does this compare with his past behavior? Restlessness, anxiety, and confusion generally indicate inadequate oxygen levels, while drowsiness, stupor, and lethargy are early indications of increased CO_2 levels.

Having gathered the data which will construct a general framework for the nurse, more specific observations can now be made. These, of course, relate to the quality of the respirations themselves—What is the rate and are the respirations deep or shallow? These two questions must be asked in conjunction with each other; a slow but somewhat deep respiratory pattern is quite normal during bedrest, while slow and shallow respirations probably indicate inadequate elimination of CO_2 and perhaps a depressed respiratory center. What is the respiratory pattern—is it fairly regular and even, or does the patient exhibit Cheyne-Stokes or Kussmaul respiration? The Cheyne-Stokes pattern is one in which respirations are first slow and shallow, gradually increasing in depth, followed by a period of 10 to 20 seconds of apnea, then beginning slowly and shallowly again. It is characteristic of late stages of central nervous system diseases and circulatory diseases, and is often seen in the terminally ill. Kussmaul respirations are very rapid and deep, and are characteristic of states of metabolic acidosis, such as diabetic ketoacidosis.

In assessing pulmonary status, the nurse should also note the ease of respirations. Is the patient breathing without obvious effort, or is he using accessory muscles, such as the scalene and sternoclidomastoids? Is nasal flaring present? Of equal significance are the factors that effect this ease; does he need to sit up in bed in order to breathe, can he speak a full sentence without taking a breath every few words, does he become short of breath with very little activity?

A very specific observation that is helpful in pinpointing problems is the distribution of ventilation. Does the patient move all portions of his thorax equally with each breath, or does one side rise and fall more than the other? This may be the first indication of a small pneumothorax or consolidating atelectasis. In noting this, it is often helpful for the nurse to place her hands on either side of the chest to feel the excursion.

The fourth area of inquiry concerns the patient's color. This should be among the last of observations made because it can be the most misleading and is also the last parameter to change when respiratory distress occurs. It is misleading because, in addition to the wide variety of skin tones in normal individuals, many variables which are not directly related to respiratory status affect skin color. Cyanosis is an indication of reduced oxygen content in capillary vessels, and this may occur as a result of varying factors. Vasoconstriction associated with anxiety, cold, or use of vasopressors will reduce circulation to the skin and may cause a cyanotic appearance; any obstruction, such as atherosclerotic plaques, can also contribute to cyanosis.

The fact that cyanosis is a very late change is related to the ability of hemoglobin to maintain relatively high saturations until the pO_2 drops below 60 mm. Hg. Until the O_2 content of arterial blood drops to almost half of the normal level ($pO_2 = 100$), hemoglobin will still carry relatively normal amounts of oxygen to the peripheral tissues. Consequently, when cyanosis occurs as a result of respiratory failure, it is an indication that there is a very serious interference in either oxygen diffusion or transport.

A second color change that is often overlooked is that of reddening or flushing. This occurs with high pCO_2 and is a result of the direct vasodilating effect of CO_2 on local blood vessels. It is an indication that the individual is not eliminating CO_2 sufficiently because of decreased ventilatory rate or volume.

Miscellaneous observations that should not be overlooked relate to the amount and kind of secretions. Color, consistency, and the ease or difficulty with which the patient clears secretions are all important observations. The patient himself is a valuable source of data in confirming whether or not he has more or less secretions than usual or more or less difficulty in clearing them.

Auscultation is the second skill which is essential for the critical care nurse. For the beginning practitioner, the emphasis should be on learning what normal lungs sound like and being able to recognize a deviation from normal. Training films with audio components are helpful aids initially in learning to listen to breath sounds, but there is no substitute for clinical practice in this skill.

Having firmly established what lungs without pathology sound like, the nurse next focuses on three observations. First, are breath sounds present, to an equal degree, on both sides of the chest? Keeping in mind that a decrease in loudness indicates a decrease in airflow, the nurse listens over all lobes, anterior and posterior, comparing left with right each time. In the peripheral regions airflow should be heard, but will be softer, with less pause between inspiration and expiration (vesicular sounds). Over the very large airways, the sound is louder and rougher, with an obvious pause between inspiration and expiration (bronchial sounds). To obtain comprehensive data, it is essential that the nurse listen to the posterior chest of the patient on bedrest in order to detect secretions pooled or effusions that have planed posteriorly. It is also important in detecting decreased breath sounds to have the patient take a deep breath; the sounds produced with a deep breath should be 2 to 3 times as loud as with normal breathing.

In listening to the chest, the nurse is also trying to establish whether or not the airways are obstructed or narrowed with secretions. In essence, she is next asking, are the breath sounds wet or dry and are abnormal sounds present? The term *rale* is used to refer to the sound of air moving through secretions; *rales* may be fine, moist sounds, perhaps crackling, heard primarily on inspiration, or may be coarser, more bubbling, depending on the size of the airway with secretions. *Rhonchi* are sounds produced more loudly during expiration, are of a lower, rumbling quality, and indicate consolidated secretions or a narrowed airway. Rhonchi clear with coughing, rales do not. A wheeze is sometimes considered a kind of rhonchus.

As can be seen, there is no universal, clear-cut distinction between terms. The reader will undoubtedly be able to find discrepancies between this text and others in the definition of rales, rhonchi, and wheezes. What is important, in fact, essential, is that the way in which the nurse communicates to colleagues, whether in writing or orally, be clear and meaningful. If the nurse chooses to use the terms rales and rhonchi, she must be certain that the listener/reader has the same understanding of these terms as she does. Because this is difficult, if not impossible, to insure, given the number of individuals involved in the care of any one patient, it is recommended that communication avoid these terms and instead include a more comprehensive description of breath sounds heard, including a comparison with the past and specification of all parameters. The following is an example of such charting:

> Breath sounds heard in equal volume on both sides of chest, but diminished posteriorly and on deep breathing. Moist crackling heard on periphery of both right and left lower lobes, and occasional wheezing on forced expiration. Crackling and wheezing do not clear with cough, and are more pronounced than yesterday.

Pulmonary Function

The second method of assessment involves pulmonary function measurements. This portion of assessment examines the mechanics of ventilation, or the ability to move air in and out. Pulmonary function testing is an essential part of the diagnostic and on-going phases of respiratory care, and the critical care nurse should be familiar with the more common measurements. Before discussing normal or expected values, however, it must be emphasized that there is no single set of "normal" values that will be valid for all individuals. Age, sex, body size, and position all affect the values obtained. For example, the total lung capacity (TLC) for a 20-year-old male, 6', 6" tall, is 7.5 liters; the TLC for a 70-year-old-female, 5' tall is 3.5 liters.

Figure 3-7 is a schematic representation of average values for pulmonary function tests. As can be seen, the measurements can be thought of as series of *volumes* and *capacities*.

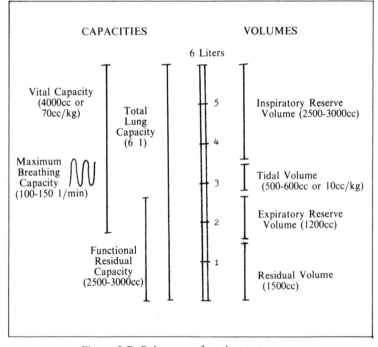

Figure 3-7. Pulmonary function tests.

Tidal Volume (TV) is the amount normally inhaled or exhaled with each breath.

Inspiratory Reserve Volume (IRV) is the amount that can be voluntarily inhaled in addition to the tidal volume.

Expiratory Reserve Volume (ERV) is the amount that can be voluntarily exhaled after exhaling the tidal volume.

Residual Volume (RV) is the amount remaining in the lung after maximal expiration, or after exhaling the expiratory reserve volume. If the lungs were to completely empty with each breath, it would require tremendous effort to re-expand the alveoli each time, just as it is much harder to inflate a balloon when it is completely empty than it is to further inflate once some air is in it. This is a protective mechanism which is altered in many disease states.

Vital Capacity (VC) is the maximum amount that can be exhaled after a maximum deep breath has been taken. It is the sum of the inspiratory reserve volume, tidal volume, and expiratory reserve volume.

Functional Residual Capacity (FRC) is the total amount remaining in the lungs after a normal expiration. It is the sum of the expiratory reserve volume and residual volume.

Minute Volume. There are three other tests of pulmonary function, which are related to time. These are minute volume, maximum breathing capacity, and timed vital capacity (also called forced expiratory volume). *Minute volume* is the total amount exhaled or inhaled in one minute during normal or quiet breathing. The average value is 7-9 liters.

Maximum Breathing Capacity is the maximum amount that can be exhaled or inhaled on forced ventilation in one minute. Average range is 100-150 liter/minute.

Timed Vital Capacity is the percentage of the vital capacity that can be forcibly exhaled in 1, 2, and 3 seconds. Average values are 80% in 1 second, 85-90% in 2 seconds, 95-100% in 3 seconds.

Of all of these measurements, the two most accessible and most valuable to the nurse are tidal volume and vital capacity. Tidal volume yields information concerning the adequacy of ventilation at the moment, and also provides an easy means to determine trends, such as the patient who is tiring and whose respirations are slowly becoming inadequate. Vital capacity is an indicator of the patient's ability to periodically take deep breaths, necessary to keep alveoli expanded, and ability to cough, which also requires a deep breath. Both of these measurements are easily obtained at the bedside by use of a respirometer (Figure 3-8).

As mentioned earlier in the chapter, with each respiratory cycle, the lungs do not empty and fill completely with fresh air. This is in part due to the existence of the residual volume, and in part related to *dead space.* Dead space is that portion of the tidal volume that is taken in, but not exposed to a blood supply for gas exchange With each breath, the conducting airways (trachea, larynx, bronchi, broncioles) fill with air, but diffusion takes place only in the alveoli; this anatomic dead space is usually expressed as a ratio compared to tidal volume: 0.3. Normal dead space is estimated as one ml. per pound of body weight. For a 150 pound adult, lying in bed, this ratio could be calculated as:

$$\frac{V_D}{V_T} = \frac{150 \text{ ml.}}{450 \text{ ml.}} = 0.3$$

Actual dead space measurements involve a comparison of CO_2 content of arterial blood and CO_2 content of expired air; an increase is termed physiological dead space, and can be the result of any disease state which prevents a ventilated alveolus from being perfused, such as a pulmonary embolus.

Negative Inspiratory Force is another commonly used pulmonary function test. It involves the measurement of the negative pressure developed when the individual attempts to inspire against a closed airway, with a pressure gauge in line. It provides an estimate of strength; -30 to -40 cm. H_2O is considered normal, and -20 cm. minimal.

Compliance is the last function with which the nurse should be familiar. Compliance refers to the expansibility or distensibility of

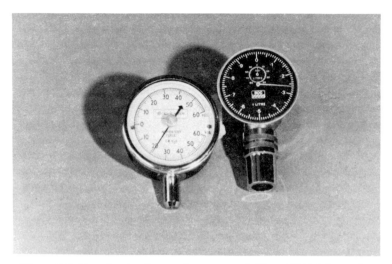

Figure 3-8. Negative inspiratory force meter (left) and Wright's respirometer.

the lung. The elastic tissue within the lung provides a constant force which tends to keep the lungs collapsed; the ability of the lungs to overcome this force—the ability of the lungs to expand or distend— is referred to as compliance. It is defined as the volume increase in the lung for each unit of pressure change in the lung, and the average value for the adult is 130 ml./cm. H_2O pressure. That is, the amount of pressure necessary to raise a column of water one centimeter high will be sufficient to increase lung volume by 130 ml.

Effective compliance used with patients undergoing mechanical ventilation, can be measured by dividing tidal volume by the peak airway pressure; the average value for the ventilated patient is 50 ml./cm. The compliance is an indication of the amount of work involved in breathing; it decreases normally with age and as larger volumes are inhaled. A decrease in compliance is also caused by many disease states which increase the stiffness of the lung or provide obstruction to lung expansion, such as tumors.

Arterial Blood Gases

Assessment of levels of oxygen, carbon dioxide, and acid-base status by analysis of arterial blood gases is the third essential portion of respiratory assessment. The intent of this section of the chapter is not to provide any kind of in-depth discussion of acid-base reactions; for this the reader is referred to any text on acid-base physiology or basic chemistry. The purpose of this section is to review certain facts which will enable the nurse to make valid interpretations of arterial blood gases and utilize this information as part of her data base.

Before examining acid-base reactions and pH, the significance of arterial pO_2 and pCO_2 will be discussed. Normal pO_2 level is between 90-100 mm. Hg (Table 3-2). There are several ways in which the pO_2 level may become abnormally low. First, the intake, or FiO_2 (fraction of inspired oxygen) may be abnormally low, although this is rarely seen. Second, there may be an adequate concentration of oxygen available, but inadequate amounts may be taken in. Third, adequate concentration and amounts may be taken in but inadequate diffusion from the alveoli into the blood occurs because of some obstruction in the alveoli, such as fluid or secretions, or in the capillary, such as a pulmonary embolus. By utilizing other facets of assessment, such as pulmonary function testing or auscultation of breath sounds, the critical care nurse can identify the cause of the hypoxemia.

Analysis of pCO_2 levels is somewhat more complex than analysis of pO_2. A general rule of thumb, however, for the beginning practitioner, is that pO_2 yields information concerning both the ventilatory or mechanical part of respiration and the gas diffusion aspect, while pCO_2 yields information only about the mechanical aspect. Carbon dioxide is constantly produced as a by-product of metabolism; it is the job of the lungs to eliminate this CO_2 through respiration. Hypoventilation will result in a build-up of CO_2 and hyperventilation will cause abnormally low pCO_2s. The pCO_2 and pO_2 have no direct relationship; that is, an abnormal pO_2 does not cause an abnormal pCO_2, although both may vary in response to the same stimulus or as a result of the same disease. The additional factor that must be considered is the way in which CO_2 production may vary and the interaction of CO_2 and pH.

In order to discuss pH, certain terms must be defined. First, it may be recalled that an *acid* is defined as any substance which is capable of donating a hydrogen ion; a *base* is any substance which is capable of accepting a hydrogen ion. The acidity of solutions are

TABLE 3-2

Arterial and Venous Blood Gas Values

	Arterial	Venous
pH	7.35-7.45	7.35-7.45
pO_2	80-100 mmHg	40 mmHg
pCO_2	38-42 mmHg	45 mmHg
HCO_3	23-25 mEq/l	
O_2 sat.	95-98%	40-70% (varies with site of sample)

measured by the concentration of hydrogen ions; the greater the free hydrogen ion concentration, the greater the acidity. Acidity is usually expressed in terms of pH. The pH is obtained by taking the negative logarithm of the hydrogen ion concentration; it is merely a convenient way to express acidity rather than dealing with the actual measurement of hydrogen ions, which would involve very small numbers and exponents (for example, the hydrogen ion content of blood at a normal pH of 7.4 is 0.000,000,039 moles per liter). The lower the pH, the greater the acidity, and the higher the concentration of hydrogen ions. The higher the pH, the lower the acidity and concentration of hydrogen ions. A pH of 7.0 is considered neutral; it contains equal concentrations of acids and bases.

A buffer is any substance which is capable of either combining with hydrogen ions to reduce the acidity and raise pH, or releasing hydrogen ions to increase the acidity and lower pH. Buffering systems are responsible for maintaining the pH of body fluids at a relatively stable level. Hydrogen is constantly liberated, in addition to CO_2, by metabolic processes and buffering systems are constantly operating in order to maintain blood pH between 7.35 and 7.45. Although there are several buffer systems which operate in the body, the lungs and kidneys are the major source of buffering; the lungs buffer by regulating CO_2 content, and the kidneys buffer more slowly than the lungs by regulating the bicarbonate content of the blood.

In the normal dynamic state which exists in the body, an equilibrium is maintained with the reaction shown in Figure 3-9.

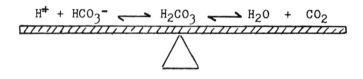

$$H^+ + HCO_3^- \longrightarrow H_2CO_3 \longrightarrow H_2O + CO_2$$

Figure 3-9.

As mentioned earlier (p. 205), this reaction takes place within the erythrocyte, aided by the enzyme carbonic anhydrase. For purposes of understanding, this equation can be viewed as a balance, with H_2CO_3 the mid-point, and equal "weights" or amounts on each end. A basic law of chemistry is that when a state of equilibrium is disturbed, the chemical reaction will proceed in the direction that will restore the equilibrium. Thus, if we add to one side of the equation, the reaction will proceed toward the opposite side in order to equalize the "weight," as shown in Figure 3-10.

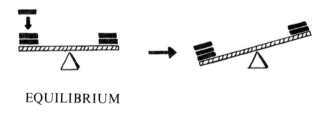

EQUILIBRIUM

IN ORDER
TO RESTORE
EQUILIBRIUM:

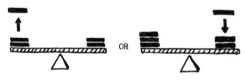

Figure 3-10.

Respiratory Acidosis

The patient who hypoventilates can serve as the first example. This patient, breathing too slowly, too shallowly, or both, is not eliminating carbon dioxide as fast as it is formed; hence, the CO_2 content increases as shown in Figure 3-11.

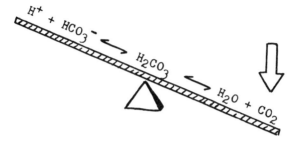

Figure 3-11.

The right side of the reaction now "outweighs" the left; the reaction will then shift to the left in order to restore equilibrium, causing an increase in the hydrogen ion content, and a fall in pH as shown in Figure 3-12.

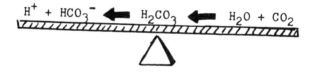

Figure 3-12.

Typical arterial blood gases of this state would be:

$$pH: 7.2 \qquad pCO_2: 60 \qquad HCO_3^-: 26$$

This is termed *respiratory acidosis; respiratory,* indicating that the cause is related to the ventilation pattern, *acidosis,* indicating that the pH is below normal. Note that the pO_2 was not included in the sample blood gases; it is irrelevant and could be quite low if the patient were hypoventilating room air, or near normal if the patient were receiving supplemental oxygen.

The primary buffering system of the body in this case would operate within the kidney. In respiratory acidosis the kidney will conserve the bicarbonate ion in order that it may combine with the excess free hydrogen and restore the pH to normal. This state is referred to as *compensated respiratory acidosis,* and typical blood gases would be: pH: 7.4; pCO_2: 60; HCO_3^-: 37. Note that the bicarbonate level is elevated, the pCO_2 elevated (because we haven't *corrected* the problem, only *compensated* for it), and the pH returned to normal.

Respiratory Alkalosis

Hyperventilation will produce exactly the opposite situation. In this case the patient is breathing too rapidly, too deeply, or both; CO_2 is eliminated faster than it is produced, and the CO_2 content becomes less, in relation to the other side of the equation as shown in Figure 3-13.

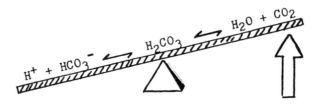

Figure 3-13.

The left side of the reaction now "outweighs" the right, and the chemical reaction will proceed toward the right as shown in Figure 3-14.

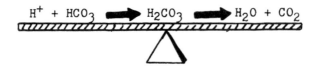

Figure 3-14.

The free hydrogen ions will be utilized as this reaction proceeds and the pH will rise. ABG (arterial blood gases) that would be seen in this example are:

$$\text{pH: } 7.5 \quad pCO_2: \ 28 \quad HCO_3^-: 24$$

When *respiratory alkalosis* occurs, the kidneys again act as the buffering organ and excrete bicarbonate, in an attempt to shift the reaction back to the left. ABG typical of compensated respiratory alkalosis, are:

$$\text{pH: } 7.4 \quad pCO_2: \ 30 \quad HCO_3^-: 18$$

Metabolic Acidosis and Alkalosis

States of metabolic acidosis and alkalosis result when the hydrogen ion content is altered not because of an abnormal ventilatory pattern, but because of the addition or build-up of free acids within the body or depletion of acid or base content. When metabolic factors cause a pH abnormality, the lungs act as the buffering organ by increasing or decreasing the CO_2 content. Because the lungs can respond to alterations in pH almost immediately, in contrast to the kidney which requires several hours, uncompensated states of metabolic acidosis or alkalosis are infrequently seen.

A common cause of metabolic acidosis is uncontrolled diabetes, in which the abnormal metabolism occurring with insulin lack leads to ketoacidosis. The metabolic processes lead to the addition of free hydrogen in the blood, lowering the pH. The lowered pH acts as a respiratory stimulant, and the lungs immediately begin to buffer by eliminating more CO_2, as represented in Figure 3-15.

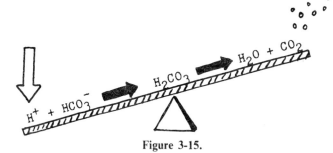

Figure 3-15.

As the pCO_2 falls below normal, then, the reaction shifts to the right, and the hydrogen and bicarbonate content are reduced. Blood gases that would be seen in this state are:

$$\text{pH: } 7.20 \quad pCO_2\text{: } 30 \quad HCO_3^-\text{: } 12$$

Metabolic alkalosis is again, just the opposite. When the hydrogen ion concentration is reduced, as the result of severe vomiting or diarrhea, for example, the pH rises; the higher pH acts as a respiratory depressant and the lungs immediately reduce CO_2 elimination. With hypoventilation the pCO_2 will increase, causing the reaction to shift to the left, thus partially restoring the hydrogen ion content as shown in Figure 3-16. The ABG would then be: pH: 7.50, pCO_2: 45, HCO_3^-: 35.

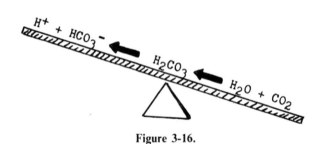

Figure 3-16.

The fourth and last portion of assessment of the patient with respiratory failure consists of miscellaneous tests and measurements, listed below.

Daily Weight

The importance of obtaining a daily weight of the patient cannot be over-emphasized. Even the most careful and scrupulous attention in recording intake and output will result in an inadequate representation of the patient's fluid balance. Consider the following sources of fluid gain or loss which cannot be measured: insensible loss (this averages 300-500 cc. per day, but can double in the presence of fever and is reduced in the intubated patient), respiratory therapy (respirators, with and without ultrasonic humidification, can contribute as much as several hundred ccs to the patient's fluid balance), intravenous fluids (manufacturers state that the content can vary as much as 100 cc. per 1000 cc. container), vomiting, and diarrhea. It can readily be seen that immeasurable sources of fluid gain or loss can change the intake and output balance by as much as 1000 cc. per day. Consequently, the only valid method to determine the state of hydration, which is essential in respiratory care, is to utilize daily weights.

Chest X-ray

Any patient in the acute phase of respiratory distress should have a chest x-ray taken daily. Minor changes or trends can be difficult to identify through physical assessment until symptoms are produced, but the x-ray can often demonstrate these changes before the symptoms occur and the treatment regime can thus be altered appropriately.

Tracheal Aspirate

The patient with respiratory disease is at increased risk of developing infection, both because his resistance as a host is reduced, and because treatment regimes unfortunately usually increase the potential sources of infection, such as ultrasonic nebulizers, suction catheters, etc. The intubated patient is especially susceptible because the normal protective mechanisms in the airway are bypassed by the endotracheal or tracheostomy tube. Sputum specimens should be obtained at least every other day for culture and sensitivity and Gram stain.

Fiberoptic Bronchoscopy

Bedside bronchoscopy can be used both as a diagnostic tool and as a therapeutic measure. In the past, because the only bronchoscope available was a rigid instrument, bronchoscopies were performed only in the operating room, where sedation and anesthesia could be readily employed and controlled lighting and positioning were available. Since the advent of the flexible fiberoptic bronchoscope, this procedure is easily carried out at the bedside (Figure 3-17.)

The bronchoscope is inserted through the airway, in a similar

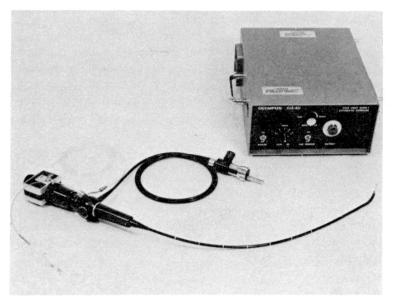

Figure 3-17. Fiberoptic Bronchoscope (Courtesy of Olympus Corporation of America, New Hyde Park, New York).

manner to inserting a suction catheter. It can be passed through the endotracheal or tracheostomy tube in the intubated patient or through the nose, with the aid of a nasal airway. The bronchoscope has its own light source; the reflected light beams enable the operator to visualize the respiratory tract and determine the location of the bronchoscope as it is advanced. The tip of the instrument can also be directed in order to move the catheter into the various bronchial segments.

In addition to inspection of the respiratory tract through visualization, suction is usually applied to the lumen of the bronchoscope and secretions that have accumulated can thus be cleared. Brush biopsies can also be obtained through bronchoscopy.

The role of the nurse when a bronchoscopy is performed begins with preparation of the patient. In addition to explanations and reassurance, mild sedation is sometimes helpful; a bronchoscopy is not painful but will cause the patient to cough and is uncomfortable. While the bronchoscope is in place, the patient's airway is partially occluded; for this reason, a high FiO_2 is usually desirable to reduce hypoxia. Careful monitoring of vital signs, particularly the cardiac rhythm, is also part of the nurse's responsibility.

RESPIRATORY FAILURE

In discussing pulmonary disease, there are several ways to classify the disorders: acute vs. chronic, according to system (neuromuscular, musculoskeletal, respiratory, CNS), or, the most common, obstructive vs. restrictive. Before elaborating on the latter method of classification, there are several general principles which will aid the reader in understanding the pathophysiology.

First, when actually caring for the patient, it is useful to keep in mind that there are few patients with a "pure disease"—most have elements of several pathological processes occurring simultaneously. Second, each disease entity consists of a battery of characteristic processes or abnormalities, and is thus more of a syndrome, with each individual patient exhibiting only some of the potential signs and symptoms. Third, all respiratory diseases may be viewed as producing symptoms either by way of abnormal mechanics and/or an abnormal ventilation/perfusion relationship.

Assessment of lung mechanics was described earlier under *pulmonary function*. In addition to changes in the amount of air exchanged with the atmosphere, the concept of *dead space* was discussed. Increase in dead space above the normal 0.3 represents one kind of abnormal ventilation/perfusion relationship. The other source of this abnormality is represented by the concept of *shunt*.

For ideal gas exchange to take place, every alveolus would be ventilated, and every ventilated alveolus would have a capillary blood supply for diffusion to take place. However, even without lung disease, there is not perfect equality in regard to ventilation/perfusion. First, there is the effect of anatomic dead space. In addition, body position causes an inequality; the most dependent portion of the lung tends to receive the greatest blood flow simply because of the effects of gravity, while the uppermost portion tends to receive the greatest air flow.

Shunt is defined as an area that is perfused but not ventilated, just the opposite of dead space. *Anatomic shunting* is caused by the small portion of the cardiac output that bypasses the pulmonary capillary bed, and returns to the left side of the heart via the bronchial and pulmonary veins. *Physiologic shunting* occurs when there are alveoli which receive normal perfusion but which are not ventilated, such as occurs with pooled secretions, atelectasis, or pneumothorax. Capillary shunting has been defined as existing when perfusion is normal and ventilation is zero; when the interference is less absolute, and a certain degree of shunting is present, *venous admixture* is said to occur.[10] This refers to the fact that venous blood, coming from the right side of the heart, returns to the left side and mixes with arterial blood without ever having become oxygenated.

Shunting can be estimated by administering 100% oxygen and measuring alveolar-arterial oxygen difference ($AaDO_2$). Normally, this difference should be only 30-40 mm. Hg; this corresponds to the 2-4% of cardiac output involved in anatomic shunting. After abdominal surgery, when hypoventilation and atelectasis are common problems, the $AaDO_2$ often rises to 300 mm. Hg (15%) and in respiratory failure reaches 400 mm. Hg (20%).[3]

This relationship of ventilation to perfusion is represented by the symbols V/Q (V = ventilation, Q = blood flow), and the normal ratio is 0.8. Figure 3-18 demonstrates a normal V/Q relationship, the effect of a dead space unit, and a shunt unit.

Obstructive vs. Restrictive Conditions

The most common way to classify respiratory disorders is to characterize each as either an obstructive or restrictive problem (Table 3-3). Obstructive diseases are those in which there is no re-

TABLE 3-3

Common Obstructive and Restrictive Disorders

Obstructive	Restrictive
Asthma	Atelectasis
Bronchitis	Kyphoscoliosis
Emphysema	Myasthenia Gravis
Cystic fibrosis	Guillain-Barré Syndrome
Large airway obstruction,	Pneumothorax
secondary to trauma,	Pulmonary edema
tonsilitis, cancer	ARDS
	Pleural effusion
	Cancer
	Obesity
	Tuberculosis

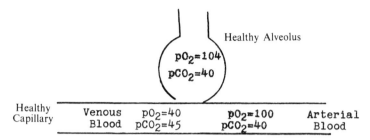

NORMAL VENTILATION/PERFUSION RELATIONSHIP

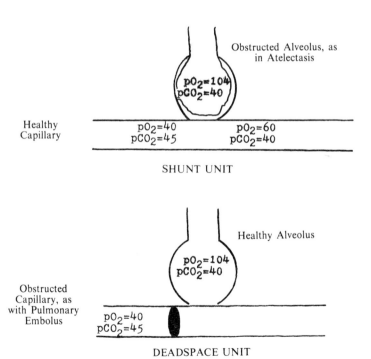

Figure 3-18. V/Q Relationships.

duction in thoracic excursion, but some interference with the movement of air and exchange between the atmosphere and blood supply. This would include the chronic obstructive lung diseases (COPD), asthma, bronchitis, emphysema, cystic fibrosis, and obstruction in the upper respiratory tract. Restrictive diseases are those in which there is a reduction in total lung capacity; included in this category are musculoskeletal diseases affecting the chest (kyphoscoliosis), neuromuscular diseases (Guillain-Barré syndrome, myasthenia gravis), CNS depression (anesthesia or drug induced), pneumothorax, pulmonary edema, and the adult respiratory distress syndrome (ARDS). The more common disease entities of each category will be briefly described before discussing nursing intervention.

Chronic Obstructive Pulmonary Diseases (COPD)

COPD has become one of the nation's largest health care problems, having increased 224% as a cause of death in the past 20 years.[4] Cigarette smoking, air pollution, and the rise in all chronic diseases, associated with our increased ability to prolong life into old age, have all contributed to this rise.

Asthma is characterized by episodic periods of bronchospasm during which there is contraction of the smooth muscles of the bronchi and bronchioles. It is associated with mucosal edema, and increased secretion production and secretion thickness, all of which produce narrowing of the airways, which causes the wheezing characteristic of this disorder. The etiology of asthma is thought to be primarily related to a hypersensitivity of the airway to a variety of allergens or stimuli, and the actual attacks may be precipitated by exposure to the allergen, by respiratory infection, or psychological stress.

Changes in pulmonary function associated with asthma are temporary increases in FRC, decreased flow rates, and decreased vital capacity. The earliest blood gas abnormality is hypoxemia; the pCO_2 is also often low, as the patient attempts to increase his minute ventilation in order to get more oxygen. In fact, when the pCO_2 of the asthmatic begins to rise, this is an indication that he is tiring and becoming unable to compensate.

These deviations are usually temporary and occur only during the attack. There may be eventual hyperinflation of alveoli and smooth muscle hyperplasia, but there is not usually any destruction of the lung tissue itself. In this sense asthma is quite different than emphysema and bronchitis.

Medical intervention centers around the use of bronchodilators. Steroids, supplemental oxygen, and mechanical intubation are necessary for prolonged, severe attacks (status asthmaticus), and the clearing of mucus plugs is of extreme importance when respiratory failure occurs.

Chronic bronchitis is a progressive disease characterized by hyperplasia of the mucus secreting cells in the bronchial tree. This hyperplasia leads to increased mucus production, which interferes with oxygen diffusion, producing local vasoconstriction and increased pulmonary resistance, eventually leading to cor pulmonale, right-sided heart failure.

Because of the cyanosis caused by bronchitis, and the peripheral edema associated with heart failure, patients with this disorder are characterized as "blue bloaters." Bronchitis occurs most commonly in men, ages 30-60, and is associated with respiratory infection and with cigarette smoking. The bronchitic patient demonstrates decreased flow rates, decreased vital capacity, normal residual volumes, mild hypercarbia and marked hypoxemia.

Treatment is aimed at removal of secretions. IPPB, suctioning, postural drainage and clapping, and mucolytic agents are all part of therapy. When positive sputum cultures are present, appropriate antibiotics are given.

Emphysema is the most common type of lung disease. It is an irreversible condition in which there is progressive destruction of the walls of the alveoli and reduction in the amount of connective tissue; consequently there is an increase in the size of the airway below the terminal bronchiole and loss of elastic properties of the lung. The capillary beds of the involved alveoli are also destroyed.

The emphysematous patient, called the "pink puffer" because of the flushing caused by hypercarbia, is persistently short of breath, with neck vein distention, and a barrel chest, reflecting the severe over-distention of airways. The patient will often have adopted a "pursed-lip" type of breathing in which he exhales slowly in order to prevent the collapse of small bronchioles. The hematocrit is often high in emphysema because of hypoxic stimulation of the bone marrow. Increases in FRC and total lung capacity, decreases in VC and FEV, severe hypoxemia and hypercarbia are all common findings.

Treatment starts with low-flow oxygen, carefully titrated according to blood gas results, because these patients' respiratory stimulus is primarily the pO_2, having become unresponsive to chronically elevated pCO_2. Pulmonary toilet, chest physiotherapy, and supportive care (e.g. nutritional supplements) are usual components of therapy.

In any of the chronic obstructive diseases, every effort is made to avoid mechanical ventilation, for several reasons. First, progress in the presence of chronic diseases is slow; prolonged periods on the ventilator may be necessary. Because of the reduced ventilatory capacity of COPD patients, weaning from ventilator support is often very difficult and sometimes impossible; even control of parameters is more difficult because the patient is accustomed to such "abnormal" states. Lastly, a very serious question must be asked—is it possible *and* worthwhile to the patient and significant others to attempt to reverse or stop the acute episode, which may be the inevitable terminal phase of this chronic disease?

Adult Respiratory Distress Syndrome (ARDS)

Of the restrictive diseases, one of the most commonly seen in the Intensive Care Unit is the Adult Respiratory Distress Syndrome (ARDS). This syndrome has, in the past, been given various names, including shock lung, wet lung, stiff lung, and low-flow syndrome, but it is now believed that all of these terms describe the same entity. The hallmark of this condition is a progressive fall in pO_2 which is refractory to increasing FiO_2. It is thought that the major etiologic factor is a reduction in surfactant production, which is a response of the alveolar Type II cells, which produce surfactant, to a variety of harmful states, such as the reduced perfusion of shock, the deposition of debris in the lung from multiple blood transfusions, and acute chemical injury of the capillary membrane. The reduction in surfactant leads to alveolar collapse, which in turn produces increased shunting, hypoxemia, decreased compliance, and an increase in the work of breathing.

The classic picture of the patient with ARDS is one in which the patient is admitted to the ICU following a major trauma. Initially ventilation appears adequate; progressive hypoxemia appears within 2-3 days and does not respond to increasing oxygen therapy. Some atelectasis is evident on x-ray, but it is not until the 4th or 5th day that the x-ray shows the diffuse white-out, similar to pulmonary edema, characteristic of this disease. Usually before this is documented on x-ray, the patient has progressed into frank respiratory failure and has required mechanical ventilation.

Treatment must include ventilator support with positive end expiratory pressure (PEEP), which will be discussed later. Steroids are frequently employed, although there is no definitive evidence that they have any beneficial effect, diuretics administered to reduce the interstitial edema, and fluid therapy carefully restricted.

Pulmonary edema: another common type of restrictive respiratory disease. This condition is classified as restrictive because the presence of fluid in the interstitium reduces compliance and in this way restricts expansion.

Pulmonary edema may be viewed as the consequence of the heart's inability to circulate the intravascular volume, regardless of whether this is due to fluid overload or left heart failure. As the output of the left heart fails to adequately circulate sufficient volume, the pressure increases in the pulmonary capillary bed; when this pressure exceeds serum osmotic pressure and the hydrostatic pressure on the opposite side of the capillary membrane, fluid leaks into the interstitial spaces of the alveoli. In addition to reducing compliance, diffusion is blocked.

The signs and symptoms of frank pulmonary edema are easily recognized and not easily forgotten. The patient becomes extremely apprehensive, breath sounds become quite wet, and copious, frothy, pink-tinged secretions are present. The patient is usually tachycardic, tachypneic, and hypotensive.

Digitalization, diuretics, and oxygen are administered immediately. Sedation is sometimes required, and in the presence of severe failure, rotating tourniquets may be used to reduce circulating blood volume. Mechanical ventilation may be required in order to improve oxygenation and manage secretions.

Pneumothorax: while not a disease, is a condition which causes a restriction in lung expansion. Pneumothorax literally means air within the thoracic cavity; this occurs when there is a communication between the pleural cavity and the atmosphere, as occurs with a stab wound, or rupture of a lung bleb. As was described earlier, the pleural space normally maintains a slightly negative pressure; when the intactness of either the parietal or visceral pleura is disrupted, air enters. Once the pressure within the pleural cavity is equalized, there is no longer any force holding the lung to the thoracic cage, and that portion of the lung will not expand with inspiration. The pneumothorax may be quite small and self-limiting, or may be large enough to significantly interfere with ventilation. A *tension pneumothorax* exists when there is air leakage into the pleural space without an avenue for air escape. The pressure within the pleural space then exceeds atmospheric pressure and causes a progressive collapse of lung tissue; the accumulation of air may be large enough to shift the mediastinal structures, the heart and great vessels, and cause arrythmias, shock, and cardiac arrest.

The only treatment for a pneumothorax is the insertion of a chest tube. The chest tube may lead to a water seal bottle only, or may also have suction applied in addition to the water seal bottle (Figure 3-19). Closed chest drainage allows air and fluid to be drained from the pleural space while preventing additional air from entering. As was described, during inspiration, as the chest wall and parietal pleura are pulled away from the lung and visceral pleura, intrapleural pressure becomes more negative and a vacuum is created; air would then enter the pleural space through the chest tube, but the layer of water at the end of the tube prevents this. During expiration, the chest wall and lungs recoil and intrapleural pressure increases; this facilitates the movement of air and fluid out through the chest tube. A common observation made is to have the patient cough and observe for the presence of bubbling in the chest tube bottle, indicating that some air is still present in the pleural cavity.

The proper functioning of the chest tube is the responsibility of the nurse. Measures to insure this, such as preventing kinking of the tubing or dependent loops of tubing, safely securing the bottle below the level of the chest, and adequate observation are of extreme importance. The amount and color of drainage should be carefully recorded, in addition to the presence or absence of bubbling or fluctuation of the water level in the tubing. Transporting the patient with a chest tube, from the recovery room to the ICU, for example, poses an additional risk and the need for extra caution. Chest tube clamps

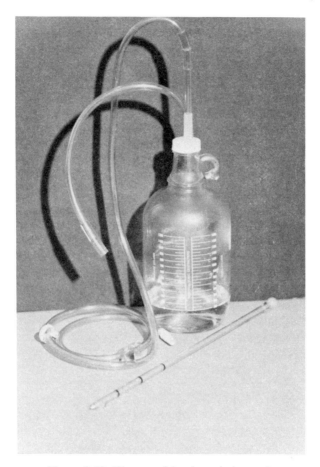

Figure 3-19. Water seal bottle and chest tube.

should be at the bedside at all times; however, an actively draining chest tube, that is, one in which there is fluctuation of fluid in the tubing or bubbling in the bottle, should *never* be clamped, even when moving the patient. This could create the situation described earlier, a tension pneumothorax.

Pulmonary embolus: the last condition to be discussed is one which is all too familiar to ICU staff. A pulmonary embolus is caused by an obstruction, usually a blood clot, which has lodged in the pulmonary vascular bed. The most common source of these thrombi is the peripheral circulation, particularly the deep veins of the lower extremities. It has been estimated that pulmonary emboli occur in as many as 15% of all hospitalized patients, according to autopsy findings, but that only 50% of these are diagnosed at the time they occur.[16]

The effect of an obstruction to perfusion is an increase in physiologic dead space. Depending upon the degree of obstruction, there will be hypoxemia and also a reduced pCO_2 if the patient hyperventilates. As with pulmonary edema, the patient is often anxious, tachypneic, tachycardic, and may be hypotensive if there is a significant reduction in blood return to the left side of the heart. In addition, pain and fever are often present. With large emboli, an ECG may reflect right-sided strain. Chest x-ray, lung scan, and pulmonary angiography will yield definitive evidence as to the location and severity of the embolus.

Anticoagulation is the major component of therapy. Intravenous heparin is administered immediately, and oral anticoagulation therapy started within several days. The patient is usually restricted to bedrest and oxygen used to reduce the hypoxemia. Surgical removal of the clot, embolectomy, may be necessary in severe cases. Mechanical ventilation is not usually indicated, except in the presence of very low pO_2s.

INTERVENTION

Intervention always begins with an accurate assessment. There is no patient care measure that is dictated solely by diagnosis or any one laboratory finding; observation and clinical judgment based on all available data serve to direct therapy and specify intervention. In order to discuss the nursing care of the patient with disorders of the respiratory system, the common methods of intervention and usual indications for each will be presented, beginning with the nonintubated paitient.

The goal of all respiratory care is to maintain ventilation in order to insure adequate oxygenation of tissues. In the nonintubated patient this care usually has two specific aims: to assist in the mechanical portion of respiration, and to maintain a patent airway, including the small airways.

Often the simplest of nursing care measures are the most effective if used early. There are four measures which will assist the patient with compromised pulmonary function in maintaining adequate exchange. First is positioning: an upright position will prevent the abdominal contents from impinging on chest excursion and the head of the patient's bed should be kept elevated to the degree of comfort. When resting, elevating the shoulder girdle by having the patient sit upright and leaning his arms on a bedside table raised to chest height will also reduce the work of breathing. It is essential that the respiratory patient not become overly fatigued; finding a position which will allow him to breathe adequately while resting comfortably is a significant part of avoiding the need for intubation and mechanical ventilation.

Teaching is an often neglected tool in the Intensive Care Unit. Patients can be taught breathing patterns and exercises which will increase their ventilatory capacity, and this intervention should not be reserved for the rehabilitative phase of respiratory care. As with any kind of teaching, a plan should be made which begins with an approach designed to elicit patient understanding and cooperation. With the patient sitting upright, the nurse can first demonstrate the various portions of the lung to be expanded by having the patient place his hands over his ribs, over the sternum, and then under the axilla as he takes several breaths. Some patients can be taught to consciously control and increase expansion of each area, or at least each side; most patients readily see how ventilatory volume can be increased voluntarily. With the surgical patient, the use of adequate pain medication and incisional support is a necessary adjunct to teaching.

Diaphragmatic or augmented abdominal breathing is taught with the patient lying in bed, with knees flexed. He is instructed to take in as much air as possible, hold his breath for a moment, then exhale through pursed lips, in order to achieve a slow air flow with low turbulence. As he exhales, he is asked to contract his abdominal muscles in order to elevate the diaphragm and assist lung emptying. Placing books or the patient's hands on his abdomen will help this.

Many commercial devices are available which assist in either the inspiratory or expiratory phase of respiration. Use of devices such as blow bottles enable the patient to generate high intra-alveolar pressures as he attempts to exhale against resistance; it is thought that this promotes alveolar expansion. IPPB is the best known inspiratory device. Intermittent positive pressure machines deliver air to the patient at a pre-set pressure, with the patient initiating or "triggering" each breath as he begins to inhale. IPPB can be quite beneficial and is often used to deliver medication such as bronchodilators; however, there are several precautions which must be observed. First, IPPB machines have been implicated in the transmission of bacteria; respiratory patients receiving IPPB should each have their own machine, in addition to having mouthpiece and manifold changed daily. Second, in order to benefit from IPPB, the patient must be taught to breathe with the machine, and "accept" the deep breath delivered. Gastric dilation sometimes occurs because the patient swallows air during the treatment. The hyperventilation achieved with a successful treatment can be quite fatiguing and adequate supervision is necessary to insure that the patient stops every few minutes to rest. More recently, the incentive spirometer has been used in clinical practice; this device assists patients in performing an inspiratory-hold maneuver.

The second aim of respiratory care with the nonintubated patient is to maintain a patent airway, which usually involves the adequate removal of secretions. The best and most effective way to clear secretions is to cough; the ideal situation then is to be able to assist the patient in coughing, rather than having to utilize artificial means. In addition to teaching and adequate pain medication, of major importance in helping the patient to clear secretions by coughing is adequate humidification. Again, the patient's own mechanisms are much more successful than ours, and the best way to liquify secretions is to adequately hydrate the patient. In the presence of dehydration, secretions are thick, tenacious, and difficult to clear, even with suctioning.

Postural drainage and clapping are techniques with which the ICU nurse must be comfortable, even if the services of a licensed physical therapist are available. Most hospitals cannot provide P.T. around the clock, and the nurse must be able to continue treatment, if needed, during the evening and night shifts. Postural drainage involves positioning the patient in ways which will promote the movement by gravity of secretions into the upper respiratory tract, where they can be easily coughed out. Positions chosen are based on segments of the lung which are involved in disease; the condition of the patient in the Intensive Care Unit adds an additional factor, usually a limitation, in choosing postural drainage positions. The six most commonly used positions and the areas of the lung drained by each are described on the following page.

1. *Supine:* lying flat, knees elevated: anterior segments of right and left bronchus.
2. *Prone:* hips elevated: posterior portion of lower lobes.
3. *Supine:* head and chest elevated: apical segment of right and left upper lobes.
4. *Lying on right side:* at least 45°, hips elevated: right lower lobe, lateral segment.
6. *Sitting in a chair, leaning forward:* posterior segment of upper lobes.

Clapping and vibrating is done with the patient in the postural drainage positions and facilitates the loosening of secretions. Clapping, or percussion, is done by placing the hands in a cupped position, with the fingers and thumb closed; the wrists are then flexed and extended. The sound produced should be a muffled, hollow sound, produced by air trapped between the hand and the patient's chest; a flat, slapping sound is an indication of incorrect technique. Clapping is always done over a sheet or the patient's gown, never on bare skin.

Vibrating is done by placing the palm of the hand on the chest wall, holding the arm rigid, and vibrating the hand rapidly while exerting gentle pressure on the chest. The patient is instructed to take a deep breath and vibration is applied during expiration. It should be emphasized that none of these measures, positioning, IPPB, clapping or vibrating, is effective by themselves; the patient must then cough to remove the secretions, or they must be cleared with suctioning.

Tracheal suctioning is a very efficient, but traumatic procedure for most patients. The nurse should not hesitate to use it when indicated, but only after other measures to assist the patient to cough have failed. Often it is necessary because the patient has become too fatigued or is too weak to generate an effective cough.

Suctioning is a sterile procedure—there are no exceptions to this. Sterile catheter, gloves, rinse solution, and lubricant are necessary; none of these components is re-used—soaking the catheters or using rinse solution from a covered basin that remains at the bedside is not adequate. The sequence of actions in the suctioning procedure is as follows:

1. Prepare the patient. This includes explaining what will be done

and positioning the patient in a sitting position, with a pillow behind his shoulders and his head tilted back in order to facilitate easy access to the trachea.

Some clinicians recommend the practice of turning the patient's shoulders to the left and his head to the right to facilitate entering the left bronchus, and turning shoulders to the right and head to the left to facilitate entering the right bronchus. However, there is no objective evidence that this technique increases the ability to direct the catheter into either side; bronchoscopy remains the only way to be certain which bronchus is entered. In the majority of patients, the right main-stem bronchus is suctioned far more often than the left, because of the anatomical differences; this is part of why postural drainage and clapping are such important adjuncts to suctioning.

2. Hyperoxygenate with 100% oxygen. This is best accomplished by holding an anesthesia bag or ambu bag with attached oxygen lightly over the face and asking the patient to take 5 or 6 deep breaths. When suctioning secretions from the airway, oxygen is also removed and the pO_2 drops; if the patient already has a low pO_2, cardiac arrhythmias, such as ectopic beats and bradyarrhythmias, may result.

3. The catheter, lubricated with water or a water-soluble lubricant, is inserted into the nares, back and downwards. For most adults, a size 14 French, 14 inches long, is appropriate. When inserting the catheter, no suction is applied, to avoid removing the air in the upper airways and causing mucosal damage. As the catheter reaches the epiglottis, resistance will be felt; at this point the patient should be asked to take a deep breath and cough. This will usually open the epiglottis and allow the catheter to be advanced into the trachea. The tongue sometimes serves as an obstruction to the trachea, and having the patient stick his tongue out is also helpful; with an uncooperative patient, it may be necessary to grasp the tongue with a 4 x 4 gauze pad and pull it forward. If the nurse has succeeded in getting the catheter into the trachea, the patient will usually begin to cough, and air can be heard whistling back through the catheter.

4. Once in the trachea, suction is applied to the catheter, the catheter rotated and withdrawn. To minimize trauma to the tracheal mucosa, the suction should not exceed −80 cm. H_2O. If secretions are thick, 3-5 cc. of saline can be instilled through the catheter prior to suctioning. If it was very difficult to direct the catheter into the trachea, rather than withdrawing the catheter each time as suction is applied, the catheter can be left in the trachea, suction applied for 5 seconds, then disconnected and low flow (2 liters/min.) oxygen connected to the catheter to re-oxygenate the patient, and suction then attached again.

5. When the catheter is removed, it should be rinsed in sterile water before using again; 100% oxygen is administered prior to additional suctioning, and upon completion of the procedure.

If repeated suctioning is required, leaving a nasal airway in place will protect the nasal passages from excessive trauma. However, even when the measures mentioned are used to minimize trauma to the patient, the effort of the induced coughing and the discomfort make this procedure unpleasant, at the least, and suctioning should be carried out only when there is a definite indication.

The Intubated Patient

Despite the most well-planned and skillfully executed care, a certain percentage of patients will require intubation and mechanical ventilation for treatment of respiratory disease. Criteria for the institution of mechanical ventilation will depend on the overall condition of the patient and underlying pathology, but the following guidelines are generally recognized as indications for intubation:[1]

Indications for Mechanical Ventilation
1. Vital capacity < 10 cc./kg. body weight
2. pH < 7.25
3. Alveolar-arterial oxygen tension difference > 350 mm. Hg
4. pO_2 < 50 mm. Hg breathing room air
5. pCO_2 > 50 mm. Hg

Note that these criteria apply to adults only, and that #4 and #5 are not valid for the patient with chronic, compensated hypercarbia, such as the emphysema patient.

The patient who is being maintained on mechanical ventilation provides one of the most frequent and most challenging of nursing responsibilities in the Intensive Care Unit. First and foremost of the tasks confronting the nurse caring for the intubated patient is that of providing emotional support. Consider the effect of having an endotracheal tube inserted, having every breath delivered by a very strange and complex machine, and being unable to ask questions, complain, or even call for help! Support begins with a calm, reassuring approach; explanations are essential and should be repeated each time the nurse intervenes, e.g., each time she suctions the patient. Anger, frustration, and fear are all common reactions on the part of the patient. Knowing what to expect will reduce stress to some extent, particularly in terms of predictable sensations. For example, the patient will be much less frightened if he knows that it will make him cough when the endotracheal tube is moved, that he may momentarily feel as if he is choking when he is suctioned, that hyperventilating him with an anesthesia bag will make him feel like he is taking a deep breath.

One of the most difficult aspects for the intubated patient is the inability to communicate verbally. Pad and pencil or some sort of writing material should be offered to every patient. Not all patients, however, are comfortable with writing or are able to express their needs in writing, and these patients depend upon the nurse to identify needs, feelings, and concerns, and then verify these by asking the patient.

Fright is often relieved by giving the patient a means to summon help. Call lights are sometimes neglected in the belief that the patient is in constant attendance by the staff; unfortunately, this knowledge reassures only the staff. In addition to call lights, commercial devices are available which work in line with the call system but consist of a small magnetic pad that only requires a slight press of a finger or even the patient's head, for use with quadriplegic patients or patients in restraints.

The Ventilator

Ventilators themselves vary considerably according to manufacturer; each has somewhat different controls, alarm systems, advantages, and disadvantages. In describing characteristics, ventilators are usually categorized as either pressure pre-set ventilators, or volume pre-set ventilators. Pressure pre-set ventilators are those designed to deliver gas until a certain pre-determined pressure, e.g., 30-40 cm., is reached in the system; the volume that is delivered is incidental and depends entirely upon the pressure limit and compliance of the patient's lungs. Volume ventilators are those which will deliver a certain pre-determined volume of gas to the patient, e.g., 800-900 cc., utilizing as much pressure as is required in order to do so.

Regardless of the specific ventilator used, there are certain features, or parameters, of which the nurse must be aware at all times. Most often it is the physician's responsibility to actually determine the proper settings and order these in writing; however, it is part of the nurse's role to know what these settings are, to assess the effectiveness of the ventilator with these given settings, and to identify the need for readjustment.

Tidal volume is certainly among the most significant of ventilator parameters. It should be viewed in conjunction with the patient's respiratory rate in evaluating adequacy of minute volume. That is, if the tidal volume is too low, the patient will breathe more rapidly in order to achieve an adequate minute volume (TV x rate = minute volume); if the TV is too high, the patient will breathe more slowly, or may not trigger the ventilator at all, which is a reflection of lowered pCO_2 and inadequate respiratory stimulus. A tidal volume of 10-15 cc./kg. and a rate of 15 is usually adequate when initiating ventilation.

"Triggering" the ventilator is a phrase used to indicate that the patient is controlling or stimulating each breath. In general it is preferable to allow the patient to initiate each respiration, rather than having the ventilator control respirations entirely. This is more comfortable for the patient and results in easier weaning. This aspect of ventilation is usually determined by a sensitivity setting on the ventilator.

Oxygen percentage is the third essential parameter, in addition to tidal volume and rate. The guiding principle is to use the lowest FiO_2 which will achieve an acceptable pO_2. It is appropriate to view oxygen as a drug in this sense; just as there is one appropriate dosage of a given drug for an individual patient, there is one appropriate oxygen level, and it is never justified to administer "a little extra." A rule of thumb for determining initial FiO_2 is:[11]

$$\frac{AaDO_2 + 100}{\text{atmospheric pressure}}$$

For example, if the $AaDO_2$ is 350, the calculation would be: $350 + 100 = 450 \div 760 = .5$, or 50% O_2. This will usually result in a somewhat high pO_2, which can subsequently be lowered by gradually decreasing the FiO_2.

Pressure gauges will reflect the amount of pressure actually being utilized; it is a reflection of the compliance of the patient's lungs. A gradual increase in the system pressure of a volume ventilator, or a gradual decrease in the tidal volume of a pressure ventilator denotes decreasing compliance; this could be caused by several changes, such as worsening of pulmonary edema, pneumothorax, or inspissated secretions, all of which increase resistance to lung expansion.

Peak flow determines the speed or rate at which the gas is delivered. It must be adequate in order to allow the patient to breathe in a normal rhythm, which is to have twice as long for expiration as for inspiration. An abnormal I:E ratio is effected by the interaction of flow rate, respiratory rate, and tidal volume. Consider the following example:

> Pre-set tidal volume = 800 cc.
> Flow rate: 24 liters/min.
> Respiratory rate: 20/min.
> 20 respirations/min. = 3 sec./respiratory cycle
> 24 liters/min. = 400 cc./sec.

A TV of 800 cc. then requires 2 seconds to deliver (400 cc. per second). In order to have 20 breaths per minute, each respiratory cycle can only last 3 seconds; if 2 seconds are utilized in inspiration, expiration can only last 1 second. The I:E ratio is then the reverse of normal. To correct the situation, the peak flow rate must be increased to at least 48 liters per minute.

An additional observation which should be part of the nurse's continuous assessment is the temperature of the gas delivered. Most ventilators have a thermometer installed in the inspiratory line; this should read close to body temperature, or 37° C. If not, an adjustment needs to be made in the heating element of the cascade.

It is the nurse's responsibility to maintain mechanical ventilation in a safe and effective fashion. In addition to knowledge of the basic principles of ventilation, this requires a knowledge of the hazards. Overconfidence or complete reliance on alarm systems and the proper functioning of equipment will inevitably result in a disastrous outcome for the patient. There is no substitute for close observation of the patient. A cardinal rule in the care of the ventilated patient is that if the patient begins fighting the respirator, having labored respirations, or any kind of respiratory difficulty, disconnect him from the ventilator and manually bag-breathe the patient until the cause of the problem can be ascertained.

A not uncommon complication of mechanical ventilation is pneumothorax. The increased airway pressure caused by the use of positive pressure ventilators is sometimes sufficient to cause rupture of blebs or tears in friable pleural membranes. Signs and symptoms of this are sudden respiratory distress, absent breath sounds, tachycardia, and restlessness. Treatment consists of the insertion of a chest tube which must be done immediately.

An even more frequently occurring hazard is infection. Most respiratory infections are the result of transmission of organisms by contact, rather than air-borne transmission. This means that high infection rates are a serious indictment of technique in the ICU. Daily tracheal aspirate cultures in addition to routine surveillance of respiratory therapy equipment should be standard procedure in the ICU.

Positioning

The importance of position changes in the respiratory patient has been discussed earlier. Intubation and use of a ventilator are *not* contraindications to getting the patient out of bed and into a chair. Although this often requires a certain amount of ingenuity on the part of the nurse, especially in working with the patient with many tubes, catheters, and monitoring cables, assisting the patient to get out of bed will be rewarded with increased ventilatory capacity and an increased sense of well-being on the part of the patient.

Airway Maintenance

Protection and maintenance of a patent airway in the intubated patient has two essential components—proper cuff management and suctioning technique. The advent of low pressure cuffs on endotracheal tubes has simplified care and reduced the risk of mucosal damage and tracheal erosion. The new low pressure cuffed tubes are characterized by a softer plastic construction, are more compliant, and have large residual volumes; when inflated with air sufficient to create a seal between the tube and tracheal wall, they exert 20-70 mm. Hg pressure, in comparison to the older "hard cuff" tubes which exerted 70-240 mm. Hg pressure.[14]

A great deal of controversy has centered around the practice of deflating the cuff every hour for two or three minutes. There is currently no objective evidence that this practice serves any purpose. Therefore, it is recommended that the cuff on the endotracheal tube be deflated once or twice per shift, to insure that the proper inflation volume is used, and that hourly deflation be avoided.

Proper inflation volume is that volume which creates an effective seal between tracheal wall and endotracheal tube. Effective may be defined as an intracuff pressure of at least 25 cm. H_2O (the pressure necessary to prevent the aspiration of fluid past the cuff)[2] and permit positive pressure ventilation without loss of tidal volume. This is achieved by first aspirating the cuff to insure that it is completely deflated, then gradually inflating it until no leak of air is heard or felt around the tube. The "minimum leak" is then obtained by withdrawing 1/2 cc. of air after the seal is obtained; this guarantees that the absolute minimum amount of pressure is being generated against the tracheal wall.

The principles of suctioning the intubated patient are identical to those guiding the suctioning of the non-intubated patient. Sterile technique and adequate oxygenation are mandatory. Patients should be suctioned as often as necessary, probably at least every 2 hours for most patients.

Fluid and Electrolyte Balance

Several additional considerations are warranted in evaluating the fluid and electrolyte status of the ventilated patient. The increased intrathoracic pressure associated with mechanical ventilation may cause a temporary reduction in venous return and cardiac output; this is in turn, sometimes associated with inappropriate secretion of antidiuretic hormone (ADH). This will result in sodium and water retention and decreased urine output. This must not be interpreted as intravascular volume deficit; it is normally a self-limiting phenomenon and fluids should be restricted.

In caring for the patient with chronic lung disease, the nurse should be alert to signs and symptoms of potassium and chloride deficit. These patients are frequently on diuretics to manage the heart failure associated with their disease; they often will come to the hospital with dehydration and hypokalemia, having reduced their dietary intake of water and potassium as they began to feel ill. Adequate chloride levels must be maintained in order that the normal buffer system be able to operate in the RBC, through the mechanism of the chloride shift. Chloride levels may be reduced in the presence of alkalosis; chloride is excreted in place of hydrogen when the concentration of free hydrogen is low.

Positive End Expiratory Pressure (PEEP) is the technique of maintaining positive pressure at the end of the respiratory cycle. Normally, at the end of exhalation, airway pressures return to atmospheric pressure; with PEEP, 2-30 cm. H_2O pressure is maintained constantly by the ventilator. The effect of this is to increase functional residual capacity and prevent the collapse of many alveoli. The addition of PEEP makes it possible to achieve acceptable pO_2 levels with a lower FiO_2, by facilitating the exchange of gases in alveoli kept open during expiration. It may be used any time it becomes necessary to administer 60% or greater FiO_2, and is an essential component of therapy in Acute Respiratory Distress Syndrome.

The problems associated with the use of PEEP are related to the increased intrathoracic pressure it causes. The risk of tension pneumothorax is many times greater when PEEP is used, as is the incidence of subcutaneous emphysema. Venous return to the heart is also impeded, particularly if the patient is not well hydrated. Some patients who have been ventilated with high levels of PEEP (20-30 cm.) while conscious, have complained of discomfort and a feeling of tightness in the chest.

When using PEEP it should be remembered, particularly in very severe disease conditions, that when the patient is disconnected from the ventilator for suctioning, the positive pressure effect is lost. Consequently, alveolar collapse may occur and, although manually bag-breathing the patient with 100% O_2, precipitous drops in pO_2 may result. In these cases, it is more advantageous to increase the FiO_2

of the ventilator to 100% and place the patient back on the respirator between each suctioning.

WEANING

The criteria for weaning the patient from ventilatory support are just the opposite of those for initiating support; i.e., a pH above 7.25, VC above 10 cc./kg., and AaDO2 less than 350 on spontaneous breathing. There are numerous alternative ways in which to wean a patient, but generally the patient is allowed to breathe spontaneously with supplemental oxygen; blood gases and pulmonary function are then evaluated after 5-15 minutes. The specific plan for weaning will depend on several variables.

First, the patient's overall condition must be relatively stable if the weaning is to be successful. If fluid balance, cardiac hemodynamics, or neurological function are questionable, weaning should be postponed. Second, the longer the patient has been maintained on the ventilator, the more gradual should be the weaning. Third, weaning will usually be poorly tolerated in the presence of untreated or complicated abdominal disease, such as severe abdominal distention or sub-diaphragmatic abscess, which will significantly interfere with ventilatory capacities. A fourth factor which must be considered is the patient's emotional readiness to relinquish ventilator support. The nurse can often intervene in assisting the patient to become ready in providing him with explanations of the plan, including the rationale, and by providing the reassurance and close attention he will need.

The most common plan for weaning after prolonged ventilation involves short periods of spontaneous breathing alternating with periods back on the ventilator. The length of time the patient breathes on his own is then gradually increased; for example, the first day the patient would be off the ventilator for 15 minutes every 2 hours, on the second day he would be off 30 minutes every 2 hours, and on the third day, off the ventilator for an hour or 2 at a time. Weaning is stopped at night in order to allow for sleep. The purpose of this method is to allow the patient to gradually increase strength and become accustomed to breathing spontaneously. When the patient has demonstrated the ability to maintain adequate respirations for 8-12 continuous hours, he is then extubated.

An alternative method involves the use of Intermittent Mandatory Ventilation (IMV). With this technique an oxygen reservoir is connected to the inspiratory line of the ventilator with a one-way valve and the rate and sensitivity settings decreased. When the patient begins to take a breath, then, rather than triggering the respirator, he breathes spontaneously from the reservoir bag. In addition to this spontaneous breathing, a minimal number of breaths are delivered by the ventilator. In this way the patient begins to breathe on his own without having to be completely disconnected from the ventilator. Initially the ventilator rate can be set close to his normal rate, e.g., 10-12, so that most inspirations are ventilator-supplied, and as the patient's condition improves, the number of ventilator breaths is reduced. In addition to the increased safety of having a certain number of respirations each minute guaranteed by the ventilator, it can be a more gradual method of weaning, and is sometimes better tolerated emotionally by the patient.

Continuous positive airway pressure (CPAP) is a maneuver similar to PEEP, in that it is used to prevent the collapse of aveoli, but CPAP is used with spontaneous breathing, rather than mechanical ventilation. As a step in the weaning process, the patient may be disconnected from the ventilator and allowed to breathe spontaneously; the endotracheal tube is attached, with a t-piece or similar equipment, to wide-bore tubing with a Y-connector and one-way valve. At one end of the Y-connector is an oxygen reservoir, providing the appropriate FiO_2 under pressure for inspiration. At the other end of the Y is the expiratory port, which is partially occluded. The partial occlusion, which can be accomplished with a water-seal device, serves as positive pressure against which the patient must breath during expiration. This resistance serves to generate a higher intrathoracic pressure, which is maintained throughout the respiratory cycle.

TRACHEOSTOMY

Tracheostomy is indicated when it is established that prolonged intubation and mechanical ventilation will be required. There are no absolute criteria in terms of the number of days of intubation after which a tracheostomy should be performed, but it is usually considered if ventilation is required beyond 1-2 weeks. Before the advent of soft endotracheal tubes and high compliance cuffs it was common to elect tracheostomy after 3 days of intubation, but this is no longer required.

The disadvantages of tracheostomy in comparison to endo-tracheal intubation center around the fact that it is an operative pro-cedure. It is often viewed as a poor prognostic sign by the patient and family. The open wound offers an additional site for infection. A small percentage of patients do experience delayed wound heal-ing, scar formation, and tracheal stenosis.

The advantages of tracheostomy far outweigh the disadvan-tages, however, if intubation must be prolonged. A tracheostomy tube is much more comfortable for the patient; it avoids the necrosis of the nares sometimes associated with nasal endotracheal tubes and the skin breakdown caused by the ties on oral endotracheal tubes. Patients are more easily and safely ambulated with a tracheostomy. The danger of laryngeal damage caused by movement of the endo-tracheal tube is avoided. The patient with a tracheostomy can eat, avoiding the need for hyperalimentation or tube feedings.

The principles of airway maintenance; e.g., in terms of safety or suctioning technique, are the same. In addition, strict aseptic tech-nique must be used in caring for the tracheostomy wound. Sterile dressing changes using a povidone-iodine solution to clean the wound, should be done at least once every 8 hours.

EXTUBATION

When the patient is extubated, it is tempting to think of the job as completed, and well done! However, a great deal of intervention is still required, particularly if the patient has been ventilated for a prolonged period of time. It is more appropriate to think of respira-tory care on a continuum, with independent functioning at one end and mechanical ventilation at the other, as shown below.

Adequate function; no inter-vention	Somewhat reduced respiratory function; intermittent treatments required	Significant impairment; intensive nursing intervention required	Inadequate respiration; intubation and mechanical ventilation required	Severely compromised function; mechanical ventilation with PEEP required

The patient who is extubated can not go from a state of sup-ported ventilation to one of independent respiratory function; rather, he must pass through the successive levels. Initially a great deal of intervention is required, including most of the specific measures used prior to intubation, such as suctioning, postural drainage and clapping, etc. The ease with which the patient is able to do this is primarily a function of the skill and efforts of the critical care nurse.

REFERENCES

1. Bushnell SS: *Respiratory Intensive Care Nursing.* Little, Brown, and Company, Boston, Mass., 1973.
2. Carroll RG and Grenvik A: Proper use of large diameter, large residual volume cuffs. *Critical Care Medicine* May-June: 153-154, 1973.
3. Codd J and Grohar ME: Postoperative pulmonary complications. *Nursing Clinics of North America* 10:5-15, 1975.
4. Comroe JH: *Physiology of Respiration.* Year Book Medical Publishers, Inc., Chicago, Ill., 1965.
5. Fitzgerald LM and Huber GL: Weaning the patient from mechanical ventilation. *Heart and Lung* 5:228-234, 1976.
6. Gracey DR: Adult respiratory distress syndrome. *Heart and Lung* 4:280-283, 1975.
7. Guyton A: *Textbook of Medical Physiology.* 5th Ed. W.B. Saunders, Philadelphia, Pa., 1976.
8. Hudak CM, et al.: *Critical Care Nursing.* J.B. Lippincott, Philadelphia, Pa., 1973.
9. Robertson KJ and Guzzetta CE: Arterial blood gas interpretations in the respiratory ICU. *Heart and Lung* 5:256-260, 1976.
10. Shapiro BA, et al.: *Clinical Application of Respiratory Care.* Year Book Medical Publishers, Inc., Chicago, Ill., 1975.
11. Skillman JJ, ed.: *Intensive Care.* Little, Brown, and Company, Boston, Mass., 1975.
12. Vander AJ, et al.: *Human Physiology.* 2nd Ed. McGraw-Hill, New York, 1975.
13. Wade JF: *Respiratory Nursing Care.* 2nd Ed. C.V. Mosby, St. Louis, Mo., 1977.
14. Wen-Hsein H, et al.: Pressure dynamics of endotracheal and tracheostomy cuffs. *Critical Care Medicine* July-August:197-202, 1973.
15. West JB: *Respiratory Physiology.* Williams and Wilkins Company, Baltimore, Md., 1974.
16. Wyper AM: Pulmonary embolism—fighting the silent killer. *Nursing '75* October: 31-38, 1975.

SELECTED READING LIST

Specific Disease Entities

Bone RC: Treatment of adult respiratory distress syndrome with diuretics, dialysis, and positive end expiratory pressure. *Critical Care Medicine* 6:136-139, 1978.

Cook W: Shock lung: etiology, prevention, and treatment. *Heart and Lung* 3: 933-938, 1974.

Cunningham JH, Richardson RH, Smith JD: Interstitial pulmonary edema. *Heart and Lung* 6:617-623, 1977.

Fitzmaurice JB: Current concepts of pulmonary embolism: implications for nursing practice. *Heart and Lung* 3:209-218, 1974.

Meador B: Pneumothorax. *Nursing '78* 8:43-45, 1978.

Michaelson ED: Oxygen therapy and delivery in obstructive pulmonary disease. *Heart and Lung* 7:627-633, 1978.

Intubation and Mechanical Ventilation

Adlkofer Sr. RM, Powaser MM: The effect of endotracheal suctioning on arterial blood gases in patients after cardiac surgery. *Heart and Lung* 7:1011-1014, 1978.

Fitzgerald LM: Mechanical ventilation. *Heart and Lung* 5:939-949, 1976.

Gallagher TJ, Civetta JM, Kirby RR: Terminology update: optimal PEEP. *Critical Care Medicine* 6:323-326, 1978.

Petty TL: Complications occurring during mechanical ventilation. *Heart and Lung* 5:112-118, 1976.

Powaser MM, et al: The effectiveness of hourly cuff deflation in minimizing tracheal damage. *Heart and Lung* 5:734-741, 1976.

Selecky PA: Tracheostomy: a review of present day indications. *Heart and Lung* 3:272-284, 1974.

General Nursing Care

Bendixen HH, et al: *Respiratory Care.* CV Mosby, St. Louis, Mo., 1965.

Keyes JC: Blood gases and blood gas transport. *Heart and Lung* 3:945-954, 1974.

Tinker JH: Understanding chest x-rays. *American Journal of Nursing* 76:54-58, 1976.

CHAPTER 4

Care of the Patient With Renal Problems

by Sharon Hudec Conway, RN, MSN

Much of how a person feels is dependent upon the sensitive balance between fluid and electrolytes. However, this balance is not dependent upon any one organ, but upon the interrelationship and interdependence of four systems: the cardiovascular system, the renal system, the nervous system, and the endocrine system. The cardiovascular system contains a network of capillaries that filters the blood and sustains the pressure necessary to filter the blood. The nervous system provides the innervation necessary to control urination and maintain vascular tone. The endocrine system responds to changes in pressure in the capillary system by secreting aldosterone and the antidiuretic hormone (ADH), which in turn affect kidney function. Finally, the renal system provides the organs necessary to filter the blood, form the urine, absorb necessary fluid and electrolytes, and excrete the urine.

This chapter will explain in more detail how the sensitive balance of fluid and electrolytes is maintained. It will be presented using the framework of the nursing process: assessment, plan, intervention, and evaluation. Basic physiological principles will be given in the first section in order that an accurate assessment can be made. The second section will present clinical guidelines to help the nurse assess the fluid and electrolyte balance of the patient. Finally, nursing interventions that can be planned in dealing with fluid and electrolyte imbalances will be explained.

BASIC PHYSIOLOGICAL PRINCIPLES
UNDERLYING FLUID AND ELECTROLYTE BALANCE

Composition of the Body Fluids

A normal 70 kg. man contains approximately 40 liters of body water, which is equivalent to 57% of the total body weight. A heavier person may contain less water (approximately 45%), just as a lighter person may contain more water (a newborn infant's body is 75% water). This body water is categorized as intracellular fluid and extracellar fluid. For the normal 70 kg. man, 25 liters of water out of the 40 liters is contained within the intracellular fluid space. The extracellular fluid is composed of interstitial fluid, fluid of the gastrointestinal tract, and fluid in the potential spaces. The extracellular fluid totals 15 liters. Blood contains both extracellular fluid, plasma, and intracellular fluid, the fluid found within the red blood cells.

As can be seen from Figure 4-1, the extracellular fluid consists of:

1. large quantities of Na^+, Cl^-, and HCO_3^-.
2. small quantities of K^+, Ca^{++}, Mg^{++}, PO_4^-, SO_4^-, and organic acid.
3. large amount of protein within the plasma.

The intracellular fluid space consists of:

1. large quantities of K^+ and PO_4^-.
2. moderate quantities of Mg^{++} and SO_4^-.
3. large amount of protein.
4. small amount of Na^+ and Cl^-.
5. almost no Ca^{++} ions.

Basic Principles of Osmosis and Osmotic Pressure

The basic principles of osmosis and osmotic pressure can be handled by defining certain terms. The definitions are presented in terms of the body fluids.

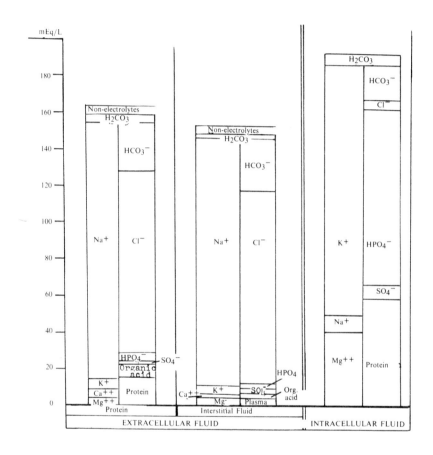

Figure 4-1. Composition of extracellular and intracellular fluid. (From: Goldberger E: *A Primer of Water, Electrolyte, and Acid-Base Syndromes.* 4th Ed. Lea and Febiger, Philadelphia, Pa., 1970, p. 4. Used with permission.)

1. Osmosis: The movement of water through a semipermeable membrane from a greater concentration to a lesser concentration.

2. Osmotic Pressure: The amount of pressure required to exactly oppose the osmosis.

3. Osmolality: The number of osmotically active particles per kilogram of water.

4. Hydrostatic Pressure: Force exerted by the fluid against the wall of the chamber in which it is contained. It is the weight of the blood against the capillary wall and the force by which the blood flows.

5. Isotonic Solution: Solution containing same number of osmotically active particles. Addition of this solution does not change the osmolality of the extracellular fluid, and results in no osmosis. Only the extracellular fluid volume is increased when isotonic fluid is given. 0.9% saline is an example of an isotonic solution.

6. Hypertonic Solution: Solution which contains a greater number of osmotically active particles, thus increasing osmolality and causing movement of H_2O out of the cell *into* the extracellular fluid.

7. Hypotonic Solution: Solution containing fewer osmotically active particles. Addition will cause osmolality to decrease, causing the osmosis of water from the extracellular fluid into the cell.

Among the different factors that change the osmolality of the extracellular or intracellular fluid and cause osmosis are the ingestion of water, dehydration, the administration of intravenous solutions, large losses from the gastrointestinal tract, profuse diaphoresis, or a large volume of fluid lost in the urine.

Anatomy of the Kidney

The kidneys lie to the right and left of the lumbar vertebrae in the retroperitoneal space of the abdominal cavity. The right kidney lies lower than the left kidney. An adrenal gland lies on top of each kidney.

The kidney consists of a cortex and a medulla; the cortex is the outer portion and surrounds the medulla. The major blood supply to the kidneys is by way of the renal artery. This artery branches out into the interlobular arteries which extend to the surface of the kidneys; branches of these interlobular arteries supply the nephrons. Branching off the renal artery, but extending inward through the kidney substance, is the arcuate artery. Veins draining the kidney follow the same patterns as the arteries and drain into the renal vein.

The functional unit of the kidney is called the nephron (Figure 4-2). There are about one million nephrons in each kidney, and each nephron is capable of forming urine by itself. The nephron unit filters the blood for the end-products of metabolism and excess nonmetabolic substances. It is composed of the glomerulus, Bowman's capsule, and a system of tubules, the proximal convoluted tubule, the descending and ascending limbs of the Loop of Henle, the distal convoluted tubule, and the collecting duct. The glomerulus, the proximal and distal tubules, and most of the Loop of Henle lie within the cortex. Within the medulla lie the deepest parts of the Loop of Henle and the collecting duct. The glomerulus is a network of capillaries that lies within Bowman's capsule and serves as the filter. The tubules and collecting ducts reabsorb essential materials.

As can be seen from Figure 4-2, blood enters each glomerulus through a branch of an interlobular artery, the afferent arteriole. The afferent arteriole branches out to become the peritubular network which extends into the cortex and medulla of the kidney. Dependent upon pressure and blood flow, the afferent arteriole controls the amount of blood that enters the glomerulus and the efferent arteriole controls the amount that leaves the glomerulus.

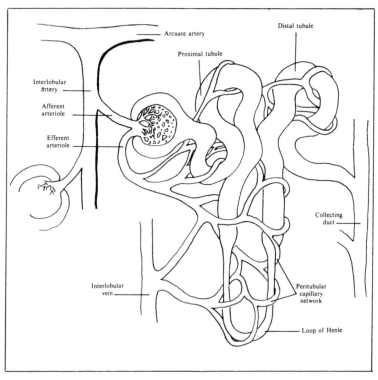

Figure 4-2. The nephron.

Process of Filtration

The main function of the kidney is to filter out and excrete the end products of metabolism, non-essential electrolytes, and non-electrolyte substances. In order for effective filtration to occur, blood flow and filtration pressure must be maintained.

The rate of blood flow through the kidneys in a healthy 70 kg. man is about 1200 ml./minute. This is about 21% of the total cardiac output. Of this 1200 ml. approximately 125 ml./minute is filtered from the glomerular capillaries into Bowman's capsule. This filtration rate, then, results in a total glomerular filtrate of about 180 liters per day. Eventually 99% of this 180 liters is reabsorbed from the lumen of the tubules back into the peritubular capillaries, leaving only 1 ml./minute of filtrate that actually forms the urine. Mechanisms effecting reabsorption will be discussed later.

The initial filtration of plasma from the arterioles into Bowman's capsule is dependent upon the effective filtration pressure that results from a balance of several forces. As stated earlier, the glomerulus lies within Bowman's capsule within the cortex of the kidney. This tuft of capillaries which branches off the afferent arteriole is a high pressure bed; the *mean* pressure of the blood flowing through the capillaries is 60-70 mm. Hg. This hydrostatic pressure *favors* movement of fluid from the capillary into Bowman's capsule. *Opposing* this is the hydrostatic pressure resulting from the fluid already in the capsule, about 14 mm. Hg.

The glomerular membrane is essentially impermeable to all plasma proteins and large molecules, including blood cells. The plasma in the capillaries thus exerts an osmotic or oncotic pressure which tends to hold fluid back or *oppose* filtration. The plasma oncotic pressure is generally considered to be 32 mm. Hg. The fluid in the capsule, on the other hand, already having been filtered, contains no large protein molecules and thus has no significant osmotic force.

Under normal conditions, the result of the interplay of these forces is a movement of fluid from the capillaries into Bowman's capsule. Figure 4-3 summarizes these pressures.

As can be seen in Figure 4-3, the plasma hydrostatic pressure is the major force which results in filtration. However, any factor which alters the pressure on either side of the glomerular membrane will affect the net filtration pressure and thus the glomerular filtration rate (GFR). Some common alterations seen in the clinical setting are listed below:

1. Increased arterial blood pressure results in a slight increase in GFR as the plasma hydrostatic pressure increases. However, this effect is limited by a compensatory automatic arteriolar constriction. Chronic hypertension, for example, is usually associated with decreases in GFR through a series of complex autoregulatory mechanisms.
2. Constriction of the afferent arteriole, as occurs in response to shock or potent vasopressors, reduces the rate of blood flow through the glomerulus, thus reducing hydrostatic pressure and GFR.

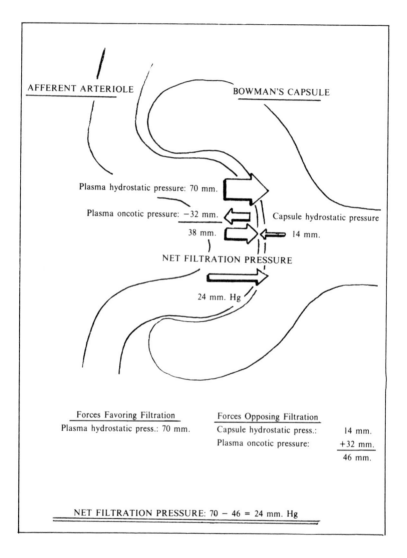

Figure 4-3. Forces favoring and opposing filtration.

3. Dilation of the afferent arteriole, as occurs in response to Dopamine administration, increases the rate of blood flow and results in an increase in GFR.

4. Constriction of the efferent arteriole presents increased resistance to the flow of fluid out of the glomeruli. This increases hydrostatic pressure and thus the GFR. Prolonged constriction, however, also results in sluggish blood flow which allows a large amount of plasma volume to be filtered into the capsule. The plasma oncotic pressure then rises as the plasma becomes more concentrated. The increased plasma oncotic pressure more strongly opposes filtration and GFR falls.

5. Increases in colloid osmotic pressure, as occurs with severe dehydration, reduce filtration rate.

6. Decreases in colloid osmotic pressure, as occurs with severe overhydration, increase GFR.

7. Increases in capsule hydrostatic pressure, as occurs with obstruction to the outflow of urine, seen with ureteral obstruction, oppose filtration and decrease GFR.

Active Transport and Diffusion

The glomerular filtrate flows through the proximal convoluted tubule, the Loop of Henle, the distal convoluted tubule, and finally the collecting duct. Throughout the tubules, water and solutes are selectively reabsorbed by two processes known as active transport and diffusion. What is not reabsorbed forms the urine and is excreted.

Active transport is the process whereby energy from a metabolic process is utilized to remove solutes, such as sodium, across the capillary membrane. Sodium diffuses easily between the lumen of the proximal tubule into the tubular cell, according to the concentration difference and electrical potential gradient. The active transport of sodium, then, occurs only on the side between the tubular cell and the peritubular fluid. Figure 4-4 illustrates this.

This process is a repetitive one. Once sodium is actively transported out of the cell into the peritubular fluid, the concentration of sodium inside the cell decreases. Because there is a lower concentration of sodium ions inside the cell, sodium can continue easily to diffuse from the lumen of the tubule into the tubular cell. Once in-

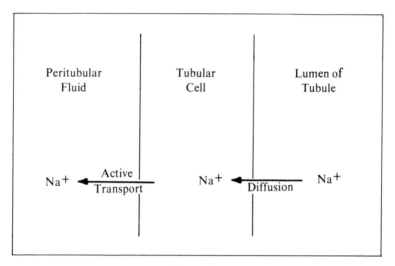

Figure 4-4.

side the cell, sodium combines with a carrier in the membrane between the tubular cell and the peritubular fluid and is then transported with this carrier across the membrane into the peritubular fluid. In addition to sodium, the other substances that are actively transported are calcium, phosphate, glucose, amino acids, and urate ions.

Diffusion can occur across both membranes (tubule to tubular cell, and tubular cell to peritubular fluid). Diffusion occurs because of differences in concentration or because of an electrical gradient difference. Active transport, however, occurs only in one direction and occurs without or against concentration differences.

Once substances have diffused or have been transported into the peritubular space, they can be reabsorbed by the peritubular capillaries, thus conserving essential elements. As can be seen from Table 4-1, all glucose, potassium, and amino acids are reabsorbed in the area of the proximal tubule. Note that most of the sodium is reabsorbed in the proximal tubule; water is also reabsorbed here since active transport of sodium is accompanied by water. This is different in the distal tubule where water and solutes are independently reabsorbed, depending on the body's needs. ADH, which will be discussed later, regulates the reabsorption of water in the distal tubule and collecting duct.

TABLE 4-1

Specific Sites of Reabsorption

Proximal Tubule	Loop of Henle	Distal Tubule	Collecting Duct
65% of Na^+ and water reabsorbed (ADH not required). All glucose, K^+, amino acids, HCO_3^-, PO_4^-, urea	Na^+ reabsorbed from ascending limb.	Na^+ reabsorbed water reabsorbed (ADH required). K^+, urea secreted H^+ secreted NH_3^+ secreted	Na^+, K^+, H^+, NH_3^+ may be excreted or reabsorbed. Water reabsorbed (ADH is required).
H^+ is secreted. Foreign substances secreted.			
Fluid is isotonic as it leaves.	Fluid is hypotonic as it leaves.	Fluid is hypotonic or isotonic as it leaves.	Final concentration occurs.

ALDOSTERONE FEEDBACK

Regulation of Sodium

Sodium is the main electrolyte in the extracellular fluid space. It must be regulated in order to maintain the fluid and electrolyte balance. Sodium is regulated by aldosterone, a hormone secreted by the adrenal gland. Aldosterone is responsible for 95% of all the sodium that is reabsorbed along the entire system of tubules. If aldosterone were not secreted, the kidneys would lose 15-30 Gm. of sodium a day, causing sodium and chloride to be depleted within a few days. The rate of aldosterone secretion can be increased greatly if:

1. There is reduced sodium in the extracellular fluid.
2. There is a high potassium concentration in the extracellular fluid.
3. The cardiac output is decreased.
4. Hypovolemia exists.
5. Physical stress, caused by trauma or burns, is present.

The effects of aldosterone are demonstrated in Figure 4-5.
There are different theories as to how aldosterone is regulated,

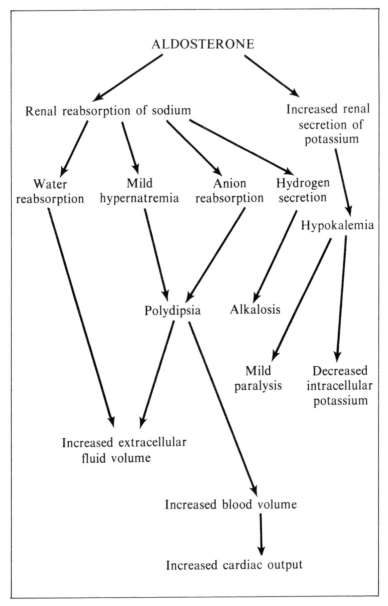

Figure 4-5. Effects of aldosterone (Adapted from: Guyton AC: *Textbook of Medical Physiology.* 5th Ed. W.B. Saunders, Philadelphia, Pa., 1976, p. 1020.

but the most widely accepted is the renin-angiotensin theory. Renin is a hormone which is secreted by the juxtaglomerular cells of the kidneys. A decreased concentration of sodium or renal ischemia resulting from reduced blood flow causes the kidneys to secrete renin. Renin combines with angiotensinogen, a glycoprotein formed in the liver, to form angiotensin I. Angiotensin I is converted into angiotensin II through the action of an enzyme. Angiotensin II causes peripheral vasoconstriction which increases arterial blood pressure, thus increasing blood flow and decreasing renal ischemia. Angiotensin II also increases aldosterone secretion, which causes the retention of sodium and water until normal levels of sodium are obtained. The peripheral vasoconstriction and increased vascular volume both result in adequate perfusion. A high level of sodium will cause renin secretion to be diminished, eventually leading to decreased sodium reabsorption. Figure 4-6 summarizes the action of renin-angiotensin.

ADH Regulation

While aldosterone is the main regulator of sodium, the anti-diuretic hormone (ADH) is the main regulator of body water. ADH is secreted by the hypothalamus and the posterior pituitary gland.

Normally, the daily intake of water is approximately 2400 cc. The daily loss of water is also 2400 cc. The loss can be broken down into:

Urine	— 1400 cc./day
Sweat	— 100 cc./day
Feces	— 200 cc./day
Skin	— 300-400 cc./day
Respiratory	— 300-400 cc./day

The urinary water loss is regulated by the action of ADH itself, the hypothalamus, the posterior pituitary gland, and the renal tubules. ADH causes reabsorption of water in the distal tubules and the collecting ducts of the kidneys. If ADH was not secreted, the kidneys would excrete 5-15 times the amount of urine usually excreted.

ADH is secreted in relation to the osmolality of the extracellular fluid. With an increase in osmolality, more ADH is secreted, and

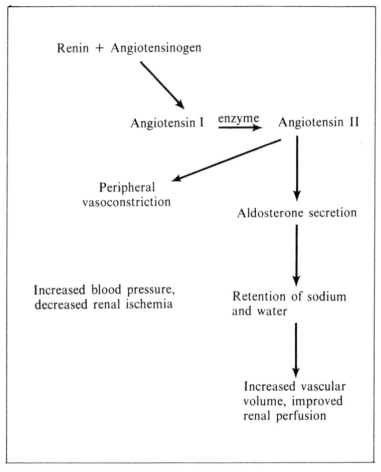

Figure 4-6. Renin-Angiotensin System.

more water is thus reabsorbed. If the osmolality is decreased, ADH secretion is inhibited, causing less water reabsorption. This effect comes about through the action of aldosterone.

As described, with a decrease in blood pressure and blood flow through the kidneys, aldosterone causes an increase in sodium reabsorption, which in turn causes the osmolality to increase. As a consequence, more ADH is secreted, causing more water reabsorption. In this way a balance is maintained between the fluid and electrolytes, and the rate of blood flow through the kidneys is increased.

When extracellular fluid (ECF) volume increases, plasma osmolality decreases, ADH secretion is inhibited, and much of the extra volume is quickly lost in the urine. However, about one-third of it remains in the plasma causing an increase in blood volume, an increase in venous return to the heart, and an increased cardiac output. The increased cardiac output increases the arterial blood pressure. With the subsequent increase in the glomerular filtration rate (GFR), the rest of the excess fluid can be excreted through the urine until the ECF and blood volume are returned to normal levels.

Regulation of Other Electrolytes

Potassium: This ion is regulated by the same mechanism regulating sodium, the aldosterone feedback mechanism. As a result of sodium reabsorption in the distal and collecting tubules due to aldosterone, there is a large quantity of positive ions being transported from the tubular cell into the peritubular fluid. Sodium reabsorption from the tubules leaves a very negative electrical potential in the lumen of the tubule. Because of this potential, potassium diffuses from the tubular cell into the lumen of the tubule in order to restore electrical neutrality. The net effect is that potassium is exchanged for sodium. In addition, potassium is directly secreted into the distal tubules and collecting ducts when there is an increased potassium level in the ECF.

Calcium: The regulation of calcium is controlled by the secretion of the parathyroid hormone. When there is a decreased level of calcium in the ECF, the parathyroid hormone acts directly on the bones to increase the reabsorption of bone salts. The bone salts release large amounts of calcium and phosphate into the ECF until a normal level is maintained. With increased levels of calcium in the ECF, calcium is excreted in the urine.

Magnesium: There is little known about magnesium regulation except that the kidneys will increase reabsorption of magnesium with decreased levels in the ECF, and will increase secretion of magnesium with increased levels in the ECF.

Chloride: The reabsorption of chloride ions from the tubules is, in part, also regulated by aldosterone, and it occurs secondarily to sodium absorption. As sodium, a positive ion, is reabsorbed, there is an electrical potential difference between the lumen of the tubule and the outside of the tubule. Sodium, a positive ion, attracts a negative ion to cross over the membrane. Since chloride is the most abundant negative ion in the tubular fluid, it is the chloride ion which is attracted. In general, negative ions, such as chloride ions, are regulated secondarily to the positive ions. When a positive ion is absorbed from the tubule, a state of electronegativity exists. To provide electrical neutrality, negative ions, primarily chloride ions, will be reabsorbed into the tubules.

Regulation of the Acid-Base Balance

The normal serum pH is 7.4. A low pH corresponds to a high hydrogen ion concentration and is termed acidosis. A pH less than 7.4 represents an acidotic state. A high pH corresponds to a low H^+ concentration and is termed alkalosis. A pH greater than 7.4 represents an alkalotic state.

The regulation of the acid-base balance is accomplished primarily by altering the H^+ ion concentration. Three major ways of regulating the H^+ ion concentration will be discussed: buffer system, respiratory regulation and renal regulation.

Buffer systems: A buffer solution consists of two or more chemical compounds that prevent drastic changes in the H^+ ion concentration when an acid or base is added to the solution. There are three main buffer systems that help regulate the hydrogen ion concentration.

The bicarbonate buffer is a weak buffering system, as its concentration in the ECF is not exceedingly great. It is made up of two elements, CO_2 and HCO_3^-. While the bicarbonate buffer is a weak one, it is an important one because the concentration of each of the elements can be regulated. The CO_2 level is regulated by the lungs, and the HCO_3^- is regulated by the kidneys.

The phosphate buffer system is also comprised of two elements, NaH_2PO_4 which is a weak acid, and Na_2HPO_4 which is a weak base. Its total buffering power is even less than the bicarbonate buffer because the ECF contains only 1/6 as much phosphate buffer as it does bicarbonate buffer. The phosphate buffer, however, is extremely important in the ICF because the concentration of phosphate is much higher here. It is also important in the tubular fluid of the kidney because the concentration of the phosphate increases in the tubules, and the tubular fluid is more acidic than the ECF.

The protein buffer is the most powerful and exists in the greatest concentration of all the buffers. Protein is composed of amino acids. These amino acids may contain free acidic radicals that dissociate into CO_2 and H^+, and free basic radicals. Thus, the protein buffer system is the most powerful one because it has the greatest capacity to react in both an acidic solution and in a basic solution, helping to neutralize each.

Each of the buffer systems are affected by the others. Any condition that changes the balance of one of the buffer systems also changes the balance of all of the others for the buffers actually buffer each other.

Respiratory regulation: In order to understand how the lungs help regulate the acid-base balance, it is important to understand the following basic formula.

$$CO_2 + H_2O \xrightarrow[\text{anhydrase}]{\text{carbonic}} H_2CO_3 \rightleftharpoons H^+ + HCO_3^-$$

Because of the many metabolic processes that are continually carried out in the body, CO_2 is constantly being formed. Carbon dioxide is transported to the lungs where it diffuses across the alveolar-capillary membrane into the alveoli and is finally exhaled out into the atmosphere.

The concentration of CO_2 increases in the ECF if the metabolic formation of CO_2 increases or if the individual hypoventilates. The concentration of CO_2 decreases in the ECF if the metabolic formation of CO_2 decreases, or if the person hyperventilates.

With a decrease in CO_2, the pH will increase. A person with normal ventilation can maintain a pH of 7.4; if the person doubles the amount of ventilation, the concentration of CO_2 decreases, and the pH increases to about 7.63. Thus, by doubling ventilation, the pH increases 0.23 pH units. Conversely, if alveolar ventilation is decreased to ¼ the normal ventilation, the pH is reduced about 0.4 pH units. Thus, the pH could decrease from 7.4 to 7.0, if alveolar ventilation was decreased by ¼.

The H^+ ion directly affects the respiratory center in the medulla, and in this way affects alveolar ventilation. If the pH is in the acidic range, the H^+ ion concentration is increased. In response, alveolar ventilation will increase to as much as 4-5 times normal to help blow off CO_2, and thereby increase the pH from the acidic range to the normal level.

If the H^+ concentration is low and the pH is in the alkalotic range, then alveolar ventilation will decrease to 50-70% of the normal. In this way, the CO_2 level increases, and the pH will decrease from the alkalotic range to the normal.

Thus, there is a feedback system in the respiratory center of the medulla that responds to changes in the hydrogen ion concentration by affecting alveolar ventilation. Ventilation decreases if the H^+ ion concentration is low in order to help increase CO_2 and decrease pH; ventilation increases if the H^+ ion concentration is high in order to help decrease the CO_2 and increase the pH. These responses cannot occur, however, if the respiratory center is depressed or damaged.

These changes can be 50-75% effective in regulating the H^+ concentration. However, if there is some other abnormality other than the respiratory system that is causing an alteration in the pH, the respiratory system cannot completely return the H^+ ion concentration back to normal. (See Chapter 3 for a further discussion of respiratory control of acid-base balance.)

Renal regulation: Whereas the lungs regulate the H^+ ion concentration by increasing or decreasing the CO_2 concentration, the kidneys regulate the H^+ ion concentration by increasing or decreasing the HCO_3^- ion concentration. These reactions involve H^+ ion excretion, sodium reabsorption, HCO_3^- excretion, and ammonia secretion into the tubules.

H^+ ion excretion begins with the CO_2 in the tubular epithelial cells. It would be helpful to review the basic formula at this time.

$$CO_2 + H_2O \xrightarrow{\text{carbonic anhydrase}} H_2CO_3^- \leftrightharpoons H^+ + HCO_3^-$$

The H^+ ion is secreted through the cell membrane into the tubular system, but the exact mechanism is not known. Eighty-nine percent of H^+ ion secretion occurs in the proximal tubule. Any factor that increases CO_2 concentration will increase H^+ ion secretion; any factor that decreases CO_2 concentration will decrease H^+ ion secretion.

Sodium reabsorption is an exchange reaction. Each time an H^+ ion is secreted, a sodium ion is reabsorbed. (Figure 4-7)

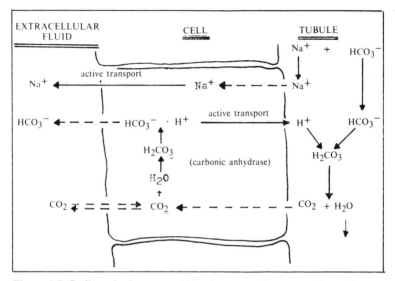

Figure 4-7. Sodium, hydrogen, and bicarbonate exchange reactions (From: Guyton AC: *Textbook of Medical Physiology.* 5th Ed. W.B. Saunders, Philadelphia, Pa., 1976, p. 492. Used with permission.)

The HCO_3^- ion is the end product of the reaction involving CO_2 and H_2O. However, the reaction is reversible and HCO_3^- can form with H^+ to make H_2CO_3, which will dissociate into CO_2 and water. The CO_2 diffuses into the peritubular fluids, and the water passes into the urine.

The bicarbonate ion, then, is continually being formed and filtered through the glomerular membrane into the glomerular filtrate. It is usually joined with sodium ions or with other positive ions (see Figure 4-7). Thus, because the HCO_3^- ions join with the H^+ ions or other positive ions, for all practical purposes HCO_3^- ions do not normally pass into the urine. They are reabsorbed from the tubules.

If an alkalotic state exists, how do the kidneys regulate the reactions to neutralize the imbalance? In alkalosis, the ratio of HCO_3^- ions to H^+ ions increases, so that the pH is greater than 7.4. Because of this, the kidneys try to increase the number of HCO_3^- ions filtered into the tubules, as compared to the H^+ ions. Since the HCO_3^- must react with an H^+ ion to be reabsorbed, all of the excess HCO_3^- ions pass into the urine and carry a positive ion with them, such as sodium. By excreting HCO_3^-, the HCO_3^- ion that is part of the HCO_3^- buffering system becomes decreased, and the alkalotic state is corrected.

In acidosis, the exact opposite of alkalosis takes place. The ratio of CO_2 ions to the HCO_3^- ions increases. The rate of H^+ ion secretion must increase more than the secretion of the HCO_3^- ion. Excess H^+ ions are secreted into the tubules without HCO_3^- attached to it. As was recently mentioned, when an H^+ ion is secreted, an Na^+ ion is reabsorbed, and an HCO_3^- ion is formed in the tubular epithelial cell. The sodium and bicarbonate ions unite to form $NaHCO_3$, which will add to the bicarbonate buffer system. The buffer system will then help to increase the pH and decrease the acidosis (Figure 4-7).

Acidosis can also be reduced by reaction of H^+ with Na_2HPO_4. This reaction proceeds as follows:

$$H^+ \; + \; Na_2HPO_4 \longrightarrow NaH_2PO_4 \; + \; Na^+$$

The NaH_2PO_4 is excreted into the urine. The free sodium radical is reabsorbed in exchange for an H^+ ion, and then combines with HCO_3^-. The resulting product is $NaHCO_3$ which adds to the buffer system and further reduces acidosis (Figure 4-8).

The final complex reaction to be mentioned in regulating H^+ ion concentration is the combination of H^+ ions with ammonia. As a result of metabolic processes, ammonia is constantly being synthesized in the epithelial cells of the tubules. The ammonia then diffuses from the cells into the lumen of tubules. In the tubules, the ammonia (NH_3) reacts with H^+ ions to form ammonium ions (NH_4^+). The ammonium radical combines with a Cl ion to form NH_4Cl, and this is excreted in the urine. In the formation of NH_4^+ from NH_3, hydrogen was secreted into the tubule in exchange for sodium. The free Na^+ is then able to combine with HCO_3^- to form $NaHCO_3$, again adding to the buffer system. The end result is

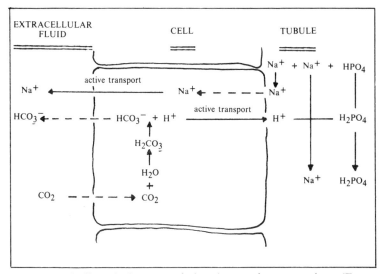

Figure 4-8. Sodium, hydrogen, and phosphate exchange reactions. (From: Guyton AC: *Textbook of Medical Physiology.* 5th Ed. W.B. Saunders, Philadelphia, Pa., 1976, p. 495. Used with permission.)

an increase in the quantity of the $NaHCO_3$ buffer system in the ECF which will help decrease acidosis (Figure 4-9).

The last renal mechanism to be discussed briefly is the counter-current system. The countercurrent mechanism is responsible for producing a concentrated urine, under normal conditions, with the help of ADH. The essential aspect of the first stage involves the active transport of sodium out of the filtrate as it passes up the ascending limb of the Loop of Henle (see Figure 4-2). As the filtrate moves up the limb it becomes more dilute because the ascending limb, while actively transporting solute out, is impermeable to water. The presence of this large amount of sodium in the interstitial fluid between the limbs then draws out both sodium and water by diffusion from the filtrate as it passes down the descending limb of the Loop. Thus the filtrate, having an initial concentration of 300 mOs, becomes first more concentrated, 1200 mOs, then more dilute, 100 mOs, prior to entering the distal tubule. It is in the distal tubule that water is reabsorbed due to the action of ADH. The resulting urine then has a concentration of 600-1200 mOs.

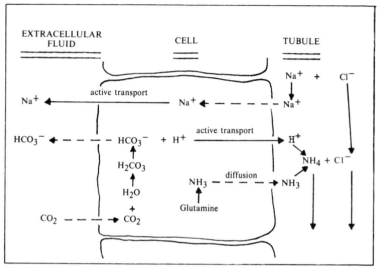

Figure 4-9. Hydrogen and ammonia reactions. (From: Guyton AC: *Textbook of Medical Physiology.* 5th Ed. W.B. Saunders, Philadelphia, Pa., 1976, p. 495. Used with permission.)

The second aspect of the countercurrent system operates in a similar fashion between the vasa recti (the blood vessels surrounding the Loop of Henle) and the interstitial fluid. Sodium and water diffuse into and out of the ascending and descending blood vessels in order to conserve sodium and maintain the concentration gradient necessary for the exchange between the limbs of the Loop of Henle. The ability to concentrate urine in this way is usually lost in renal failure and is often among the last of functions to return when recovery occurs. The reader is referred to a text on renal physiology for a more detailed explanation of this complex mechanism.

RENAL FAILURE

Pathophysiology

Renal failure is a condition in which glomerular filtration is inadequate to clear the body of its metabolic wastes, thus causing a build-up of metabolic wastes in the blood, leading to fluid and electrolyte imbalances and acid-base disturbances. Renal failure may be acute or chronic, congenital or acquired, permanent or reversible. There are many causes of renal failure, but generally, renal failure is caused by conditions that lead to decreased blood flow to the kidneys, primary damage to the kidneys, or obstruction to urinary excretion.

The kidneys have an intrinsic ability to maintain renal blood flow in order to maintain the glomerular filtration rate. A systolic blood pressure of 80-180 mm. Hg is needed to maintain glomerular filtration. When renal blood flow is decreased, changes in renal function occur. Changes in renal blood flow occur when there is a reduction in effective blood volume, a fall in cardiac output, or a decrease in systolic pressure to less than 80 mm. Hg.

There are many changes in renal function that occur. The glomerular filtration rate decreases. Renal blood flow becomes more sluggish as the amount of tubular fluid is reduced. Aldosterone responds to changes in pressure and decreased renal blood flow by increasing sodium reabsorption. Secretion of ADH causes conservation of more water. Thus, aldosterone and ADH try to increase blood volume by increasing water and sodium reabsorption. Since glomerular filtration decreases, the removal of solutes is decreased. The increased number of solutes causes the tubules to become hypertonic. To reduce the hypertonicity, more water is pulled into the tubular cells. Urine output decreases with the fall in GFR. Urine sodium also decreases. Substances such as urea and creatinine, which are normally, but poorly, reabsorbed, are excreted in large quantities in the urine as a result of increased water reabsorption.

Four categories of renal disease exist, related to the causes. They are:

1. Acute renal shutdown
2. Chronic renal insufficiency
3. Nephrotic syndrome
4. Specific tubular abnormalities

Acute Renal Shutdown

In acute renal shutdown, the kidneys cease or almost cease to function at all. Examples of conditions leading to acute renal shutdown are acute pyelonephritis, acute glomerulonephritis, or acute tubular necrosis. In acute glomerulonephritis, a large number of glomeruli become inflamed, a large number of white blood cells collect in the inflamed glomeruli, and ruptured endothelial cells block the glomeruli. The inflamed glomeruli become non-functional. The functioning glomeruli become more permeable, allowing a large quantity of protein and ruptured red blood cells to be lost into the glomerular filtrate. The glomeruli can return to normal within ten days to two weeks, including full return of function. However, the condition can also become chronic, with episodes occurring periodically. With chronic glomerulonephritis, many glomeruli are destroyed permanently.

Acute pyelonephritis is a condition in which the renal pelvis becomes infected and inflamed. It is secondary to a bacterial infection, and results in progressive destruction of the renal tubules, glomeruli, and other structures damaged by the bacteria. The infection usually starts in the medulla and works outward to the cortex of the kidney.

Chronic Renal Insufficiency

In chronic renal insufficiency, a progressive number of nephrons are destroyed to the point that the kidneys cannot function adequately. Causes leading to chronic insufficiency are: chronic glomerulonephritis, traumatic loss of kidney, congenital absence of kidney, polycystic disease, or urinary tract infection.

Nephrotic Syndrome

In the nephrotic syndrome, the glomeruli become more permeable. A large number of proteins are lost into the urine because of the increased permeability. Any disease that increases membrane permeability can cause the nephrotic syndrome. Among such diseases are chronic glomerulonephritis, syphilis, and systemic lupus erythematosus.

Specific tubular abnormalities

Acute tubular necrosis: In tubular abnormalities, there is an abnormal reabsorption and secretion by the tubules. Because of tubular disorders, active transport processes may be disturbed, and there may be deficient enzyme carriers transported in the tubules. Therefore, metabolic processes are altered. Because of the frequency of acute tubular necrosis occurring in the types of patients seen in Intensive Care Units, ATN will be discussed separately and in detail.

Acute tubular necrosis (ATN) is also referred to as acute tubular insufficiency, or acute renal failure. In ATN the epithelial cells in the tubules are destroyed. Most of the causes of ATN in the critically ill may be grouped under two main classifications: (1) nephrotoxic agents that destroy the epithelial cells, and (2) acute ischemia.

Nephrotoxic agents cause a rapid decrease in renal function. Among the nephrotoxic agents causing ATN are drugs, blood transfusions, and industrial and agricultural products. A number of antibiotics can also cause a decrease in renal function. Among them are: polymyxin B, gentamicin, streptomycin, kanamycin, neomycin, and keflin. The sulfonamides can cause crystal formation which leads to glomerulonephritis and interstitial nephritis.

Nephrotoxic agents have a direct toxicity on the epithelial cells, causing the loss of structural or functional integrity. There may also be hypersensitivity reactions, which cause an antigen-antibody response. Drugs may cause prolonged states of shock, which secondarily cause renal damage. Situations in which patients in Intensive Care Units suffer ATN related to nephrotoxic agents include barbiturate overdoses, antibiotic therapy, and allergic reactions to radiologic contrast material.

In transfusion reactions, another common nephrotoxic event, there is hemolysis of the red blood cells, and hemoglobin is released into the plasma. The hemoglobin molecule passes through the glomerular membrane into the glomerular filtrate. There is such an increase in hemoglobin in the tubules that it cannot all be reabsorbed, and the excess hemoglobin settles in the nephron causing blockage. Damage to the tubules is also caused by the release of a vasoconstrictive substance during the hemolysis of the red blood cells. Because of the vasoconstriction, there is reduced blood flow to the kidneys, leading to ischemia.

Common situations in which patients in ICU develop acute ischemia leading to ATN are: (1) hypovolemia, which produces decreased renal blood flow; (2) septic shock, which causes poor perfusion of tissues; (3) cardiogenic shock, which produces low cardiac output, decreased renal perfusion, and inadequate pressures to sus-

tain filtration; (4) severe trauma; and, (5) major surgical procedures which cause poor tissue perfusion and reduced renal blood
flow, or obstruction to flow.

The most likely cause of acute renal ischemia is severe circulatory shock. In shock, the heart is unable to pump enough blood at
sufficient pressures to supply the tissues with adequate cellular
nutrition. There is general vasoconstriction of the blood vessels as a
compensatory response in order to increase blood pressure, increase
venous return to the heart, and increase cardiac output. Blood flow
then decreases to the kidneys. Many tubules are destroyed due to inadequate blood supply and nutrition. Nephrons are then blocked by
destroyed epithelial tubular cells.

There are three specific stages classically seen in ATN. Stage I is
usually called the oliguric/anuric phase. Some patients, however,
may have ATN without having oliguria, which is usually defined as
less than 20 cc. of urine per hour. Renal damage in patients who do
not exhibit oliguria is usually reversible, symptoms are less severe,
and the disease is much less serious than the oliguric/anuric form of
ATN.

The more classic oliguric/anuric stage begins with a precipitating event followed by oliguria. During the oliguric phase, the
urine output is less than 400 cc./day. The average length of the
oliguric phase is approximately twelve days; however, it may be as
short as two or three days or as long as thirty days. The longer the
oliguria, the poorer the prognosis. During the oliguric phase, the
BUN rises 25-30 mg./100 ml. a day, and the creatinine clearance
rises 1.5-2 mg./100 ml./day. Complications occurring during this
phase are cardiac failure, pulmonary edema due to overhydration,
and death. Fluid and electrolyte disturbances encountered during
the oliguric phase are hyperkalemia, acidosis, decreased hematocrit,
and decreased hemoglobin levels.

The oliguric phase is followed by the diuretic phase, as renal
function gradually returns. The degree of diuresis depends on the
state of hydration of the patient. If the patient is volume-over-
loaded, the diuresis may be as high as 4-5 liters/day. Electrolytes,
particularly sodium, may be excreted in greater quantities, causing
sodium depletion. During the early diuretic phase, the BUN may
continue to rise; similar electrolyte disturbances which occurred
during the oliguric phase are still encountered during the diuretic
phase, particularly the early diuresis. The ability to selectively re-

absorb electrolytes and filter wastes is among the last of functions to return. During the later stages, the BUN begins to fall and eventually stabilizes near normal values.

The third stage, the final stage before recovery, is the convalescent stage. It may last a period of several months. During this phase, the BUN is stable. Urine volume returns to normal and electrolytes return to normal levels. Fluid and electrolyte administration must still be carefully monitored.

The prognosis of patients with ATN is largely determined by the primary event that led to the development of ATN. Those that developed ATN from nephrotoxic agents or simple volume depletion have a 25% mortality rate. Those that develop ATN from trauma and severe surgical complications carry a 70-80% mortality rate. Death usually results as a complication from poor wound healing and sepsis.

NURSING ASSESSMENT OF FLUID AND ELECTROLYTE BALANCE

To adequately assess the fluid and electrolyte balance of a patient, the nurse must not only look at the objective data obtained, but must also be able to explain the reason for the signs and symptoms occurring. The pathophysiological principles given in the preceding section will assist in this. Understanding basic laboratory studies, precipitating causes for certain inadequacies, and recognizing the signs and symptoms of electrolyte disturbances will also help the nurse to put the total picture of the patient together and make a complete assessment of the fluid and electrolyte balance.

Selected Renal Function Tests

There are several tests that reflect the functioning of the kidneys and should be monitored in critical patients suspected of impaired renal function. The major tests that are best reflective of renal function are: (1) creatinine clearance; (2) specific gravity; (3) urine osmolality; (4) urine electrolytes.

Creatinine clearance

The creatinine clearance is the most common test used to measure renal function; it is a useful indicator of glomerular filtration rate. Creatinine is a by-product of muscle metabolism filtered into the tubules and excreted in the urine. The amount of creatinine excreted is related to the muscle mass of the individual and should remain fairly constant, unless there is severe muscle wasting. The normal range of the serum creatinine clearance is 80-140 ml./minute, depending on the person's size and weight. This means that under normal conditions the kidneys are able to "clear" 80-140 ml. of plasma per minute of all creatinine.

In order to determine the creatinine clearance, both a urine sample and blood sample are needed. The urine is usually obtained over a twenty-four-hour period. An accurate urine collection is imperative; all urine excreted during the twenty-four-hour period must be saved. At the end of the twenty-four-hour period, a blood sample is obtained so that the serum creatinine can be measured. The normal plasma creatinine is 0.7-1.4 mg./100 ml. The normal urine/creatinine clearance is 1-10 ml./minute, and the normal urine creatinine level is 196 mg./100 ml.

The formula for determining creatinine clearance is: $\dfrac{UV}{P}$ where U = urine creatinine concentration; V = urine volume; and P = plasma creatinine concentration.

Due to kidney damage, the amount of creatinine able to be excreted or "cleared" will decrease, resulting in a rise in serum creatinine and a decrease in urine creatinine. The serum creatinine, however, is a more useful indicator of renal function in conditions such as ATN.

Specific Gravity

Specific gravity measures the kidney's ability to concentrate and dilute urine. It is dependent upon the number of particles present in solution and their size and weight. The normal specific gravity ranges from 1.010-1.025. Normally, the specific gravity is an indicator of the hydration state of the individual. A low specific gravity reflects a dilute urine which is an indication of water excess. If the specific gravity is high, the urine is more concentrated, indicative of a water deficit. In renal failure, the specific gravity remains constant as the kidneys lose their ability to concentrate the urine.

The specific gravity, however, is not always an accurate indicator of the kidney's ability to concentrate urine. A false high specific gravity will be found when substances such as protein, glucose, mannitol, or radiographic material are also found in the urine.

Osmolality

The osmolality is perhaps the best indicator of renal function. It is an expression of the total concentration of particles in solution. Unlike the specific gravity, it is not dependent on the size, molecular weight, or electrical charge of the molecule. The osmolality is expressed in units of milliosmols/kg. of solvent.

As was mentioned earlier, water can freely diffuse between blood, interstitial fluid, and tissues. A change in osmolality of one body compartment will cause a shift in body fluids so that the osmolality of the plasma remains the same as that of the other fluid compartments.

Plasma osmolality is the main regulator of the release of ADH. With a decrease in water and increase in plasma osmolality, ADH is released. In response to the secretion of ADH, the kidneys will conserve more water, and urine then becomes more concentrated. With a decrease in plasma osmalality, ADH is inhibited, and the urine becomes more dilute as excess water is excreted.

Because of renal damage, the kidneys cannot concentrate urine. Thus, the urine osmolality becomes fixed within 50 milliosmoles of the serum osmolality, determined at the same time, and the kidneys are no longer able to regulate serum osmolality by varying the amount of water loss. Serum osmolality increases when the serum sodium is increased, the blood glucose increases, or the BUN increases. Levels greater than 350 mOsm cause symptoms, and coma and death usually occur when the level is greater than 400 mOsm.

To calculate the normal osmolality, the serum sodium, urea, and glucose concentrations are needed because the major particles contributing to osmolality are sodium, urea, and glucose. The formula to calculate serum osmolality is:

$$\text{Osmolality} = 2\text{Na} + \frac{\text{BUN}}{2.6} + \frac{\text{Glucose}}{18}$$

The normal range of serum osmolality is approximately 285-295 mOsm/kg., and in the normal individual is fairly constant. The normal urine osmolality is 400-600 mOsm/kg., and should vary with changes in serum osmolality and hydration.

Urine Electrolytes

The urine electrolytes reflect the kidney's ability to excrete and reabsorb electrolytes, thus helping to regulate the electrolyte balance. The normal levels of urine electrolytes are as follows:

Sodium:	130-220 mEq./l.
Potassium:	39-90 mg./24 hours
Calcium:	100-300 mg./24 hours

Other blood tests will be monitored while the patient is in Intensive Care, but will not be as indicative of decreased renal function. Among these are:

Blood urea nitrogen (BUN):

As the nitrogenous wastes build up in the body, the BUN will begin to rise. The normal range is 5-20 mg./100 ml. For patients with renal damage, such as ATN, it is not unusual to see the BUN exceed 110.

Hematocrit

The normal hematocrit is 41-47%. Increases in the hematocrit indicate the loss of extracellular fluid. Decreases in the hematocrit may indicate increased water reabsorption for the patient with renal damage, in addition to indicating a decrease in blood cells.

Serum Electrolytes

Measurement of electrolyte changes do not yield conclusive results in terms of impaired renal function. They may be normal, elevated, or decreased, depending upon many factors. The normal levels of the most commonly measured electrolytes are:

Sodium:	135-140 mEq./l.
Potassium:	3.5-5.0 mEq./l.
Chloride:	98-102 mEq./l.
CO_2:	24-28 mEq./l.
Calcium:	9-11 mg.%

Table 4-2 outlines common alterations in electrolyte levels and the possible causes of each.

TABLE 4-2

Electrolyte Disturbances, Their Symptoms, and Their Causes

Electrolyte Disturbance	Signs and Symptoms	Causes
Hypernatremia with fluid overload	Dyspnea, edema, rales, increased JVP	CHF, renal disease, liver disease, large doses of adrenal corticoids
True hyponatremia	Lethargy, thirst, weakness, tachycardia, sunken eyes, dry mouth, poor skin turgor, high Hct., low BP, thready pulse, collapsed neck veins, postural hypotension	Vomiting, diarrhea, renal disease, diuretics without replacement, adrenal insufficiency, profuse diaphoresis
Dilutional hyponatremia	Dyspnea, edema, rales, tachycardia	CHF, renal disease, liver disease
Hyperkalemia	Weakness, ECG changes (spiked T waves, widened QRS, flattened p wave), paralysis	Renal disease, increased potassium replacement
Hypokalemia	Weakness, paralysis, hypoventilation, U waves, T waves flattened, cardiac arrhythmias, paralytic ileus	Renal disease, vomiting, diarrhea, diuretics, diabetic ketoacidosis
Hypercalcemia	Nervous system is depressed: reflexes sluggish, muscles weak; lengthened Q-T interval, anorexia, constipation	Parathyroid abnormality
Hypocalcemia	Tetany, numbness, tingling, prolonged Q-T interval, lengthened S-T segment, positive Trousseau's and Chvostek signs	Alkalosis, increased loss of calcium, inadequate intake of calcium, renal disease
Hypermagnesemia	Weakness, hypoventilation, hypotension, flushing	Renal disease, antacids
Hypomagnesemia	Similar to those in hypocalcemia	Inadequate intake, liver disease, alcoholism

Causes for Abnormal Fluid Balance

Fluid balance of the individual is dependent on sufficient water intake and adequate output. Under normal circumstances, the intake usually equals the output. The intake of water is obtained by fluids ingested, by water obtained from solids that are ingested, and from the water that results from metabolic processes. Water is excreted by the kidneys, the gastrointestinal tract, the skin, and the lungs.

Those factors that cause a disturbance in the fluid balance are (1) inadequate intake; (2) excessive losses; and (3) impaired renal function. The discussion thus far has focused on impaired renal function; however, in assessing fluid imbalance, the nurse must also consider other possible causes.

Inadequate intake

The most obvious reasons for an inadequate intake include anorexia, dysphagia, apathy, lethargy, or a coma-like state in which the individual is unable to take in any kind of oral fluid by volition.

Excessive fluids

There are several reasons why the body may lose excessive fluid. Among these are:

1. Increased perspiration: The patient may lose 500-1000 cc./day with mild to profuse diaphoresis
2. Increased gastrointestinal losses from vomiting, diarrhea, gastric suction, fistulas, and ileostomies
3. Massive fluid loss due to burns in which there may be between 1000-2000 cc. of fluid lost through the skin alone
4. Fever, which causes an increase in the metabolic rate, and increased perspiration
5. Hyperventilation
6. Tracheostomy
7. Increased metabolic rate due to activity
8. The diuretic phase of ATN
9. The administration of diuretics without adequate fluid replacement

Symptoms which the nurse may observe vary with the severity of the imbalances they reflect. However, observing certain parameters will assist the nurse in determining if the patient is fluid-overloaded or volume-depleted. These aspects are given in Table 4-3.

TABLE 4-3

Fluid Overload Versus Volume Depletion

What To Look At:	Fluid Overload	Volume Depletion
Skin	Warm, moist. May have pitting edema	Dry, poor skin turgor
Eyes	Periorbital edema	Sunken
Tongue	Moist	Dry, coated
Saliva	Excessive, frothy	Thick, scanty
Thirst	Not significant	Present
Temperature	Not significant	May or may not be elevated
Pulse	Rapid, bounding	Rapid, but weak and thready
Respirations	Rapid, slight dyspnea	Rapid, shallow
Breath sounds	Moist rales	May not be significant
Blood pressure	Normal to high	Low Orthostatic hypotension Narrow pulse pressure
CVP	Elevated	Decreased
Pulmonary artery wedge	Usually elevated	Decreased
Weight	Increased	Decreased
Urine Sp. Gr.	Decreased	Increased
Urine volume	May be increased or decreased, dependent on renal function	Decreased
Osmolality	May be increased or decreased, dependent on renal function	Increased

Assessment in ATN

Many of the patients in Intensive Care Units develop renal failure due to acute tubular necrosis. As mentioned, there are several causes for the development at ATN, and there are several tests that the nurse can utilize in determining if the patient is actually in ATN, or if the patient only has decreased renal blood flow. The decreased renal blood flow state may be temporary if progressive treatment is begun early. However, it could result in ATN if allowed to persist. The following differences, outlined in Table 4-4, assist the nurse in evaluating the renal status.

Certain systemic clinical manifestations are exhibited in acute renal failure. They include:

1. *Skin:* Rashes, itching, purpura, dryness.

2. *Neurological:* Drowsiness, confusion, convulsions, coma.

3. *Respiratory:* Hyperventilation, rales, pulmonary edema, acidosis.

4. *Cardiovascular:* Hypotension, tachycardia, increased CVP, arrhythmias, CHF, edema, pericarditis.

5. *Gastrointestinal:* Anorexia, nausea, vomiting, diarrhea, constipation, stomatitis, bloody stools, abdominal distention.

6. *Hematological:* Anemia occurring within forty-eight hours, increased white blood count, decreased platelet adhesiveness, bruises, hematemesis, abnormal coagulation factors.

Due to the increased white blood count, the patient is more susceptible to infection, and is especially more prone to respiratory, urinary, or wound infections. Because protein is not absorbed as it is normally, protein loss is excessive and the patient's wounds do not heal as well as they should. This further increases the risk of infection.

Bleeding abnormalities occurring in renal disease are a result of many factors. Anemia is present forty-eight hours after the onset of renal failure (related to bone marrow depression secondary to uremia). There is decreased platelet adhesiveness, and hypocalcemia

TABLE 4-4

Differences Between ATN and Decreased Renal Blood Flow

Test	Normal	ATN	Reduced Renal Flow
Urine volume	Approx. 1500 ml/day	Less than 400 ml/day	Less than 400 ml/day
Urine sp. gravity	1.010-1.025	1.010—remains constant	Greater than 1.020
Urine osmolality	400-600 mOsm/L	250-350 mOsm/L	Greater than 500 mOsm/L
Urine urea nitrogen	5-13 g/24 hours	200-300 mg/100 ml	Greater than 600 mg/100 ml
Urine creatinine	15-25 mg/kg/24 hours	Less than 60 mg/100 ml	Greater than 150 mg/100 ml
Urine sodium	130-220 mEq/L	30-40 mEq/L	Less than 20 mEq/L
Urine potassium	25-100 mEq/L	Decrease in oliguric ATN Increase in high output ATN	Decreased
BUN	5-20 mg/100 ml	Increased by 25-35 mg/100 ml/day	Rate of increase not as rapid as in ATN
Serum creatinine	0.8-1.4 mg/100 ml	Increases by 1-2.5 mg/100 ml/day	Rate of increase not as rapid as in ATN
Serum osmolality	285-295 mOsm/L	Varies as to hydration state	Varies as to hydration state
Response to lasix	Flow increases	None	Flow increases to greater than 40 ml/hour

may be present. In order for the clotting mechanisms to work, calcium ions are necessary. Although calcium is not a component of any of the reactions that take place in clotting, calcium acts as a cofactor. It must be present for certain steps in the clotting sequence; it is needed in the conversion of prothrombin to thrombin. Thrombin is the essential step in the reaction leading to clot formation. Although calcium is regulated mainly by the parathyroid hormone, it is also regulated, in part, by the kidney tubules. If the calcium level is low, the kidney tubules should reabsorb more calcium ions. However, in renal failure, calcium reabsorption is not totally effective, and calcium ions are lost into the urine. Hypocalcemia may result, which then may lead to bleeding abnormalities.

Acid-Base Abnormalities

Four types of acid-base disturbances may be present. They are respiratory acidosis, respiratory alkalosis, metabolic acidosis, and metabolic alkalosis. The determination of blood gases is the main indicator in assessing the acid-base balance. The blood gas determination measures the pH, pCO_2, pO_2, HCO_3^-, and oxygen saturation.

The pH measures the hydrogen ion concentration. It reflects the degree of acidosis or alkalosis and the compensatory mechanisms involved in trying to maintain a balance. The normal pH is 7.4

The pCO_2 measures the adequacy of the ventilatory volume. The normal pCO_2 is 35-45 mm. Hg. The pO_2 is a measure of oxygenation, and the normal level is 80-100 mm. Hg. The O_2 saturation indicates how much oxygen is combined with hemoglobin; the normal oxygen saturation is 97.5%.

As was discussed earlier, the body depends on the kidneys and lungs to regulate the acid-base balances. The level of CO_2 is regulated by the lungs; the HCO_3^- concentration is regulated by the kidneys. The lungs respond quickly to changes in the pH because of baroreceptors that stimulate the respiratory center in the medulla. However, the lungs cannot totally compensate for metabolic imbalances. In contrast, the kidneys react more slowly. They are effective in providing compensation for metabolic and respiratory problems.

In renal failure, the kidneys' ability to regulate the acid-base balance decreases markedly. Because metabolic and non-metabolic waste products are not adequately excreted, electrolyte imbalances occur, and there is an increase in H^+ ion concentration. The kidneys can no longer effectively compensate for changes in the acid-base balance by regulating the HCO_3^+ ion. Thus, metabolic acidosis develops in patients with renal failure.

NURSING INTERVENTION

Having given a foundation of basic physiological principles and a review of assessment parameters, it is now time to utilize this knowledge in carrying out therapeutic nursing interventions. Patients with fluid and electrolyte imbalances of a temporary nature or due to a more serious, acute event as in renal failure, require close observation of physical and psychological symptoms. It is the observation of subtle changes, the ability to make accurate judgments and take quick decisive action that is required in treating patient problems as they may occur, or preventing complications from arising.

Establishing A Baseline

Establishing a baseline of the patient's status is the first step in nursing intervention. A systems approach is one of the easiest ways to obtain the physical data needed to establish the baseline. The following data is necessary.

Neurological:

Pupil response
Response to verbal and painful stimuli
Response to verbal commands
Sensorium
Movement of extremities

Respiratory:

Rate, depth, type of respirations
Color
Symmetry of chest movement
Sputum production—type, quality, amount
Arterial blood gases
Adjunctive oxygen therapy needed or type of ventilatory
  assistance required

Cardiovascular:

Temperature
Pulse, BP, Pulse pressure
CVP readings
Pulmonary artery readings
Quality of peripheral pulses
Skin temperature; skin condition
Rhythm of heart beat or ECG pattern
Weight
Signs of edema
Bruises

Gastrointestinal:

Symptoms of nausea, vomiting, diarrhea
Palpation of abdomen
Appetite
Stools
Thirst
Breath odor
Stomatitis

Urinary:

Accurate output and intake
Results of laboratory studies indicating renal function

Psychological:

Behavior pattern
Symptoms of anxiety
Coping mechanisms noted
Response to environment
Response to medical team, family members
Sources of support utilized
Family responsibilities of patient
Financial concern

Maintenance of Cardiovascular Function

Vital signs need to be monitored and recorded frequently (every 1-2 hours, or more often) while the patient is in Intensive Care. Episodes of hypotension or hypertension need to be reported and treated, as do cardiac arrythmias. Changes in right atrial or pulmonary artery readings can be expected, and need to be recorded and reported. Pulmonary capillary wedge pressure readings below 10 mm. Hg usually indicate fluid depletion, whereas readings greater than 20 mm. indicate fluid overload. Peripheral pulse checks should be done every four hours.

The fluid intake must be carefully monitored, as well as the types of fluids given. Water ingested through solid foods must be considered as part of the fluid intake. Intravenous fluids are usually given to replace insensible fluid losses and the volume put out in urine. However, patients in acute renal failure may be limited to a total daily fluid intake of 500-600 cc. to prevent fluid overload. Sodium intake is also restricted. Patients with high output renal failure, on the other hand, must be replaced with enough fluid to prevent volume depletions.

Urine output should be measured hourly in patients suspected of any fluid and electrolyte imbalance, or patients with renal failure. Any source of output that the patient is having (N/G output, wound drainage, output from various ostomies) should also be accurately measured, recorded, and included in the twenty-four-hour total output. The specific gravity of the urine should be measured at least every four hours.

Daily weights are absolutely essential for the patient in renal failure or for any patient suspected of a fluid and electrolyte imbalance. A significant weight gain over twenty-four to forty-eight hours is a reliable indication of fluid overload. A weight loss indicates loss of excess fluid, or inadequate nutritional replacement. It must be remembered that the patient who is not receiving nourishment should lose approximately 0.5 kg./day; a stable weight indicates gradual fluid accumulation.

The skin should be observed for areas of irritation, itching, and/or breakdown. Measures to prevent decubiti should be employed, such as turning often, padding pressure areas, using waterbeds or air mattresses. Any changes in skin color should be observed. Prevention is the key in this area, and the nurse should not wait for symptoms to appear before initiating these measures in renal failure patients, who are all at increased risk.

Patients in renal failure usually develop anemia. They should be observed for signs of fatigue and given proper amounts of rest. Patients in renal failure should also be observed for bleeding because of the bone marrow failure, decreased platelet adhesiveness, and decreased RBC production. Transfusions are necessary only if symptoms occur. Only fresh blood should be given to patients with renal failure, as stored blood has higher levels of potassium, and the survival of RBCs is shorter. Iron compounds may be given to help limit the anemia.

Maintenance of Respiratory Function

Because of problems associated with acid-base disturbances caused by decreased renal function or renal failure, these patients have increased potential for developing respiratory distress. Therefore, the rate, depth, and type of respiration should be observed closely. Supportive oxygen therapy should be instituted when decreased pO_2 levels are discovered. Breath sounds need to be assessed every one to two hours. Patients who are fluid overloaded will usually have some degree of pulmonary congestion, evidenced by rales. Patients should be deep-breathed, coughed, and turned at least every two hours. Pulmonary care may need to become more vigorous if the patient is unable to effectively expectorate the secretions. Ultrasonic treatments, IPPB, clapping, and tracheal suctioning may become necessary.

Sedation and analgesics may also be necessary to decrease the pain or anxiety that is causing an increased respiratory rate. However, for patients who already have an inadequate ventilatory effort, analgesics and sedatives must be used cautiously as they may further depress the respiratory effort. This is especially true if the sensorium is already diminished secondary to uremia. In addition, the excretion of these drugs is often decreased.

Intubation and ventilatory assistance may be required for patients who are unable to sustain adequate ventilation. If this is necessary, the nurse must be aware of the settings on the respirator, and why changes in settings occur. Proper humidity must be provided. The patient should be suctioned hourly, using sterile techniques. (See Chapter 3 on Respiratory Care).

Maintenance of Adequate Nutrition

Adequate nutrition must be maintained, and this often presents a difficult problem because patients who have renal failure or electrolyte imbalance often have anorexia, nausea, vomiting, or diarrhea. The monitoring of protein, sodium, potassium, fluids, and calories is imperative.

Enough calories should be provided so that the patient's ideal weight is maintained. A high caloric intake is usual, up to 3000-3500 calories per day. The caloric intake is provided by protein, fats, and carbohydrates. The ratio of non-protein substances to protein should be 5:1.

An adequate protein intake is needed to build, repair, and maintain cells and tissues. Protein catabolism causes the release of acid metabolites and potassium ions. When renal function is decreased, there is often an increase in the products of protein catabolism, leading to increased acid-base and electrolyte imbalances. Therefore, the protein intake is regulated according to age, need of protein, and renal function. The recommended protein intake is 40-60 Gm. of essential protein a day, but will be less for a patient with decreased renal function. For patients who have an adequate protein intake, the ratio of BUN to serum increases. If the protein intake is inadequate, the serum albumin decreases.

It is important to prevent a negative nitrogen balance from developing since it will contribute to acidosis. In a negative nitrogen balance, a state of hypercatabolism exists, in which excess proteins are broken down, leading to an increase in acid metabolites and potassium levels. Anabolic agents such as testosterone may be necessary to help avoid a negative nitrogen balance.

The metabolism of carbohydrates and fats yields CO_2, H_2O, and energy, and does not increase the workload of the kidneys. Carbohydrate intake should be about 100-200 Gm./day so that proteins do not have to be utilized to provide energy. Carbohydrates also help to reduce the acid metabolites and potassium resulting from protein catabolism. The carbohydrate intake may have to be further regulated if the patient has diabetes mellitus.

Electrolytes should be supplied in the diet according to the kidneys' ability to regulate and excrete them. The normal sodium intake is 3-10 Gm./day. Sodium depletion causes hypotension, and sodium excess leads to fluid overload, which in turn may lead to cardiac complications, edema, and hypertension.

The normal potassium intake is 40-60 mEq./day. Increased or decreased levels lead to interference in neuromuscular function and cardiac arrhythmias. For patients in renal failure, potassium is usually restricted and potassium levels monitored closely.

Other electrolytes which must be controlled are calcium, phosphorus, and magnesium. Vitamins and iron also need to be supplied in adequate amounts.

For those patients unable to meet the nutritional demands through oral intake, intravenous feedings and/or nasogastric feedings may be necessary. Intravenous therapy aims at providing enough calories to minimize protein breakdown. Hyperalimentation, or total parenteral nutrition (TPN), may be necessary to provide essential amino acids and increased calories, provided in the base hypertonic glucose solution. The hyperalimentation is administered gradually so as to prevent a hyperosmolar crisis, and the administration of insulin to control the blood glucose levels may be necessary. The amount of calories provided by hyperalimentation is increased gradually until a positive nitrogen balance exists. Tube feedings are an alternate and safer route for meeting nutritional needs. (See Chaper 8 for a complete discussion of hyperalimentation and tube feedings).

Maintenance of Drug Therapy

Consideration must be given to the drugs prescribed to patients with decreased renal function. Drug toxicity is especially hazardous to the patient with uremia. Decreased renal function results in abnormal excretion of certain drugs, abnormal metabolic rates of certain drugs, and increased sensitivity to certain drugs (i.e., barbiturates).

The metabolism and excretion of certain drugs is slower for patients in renal failure, which causes some drugs to accumulate to toxic levels. Drug dosages are modified according to the patient's creatinine clearance and the drug's half-life. Drug dosages need to be modified if the serum creatinine is greater than 10 mg./100 ml. Smaller doses or an increased time interval between doses may be necessary. Determining levels of certain drugs in the blood, particularly antibiotics, is an essential part of determining appropriateness of therapy.

Antacids containing magnesium, when given to patients with decreased renal function, may lead to hypermagnesemia. If antacids are needed, it is generally best to give those containing aluminum hydroxide.

Digoxin given to patients with hypokalemia is associated with digitoxicity as renal excretion of digoxin decreases. Patients with increased calcium levels also can develop digoxin toxicity, and digoxin levels should be routinely measured. Generally, the maintenance dosage of digoxin is reduced to 2/3 normal.

Prevention of Infection

Preventing infection is a major goal for patients with decreased renal function. Good handwashing technique by personnel is vital. Proper care of wounds and incisions is imperative. Wounds should be observed for signs of redness, swelling, or any drainage. The drainage should be cultured every two to three days. Strict sterile technique should be employed in changing any dressing, including wound, IV, or arterial lines. Tracheostomy care should be given every four hours or more often, if needed. Keeping the lungs clear, in general, will help reduce the risk of a respiratory infection. Frequent mouth care is needed to prevent stomatitis. Using lemon-glycerine swabs helps to keep the pH of the mouth acidic. If the patient is able, sucking on candy or chewing gum helps to improve the taste in the mouth.

Indwelling urinary catheters should be limited to extreme emergencies. When used, a closed system of urinary drainage is a must, as well as catheter care, using a povidone-iodine solution, or soap and water at least three times a day.

Good skin care helps to prevent breakdown, prevent infection, and decrease itching. Lotions should be applied to dry skin. Pressure areas should be padded, and the pressure relieved frequently. Edematous extremities should be elevated. Changes in skin color and condition should be observed.

Monitoring Lab Studies

The results of the following tests should be monitored by the nurse:

1. Serum and urine osmolality
2. Serum and urine creatinine
3. Creatinine clearance
4. Serum and urine electrolytes
5. BUN
6. Calcium

7. Hematocrit and hemoglobin
8. Magnesium

The nurse should pay particular attention to the sodium and potassium levels.

Hyperkalemia can cause cardiac arrythmias and death if not corrected. Ways to correct, treat, or modify hyperkalemia are:

1. Correction of acidosis
2. Kaexalyte enemas
3. Hypertonic glucose and insulin given IV to move the potassium into the cells
4. Administering calcium gluconate IV to modify myocardial irritability
5. Avoiding hypercatabolic states in which potassium is released
6. Using washed packed cells if transfusions are necessary
7. Dialysis

If the patient is hypokalemic, potassium replacement is necessary.

Calcium is an antagonist of potassium because of the need for phosphorous to move potassium in and out of the cell. By increasing the calcium level, the phosphorous level decreases. With decreased levels in phosphorous, the movement of potassium may be inhibited.

If a large amount of blood is replaced, calcium may also have to be given. Giving large amounts of citrated blood may cause a decrease in the level of ionized calcium since the citrate binds the free calcium. When giving calcium, it should never be given in the same line that blood is infusing, as the calcium will cause the blood to clot.

In true hyponatremia, sodium should be replaced; sodium depletion will lead to volume depletion and hypovolemia. Hypernatremia leads to volume overload, cardiac difficulties, edema, and hypertension. Sodium and water should, of course, be restricted in fluid overload.

Acidosis or alkalosis should be corrected. Sodium bicarbonate may be given to help correct the acidosis, but is only temporarily useful. Fluid and electrolyte adjustments may help to correct the acidosis and alkalosis, but dialysis may be necessary.

Providing Psychological Support

Patients acutely ill with an electrolyte imbalance, decreased renal function, or renal failure may exhibit signs of increased anxiety and fear. The way a patient responds to acute illness will depend upon conditioning from previous life experiences, emotional resources available to him (including members of the health team and family members), defense mechanisms utilized, and the level of acceptance of the disease or condition. Feelings of powerlessness, inability to control his life or situation at the time, insecurity, and isolation underlie feelings of anxiety. Patients may respond to an anxiety situation by withdrawal or with aggressive behavior, hostility, overdependency, or depression.

Nursing intervention should be aimed at developing a therapeutic relationship with the patient. An accurate assessment of the patient's feelings should continually be made. Communication with the patient can be through verbal or nonverbal means. An environment that provides the patient with a sense of personal worth and dignity should be maintained by avoiding unnecessary exposure, using the patient's name, and giving the patient more control by allowing him to make certain decisions about his care. The patient should be told of progress in his condition, in response to his need to know he is improving. Setbacks should be explained in such a way as to offer the patient hope and motivation for recovery. Measures to provide comfort, relief of pain, normal sensory stimuli, or decreasing unusual sensory stimulation help foster a sense of trust in the patient, and a sense of well-being. Using measures to help reorient the patient or reduce confusion should be employed. The nurse must also be able to effectively handle her own emotional responses before she can help the patient and family cope with the situation.

Emotional support must also be given to the family. They often require help in handling realistic decisions that must be made. They may need support in how to relate to an acutely ill relative. They can be helped to feel that they have a therapeutic role in helping the patient recover by giving their support and encouragement to the patient, and assisting the patient when needed and as directed. Visiting hours may have to be adjusted if it has been decided that the family's presence is, indeed, most therapeutic to the patient.

DIALYSIS

Dialysis is the diffusion of dissolved particles through a semipermeable membrane separating two solutions. It is employed to rid the body of metabolic waste products and non-metabolic waste products that the body cannot eliminate due to renal failure. It removes the by-products of protein metabolism, such as creatinine, urea, uric acid, and water. It maintains or restores the body buffer system and restores the electrolyte balance in the patient.

There are two methods of dialysis: hemodialysis and peritoneal dialysis. In hemodialysis, the patient's blood flow is diverted into artificial cellophane tubing outside the body. The tubing serves as the semipermeable membrane; the patient's blood is one solution, and the dialysate solution surrounding the tubing is the other solution. In peritoneal dialysis, the peritoneum is the semipermeable membrane, and the two solutions are the patient's blood circulation in the abdominal vessels and the dialysate introduced into the abdominal cavity by way of a catheter. Advantages and disadvantages of each of the two types of dialysis is given in Table 4-5.

Dialysis is based upon the movement of particles from a greater concentration to a lower concentration. The dialysate contains an isotonic solution of electrolytes. The patient's blood has a higher concentration of particles such as urea, creatinine, and electrolytes, which, therefore, move across the membrane into the dialysate. Both red blood cells and white blood cells, serum protein, and bacteria are too large to pass through the semipermeable membrane and are retained in the patient's blood stream.

In addition to electrolytes, fluid moves across the membrane because of osmosis and hydrostatic pressure. In osmosis, there is movement of water molecules from a greater concentration to a lesser concentration. Due to hydrostatic pressure, there is movement of fluid from an area of high pressure to lower pressure.

Peritoneal Dialysis

Peritoneal dialysis is not used as often as hemodialysis. It is used, however, more often in infants, children, and patients with bleeding problems. It should not be used in anyone with recent abdominal surgery, peritonitis, or a severe hypercatabolic state, and is

TABLE 4-5

Advantages and Disadvantages of Hemodialysis and Peritoneal Dialysis*

HEMODIALYSIS	
Advantages	Disadvantages
1. Rapid treatment procedure.	1. Rapid derangement of fluid electrolyte balance possible.
2. Efficient.	2. Requires circulatory access.
3. Chronic intermittent dialysis feasible.	3. Special equipment and staff needed.
	4. Heparinization required.
	5. Technically difficult for infants and children.
	6. Blood transfusions sometimes needed.

PERITONEAL DIALYSIS	
Advantages	Disadvantages
1. Less likely to cause fluid and electrolyte imbalance.	1. Slow treatment procedure, less efficient.
2. Can be instituted quickly.	2. Danger of infection.
3. Does not require special staff or as much equipment.	3. High protein loss.
4. No heparinization required.	4. Contraindicated with abdominal adhesions, infections, and recent surgery.
5. Suitable for use with infants and children.	5. Not as satisfactory for chronic intermittent dialysis.

*Adapted from: Brundage D: *Nursing Management of Renal Problems* C.V. Mosby Co., St. Louis, Mo., 1976, p. 79. Used with permission.

absolutely contraindicated in the presence of disease of the diaphragm.

To initiate peritoneal dialysis, a catheter is placed into the peritoneal cavity. The patient should empty his bladder before the procedure starts, and the area around the umbilicus is shaved, prepped, and draped with sterile towels. A local anesthetic is used to anesthetize the area. The catheter is introduced into the abdominal cavity through a trocar and sutured into place. The catheter is then connected to the dialysis fluid inflow and outflow tubings. The dialysate is instilled at room temperature through the inflow tubing, which takes about five to ten minutes. The fluid is allowed to stay in the abdominal cavity approximately fifteen to forty-five minutes. During this time, metabolic wastes, electrolytes and water move across the semipermeable membrane (peritoneum) by diffusion, osmosis, and filtration. The drainage is allowed to drain out of the abdominal cavity by way of the outflow tract; this usually requires thirty minutes. Peritoneal dialysis for acute conditions usually lasts from twenty-four to seventy-two hours, while chronic peritoneal dialysis may last ten to twelve hours, three to five times a week. Complications of peritoneal dialysis are:

1. Peritonitis, caused by perforation of the bowel, bladder, or blood vessel, or infection by a break in sterile technique during insertion.
2. Leakage of fluid into the abdominal tissues, chest cavity, and scrotum.
3. Pulmonary complications caused by prolonged immobility during the procedure, and decreased ventilatory excursion from pressure on the diaphragm.
4. Hypovolemia that results from excess fluid being removed.
5. Hypervolemia may result from dialysis fluid being retained due to the closure of the catheter opening. Hypervolemia and hypertension may develop if not all of the fluid is removed in each cycle.
6. Pain, due to constant distention or chemical irritation of the peritoneum.

Nursing interventions required during peritoneal dialysis include:

1. Observation and recording of vital signs during dialysis. Any drastic changes should be reported.
2. Accurate intake and output of all fluids, including the dialysate. The dialysate should be kept in a separate record.
3. Daily weights are necessary, and sometimes done every 4-8 hours during dialysis.
4. Prevention of complications due to immobility. The patient should be turned frequently, and measures to prevent pressure sores should be taken.
5. Accurate measuring of outflow fluid in order to determine if it equals the fluid instilled is necessary. If the fluid is less, the cath-

eter may be buried in the omentum, or clogged. Turning the patient, elevating the head of the bed, and gently massaging the abdomen may help to facilitate drainage.
6. Observe for signs of respiratory distress.
7. The patient should be reassured frequently. Sedatives and tranquilizers may be necessary.
8. Nourishment should be given in small amounts to avoid increased distention.
9. Reduce risk of infection by proper care of the catheter. The dressing around the catheter should be changed, using aseptic technique, every eight hours, or more often if necessary.

Hemodialysis

Hemodialysis provides a more rapid, efficient treatment to remove metabolic wastes and fluids than peritoneal dialysis and is more feasible to use for chronic intermittent dialysis.

Access to the circulatory system is by way of an arterio-venous fistula or shunt. An A-V fistula is the attachment of a vein to the opening in the side of an artery. An A-V shunt is the cannulation of an artery and vein and connecting of the two cannulas. The advantages of a fistula over a shunt are that it can be used longer (average life is three to four years), requires fewer limitations of activity, and avoids the danger and complications prevalent with the use of an external shunt. The complications of an A-V fistula are hemorrhage, thrombosis, infection, and aneurysm formation.

The average life of a shunt is seven to ten months. Complications of a shunt are: local or systemic infections, reduced flow, hemorrhage, hematoma, and clotting.

The major components of a hemodialysis unit consists of a dialyzer, dialysate, and the dialysate delivery system. The dialyzer supports the cellophane tubing. Dialyzers vary in efficiency: some are designed for shorter dialysis times, removing fluid and electrolytes rapidly, whereas some are low-blood volume dialyzers which require longer run times. The dialysate is an isotonic electrolyte solution. The dialysate delivery system consists of a proportioning pump which mixes the water and dialysate concentration in proper proportion and propels the heated solution through the dialyzer.

After the dialysis system has been completely checked out, primed with saline, and anticoagulation therapy is begun to prevent clotting, the patient is connected to the machine by way of the shunt or fistula. Dialysis is continued for three to eight hours, depending upon the patient's need, and his response to treatment. To end dialysis, the arterial lines are clamped so that no more blood enters the dialyzer. Heparinization is stopped, and reversed with protamine.

Complications of hemodialysis during the acute phase of illness are:

1. Hypovolemia caused by too rapid removal of fluids.
2. Hypotension, resulting from hypovolemia, antihypertension therapy, and ultrafiltration.
3. Hypertension resulting from fluid overload and/or anxiety during dialysis.
4. Electrolyte imbalance.
5. Infection, via the shunt.
6. Bleeding as a result of excessive anticoagulation or a preexisting state contributing to the bleeding, such as an ulcer or gastritis.
7. Cardiac arrythmias, most probably due to hyperkalemia.

Nursing interventions for the care of a patient on hemodialysis include:

1. Frequent monitoring and recording of vital signs, and reporting any changes that occur. Blood pressure monitoring is especially important.
2. Weights pre- and post-dialysis.
3. Saline, plasma expanders, and blood replacement if hypotension occurs.
4. Accurate intake and output.
5. Observation of the respiratory status, administering oxygen therapy, or ventilatory support as needed.
6. Evaluation of lab studies before, during, and after dialysis.
7. Prevention of infection by:
   a) Maintaining strict aseptic technique in caring for wounds, IVs, arterial lines, or any other catheters.
   b) Strict aseptic technique in tracheal suctioning.
   c) Vigorous pulmonary care to reduce pulmonary congestion.
   d) Good oral hygiene.
8. Blood pressures should not be taken on any extremity with a shunt or fistula. Venipunctures are also not to be done in the same extremity.

9. Medications may be given during dialysis.
10. Provide comfort and emotional support to the patient.
11. Oral intake does not have to be restricted during dialysis. However, it may be more appetizing to the patient if smaller feedings are given.
12. Check connections between the cannula or fistula and machine frequently to prevent leakage.
13. Shunt care includes:
    a) Limiting the activity of the extremity for two to three days after the shunt is performed.
    b) Daily shunt care, including dressings, povidone-iodine ointment around the cannula sites, sterile 4 x 4s, and wrapping the shunt cannulas with kerlix. Enough tubing should be visible to detect clotting in the tubing.
    c) Observation of the tubing for adequate circulation includes palpation of a bruit, and checking for uniformly red blood. If clotting appears, the blood will become darker, and the serum and cells will separate. The physician should be called immediately to see if the shunt can be irrigated with a weak heparinized solution and patency restored.
    d) Observation of signs of infection around the shunt sites, including redness, swelling, tenderness, and drainage.

The patient in renal failure presents a most difficult challenge to the intensive care team because of the many complications associated with this disease entity. Treatment of renal failure, once recognized, is readily accomplished through today's advanced technololgical modalities. However, the prevention of the collapse of other body systems, such as respiratory or cardiovascular, is dependent upon accurate observation, astute judgments, and efficient institution of early measures by the nurse.

REFERENCES

1. Anderson CF, et al.: Nutritional therapy for adults with renal disease. *Journal of American Medical Association* **233**:68-72, 1970.
2. Bailey GL: Uremia as a Total Body Disease. In Bailey GL (Ed): *Hemodialysis: Principles and Practice.* Academic Press, Inc., New York, 1972.
3. Brundage DJ: *Nursing Management of Renal Problems.* C.V. Mosby, St. Louis, Mo., 1976.

4. Dolan PO, et al.: Renal failure and peritoneal dialysis. *Nursing '75* **5**:40-49, July, 1975.
5. Dossetor JB, et al. *Nephron Failure: Conservation, Substitution, and Replacement.* Charles C Thomas, Springfield, Ill., 1971.
6. Freedman P, Smith EC: Acute renal failure. *Heart and Lung* **4**:873-878, 1975.
7. Goldberg E: *A Primer of Water, Electrolyte, And Acid-Base Syndromes.* Lea and Febiger, Philadelphia, Pa., 1970.
8. Grant MM, Kubo WM: Assessing a patient's hydration status. *American Journal of Nursing* **75**:1306-1311, 1975.
9. Gutch CF, Stoner M: *Review of Hemodialysis For Nurses and Dialysis Personnel.* C.V. Mosby, St. Louis, Mo., 1971.
10. Guyton AC: *Textbook of Medical Physiology.* 5th Ed. W. B. Saunders, Philadelphia, Pa., 1976.
11. Jennrich JA: Some aspects of the nursing care for patients on hemodialysis. *Heart and Lung* **4**:885, 889, 1975.
12. Miller RB, Tassistro CR: Peritoneal dialysis. *New England Journal of Medicine* **281**:945, 948, 1969.
13. Muehecke RC: *Acute renal failure.* C. V. Mosby, St. Louis, Mo., 1969.
14. Pitts RF: *Physiology of The Kidney and Body Fluids.* 2nd Ed. Year Book Medical Publishers, Inc., Chicago, Ill., 1968.
15. Popper S: *Clinical Nephrology.* Little, Brown, and Company, Boston, Mass., 1971.
16. Shoemaker WC, Walker WF: *Fluid and Electrolyte Therapy in Acute Illness.* Year Book Medical Publishers, Inc., Chicago, Ill., 1970.
17. Smith EC, Freedman P: Dialysis—current status and future trends. *Heart and Lung* **4**:879-883, 1975.
18. Sullivan LP: *Physiology of the Kidney.* Lea and Febiger, Philadelphia, Pa., 1974.
19. Visel JM: Clinical aspects of renal biopsy. *Heart and Lung* **4**:900-902, 1975.

CHAPTER 5

Care of The Patient with Neurological Problems

by Virginia Burke Karb, RN, MSN

ANATOMY AND PHYSIOLOGY

The nervous system can be thought of as having two parts: the central nervous system and the peripheral nervous system. The central nervous system (CNS) includes the brain and spinal cord. The peripheral nervous system includes the cranial nerves, the spinal nerves, the autonomic nerves and the ganglia. For purposes of discussion, the nervous system review will begin with the bony structure, proceed through the meninges, the vascular system, the voluntary nervous system, and finish with the involuntary system. For additional detail, the reader is referred to the books listed in the bibliography.

Bony structure of skull

The skull is the bony structure that surrounds the brain. It is composed of over 25 separate bones, although after infancy the bones join and become immovable, with the exception of the mandible or lower jawbone. The larger bones in the posterior portion of the skull correspond in name with the lobe of the brain located underneath. Thus, the frontal bone, parietal bones, occipital bones, and temporal bones correspond in location to the same-named lobes of the brain. Other bones which are commonly injured in head trauma are described below. The maxilla is the upper jawbone, and the mandible is the lower. The eyes are surrounded by the frontal bone superiorly, the molar or zygomatic bone (the cheekbone) and the maxilla nasally. The nasal bone is a small bone located at the top of the nose between the right and left maxilla and the frontal bone. The sphenoid bone is located anteriorly to the temporal bone and inferiorly to the frontal bone. It extends inward from either side of the skull and contains the sphenoid sinus.

Other bony structures referred to in the skull include the sella turcica, a saddle-shaped depression on the inside of the sphenoid bone; it is the location of the pituitary gland. The foramen magnum is the opening at the base of the skull through which the spinal cord descends (Figure 5-1).

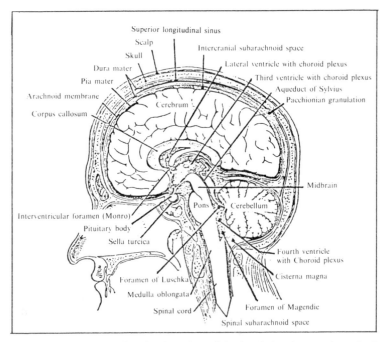

Figure 5-1. Diagram of sagittal section of the head showing cerebrospinal fluid spaces, principal structures, and meninges. (From: Carini E, Owens G: *Neurological and Neurosurgical Nursing.* 6th Ed. C.V. Mosby, St. Louis, Mo., 1974, p. 16. Used with permission.)

Vertebrae

The vertebral column consists of twenty-six individual vertebrae joined to permit movement while encasing the spinal cord within. In descending order the vertebrae include seven cervical vertebrae, twelve thoracic vertebrae, five lumbar vertebrae, the sacrum, which is one bone formed from the fusion of five vertebrae, and the coccyx, which has resulted from the fusion of four or five vertebrae. The first cervical vertebrae is also known as the atlas and the second one is known as the axis. Most of the vertebrae consist of, among other things, a body, two transverse processes, and a spine which encircle the vertebrae foramen, the opening through which the spinal cord passes.

The Meninges

The meninges are the membranous coverings of the brain and spinal cord. The dura mater serves two functions; it is the outermost layer of meninges, and it is the inner periosteum of the cranial bones. The pia mater adheres to the brain and contains blood vessels. The arachnoid mater is web-like, and lies between the dura mater and pia mater. The subdural space is between the dura mater and the arachnoid mater; the subarachnoid space is between the arachnoid mater and the pia mater (Figure 5-2).

Three extensions of the dura mater are important to know: the falx cerebri projects downward from the middle of the skull to separate the right and left hemispheres of the brain. The tentorium cerebelli separates the cerebellum from the occipital lobe. The falx cerebelli separates the two cerebellar hemispheres. Inflammation of the meninges is called meningitis. Usually only the arachnoid and pia mater are involved.

The meninges also cover the spinal cord and descend through the vertebrae. The meninges continue a few inches below the point at which the cord itself ends. This projection allows lumbar puncture into the subarachnoid space to occur without damage to the spinal cord.

The Vascular System

The major circulation to the brain comes from four arteries: the internal carotid arteries anteriorly and the vertebral arteries

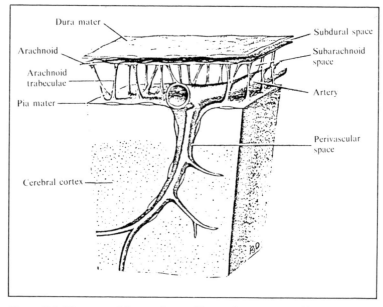

Figure 5-2. Diagram of the meninges. (From: Carpenter M: *Human Neuroanatomy.* 7th Ed. Williams and Wilkins, Baltimore, 1976, p. 16. Used with permission.)

posteriorly. These four connect with the basilar artery at the Circle of Willis. The main blood supply for the two hemispheres of the brain is from the internal carotid arteries, which each divide into anterior, middle and posterior cerebral arteries. The basilar and vertebral arteries supply blood to the brainstem and cerebellum. The venous drainage from the brain is primarily into sinuses, such as the superior longitudinal sinus, and finally into the internal jugular vein (Figure 5-3).

The arterial supply to the vertebral column is via the anterior spinal artery and two posterior spinal arteries, all of which arise from the vertebral arteries at the level of the foramen magnum. Smaller lateral spinal arteries also provide additional blood supply at each vertebral level. The venous system from the cord includes both an intradural and extradural component.

Blood supply to the meninges is via the anterior, middle and posterior meningeal arteries.

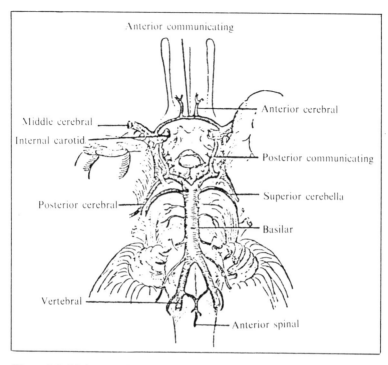

Figure 5-3. Major arterial blood supply to the brain (showing Circle of Willis). (From: Carini E, Owens G: *Neurological and Neurosurgical Nursing.* 6th Ed. C.V. Mosby, St. Louis, Mo., 1974, p. 16. Used with permission.)

Cerebrospinal Fluid

The cerebrospinal fluid, or CSF, is that clear liquid that surrounds and cushions the brain and spinal cord within their membranous boundaries. It is formed primarily at the sites of the choroid plexi located at various points within the ventricular system. Approximately 150 ml. of fluid is found within an adult. The CSF circulates in the following direction: from the choroid plexi in the lateral ventricles through the foramen of Munro, into the third ventricle, through the aqueduct of Sylvius into the fourth ventricle, to the cord via the central canal. The foramen of Magendie and foramina of Luschka in the fourth ventricle permit seepage of the CSF into the subarachnoid space around the cord and then into the subarachnoid space around the brain. It is then gradually absorbed into the venous system. Any pathology which blocks the circulation of the CSF, causes overproduction of CSF, or malabsorption of CSF can cause an excessive accumulation of fluid within (usually) the brain; this is called hydrocephalus.

In addition to cushioning the brain, the cerebrospinal fluid also serves to transmit information about changes in respiratory function, via changes in pH and/or carbon dioxide content of the CSF, to the brain.

THE VOLUNTARY NERVOUS SYSTEM

Lobes of the Brain

The cerebrum refers to the largest and most important part of the brain. It is composed of the right and left temporal lobes, parietal lobes, occipital lobes and frontal lobes. The right and left hemispheres are separated by the falx cerebri and supported posteriorly by the tentorium cerebelli (see meninges). In each person, one hemisphere is functionally more important or dominant; in the right-handed individual it is the left hemisphere. The left hemisphere is dominant for speech for over 90% of the population, regardless of handedness. A broad band of white tissue, the corpus collosum, connects the two hemispheres (Figure 5-4).

The frontal lobes are concerned with, or control personality, memory, behavior, intellectual functioning, level of consciousness, abstraction, creative thinking, judgment, and social, ethical and moral values. They also have some control over autonomic functions such as respiration and cardiovascular function. Finally, the area of the pre-central gyrus controls the motor functioning of the body, the left side of the brain controlled by the right side of the body.

The post-central gyri, which control and interpret sensation, are located in the parietal lobes directly behind the frontal lobe. Other functions of the parietal lobes include recognition of objects by shape (stereognosis), weight, size, consistency, and discrimination of fine touch.

The temporal lobes, inferior to the frontal and parietal lobes, are concerned with hearing, taste and smell, and understanding speech.

The occipital lobes, at the back of the cerebrum, contain the visual cortex (Figure 5-5).

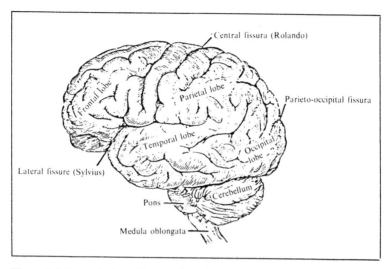

Figure 5-4. Lateral view of lobes of cerebral hemisphere. (From: Carini, E, Owens G: *Neurological and Neurosurgical Nursing.* 6th Ed. C.V. Mosby, St. Louis, Mo., 1974, p. 22. Used with permission.)

The Thalamus

The thalami are small masses of tissue which bulge into the third ventricle from either side. Their function is primarily that of relay station for sensory impulses on their way to the cerebral cortex, but they also influence primitive emotional responses such as pain, rage and fear.

The Hypothalamus

The hypothalamus lies below the thalamus. Attached to the underside of the hypothalamus via a short stalk is the pituitary gland, a major endocrine organ. Other functions of the hypothalamus include maintenance of the working state, regulation of appetite, temperature regulation, and pleasure interpretation for eating, drinking and mating.

The Basal Ganglia

The basal ganglia are paired structures, one in each hemisphere. They include the corpus striatum, the amygdaloid nucleus, and the

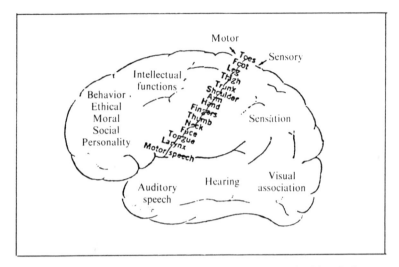

Figure 5-5. Principal functional subdivisions of the cerebral hemispheres. (From: Carini E, Owens G: *Neurological and Neurosurgical Nursing.* 6th Ed. C.V. Mosby, St. Louis, Mo., 1974, p. 23. Used with permission.)

putamen, among other structures. They function to exert a steadying influence on muscular activity.

The internal capsule is composed of ascending and descending fiber tracts. It is located near the thalamus and basal ganglia in each hemisphere.

The Cerebellum and Brainstem

The cerebellum is found just below the occipital lobes. Its primary functions are muscle coordination and equilibrium. The brainstem connects the cerebral hemisphere to the spinal cord; in fact, it merges with the spinal cord. The three sections of the brainstem have separate functions. The medulla helps regulate heartbeat, blood pressure and respirations, and influences the reflexes for coughing, vomiting and hiccoughing. The cell bodies for cranial nerves nine through twelve are located here. The pons contains the nuclei of cranial nerves five through eight. The midbrain contains the centers for cranial nerves three and four. All parts of the brainstem function to control or transmit impulses between the spinal cord and the brain.

The *cranial nerves* are twelve pairs of nerves which provide motor, sensory or mixed motor and sensory innervation to areas on the hand, neck and shoulder area. Please refer to the chart describing the function of each nerve under physical assessment section of Chapter 1. In addition, note the following anatomical and physiological correlates.

The course of the olfactory nerves carries them near the optic chiasm. Pathology associated with the pituitary gland, optic nerves or some facial-sinus injuries may result in damage to the sense of smell.

The optic nerves, for vision, traverse the brain from front to back, from the eye to the occipital cortex. Half of each nerve crosses at the optic chiasm. Again, pathology in or near the optic chiasm can affect vision, as can damage to one or both occipital lobes. Increased intracranial pressure often results in compression of one or the other, or both, of the optic nerves, which leads to swelling of the head of the optic nerve. This swelling can be seen with an ophthalmoscope, and is called papilledema.

All of the other cranial nerves eventually reach the brainstem. Various pathologies can affect nerves individually (e.g., tumors, increased intracranial pressure, inflammation) and trauma or pathology of various parts of the brainstem can manifest itself with cranial nerve dysfunction.

The Spinal Cord

As mentioned, the spinal cord extends from the brainstem downward to about the level of the second lumbar vertebra. The cord contains thirty-one segments: eight cervical, twelve thoracic, five lumbar, five sacral and one coccygeal, and from each segment come two spinal nerves, one for each side of the body. Each spinal nerve has afferent (carries impulses from the cord) fibers, and each spinal nerve innervates body muscles, and transmits sensory information from the skin, tendons, muscles, joints, and so on.

Detailed information about spinal cord function is complex and voluminous. Briefly, the impulses from and to the body from the cord are organized within the cord into various tracts which can be identified anatomically. For example, the lateral spinothalamic tract in the spinal cord transmits information about pain and temperature from the spinal nerves to the brain. The lateral corticospinal tract carries impulses downward from the brain to produce voluntary movement, that is, contraction of individual or small groups of muscles, especially those of the hands, fingers, feet and toes. What makes it more difficult to remember is that some information from the spinal nerves crosses to the opposite side of the cord from which it enters before reaching the appropriate tract, while some types of information are carried to the brain in tracts on the same side of the cord that the information enters the cord. In this latter case the information eventually crosses to the opposite side of the *brain*, but does so at the level of the medulla. Thus, the cortex in the brain regulates and receives information from the opposite side of the body, but the crossover of impulses upward or downward may take place at the level of the medulla or at the level of the spinal nerve depending on the type of impulse.

The following types of impulse cross at the level of the spinal nerve: ascending tracts for pain, temperature and crude touch and descending tract for voluntary movement of some individual muscles or small groups of muscles. The following types of information cross at the level of the medulla: ascending tracts for conscious and unconscious kinesthesia, vibration, stereognosis, deep touch and pressure, and two-point discrimination. The descending tracts which cross at the level of the medulla exert facilitory or inhibitory influences on skeletal muscles.

A final function of the spinal cord is in reflex activity. All reflexes, except those influenced by the cranial nerves, pass through the spinal cord. The reflex activity is thought of as an involuntary response to a stimulus. The knee jerk, Babinski reflex and abdominal reflex are examples.

THE AUTONOMIC NERVOUS SYSTEM

The autonomic nervous system can be thought of as automatic or involuntary. It serves many functions, including regulating contraction of smooth muscles, secretion of glands, and transmission of pain from vessels, viscera and bone. Other autonomic functions include regulation of cardiovascular reaction, gastrointestinal motility, respiration, and sweating. Much of the autonomic regulation occurs in the cortex, but much is also mediated in the hypothalamus.

There are two components to the autonomic system, the sympathetic and parasympathetic system. Structurally, the sympathetic system contains two sets of ganglia (nerve-cell bodies) located outside of the spinal cord, but anatomically close to the backbone on either side. In addition to short fibers which connect these ganglia to the cord, there are long fibers which extend from the cord to the visceral structures innervated. Conversely, the ganglia for the parasympathetic system are anatomically located near the individual viscera and glands.

Some general principles of autonomic functioning should be kept in mind.[2] The autonomic system functions to help maintain homeostasis. Most visceral effectors have both sympathetic and parasympathetic innervation, but the adrenal medulla, the sweat glands, smooth muscles of hairs and most blood vessels have only sympathetic innervation. Neurotransmitters are released at effector sites to produce the desired response. Acetylcholine is released at all autonomic synapses. Either acetylcholine or norepinephrine is released at the neuroeffector junction. Those that release acetylcholine are called cholinergic fibers; those that release norepinephrine are called adrenergic fibers. Sympathetic and parasympathetic impulses tend to produce opposite effects; in doubly-innervated effectors, it is the algebraic sum of the two impulses which produces the final result (i.e., determines which impulse will dominate).

In stress situations, the sympathetic division dominates to help the body expend effort and energy wisely. This sympathetic response causes, among other things, an increased heart rate, dilated pupils, bronchial dilation, decreased gastric motility, closed anal and urinary sphincters, and stimulates glycogenolysis to increase the blood sugar, and stimulates the adrenal medulla to release epinephrine.[2]

DIAGNOSTIC TESTS

Numerous diagnostic tests can be ordered and/or performed by the physician to confirm or further delineate a neurologic problem. The choice of test(s) depends on the presenting signs and symptoms of the patient, the suspected diagnosis, the speed with which neurologic symptoms have appeared or progressed, and the resources available. The nurse's roles are several: to prepare the client and his family through teaching, reassurance and physiological preparation before the test; to accompany and reassure the patient during the test if possible; to assist the physician during the procedure if indicated; to provide comfort and reassurance after the test; and to make appropriate, careful, and frequent observations of the client's condition after the procedure.

A brief summary of the most frequently used diagnostic tests follows. Each institution will have additional standing orders or procedures in relation to each test with which the nurse should be familiar.

Lumbar Puncture or Spinal Tap

Lumbar puncture is the insertion, under sterile conditions, of a needle into the lumbar subarachnoid space in order to (1) obtain cerebrospinal fluid for examination, (2) measure the intracranial pressure, and (3) inject medication or radiopaque substances for later x-ray visualization. The major contraindication to the test is greatly increased intracranial pressure; the rapid withdrawal of cerebrospinal fluid may cause sudden downward shift of intracranial contents with subsequent herniation of the brain, coma and death. The nurse's role includes explaining to the client and/or his family what is to be done, positioning the patient on his side or sitting as indicated, assisting the physician with the necessary equipment, and reassuring the client during the test.

After the procedure the client is usually instructed to lie flat for several hours. His vital signs, blood pressure, and level of consciousness should be monitored frequently. Fluids should be encouraged. If headache is present, have the patient remain flat or medicate him as ordered.

Ventricular Puncture or Cisternal Puncture

Cisternal or ventricular puncture is done less often now than formerly. It involves the insertion under sterile conditions of a needle into one of the lateral ventricles or the cisterna magna (below the occipital bone). The indications for these procedures are the same as for the lumbar puncture. Known increased intracranial pressure is not a contraindication. The care of the client is the same as for lumbar puncture.

Neuroradiology

X-ray films may be taken of any body area in which lesions may be demonstrable. For the nervous system, x-rays may be taken of the skull, including special views of the sella turcica, optic foramina and petrous bones. X-rays of the spinal cord are used to demonstrate suspected fractures of various vertebrae. X-rays are usually performed in the radiology department. The nurse's role would include teaching the client and/or family before the procedure and repositioning the client in his own bed after the procedure.

Myelogram

During a myelogram, air, radiopaque dye, or other contrast media is injected into the subarachnoid space via lumbar puncture. The patient is then frequently repositioned while desired x-ray views of the spinal column are obtained. This test is particularly helpful in defining tumors of the spinal column or blocks in cerebrospinal fluid circulation. The test is usually performed in the radiology department or the operating room. The nurse's role begins with teaching the client and/or family about the test to be performed. After the procedure, the client is usually instructed to lie flat for several hours; he may also complain of headache or back pain. The nurse may be able to reduce the patient's discomfort with repositioning, reassurance or medication.

Ventriculogram

Ventriculogram involves the introduction of a radiopaque dye or gas directly into one or both of the lateral ventricles via burr holes and ventricular pressure. Radiographic examination of the ventricular system can then be made. Major indications include suspected tumor, suspected cerebral anomalies, or need to visualize the ventricular system. This test is considered a surgical procedure and is usually performed in the operating room. The nurse's role includes careful patient preparation and teaching, and postoperatively, monitoring of vital signs, blood pressure, neurological status and the wound.

Pneumoencephalogram

The pneumoencephalogram involves the introduction of air or

oxygen into the subarachnoid space via lumbar puncture for the purposes of examining, via x-ray, the subarachnoid space or the ventricular system. After the introduction of the contrast media the patient is repositioned into side lying, head down and head upright positions. With the increased use of more sophisticated brain scans, this procedure is being performed less frequently. The pneumoencephalogram has serious complications associated with it, including death, and at least often causes severe, sometimes prolonged headache. The procedure is performed in the operating room.

Preoperative preparation includes client and family teaching and reassurance. Postoperatively, the client will usually be instructed to lie flat for twelve or more hours; diet may be limited to clear liquids only until nausea subsides. Frequent observations of vital signs and neurological status should be made.

Arteriogram (Angiogram)

Arteriogram is the radiologic study of the intracranial blood vessels after intra-arterial injection of a radiopaque contrast medium. The test is particularly useful for confirming aneurysms, hematomas and some tumors. An arteriogram is considered a surgical procedure and is usually performed in the operating room. Nursing care includes the teaching and reassurance of the client and his family. Post-procedure, the vital signs and neurological status of the patient should be monitored closely. In addition, the injection site or sites should be checked frequently for hematoma formation, and circulation to the extremity distal to the insertion site should be monitored by checking pulses, color, temperature, movement, and sensation frequently for the first eight to twelve hours after the test.

Scans

Brain Scan

The conventional brain scan involves the intravenous injection of a radioactive isotope, followed a short time later with the use of a rectilinear scanner to "trace" the circulation of the isotope through the brain. The test can detect tumors, infarcts and other lesions with accuracy of 40-90%, depending on location and nature of the lesion. The posterior fossa is poorly visualized in a routine brain scan. The nurse should prepare the client and his family for this painless x-ray examination with teaching and reassurance.

Computerized Axial Tomography (C.A.T. Scan)

This is also known as EMI scan, for the first manufacturers of the equipment, Electronics and Musical Instrumentation Ltd. The recently developed type of scan combines the use of the x-ray with a computer to produce serial views of the brain which are captured on Polaroid pictures. The test is noninvasive, usually requires no injections, is short and causes no client discomfort. It is more reliable than conventional scans and can accurately identify lesions in areas inaccessible by other types of scans, such as the eye and the posterior fossa. Because of its cost and size, the necessary equipment for the C.A.T. scan is presently available only at selected institutions. Because of its noninvasive nature the C.A.T. scan requires no pre- or post-procedure care other than client teaching; it may be performed on an in-patient or out-patient basis.

Radioactive Iodinated Serum Albumin (RISA) Scan

The RISA scan involves the intrathecal injection via lumbar puncture or cisternal puncture of the tracer substance, the RISA, in order to study the cerebrospinal fluid circulation. Serial scans are performed at 6, 24, and 48 hours after injection. Presently, the primary use of this scan is for the delineation of low or normal pressure hydrocephalus. Patient care is the same as that for lumbar puncture or cisternal puncture.

Indium scan

This scan is identical to the RISA scan but uses indium as the tracer substance.

Electroencephalogram (EEG)

Through the use of electrodes placed on the head, the electroencephalogram records cerebral electrical activity. Abnormalities in an individual's EEG pattern may indicate some form of lesion, e.g. infarct or tumor, or seizure activity. The test can be performed at the bedside, but usually the patient is taken to a special room where sound and activity can be controlled. If the diagnosis of seizures is confirmed via EEG, then regulation with medication can be commenced or altered. If a lesion is documented, further diagnostic studies are indicated. The test is essentially painless. Pre-procedure care involves teaching; post-procedure care includes washing the patient's hair to remove electrode jelly.

Echoencephalogram (Echo)

The echoencephalogram involves the measurement of ultrasound waves and their reflection back through the brain. The information is projected onto an oscilloscope. The test is painless and can be done at the bedside. A transducer is placed against the head first on one side, then the other, and repositioned until the oscilloscope indicates that the waves are moving to the same midline structure and at the same speed. The only information the test can give is confirmation of suspected midline shifting due to possible growing mass lesions or hematomas; usually additional diagnostic studies are needed because of frequent false positive and false negative readings. Post-procedure care would involve washing off electrode jelly, if used.

HEAD INJURY

Etiology

Auto accidents and motorcycle accidents are the chief cause of head injuries in the United States. In addition, injury to the head is often seen in battle situations, and in accidental falls. Men are the more frequent victims of craniocerebral trauma. Closed head injuries are more common in civilian life, and perforating wounds with compound fractures are more common in military situations.

Pathophysiology

Effect of Trauma

Injuries to the head can be classified in a variety of ways. Closed head injuries include those in which there is no injury to the skull (e.g., scalp laceration) or only a linear fracture of the skull. Within the category of closed head injury, patients may have no significant structural damage to the brain, and are diagnosed as having a simple concussion, or may have damage of the brain tissue, due to edema, laceration, contusions, and hemorrhage.

Simple depressed fracture implies that pieces of fragmented bone are depressed inward, but the pericranium is still intact. Compound fracture implies that pericranial tissues have been torn and that there is a direct line of communication between the lacerated scalp and the brain tissue.

Regardless of the nature of the external injury, it is the severity of the injury to the brain itself that determines prognosis and expected recovery. Classification of the bony injury is helpful primarily for determining if surgical intervention will be required.

The injury to the brain may be at the site of the trauma, or it may be on the opposite side of the skull (contrecoup injury), due to shearing forces and the bouncing of the brain within the skull. The injury to the brain may be due to edema, contusion, laceration of brain or vessels, hemorrhage, or necrosis (following penetration injuries).

In the case of head injury, several processes may occur: (a) actual structural damage to the neurons will produce changes in nervous system function as manifested by focal neurologic signs; (b) damage to vessels may cause rupture and hemorrhage of blood into the brain or compartments within the skull; (c) destruction of brain tissue will result in necrosis of tissue; (d) a reactive edema, or cerebral edema, will occur. The edema worsens for 48 to 72 hours posttrauma, then gradually subsides.

All of the above physiological changes contribute to altering neurologic function and/or increasing the intracranial pressure (see section on intracranial pressure). Changes in function due to cerebral edema and increased intracranial pressure may completely disappear in time; neurologic changes due to actual tissue destruction will remain. It is not possible to determine the specific causes of an individual patient's neurologic signs (i.e., damage or pressure) but treatment is usually initiated with the goal of reducing edema and preventing any worsening of patient condition.

Signs and symptoms of head injury vary from slight headache to coma and death. Most frequently, the individual will manifest changes in level of consciousness, or loss of orientation to his surroundings or time. There may be confusion, dizziness, nausea, vomiting, hemiplegia, aphasia, cranial nerve palsies, and other focal neurologic signs. There may be loss of memory of events just preceding the injury (retrograde amnesia).

Effects of Alcohol

If the patient ingested alcohol just prior to sustaining head injury, two problems may occur. First, any alteration in level of consciousness, headache, vomiting and some other signs may be due to alcohol ingestion or head trauma or both. Second, the ingestion of alcohol delays the onset of cerebral edema by two to three hours, but the cerebral edema persists significantly longer.[41]

Diagnostic studies which may be helpful in determining the extent of injury include skull and neck x-rays, echoencephalogram, arteriogram, occasionally lumbar puncture and electroencephalogram.

Complications

Numerous complications can occur as a result of head injury.

Extradural Hematoma

Extradural hemorrhage (i.e., into the extradural space) is usually caused by rupture of the middle meningeal artery, or from one of the dural sinuses. The hematoma is often quite large. In a typical case the patient suffers some form of head trauma, loses consciousness for a short period, again becomes lucid, then subsequently loses consciousness again. Diagnosis is made by clinical history and x-ray evidence of arterial or sinus tear. This is the most fatal complication, but fortunately occurs rarely.

Subdural Hematoma

Subdural hemorrhage is bleeding between the dura and arachnoid. It is usually caused by small vein rupture, and may be bilateral. Because the bleeding is venous in origin, the intracranial pressure increases slowly as a result of the enlarging hematoma, symptoms not appearing until a few days after injury. The symptoms are the same as for any slowly growing mass lesion: headache, unequal pupils, alterations in level of consciousness, extremity weakness on the side opposite of the hematoma, and so on. Arteriogram, echoencephalogram, and careful observation of the patient are helpful in diagnosing it. Treatment consists of drilling burr holes over the hematoma and draining it.

Intracerebral Hematoma

Intracerebral hemorrhages are usually small, and multiple ones may occur. Because of location, many cannot be removed.

Rhinorrhea and Otorrhea

Rhinorrhea or drainage of cerebrospinal fluid through the nose may occur after fracture of facial bones in sinuses. The problem is not the drainage itself, but the possible meningitis that can occur if the CSF is contaminated. Otorrhea is similar to rhinorrhea, but is drainage of cerebrospinal fluid through the ear.

Diabetes Insipidus

Diabetes insipidus is a condition of high urine volume of low specific gravity (1.000-1.005). It is caused by a (usually temporary) deficiency of antidiuretic hormone (ADH), which is stored and secreted in or near the pituitary gland. This ADH insufficiency is due to manipulation or damage to the pituitary gland, which in turn is due to trauma to the gland or to compression of the gland from the increased intracranial pressure. If not treated, the condition can result in gradual weight loss and severe electrolyte imbalance. In the acute care situation, diabetes insipidus can be controlled by the administration of Pitressin or Pitressin Tannate in oil.

Inappropriate ADH

Inappropriate ADH is a syndrome of excessive secretion of ADH. It may be seen in patients with head trauma, tumors, meningitis and a variety of other conditions. In this syndrone, the excessive ADH secretion reduces urine output and increases urine concentration. If fluid intake exceeds fluid output, a positive water balance ensues in which there is weight gain and dilution of body fluids, one aspect of which is a fall in sodium concentration. The increased fluid volume results in increased kidney perfusion, but since the plasma volume is overexpanded, tubular reabsorption of sodium and chloride is decreased, so large amounts of sodium can be lost in the urine. Thus, this syndrome is characterized by hyponatremia and hypochloremia, normal cardiovascular function as manifested by normal blood pressure and normal skin turgor, normal renal function as manifested by a low BUN and serum creatinine, normal adrenal cortical function, and a urine sodium excretion as high as dietary sodium intake.

Symptoms include headache, mental sluggishness, nausea, vomiting, alterations in level of consciousness, convulsions, coma, and death. The hyponatremia is usually asymptomatic until it falls below 120 mEq. per liter. Administration of sodium does not help, except on an emergency or temporary basis. Restriction of fluid intake will help correct the physiologic manifestations.

Neurosurgery

Many of the procedures done in neurosurgery can be thought of as forms of head injury. Three procedures will be mentioned. In performing burr holes, small (1-2 cm. or smaller) holes are drilled through the skull in order to provide access to the meninges or to provide needle injection sites to various parts of the brain.

Craniectomy is the removal of some of the skull bone, occasionally to relieve excessive pressure within the skull.

Craniotomy is the term applied to any neurosurgical operation in which a piece of the skull is removed, direct access to the brain is provided, and manipulation of the brain for the purpose of excising lesions or masses, repairing aneurysms, removing foreign matter such as bone fragments, and so on, is done. Obviously, a craniotomy can be analogous to a head injury. Both in head injury and in craniotomy, damage to the brain may occur, cerebral edema does occur, and intracranial pressure rises. In a neurosurgical situation the patient must undergo anesthesia which complicates management.

Because of the similarities between craniotomy and head injury a special section devoted to the patient undergoing craniotomy will not be done. Assessment of and interventions for the head injured patient and the neurosurgical patient are the same.

Assessment

Regardless of whether a patient has undergone craniotomy or sustained a head injury, a total body assessment is required to give the nurse baseline data from which to make later observations and comparisons. See also the section on intracranial pressure.

The first area of assessment should be respiratory function. Hypoventilation often indicates upper airway obstruction, which can often be cleared by repositioning and suctioning. Bagging and suctioning can increase intracranial pressure briefly, but the respiratory acidosis produced by hypoventilation may lead to cerebral hypoxia. Hyperventilation can lead to respiratory alkalosis, which causes vasoconstriction and may lead to cerebral ischemia.

Of course, alterations in respirations may be due to actual compression or damage to the respiratory centers in the brainstem. Cheyne-Stokes respiration, that is, respirations of increasing depth followed by periods of apnea, are often indications of moderate to severe intracranial pressure elevations. Changes over time of the respiratory pattern may be indications of increasing intracranial pressure in the head injured patient.

The next area of assessment should be the neurologic system. This should include evaluation of level of consciousness, orientation, memory and other aspects of higher level functioning. This includes a determination of the appropriateness of the patient's responses. If the patient cannot speak, it will be necessary to look at body movements: are they purposeful, or random? It may only be possible to test for deep pain response.

Pupillary response is especially important. Compression of cranial nerve III by growing mass lesions or cerebral edema and pressure will cause a decrease in the transmission of impulses to the pupil, resulting in pupillary dilation, or unequal pupillary response to light. Some discretion about whether to test *all* of the cranial nerves should be used. Assessing facial symmetry (C.N. VII), ability to stick out the tongue in the midline (C.N. XII) and eye movements (C.N. III, IV and VI) may be particularly helpful.

The next area of assessment is usually motor ability. Check for equality of strength, looking at right versus left and upper extremity versus lower extremity. Unless the nurse has the time, it is usually not necessary to do a detailed examination of such things as vibration sense, sensory equality, deep tendon reflexes, and so on. It may be helpful to monitor the Babinski reflex.

In the unconscious patient, two kinds of abnormal responses to pain may be seen. In *decerebrate rigidity,* the patient has opisthotonus, with all four limbs extended, head erect and jaws closed. The arms are internally rotated at the shoulder, extended at the elbow and hyperpronated, with the fingers extended at the metacarpophalangeal joint and flexed at the interphalangeal joints. The legs are extended at the hips, knees and ankles; the toes are plantar flexed. In *decorticate rigidity,* the positioning is the same as above except the arms are semiflexed. Both situations are indicative of a loss of the cerebrum's ability to inhibit primitive reflexes. These responses are usually seen only in the critically ill neurologic patient.

In recording information about the neurologic exam, the more precise and clear the description of objective data is, the more helpful it is to later observers.

The next area of assessment should be vital signs. Temperature elevations are occasionally due to actual neural damage to or compression of the temperature regulating center, but are more often due to infection. Slight temperature elevation (.5 to 1°C) may be due to meningeal irritation from blood.

Pulse as an indicator of cardiac function is important, but also as an indicator of cerebral functioning. Traditionally, increasing intracranial pressure produces a slowing of the pulse. Respiration has already been discussed. Blood pressure should be monitored carefully. Again, an increasing blood pressure with a widening pulse pressure may be indicative of increasing intracranial pressure. An isolated blood pressure reading without other patient data is not helpful, since treatments, moving in bed, and many other variables can raise the blood pressure. In order to adequately perfuse the brain, the arterial pressure must be greater than the intracranial pressure.

If direct measurement of intracranial pressure is being done, it should be assessed regularly.

The nurse should assess the patient for any undiagnosed trauma. It is easy, when there are known severe head injures, to overlook trauma to long bones, ribs, and so on. The other signs the nurse should be familiar with are Battle's sign and signs of meningeal irritation. Battle's sign, or subcutaneous blood (a bruise) over the mastoid area is suggestive of a basal skull fracture. Signs of meningeal irritation include a stiff neck when neck flexion is attempted or pain and resistance on straight leg raising. In the head injured this irritation is usually caused by blood in the subarachnoid space. Do not bend the neck unless it has been confirmed that there is no spinal cord injury.

Drainage from the nose or ear should be noted. Test nasal drainage for glucose—nasal mucus has no sugar, cerebrospinal fluid contains glucose. Ear drainage may be mixed with blood. If the ear drainage dries on the pillow or a dressing with a pale yellow halo around the center blood-colored spot, there is a good chance that there is cerebrospinal fluid mixed with the blood.

Quantity and character of drainage from head wounds or surgical incisions should be monitored regularly.

Interventions

Many nursing interventions in caring for the neurosurgical patient are related to maintenance and/or restoration of normal intracranial pressure. Consequently, these interventions will be discussed under a separate heading.

Head dressings can be reinforced or changed if needed. Sterile technique should be maintained in applying new dressings. If drains are in place, as might be after burr holes for subdural hematoma, care should be taken not to remove them. Many physicians prefer that wounds with drains in place have dressings reinforced only, not changed, until the drains are removed.

Sutures will remain in place a week to ten days. The head dressing can usually be removed and left off after four to five days. For aesthetic reasons the patient or family may prefer that a dressing or cap be left on. Also, the sutures sometimes "catch" on the sheets, and for that reason a small dressing may be desired to prevent this. Once sutures are removed the head can usually be washed as usual.

Many neurosurgical procedures will necessitate removing all of the patient's hair. Hair should not be discarded without the patient's approval. If a portion of the hair is left in place, many patients prefer it to be clipped short rather than left long in sharp contrast to other bald areas.

If a portion of the skull has been removed during neurosurgery a "window" to the brain has been created. If intracranial pressure is elevated, the skin flap may appear and feel tense and taut; as intracranial pressure drops the flap will become softer and less tense. It does no harm to touch the skin flap, but injury to the brain below should be prevented. At a later date surgery can be done to repair an unattractive skull defect.

Pain medication is administered cautiously to the neurosurgery patient. Morphine, Demerol and Talwin are usually avoided. Low dose codeine is usually satisfactory.

Restlessness can be a problem. Sedation, because of the effect on the nervous system, is usually avoided. Careful padding of the side-rails may be helpful. Restraints should be avoided if possible; struggling against the restraints can increase intracranial pressure. If the patient is pulling at his various treatment and monitoring tubes, the application of mitts to his hands may be satisfactory for preventing him from removing these tubes.

Frequent reorientation of the patient to his surroundings is usually necessary. The patient's family may need some emotional preparation before seeing the patient. In addition, the family should be reminded that the patient has virtually no control over bizarre behavior which may be seen after head injury. Careful explanation of nursing actions is helpful to patient and family.

If otorrhea and/or rhinorrhea are present, the ear or nose can be *loosely* packed or dressed to absorb drainage. Do not irrigate the ears. Dressings should be sterile, especially if there is a chance that drainage is CSF.

Intake, output, specific gravity of urine, and weight should be monitored carefully.

INTRACRANIAL PRESSURE

Etiology and Pathophysiology

The brain is enclosed in the rigid bony box, the skull. Within the skull, intracranial volume is the sum of the volumes of the brain tissue, the cerebral blood flow and the cerebrospinal fluid. The Munroe-Kellie Hypothesis states that "an increase in the volume of any one of the contents of the cranium is usually accompanied by a reciprocal change in the volume of one of the others."[38] Thus, an enlarging tumor, for example, must either decrease the volume of cerebrospinal fluid or the cerebral blood flow, or increase the pressure of the contents within the skull, or ultimately force some of the contents of the skull out, as through the foramen magnum.

In fact, two events occur simultaneously: an increase in volume of any one of the intracranial contents increases the intracranial pressure and decreases the volume (slightly) of the other intracranial contents. Actually, shifting of brain contents is a late stage of intracranial manifestation. The objective parameter used to monitor the equilibrium within the skull is the intracranial pressure.

The normal intracranial pressure is 50-180 mm. H_2O (approximately 4-13 mm. Hg) and is usually determined by measuring the ventricular fluid pressure. It is easy to think of intracranial pressure (ICP) as a relatively stable, unchanging value since the most frequently seen measurement analogous to it is the opening pressure during lumbar puncture, a one-time measurement. [Both ventricular fluid pressure and lumbar cerebrospinal fluid pressure are essentially the same, but represent measurements at different points in the circulating system of cerebrospinal fluid (CSF)]. Depending on patient condition, position, presence of injury or block, etc., they may be the same at any one moment or different. When monitoring intracranial pressure when an elevation is suspected, lumbar puncture is avoided to prevent the sudden withdrawal of CSF, which would lower the pressure in the spinal subarachnoid space and precipitate sudden downward shifting of intracranial contents, or herniation.

Intracranial pressure is changing all the time. Systemic blood pressure variations may cause normal fluctuations up to 11 mm. Hg, and respiration causes slight variations in pressure. Activities such as the Valsalva maneuver (forced expiration against a closed glottis, as used when straining for bowel movement), tracheal suctioning, and moving around in bed can cause transient spikes in pressure as high as 800 mm. H_2O (60 mm. Hg). These frequent but short spikes in pressure are normal.[36]

Problems with intracranial pressure occur with sustained pressure peaks of up to 1360 mm. H_2O (100 mm. Hg), which last five minutes or longer.[36] In these instances of sustained increases, the increased ICP causes a decrease in the cerebral blood flow, which in turn causes inadequate perfusion and hypoxia. The hypoxia increases the $PaCO_2$ and decreases the pH, which in turn results in vasodilation and edema. Of course the edema further increases the ICP. In addition, actual compression of neural tissue can occur as ICP rises. Ultimately, the brain will push downward through the only escape valve present, the tentorial notch, and herniation will occur.[38]

In order to maintain adequate cerebral functioning, an adequate cerebral perfusion pressure must be maintained. Cerebral perfusion pressure (CPP) is the difference between the mean arterial pressure (MAP) and the intracranial pressure (ICP). The MAP is usually slightly less than the average of the systolic and diastolic pressures; for ease of computation, the mathematical average can be used. The CPP should be maintained above 60 mm. Hg; a CPP below 30 mm.

Hg may be incompatible with life.[50] An example:

ICP = 80 mm. Hg (1088 mm. H_2O)
BP = 170/110 mm. Hg
MAP = 130-140 mm. Hg
CPP = MAP - ICP
40-50 = (130-140) - 80
1 mm. Hg = 13.6 mm. H_2O
Calculation must be done using same units.

Thus, although the ICP and MAP are both elevated, an adequate cerebral perfusion is barely being maintained, and reduction of the blood pressure without reduction of the ICP would be inappropriate, if not disastrous.

Clinical manifestations of increasing intracranial pressure include headache, deteriorating level of consciousness, alterations in pupillary size and reaction, and changes in motor ability. The classic objective parameters include an increasing systolic blood pressure (an autoregulatory attempt to maintain cerebral perfusion), widening pulse pressure, decreasing pulse (due to vagal stimulation from the increased pulse pressure and carotid baroreceptor stimulation due to increased systolic pressure) and some respiratory changes. In the unconscious patient there may be increasingly inappropriate responses to painful stimuli or abnormal posturing (decorticate or decerebrate rigidity). Unfortunately, there is not a good correlation between changes in the clinical picture and actual values of intracranial pressure. While it is true that as the patient's ICP continues to rise, the clinical picture will continue to deteriorate, each patient can tolerate actual levels of ICP differently. Also, the changes in vital signs are often a late sign of ICP changes.

Causes of increased intracranial pressure include cellular hypoxia, cerebral edema, increasing mass lesions such as hematoma, tumor or abscess, or blocks in CSF circulation. Recall, too, that normal activities such as the Valsalva maneuver, *superimposed* on already increased ICP, further increase the ICP.

Assessment

In assessing the patient for his level of intracranial pressure, the nurse must consider a variety of variables. If there is a monitoring system available for the actual measurement of ICP, so much the better. Careful, accurate measurements should be made, taking care to use the monitoring system correctly. Principles of ICP monitoring are discussed below. Actual measurement should not be evaluated without also considering patient activity, blood pressure, and position.

At the time the intracranial pressure is measured, the blood pressure and pulse should be obtained. Ideally, intra-arterial pressure should be monitored, but if this is not possible, the usual sphygmomanometer reading can be made. It is important to recognize the relationship between blood pressure and intracranial pressure.

Other vital signs should be measured also, although temperature will usually not change too drastically, and usually only needs to be taken every two hours.

It is very important to carefully assess the neurologic status, but especially in those institutions where direct monitoring of ICP is not possible. In particular, the nurse should look at level of consciousness, pupillary changes, changes in motor function, and response to pain.

Interventions

Nursing interventions in relation to increased ICP fall into two categories: prevention and treatment. Prevention will be discussed first.

It is important to maintain a patent airway so that hypoxia from a respiratory source can be prevented. It may be necessary to suction a patient to do this, which increases ICP, but efficient suctioning to maintain an airway is of high priority and should not be omitted. Bagging with high concentration oxygen before and during suctioning will help prevent momentary hypoxia.

Position the patient carefully and reposition frequently. Elevating the head 15-45° if possible will promote gravity drainage. Try to prevent neck flexion, especially if the flexion would produce venous obstruction resulting in increased ICP.

Prevent the Valsalva maneuver as much as possible. Administration of stool softeners (with physician consultation) and regulation of diet can reduce the need to strain at stool. Instructing the patient to exhale during bowel movements and during position changes in bed will prevent the Valsalva maneuver.

Isometric exercises are contraindicated. The nurse should do passive range of motion exercises to the patient to maintain joint function.

In treating the patient with known increased ICP, the above mentioned interventions can still be utilized. In addition, other approaches will be necessary.

Pharmacologic intervention is helpful in decreasing intracranial pressure. Administration of dexamethasone (Decadron), a glucocorticoid, has been helpful. The nurse should be alert to the possibility of gastric irritation and ulceration; antacids or frequent small feedings may be ordered also. Remember to check stools for occult blood. Also, as the dosage is reduced, the patient may temporarily worsen slightly.

Mannitol and urea, osmotic diruetics, may occasionally be administered. The drugs are used primarily in crisis situations as they do not have a long-term effect, are usually given intravenously, and are often followed by a rebound period of patient deterioration when stopped. Intake, output, and weight should be monitored, in addition to electrolytes. Usually, a Foley catheter is necessary.

Slight hyperventilation to a $PaCO_2$ of 25-30 mm. Hg will cause vasoconstriction and reduce ICP by decreasing the cerebral blood flow, and thus is often desirable. However, if the $PaCO_2$ drops too low, a shift of the oxyhemoglobin dissociation curve will occur resulting in cerebral edema. Frequent assessment of arterial blood gases is important, and interventions based on blood gases should usually be determined in consultation with the physician.

Changes in temperature due to nervous system injury alone are unusual. If the patient is febrile, a careful search should be made for possible infections. Regardless of the cause of the fever, the usual choice is to decrease the patient's temperature, at least until normothermia is reached. An increased temperature places increased tissue demands for oxygen upon the system and can further damage the already compromised brain.

Usual nursing measures for temperature reduction include administration of antipyretics, ice bags, tepid baths, and cooling the environment. In addition, many hospitals now use hypothermia units, or electrically controlled units that can provide heat or cooling. Remember to assess any patient being cooled for adequate capillary refill of fingers and toes, and monitor for frostbite. Hypothermia mattresses cool large skin surfaces, and these surfaces are more vulnerable to pressure sores and decubitus formation. Cold is also drying to the skin; skin should be kept clean, dry, inspected frequently, and lubricated as needed. It is important to turn the patient regularly. Shivering is a protective mechanism of the body to increase temperature. Shivering should be prevented by cooling more slowly, by cooling intermittently, or by administration of chlorpromazine (Thorazine), or promethazine (Phenergan). The temperature should be monitored carefully during any prolonged measures for cooling. Finally, if cooling below normothermia is required, careful cardiac monitoring should be done. Below 35°C, cardiac arrhythmias are not uncommon.

Direct Measurement of Intracranial Pressure

It is not possible to discuss in detail the variety of devices used for monitoring the intracranial pressure. A few devices will be briefly described, and a few general principles of care will be outlined. One of the simplest devices consists of a direct tube connection between a manometer and the cerebrospinal fluid, via burr hole entry through the skull. More sophisticated devices use transducers, which are either directly implanted under the scalp, or which are connected to a ventricular cannula.

Each system has advantages and/or disadvantages in terms of ease of implantation, ease of infection, accessibility, accuracy of ICP reading, and so on. The nurse should review carefully the devices used in her institution in order to understand the positive and negative features of each system.

The following principles of care should be followed. Strictest asepsis should be used in manipulation of equipment, tubes, or monitors which have direct access to the cerebrospinal fluid. If open devices such as manometers are used, overflow of the manometer should be prevented. If the manometer overflows it should be changed. If tubes containing CSF disconnect they should be replaced if possible, or connections cleaned carefully before reconnecting.

For many systems, having the patient's head at the level of the transducer or at the zero point of the manometer is crucial to accurate readings over time. Ideally, the measurement should be taken while the patient is at rest, and not immediately after coughing, suctioning, repositioning, or other activities which elevate intracranial pressure. The reading should fluctuate slightly due to respiration and pulse; if it does not, there may be a malfunction of the system.

In open systems, where there is direct access to the cerebro-spinal fluid, specimens of CSF should be sent regularly for culture. Inspect the CSF regularly. The appearance of blood, cloudy CSF, particulate matter or bubbles, if not present earlier, should be investigated and the physician should be notified.

Intraventricular cannulae should never be flushed directly into the ventricle. Recalibration of the zero point should be done every four hours if the measuring device can be recalibrated. If there is an alarm system on the device to warn of dangerously high ICP levels, the alarm should be used and not turned off.

It should be determined in consultation with the physician if there are to be values for the ICP above which, or below which, emergency measures should be instituted or the physician called. If the intracranial pressure remains unchanged, but objectively the patient is deteriorating, the physician should be called; it may be that the equipment has failed.

Changes in treatment plans by the nursing and/or medical staffs may be based on changes in ICP values. Blood pressure, neurologic status, level of activities, and medications the patient is receiving must be included in the evaluation of changes in ICP prior to making decisions regarding treatment.

Ventricular Fluid Drainage System

Several situations might necessitate the use of an external drainage system for drainage and collection of cerebrospinal fluid. These situations include: occlusion, malfunction or infection of an internalized shunt (usually for hydrocephalus), and increased intracranial pressure due to occlusion of the CSF circulatory system, head trauma, tumor, or intracranial hematoma. The CSF can be drained from one of the lateral ventricles or from the lumbar subarachnoid space. The care of the patient in both situations is essentially the same. For that reason, only ventriculostomy will be discussed.

For direct ventricular drainage, the physician usually inserts a cannula, under sterile conditions, into one of the lateral ventricles. The tube provides access to the CSF and the ventricle for the purpose(s) of collection of CSF, introduction of air, dye or medication into the ventricle, and monitoring of intraventricular pressure. A one-way pressure regulating valve is usually connected to the ventricular cannula, and the collection system is placed distal to the valve. The valve does two things: (a) CSF can only flow one way, i.e., out of the ventricle; and (b) the CSF must reach a certain pressure before the valve will permit the CSF to drain. The physician chooses the particular valve and its required pressure based on the anticipated intracranial pressure, patient condition, age, and desired purpose of the system. Proper functioning of the valve will help to reduce contamination of ventricular fluid and prevent overdrainage of the ventricles.

In most systems, the drainage of the CSF is controlled in two ways. First, the valve, already discussed, partially regulates drainage. Second, the level of the collection bottle or bag can be used. If the collection bag is at head level, the drainage of CSF is controlled only by the valve. If the collection bag is below head level, drainage of CSF is increased because of gravity and pressure gradients. If the bag is above the level of the head, then the CSF pressure required to force fluid into the bag is increased, and CSF drainage is decreased. All three situations presuppose that the valve is at head level (it is usually taped into place).

The patient situation may be managed in one of three ways. One way is to keep the collection receptacle always at head level. Thus, any CSF that drains into the collection bottle represents displaced CSF that drained when the intracranial/CSF pressure exceeded the valve pressure.

In other situations, the goal may be to manipulate the level of the drainage bag so that a predetermined amount of CSF is drained over 24 hours. For example, perhaps the goal is to restrict CSF drainage to 120 cc. per 24 hours. This is equivalent to 5 cc. per hour, or 20 cc. every four hours. The nursing staff must then judiciously move the collection receptacle every two to four hours to regulate drainage.

Finally, the drainage of CSF may be determined by intracranial pressure measurement. This patient situation requires that some device must be in place to measure ICP. If ICP is above a predetermined level, the drainage system is unclamped or the bag lowered; if ICP is below a certain level the system is clamped or the level of the bag is raised.

Obviously, all situations of open ventricular drainage require careful and frequent monitoring. Too much drainage of CSF can precipitate subdural hematoma. Too rapid drainage can precipitate brain collapse and subarachnoid hemorrhage.[9] If the patient is allowed out of bed, the drainage system should be temporarily clamped while he is up.

Prevention of infection is of prime importance. Dressings around scalp insertion sites should be kept clean and changed using aseptic technique. The system should remain closed; if necessary, clamp the system closed. Do not open the system unless absolutely necessary.

If,connections in tubing separate, the collection system should be replaced. Sending specimens of CSF for culture on a random basis may be done. If the whole drainage system is changed, daily care should be taken to maintain asepsis.

Explain to the patient what is going on. Teach him not to touch the catheter or connections. Observe the patient carefully and frequently. Regardless of the orders concerning the ventriculostomy, any sudden, unexpected change in the patient's condition should be reported immediately to the physician.

SEIZURES

Etiology and Pathophysiology

The exact pathophysiology of seizures is unknown. It is known that seizures can be caused by anoxemia, metabolic disturbances, and structural lesions in the brain and associated with the ingestion of a variety of drugs and toxic substances. In fact, though, the exact cause of seizures in most patients is idiopathic.

In the intensive care situation, however, the incidence of seizures increases because of the kinds of neurologic conditions treated there. Some conditions frequently accompanied by seizures include meningitis, cerebral trauma, metabolic disturbances or intoxication with such things as alcohol, water and uremia, cerebral edema, carbon monoxide poisoning, anaphylaxis, tetany, insulin shock, and drug overdose.

A seizure or convulsion is defined as a "paroxysmal disorder of the nervous system characterized by recurrent attacks of alteration of consciousness, with or without convulsive movement."[34] Seizures are classified according to their manifestations as well as according to the kind of neuronal discharge present. Thus, generalized seizures, in which the site of the abnormal discharge cannot be pinpointed, include grand mal and petit mal. Focal seizures, in which the site of brain pathology can be pinpointed, include psychomotor, myoclonic, and jacksonian.

Any abnormal or unexpected patient activity, whether it involves muscles twitching, loss of consciousness, periods of abnormal response, etc., should be observed carefully and reported to the physician as it is not always possible to diagnose all kinds of seizures quickly and accurately. A brief description of some kinds of seizures follows.

Grand mal seizures are the most common kind of seizures. They are characterized by a tonic phase followed by violent clonic movements. They may last less than a minute or longer than 30 minutes. During the attack, the individual may bite his tongue, urinate or defecate. During the tonic phase, breathing almost ceases; the patient may become cyanotic. Some patients report an aura, or warning, before the seizure, during which there are strange feelings, tastes, smells or noises. Some patients seem to cry out as the seizure begins; this occurs as air is forced quickly out of the lung during the first tonic spasm. After the seizure, the patient may regain consciousness briefly, then lapse into sleep. He will not remember his seizure. Even up to several hours after the seizure, the patient may be drowsy, disoriented, complain of a headache. This is referred to as the post-ictal period.

In petit mal seizures, the individual loses consciousness for a period of seconds. In the child these are often diagnosed after someone, often a teacher, complains of frequent "staring spells." Another name for these is absence seizures.

Myoclonic seizures are involuntary contractions of the muscles of the arms, legs and trunk. The individual usually remains conscious.

In psychomotor seizures, or temporal lobe epilepsy, the patient, after a brief lapse of consciousness, begins to engage in seemingly purposeful activity such as lip smacking, disrobing, and in some rare instances, some destructive behavior. These activities are non-volitional.

In jacksonian seizures, the muscle spasm starts in one place, such as the thumb, or the lip, and then "marches" along the limb and body to involve half or all of the body.

Status epilepticus is a continuous series of seizures, usually grand mal, in which the patient does not regain consciousness between seizures. This is usually an emergency condition.

Assessment

Careful observation of the patient is usually the best thing for the nurse to do. Any patient having a (possible) seizure should be observed, keeping in mind the following types of information which should be recorded afterwards.

Presence and kinds of motor activity
Length of seizure activity or unusual activity
Presence of tongue biting, urinary or fecal incontinence
Position of head and/or eyes if they can be seen
Presence of aura or cry
Vital signs (see interventions)
Occurrence of injury during the seizure

Behavior after the attack:

Level of consciousness and degree of orientation
Ability to move all extremities
Complaints of pain or unusual feelings
Description of anything patient might remember about his "episode"

Interventions

One of the most difficult tasks of a nurse is to refrain from doing all she would like to do during a seizure, especially a grand mal seizure. In order of importance the nurse should do or not do the following:

1. Do not leave the patient.
2. Protect the patient from injury by easing him to the floor if he is in danger of falling, or putting side rails up if he may fall out of bed; cradle the head or put a pillow under it to prevent banging of

the head if he is on the floor; lower the head of the bed if appropriate. Do not try to restrain the patient.

3. If possible, turn the patient on his side to prevent aspiration of vomitus. This may take some help as it is usually not possible to turn only the head. Suction if necessary, but remember that the patient is barely breathing during the seizure. It is necessary to prevent aspiration and maintain a clear airway, but the seizure patient is at increased risk of becoming hypoxic during suctioning.

4. If the mouth is open or can be easily opened, remove food and/or loose false teeth. Put a padded tongue blade or a corner of a towel between the teeth to prevent tongue biting. *Do not* forcibly try to open the mouth already clenched tightly closed. Do not force any objects in through clenched teeth—it is easy to break teeth and injure the patient. Do not ever put fingers between the patient's teeth as a serious injury to the fingers can result.

5. Consciously observe all aspects of the seizure, including duration, for later recording.

If the patient has a history of seizures or has had one already, a few additional measures can be instituted. Side rails and, if necessary, the head of the bed can be padded. Refrain from taking temperatures orally until control of the seizures is achieved.

It may be possible to take vital signs during a seizure, but this is usually of less help in confirming the diagnosis than is careful observation.

The question of padded tongue blades at the bedside is a recurrent one. In the majority of cases the seizure begins so quickly that there is little time to get the tongue blade in place before the jaws are clamped shut. It does no harm to have the tongue blade ready, but it is often not possible to use it and it may be upsetting to some patients and families.

If a patient with an oral endotracheal tube in place is having seizures, it may be appropriate to keep something firm between the teeth at all times, since it is possible for the patient to close off the endotracheal tube in rare instances. A hard rubber airway may be used for this purpose.

Putting side rails up or down during the seizure depends on the risk to the patient. Of first priority is preventing a fall to the floor. If the patient is injuring an extremity on the side rail, and the rail can be safely lowered without allowing the patient to fall, then it should be.

For a patient with frequent seizures it may be appropriate to keep Dilantin, Valium or sodium phenobarbital at the bedside.

A few cautions about anti-seizure medications will be mentioned. Phenytoin (Dilantin) is best absorbed orally; intramuscular injection is not appropriate because the diluent can crystallize in the tissue, resulting in poor and erratic absorption. Intravenous Dilantin, when given direct IV push, is acceptable; it should not be given slow IV drip because of incompatibility with most IV solutions. It is necessary to keep in mind cardiac effects of Dilantin when giving it IV push. Of greatest concern is precipitation of arrhythmias and asystole. It should be given very slowly, over several minutes, with cardiac status being monitored with ECG machine or cardiac monitor.

Diazepam (Valium) is the drug of choice for status epilepticus. It is given intravenously. The patient's respiratory status must be monitored closely. In some cases the physician may choose a drug with fewer mental clouding effects for treatment of status epilepticus.

Sodium phenobarbital remains an excellent anticonvulsant whether used alone or in combination with other drugs. Again, the side effect of sedation makes it undesirable in some situations.

SPINAL CORD INJURY

Etiology

In order of frequency, spinal cord injuries are caused by auto accidents, water accidents (diving), gunshot wounds, motorcycle accidents, falls, and miscellaneous other accidents. Men are more frequently involved than women, and the majority of these men are between the ages of 15 and 19.

Pathophysiology

Spinal *cord* injury is usually related to the degree of vertebral injury. Simple vertebral fractures, perhaps caused by a direct blow to the back or a gunshot wound, are fractures usually of the spinous or transverse processes of the vertebra; usually there is no cord compression. In a compression fracture, as might be seen after a direct blow to the head, a diving accident, or in hyperflexion injuries, the vertebral body is compressed, decreasing the anterior height of the vertebral body, with or without neural compression. In dislocation fractures, the vertebral facets dislocate, either unilaterally or bilaterally. On x-ray view, the laminae would appear to be out of line. Damage to the cord may or may not occur. In the teardrop fracture, a piece of the vertebral body breaks off and may lodge in or near the cord; the vertebrae are also often dislocated at this time. This injury occurs with acute flexion of the spinal column, usually the neck, and is associated with spinal cord damage.

Regardless of the nature of the body trauma, it is the extent of damage or injury to the spinal cord which is of most concern. The spinal cord may be completely transected, partially transected, have a foreign body lodged in it, or be compressed. Of immediate concern when spinal cord injury is suspected, is immobilization of the patient in order to prevent progression of an incomplete lesion to a complete transection.

The following four parameters are evaluated to determine the extent of injury: paralysis of voluntary muscles below the level of the lesion, lack of sensation below the level of injury, lack of reflexes, and urine retention. Cord concussion, without transection, may be the only injury, but this may manifest itself with complete loss of function initially, with function returning gradually over the next several hours or days. The parameters usually tested for possible presence of or return of function, especially in the early post-trauma period, are sensation in the perianal region and motor function of the lower extremities. If neurologic function can be demonstrated in these areas, the patient is said to have sacral sparing. This sparing indicates that function in at least some of the long tracts of the cord has remained, and the prognosis for recovery is much better. If, by 24 hours post-injury, no sensory or motor function has returned, and there is no sacral sparing, the lesion is felt to be complete and the outlook for functional recovery is grim.

In addition to the degree of cord damage, it is also important to consider the level of the injury. The lower the level of injury, the better the prognosis for the patient, both in terms of his survival of the acute period and in relation to ultimate degree of rehabilitation.

Injury to the sacral level results in loss of innervation to the anus, penis, vagina and bladder. Injury at T_{11} or below usually means that functional walking will be possible after much rehabilitation. As the level of injury ascends the spinal cord, the amount of patient mobility and sitting balance decreases. A T_1 injury will still permit patient independence via wheelchair, but much more training will be needed for activities of daily living, transfer and maintaining balance.

Injuries above the C_8 level result in decreased upper extremity function and the possibility of complete independence is limited. Two easily remembered landmarks for cord function are the nipple line (in males) which is innervated by the T_4 nerves, and the navel, which is innervated at level T_{10}.

Spinal shock is the name applied to the period of time from the injury, when all function distal to the level of the injury ceases, until the reappearance of muscle reflexes. The spinal shock phase may last only a few hours, a few weeks, or as long as six months. The first reflexes to reappear are usually the bulbocavernous reflex (contraction of the external anal sphincter when the glans is compressed or the Foley catheter is tugged) and the perianal wink (contraction of the external anal sphincter when the perianal region is pricked with a pin).

Initially the paralysis experienced by the patient is flaccid. As reflexes begin to return, nerves stimulated in various parts of the body will transmit impulses to the spinal cord. If they are below the level of the lesion, the impulses are sent back to the area of initial stimulation causing muscle stimulation, and thus spastic paralysis. This is rarely a problem in the acute post-trauma period. While on the topic of reflexes, it should be noted that manipulation of the penis while washing the penis, catheterizing, or by manipulating the urinary catheter may cause an erection in the male. This is only a reflex response, and cannot be controlled by the patient.

One final type of lesion is the transverse hemisection of the cord, in which only the right half or the left half of the cord is cut. The clinical picture is called the Brown-Sequard Syndrome. On the side of the cord injury, the patient has paralysis due to loss of voluntary movement, loss of vibratory and position sense and loss of autonomic function. On the side opposite the side of the lesion, the patient loses pain and temperature sense below the level of the lesion.

Diagnostic studies used by the medical team to confirm spinal cord injury will include x-rays and perhaps lumbar puncture. Myelogram is often not required.

Complicating Situations

Any spinal cord injury is a serious and long-term problem for the patient. There are several factors which can complicate the situation.

The diaphragm is innervated by the phrenic nerves which leave the cord between C_{3-5}. Transection of the cord at this level almost always results in severe respiratory distress requiring intubation or tracheostomy and ventilatory assistance. The movement of the diaphragm accounts for about 80% of the ventilatory effort; the remaining muscles of inspiration, the intercostals, account for 20%. Loss of part or all of the intercostal innervation (injury at T_{1-12}) may cause some decreased respiratory functioning, but the problem is not as severe as it is when injury occurs at C_{3-5}. The abdominal muscles, and to some degree the intercostals, are needed for effective coughing: injury below T_{12} will still result in potential for respiratory problems because cough is diminished.

Edema to the cord at the site of injury is known to occur and may increase for 1 to 48 hours after injury. This edema often masks the exact damage to the cord. The danger is that the edema, which is increasing within the confines of the backbone, may rise and compress the cord at a higher level. Thus, it is possible for swelling at the site of a C_8 injury to result in compression at C_5 or $_6$, and cause some diaphragm failure. Usually the edema is temporary and after four or five days will subside without permanent effect.

The need for surgery may be a complicating factor to the spinal cord injured patient who is obviously already compromised. Surgery to the cord may be indicated when (a) there is an open fracture at the site of the spinal cord injury; (b) a dislocation cannot be reduced by closed methods; (c) a lesion thought to be incomplete seems to be progressing; (d) bony fragments are thought to be present in the spinal canal; (e) there is known block of the subarachnoid space. In addition, of course, other fractures and injuries sustained at the time of the initial trauma may require surgery, with its associated hazard of general anesthesia.

Some hypotension occurs with most spinal cord injuries because of loss of vascular tone. Extremely pronounced or severe hypotension is dangerous to any patient, but especially if associated with cardiovascular disease or other problems. The level of injury influences hypotension as does the presence of other injuries (i.e., hypovolemic shock may be present due to blood loss associated with other fractures or injuries).

In spinal cord injury, the ability to sweat is lost below the level of the lesion. Thus, an important method of temperature control is lost. The patient's temperature should be monitored carefully, and if it rises, measures should be taken to decrease it.

Assessment

The need for a careful initial total body assessment cannot be overemphasized. Ideally, the nurse and physician should work together on this since the nurse must know the degree and level of injury the medical team feels the patient has. Also, the nurse should know of any reflex or motor activities that deserve special attention. Finally, the degree of back or neck mobility to be permitted should be clarified before nursing actions are instituted.

Please refer to the chapter on patient assessment. The nurse should do careful and frequent assessments of respiratory function, especially if a high cord lesion is suspected. In addition, careful monitoring of the cardiovascular system should be done, including rate, rhythm and quality of pulse, color and blood pressure. Usually the patient will be placed on a cardiac monitor. Temperature should be watched carefully.

Injury to the spinal cord results in decreased motility to the gastrointestinal tract. The patient will of course be NPO initially, but regular monitoring for the presence of bowel sounds and passing of flatus is important. The bladder will usually be flaccid and the patient will have no sensation when the bladder is full. Close monitoring of intake and output is important.

Careful assessment for the purpose of discovering undiagnosed injuries should be done regularly the first few days. This would include a careful examination of the level of consciousness, pupillary response and other parts of the cranial check to determine if head injury has occurred.

Once the nature of the injury has been determined, it is usually possible to condense the assessment to focus primarily on acutely involved systems. For example, if it has been decided that complete transection has occurred at the T_1 level, it serves little purpose to spend a lot of time repeatedly testing lower extremity function. Once a day, or once a shift, a complete neuroexam can be performed to maintain baseline data, but the nurse's time can better be spent evaluating the respiratory function and preventing complications.

Intervention

It is not an overstatement to say that the quality of nursing care will determine the long-term prognosis for the patient with a spinal cord injury. Goals fall into the following general areas:

1. The patient will not sustain progression of his lesion.
2. The patient will not develop complications related to the respiratory system, the cardiovascular system, the integumentary system, the renal system, the gastrointestinal system, or inadequate nutrition.
3. The patient and his family will be supported as they begin to deal with the emotional impact of the spinal cord injury.

As alluded to earlier, it is necessary to have a clear understanding of the amount of back or neck movement the patient can tolerate. Usually the patient will be put into traction, either with Crutchfield tongs, or their equivalent. The tongs permit turning from side to side in a bed, or can be adjusted to fit a Foster or Stryker frame to permit turning from back to front. In some situations a halo cast can be used which immobilizes the head in relation to the body and permits greater movement in bed. For certain low back injuries, casts, careful immobilization in bed, or a Foster or Stryker frame without traction may be all that is needed.

In relation to the immobilization situation, remember that the body should be kept in direct alignment with the head and neck, and the nurse should request adequate assistance in attempting to move or transfer the patient. The skin around any tongs or screws into the head should be cleaned at least every eight hours with a dilute hydrogen peroxide solution. This cleaning is often followed by the application of a small amount of a povidone-iodine cream. If the patient has long hair, he/she may permit one to trim it since it will be difficult to wash, will frequently fall over the tong sites, and will fall in the patient's face. The tongs or screws should regularly be examined to make certain they are still securely placed and not coming loose.

If the patient can survive the initial post-trauma period, the next greatest problem is preventing complications. After the acute phase of injury, death in the spinal cord injured is usually due to infection: respiratory, kidney or bladder, and decubitus ulcer.

Respiratory function

The prevention of respiratory complications is the same as for any immobilized patient. Remember, though, that this patient may not be able to cough so that the clearing of secretions may become a nursing function, via suctioning. If the patient requires the use of a respirator, the usual care required for the respiratory system-impaired client would be appropriate. Remember that the spinal cord injured patient often cannot move his hands. He therefore may have difficulty getting the nurse's attention if the respirator becomes disconnected or malfunctions. He is totally dependent on the nurse to maintain respiratory function.

Integumentary and musculoskeletal

The maintenance of skin integrity and the prevention of decubiti must be a major nursing function from the moment the patient enters the intensive care setting. Every decubitus that is allowed to develop increases the patient's hospital bill by $10,000 to $15,000 by prolonging the stay. In addition, the scar tissue formed after an ulcer heals is more fragile than normal healthy skin, making the possibility of repeated skin breakdown greater.

The patient must be turned religiously every two hours or more often, and his skin inspected regularly. It is important to note that since the patient cannot feel how he is positioned, he also cannot feel pressure developing and will almost never request to be turned. Patients on turning frames are often uncomfortable and/or uneasy when face down. This discomfort can be relieved by better padding around the face and neck, by reassuring the patient and checking on him often, and by identifying yourself when approaching him when face down. Some nurses have even put their names on the toes of their shoes so the patient could identify them. The actual turning of the frame can be anxiety-producing, too. If the nurse is uneasy with the equipment the patient can usually detect this and may not want to turn. Finally, do not attempt to turn the patient at night without waking him; the patient may waken and be frightened during the turn or disoriented after the turn.

Turning is important, but so is the position of the body at all times and the surfaces on which the patient must lie. Obviously clean, dry, wrinkle-free sheets should be next to the skin. When the patient is on his back adequate pillows, sand bags, and trochanter rolls should be used to keep the feet straight up (prevention of foot-drop) and the legs straight (prevention of external rotation of the hip). Hands should be wrapped around a small handroll or placed in splints to maintain a functional hand position. If a Foley catheter is being used, it should be taped or secured to the abdomen of the male and the inner thigh of the female. Anti-embolism stockings are often ordered for the patient. These must be removed every eight hours to allow for careful inspection of toes and heels. Sheepskin elbow and heel pads may be indicated.

If the patient can be positioned on his side remember to: (a) use a small pillow under his head, (b) pad between bony prominences that may rub, such as knees and ankles, (c) assess carefully the position of the lower shoulder and arm, and (d) keep the head, neck and back in straight alignment.

When the patient is prone, the feet should be allowed to hang over the edge of the frame or mattress in order to prevent footdrop. Careful padding with pillows is usually needed for the whole front side of the patient. In the male, the penis should not be compressed; in the female the breasts should not be compressed. As mentioned earlier, careful padding of the forehead and chin (jaw) should be done when the patient is prone. Finally, always observe the patient and decide if you could maintain that position comfortably for two hours before leaving and assuming that he can.

Even in the patient with flaccid paralysis, maintenance of joint range of motion exercises should be done regularly. It may be help-ful to consult with the Physical Therapy Department even in the in-tensive care setting to collaborate on any unique positioning prob-lems the patient has.

Since the patient has no sensation below the level of cord tran-section, the application of heat or cold poses a great threat. The nurse should be extremely careful not to burn the patient or apply ice without adequate padding.

The Renal and Gastrointestinal Systems

In developing a plan of care for management of bowel and blad-der function, it is helpful to collaborate with the nursing staff on the general medical-surgical unit(s) where the patient may go after leaving the intensive care setting, in addition to the rehabilitation units or facilities in the area, to determine, if possible, one routine. In this way the established routine can be started immediately after admission and can be continued until discharge.

Presently, the first choice for bladder management is intermittent catheterization, and the second choice is indwelling catheterization. Needless to say, strictest aseptic technique should always be used when inserting a catheter. In both cases a fluid intake of 3,000 to 5,000 cc. per 24 hours should be maintained. There is some discussion about whether certain types of fluids should be excluded, e.g., milk, orange juice, beer, and other fluids encouraged, e.g., cranberry juice. A decision about types of fluids to be used should be made by the medical and nursing staffs together. Intake and output should be monitored closely.

It is also desirable to have an agreed upon pattern for bowel retraining, and the sooner it is started, the better. Bowel programs vary, but include some common features. The best time to schedule the planned bowel evacuation is a time suitable for the patient at home (if it is possible to determine this in the early post-injury period). Determine if any activities or foods stimulated bowel movement at home, such as drinking coffee or fruit juice just before bowel evacuation and, if possible, include these stimulators in the bowel program. Adjust the diet to facilitate regular bowel movements: adequate fluids, inclusion of roughage, addition of prune juice, and so on. Determine if a bowel movement is to be precipitated daily or three days a week; if the latter, decide which days and stick to the plan. Initially, use a bisacodyl suppository to stimulate the evacuation. In time, glycerin suppositories can be used instead. Refrain from using enemas unless absolutely necessary. It is difficult to imagine developing a bowel retraining program in the immediate post-injury period, but if the patient is to remain in the Intensive Care Unit even as long as three weeks, plans for a bowel program will be needed.

An emergency problem that may occasionally arise even in the intensive care situation is autonomic hypertension: severe headache, blurred vision, bradycardia, nausea, chest pain, nasal congestion, and vasodilation above the level of the lesion, and pilomotor spasm. It is an excessive autonomic response to normal stimuli, and usually occurs in patients with lesions at T_8 or higher.[15]

The trigger stimulus is caused by distention or contraction of the viscera, as with distended bladder, distended rectum, pressure on the glans penis, or uterine contraction in the pregnant female. It is usually not a problem until reflexes begin to reappear, as when bladder tone returns. Immediate treatment includes removing the trigger stimulus: check for catheter patency, and irrigate the catheter or replace it if necessary. Elevate the head of the bed, if condition permits, and monitor vital signs. If the cause is fecal impaction, Nupercaine ointment (dibucaine HCl) or its equivalent should be applied to the anus and about an inch into the rectum. This will prevent the insertion of the suppository or the manual disimpaction from stimulating the sympathetic system even more. Pharmacologic intervention in the form of antihypertensives or adrenergic blocking may be necessary.

Not all patients have autonomic hyperreflexia, but in those who do, it is usually a chronic problem, so the patient and staff should be alerted and measures to prevent recurrence should be employed.

Nutritional Status

Initially, the spinal cord injured patient will be kept NPO. After the patient's condition stabilizes and bowel sounds are again present, oral intake may resume. It is difficult to drink fluids while flat, so a nasogastric tube may be inserted for a time before an attempt is made to feed a semi-solid, soft, or regular diet. Any accepted regime for diet advancement is fine, so long as the patient is monitored carefully; he usually must lie flat, and often cannot cough effectively.

Eventually the rehabilitation team can work with the patient to decide on an appropriate weight goal and develop any special diets needed. The patient should not be expected to lose weight in the immediate post-trauma period. The diet should be high in protein, probably low in fat, with determination of appropriate caloric, carbohydrate and fluid needs. Consultation with a dietician will be helpful.

Emotional Support

Just as the physical needs of the spinal cord injured patient are enormous, so are the emotional. It is not unusual to find that the patient, his family *and* the nursing staff have initial feelings of shock, disbelief and denial, particularly if the patient is an otherwise healthy and attractive young male. It will take everyone time to adjust.

Even the almost obvious aspects of good emotional support should not be omitted. Tell the patient and his family what procedures you are doing and why. In his dependent and defenseless state, the patient may be easily startled and frightened. Be sure to speak to him before touching him if he cannot see you, so that he will not be startled by your presence.

Do not destroy the patient's hopes, especially if the extent of injury is not clearly defined or severe edema is clouding the picture, but at the same time do not be falsely optimistic, or unrealistic. Try to be honest with the patient and his family, but gently so. Answer questions as they ask them. The sensitive nurse can usually determine when the patient or his family needs additional information or more specific details. The patient and family often do not recall at a later time information about prognosis which was given to them in the first few hours after injury while they were in shock. Both the patient and family need time alone with the nurse. Other resources available include the Chaplain and Social Service.

As the patient slowly begins to see and understand his injury, he may have many questions about the future: his job, his family, his role in society, his level of activity, and sex. The nurse's role is to (1) allow the patient to verbalize concerns, (2) answer questions she can answer honestly, (3) consult other appropriate resources or indicate that they will be available after the patient's condition improves (e.g., Vocational Rehabilitation).

Finally, help the patient to become better adjusted to his environment and help to reorient him. Prism glasses for the patient required to lie flat on his back will help. Television or radio, even in the Intensive Care Unit, may be a welcome distraction for him, but remember that few people enjoy them for 18 continuous hours. Assuring him a restful night's sleep and orienting him to day and time are important also.

NEUROMUSCULAR DISORDERS

The two neuromuscular problems seen most often in the intensive care situation are myasthenia gravis and Guillain-Barré Syndrome. The etiology, pathophysiology, complications and assessment of each will be discussed separately; nursing interventions will be discussed together for the two diseases.

Etiology and Incidence of Myasthenia Gravis

Myasthenia gravis is a disease of voluntary muscle weakness. It is insidious in onset, and is found most often in women in their twenties and men in their fifties and sixties. Approximately two-thirds of diagnosed cases are female. The disease is non-hereditary and may be an auto-immune disease.

Pathophysiology of Myasthenia Gravis

In normal individuals, the transmission of impulses from the end of a nerve to the motor end-plate of the muscle is via the transmitter substance acetylcholine (ACh). The ACh is released from the nerve ending, moves to the end-plate causing depolarization (and thus muscle contraction) and is quickly broken down into acetate and choline by cholinesterase.

In myasthenia, one of three problems may exist; (a) too much cholinesterase is present (thus destroying ACh too quickly); (b) too little ACh is released (thus there is insufficient depolarization of the end-plate); or (c) the end-plate is no longer sensitive to ACh. Probably, too little ACh is released.

The patient with myasthenia, then, presents with muscle weakness, and each patient may have different muscles involved to a different degree. The clinical picture is one of ptosis, diplopia, difficulty in breathing, a high-pitched nasal voice, difficulty in holding up the head, and drooping of the face with difficulty smiling.

The patient with early disease is usually not actually ill. The diagnosis will be confirmed, usually with a Tensilon test (see p. 352), and a program of pharmacologic regulation will be instituted. The course of the disease is one of remissions and exacerbations, the latter being triggered by such things as stress, other illness, changes in activities, poor adherence to the treatment program, and unknown stimuli. An acute exacerbation may manifest itself as myasthenic crisis, a life-threatening situation in which the patient presents with respiratory failure and acute difficulty swallowing, resulting in inability to handle secretions. The patient in crisis will usually require some form of mechanical respiratory assistance.

The course of the disease varies with each individual; a patient with only ocular involvement or a generally mild case may live many years, and actually never view the disease as a major problem. Other individuals may have more serious cases which progress rapidly, and even with strict adherence to a complicated regime may never be without some generalized weakness and reduced ability to function. In addition, some patients seem to quickly become refractory to the usual pharmacologic regime, and thus are more difficult to manage. Death is often due to infection and/or associated respiratory failure.

Some patients show improvement after removal of the thymus gland. This is probably due to the apparent relationship between the thymus gland and the immune response. It has also been noted that there is an increased incidence of thymomas in myasthenic patients.

Diagnosis, Pharmacologic Treatment and Complications of Myasthenia Gravis

Drug treatment of myasthenia involves two groups of drugs: anticholinesterases and steroids.

Anticholinesterases act to destroy cholinesterase, and thus permit more of the ACh to reach the end plate. The choices in this category vary in their dosage, form, potency, and duration of action. Edrophonium chloride (Tensilon) is administered intravenously and is of short duration; neostigmine bromide (Prostigmin), pyridostigmine bromide (Mestinon), and Ambenonium chloride (Mytelase) are the drugs usually used for day-to-day management because of their longer duration.

The Tensilon Test

Because of its short duration, Tensilon is used to help confirm the diagnosis and, in the already diagnosed patient, to monitor the level of control achieved by the treatment regime. The Tensilon is administered intravenously to the symptomatic patient. Almost immediately there is improvement of symptoms in the under-medicated patient: ptosis may disappear, muscle strength increases, activity to swallow improves, the patient can swallow and speak. This is a *positive* Tensilon Test. The effects are only momentary.

In the patient overmedicated with anticholinesterases, administration of Tensilon will cause the patient to complain of nausea, vomiting, abdominal cramps, dysphagia, and so on. This state is called the cholinergic state, and the results indicate a *negative* Tensilon test. Atropine sulfate can be administered to reduce symptoms if the response to the Tensilon was severe. The Tensilon test is a helpful tool for the physician in determining the

TABLE 5-1

Comparison of Signs and Symptoms of
Myasthenic States and Cholinergic States[26,37]

Group of Symptoms	Myasthenic Crisis (undermedication)	Cholinergic State (overmedication)	
Central Nervous System	anxiety, psychomotor restlessness	irritability, restlessness, insomnia, headache, mental clouding, anxiety, dysarthria	
Ocular Symptoms	ptosis, diplopia		
		Muscarinic-like symptoms (vagotonic)	Nicotinic-like systems (para- lysis of ganglia)
Bulbar Symptoms	dyspnea, dysarthria, dysphonia, difficulty chewing		"thick tongue," dysarthria, dysphagia, difficulty chewing, dyspnea
Gastro-intestinal Symptoms		salivation, anorexia, nausea, vomiting, abdominal cramps, diarrhea	
General Muscle Symptoms	generalized weakness, dyspnea		fasciculations of eyelids, face, neck, legs; generalized weakness, spasms
Miscell-aneous		increased bronchial secretions, lacrimation, perspiration, miosis, blurred vision	

treatment plan. It may be necessary to repeat the test every several hours. It is necessary, then, for the nurse and the patient to know the difference between undermedication (a myasthenic state) and over-medication (a cholinergic state). The differences are outlined in Table 5-1.

As mentioned earlier, administration of atropine sulpate will help reduce symptoms of cholinergic crisis. The following should be kept at the bedside of the myasthenic: vials of Prostigmin, Tensilon, and atropine; tuberculin syringes, alcohol swabs and a tourniquet. Finally, it is extremely important to give anticholinesterases on time. Delay of even five minutes might mean that the patient is no longer able to swallow.

Steroids can be used as an adjunct to anticholinesterase therapy, but are usually withheld until the other group of drugs is no longer providing adequate relief of symptoms. Because of the problems associated with long-term steroid therapy, most physicians would prefer not to use this choice of therapy. The exact mechanism of improvement is not clearly understood. Prednisone or ACTH gel may be given on a daily basis, or in regimes of every-other-day therapy, or periods of therapy interspersed with periods of no steroid therapy. For some unclear reason, patients may initially exacerbate on steroids before going into remission.

Finally, the following drugs or groups of drugs should be avoided or given cautiously to the myasthenic: neuromuscular-blockage agents (curare, pancuronium bromide), central nervous system depressants (morphine, some barbiturates and tranquilizers), quinine and quinidine, ether, procainamide, enemas (in some patients), aspirin, and some antibiotics (streptomycin, kanamycin, gentamicin and the tetracyclines). Hypokalemia may increase muscle weakness also.

Assessment of the Myasthenic Patient

The myasthenic patient in the intensive care situation is often in pending respiratory failure. The area of greatest need, the respiratory system, requires the first and most thorough assessment (see Chapter 3).

If the patient is in severe myasthenic crisis, she may be so weak as to be unable to even speak. The nurse must assess only objective data. As the patient improves, she will often be able to assist in the gathering of data. Parameters important to assess in the myasthenic include: vital capacity, ability to swallow, ptosis, diplopia (subjective), muscle strength.

Vital capacity is used as a measure of respiratory muscle strength. Each patient will have her own "normal" range of vital capacity. In conjunction with the physician, then, the danger point for each patient, below which the physician should be called or emergency measures instituted, should be determined. Thus, an elderly female may be at the point of respiratory failure with a vital capacity below 1.0 liter; a 25-year-old male may be in danger with a vital capacity below 2.5 liters. The vital capacity can be used as a guide to the degree of improvement in the patient on a mechanical respiratory-assistive device.

It would be expected that the patient would be the weakest just before receiving the next dose of anticholinesterase medication. This, then, would be the best time to measure vital capacity.

Ability to swallow often cannot be measured in the acutely ill individual, but as she improves, can also be a guide. One way to measure it is to rank the ability to swallow on the following scale (or its equivalent):

$$0 = nothing$$
$$1 = saliva$$
$$2 = liquids$$
$$3 = puree$$
$$4 = dental\ soft$$
$$5 = normal[26]$$

As the patient learns the system she can probably tell you immediately when asked. Pills should only be administered at a grade 3 or above; below 3 the patient may be able to take the crushed pills or liquid dosage forms. It is important to know the ability to swallow before arriving at the bedside with an inappropriate pill or capsule. If the drug to be administered is an anticholinesterase, the delay caused by having to crush the pill may mean the patient will lose even more of the ability to swallow. If swallowing in general is a problem for the patient it may be possible to change the hours of medication administration so that anticholinesterases are administered approximately one hour before meals so that the patient can eat.

Ptosis can be evaluated objectively, and degree of ptosis measured as severe, moderate or slight. The patient herself can be asked if diplopia is present. Muscle strength can be evaluated by measuring hand grip strength. The parameters considered most helpful are the vital capacity and ability to swallow.

Finally, the nurse should assess to see if the expected result of anticholinesterase medication is occurring. If not, readjustment of the medication schedule may be necessary.

Etiology and Incidence of Guillain-Barré Syndrome

The etiology of Guillain-Barré Syndrome (GBS), or infectious polyneuritis, is unknown. In about two-thirds of the patients the onset of symptoms is preceded by a history of upper respiratory infection. Recently it has been linked to swine flu immunization. Except for the possible link to the swine flu virus, it is thought not to be related to viral or bacterial infection, metallic poison or alcohol consumption.

Males and females are equally affected, and the disease can occur at any time in life, including childhood.

Pathophysiology of Guillain-Barré Syndrome

The only pathologic changes found in patients with GBS are some degenerative changes in spinal and cranial nerves. The patient usually presents with muscle weakness, most commonly of the lower extremities. This weakness often increases in an ascending fashion, until the trunk, all four extremities and some of the cranial nerves are involved. In other cases it will stop at any point in the ascending process.

The course is one of increasing paralysis over a period of several hours to a week or more, a plateau period during which the paralysis stops ascending and remains stable (lasting days to weeks), and a gradual recovery period, often lasting for months. The paralysis is flaccid. The muscles, even though paralyzed, are often tender, and even slight pressure may cause discomfort. Tendon reflexes are diminished or absent. Occasionally a low grade fever is present (cause unknown).

Involvement of the vagus nerve (cranial nerve X) is thought to be the cause of sympathetic nervous system involvement. These symptoms include fluctuating blood pressure, especially orthostatic hypotension, facial flushing and generalized sweating and warmth, and bradycardia or tachycardia.

Cerebral function is usually maintained and the patient is conscious, alert and can hear. In severe cases cranial nerve involvement may result in diminished or absent gag reflex and corneal reflexes.

Diagnosis is made on the basis of the clinical picture and lumbar puncture results. In many cases the cerebrospinal fluid pressure is elevated as is the CSF protein level.

Treatment is nonspecific and symptomatic. In several weeks the paralysis will begin to disappear, usually starting from the head and moving downward. Residual effects are rare, but in prolonged courses the flaccid paralysis may have lead to moderate muscle atrophy requiring rehabilitation and an extensive program of physical therapy.

Complications of Guillain-Barré Syndrome

Death may occur in 15 to over 50 percent of cases. Though death is attributed to GBS, it is often due to respiratory failure with intercurrent infection. In patients with marked sympathetic involvement the bradycardia and/or postural hypotension may be difficult to manage.

Assessment of the Patient with Guillain-Barré Syndrome

As has been repeated throughout the chapter on neurologic problems, assessment of the respiratory status is of prime importance. This assessment includes vital capacity and/or tidal volume in association with other objective data (see Chapter 3).

In addition, cardiovascular status should be monitored, with special attention to pulse, blood pressure, and cardiac rhythm (a cardiac monitor is usually used until the patient is thought to be stabilized).

Neurologically, the progression of the paralysis, though slow, can usually be monitored by requesting the patient to perform various tasks, depending on the level of paralysis, e.g., move the hands, blink the eyes, and so on. Unlike patients with many other neurologic problems who present with completed symptomatology, the GBS patient may present relatively well, and there may be time to do a thorough history and assessment as a baseline before the patient becomes acutely ill.

Interventions for Patients with Neuromuscular Disorders

Although patients with the two diseases discussed under the section of neuromuscular disorders have different prognoses and pathologies than patients referred to under the section on spinal cord injury, the care of the dependent patient is essentially the same. (Please refer to the section on nursing intervention under spinal cord injury.)

It is very important to develop a means of communication with patients with myasthenia or GBS if these patients have disease so severe they are unable to speak. In contrast to the patient with spinal cord injury, the myasthenic or the GBS patient still has the sensations of touch, pressure and pain. He can tell you if positioned incorrectly, or if he feels constipated, or that he needs his position changed.

Patients with neuromuscular disorders need aggressive pulmonary management, including aseptic suctioning technique. See Chapter 3.

Frequent turning, range of motion exercises and careful positioning are important. Especially for the patient with GBS, encouragement to persist in exercises and use of assistive devices such as splints are helpful. Both the myasthenic and the GBS patient fatigue easily so conscientious development of a plan for rehabilitation with the P.T., O.T., and nursing staffs is essential.

Urinary management usually involves offering the bedpan/urinal as requested or inserting a Foley catheter until the patient is stronger. Patients should have bowel status monitored, and bowel management programs instituted as needed.

Monitoring eye function in these patients is important. The myasthenic may have severe ptosis, preventing vision. Little can be done except to remember that closed eyes do not mean the patient is necessarily asleep, not interested, or not alert. The patient with Guillain-Barré, on the other hand, may be unable to close his eyelids. Use of artificial tears to prevent corneal drying and use of eyepatches to prevent corneal scratching may be necessary.

If hypotension is a problem with the patient with Guillain-Barré Syndrome, it may be necessary to keep the patient flat or in the Trendelenburg's position. Unfortunately, this position may make respiratory care more difficult.

CEREBROVASCULAR DISORDERS: ANEURYSM AND STROKE

Etiology of Aneurysms

An aneurysm is an abnormal dilation or outpouching of the arterial wall, usually due to a congenital defect in the wall, a degenerative process, or both. The defect is usually of the muscle layer of the vessel. Aneurysms most frequently occur at the bifurcation of a vessel or at the point where two vessels join, and most often occur at the Circle of Willis.

Different kinds of aneurysms occur, but the most common is the Berry aneurysm, which is shaped like a small sack or pouch. Women are affected more frequently than men (ratio 3:2) and the most frequent age is early fifties.

Pathophysiology of Aneurysms

The classic picture associated with aneurysm pathology is the subarachnoid hemorrhage. In this situation the aneurysm ruptures, causing hemorrhage into the subarachnoid space. The patient complains of sudden, severe headache, nausea and vomiting. Deteriorating level of consciousness, coma and death may ensue. A grading system has been developed to classify the patient according to severity of bleed and surgical risk (Table 5-2).

An additional grade is given for age over fifty, and an additional grade is given for presence of serious medical conditions such as heart, kidney, liver, or lung involvement. Remember that the grading system is a guide, but in general, the lower the grade the better the prognosis for that patient and the better the surgical risk. Presently, most physicians wait until the patient improves (reaches a lower grade) before performing surgery, but again, the higher the grade, the longer the wait until surgery can be performed.

The major treatment, surgery, has already been mentioned. There are two major periods in the care of the aneurysm patient. Before surgery, prevention of re-bleed and complications associated with bedrest are important. The second phase is the postoperative period.

Various surgical therapies can be used depending on the size, location and kind of aneurysm. These include ligating and wrapping it, or applying a clip to the neck of the aneurysm to obliterate it; the latter choice is preferred.

The diagnosis of aneurysm is confirmed by arteriography and lumbar puncture. In rare instances, a CAT scan may also provide some additional helpful information. When the lumbar puncture is done there will be gross blood in the CSF.

TABLE 5-2

Classification of Subarachnoid Bleeds[21]	
Grade I:	Minimal bleed. Alert, no neurologic deficit, no signs of meningeal irritation
Grade II:	Mild bleed. Alert, minimal neurologic deficits such as stiff neck, third nerve palsy
Grade III:	Moderate bleed. Drowsy or confused, stiff neck with or without neurological deficits
Grade IV:	Moderate or severe bleed. Stupor to coma with some purposeful movements. May or may not have major neurological deficits
Grade V:	Severe bleed. Coma and decerebrate movements
Grade VI:	Moribund patient

Complications of Ruptured Cerebral Aneurysm

The most serious complication, of course, is death due to the growing subarachnoid hemorrhage. In most cases, however, the initial hemorrhage reflects rupture of the aneurysm with some oozing of blood (the formation of the hematoma). This subsides slowly. The chance of re-bleed is high, however, and usually occurs within a week to fourteen days after initial hemorrhage. A re-bleed into an already compromised brain can, of course, be disastrous. Thus, the risk of re-bleed must be weighed against the grade or severity of the patient on admission to determine whether and how long to wait before initiating treatment.

Another complicating factor is vasospasm, or spasm (contraction) of the cerebral vessels. The problem is that vasospasm may make angiography difficult to perform, diagnosis more difficult to make, and patient symptoms a little more severe. If prolonged, it can result in cerebral ischemia.

There is no way to determine at the time of admission of the patient the extent of permanent neurologic damage, if any. Neurologic signs due to increased intracranial pressure will usually disappear. Signs due to actual bleeding and compression by the clot may or may not disappear.

Increased intracranial pressure always develops to some degree, but may be a serious problem in some patients (see section on intracranial pressure). Diabetes insipidus and inappropriate ADH have been associated with aneurysm patients (see section on complication of head injury).

Finally, hydrocephalus as a result of blockage of CSF circulation may occur. It may be severe enough to necessitate insertion of a ventriculoperitoneal shunt.

An arteriovenous malformation (AVM) may present as an aneurysm. An AVM is an abnormal collection or growth of arteries or veins, usually reflecting some abnormality in fetal development, in which one or more connections allow the abnormal shunting of blood from the artery directly to the vein. The AVM may produce symptoms either from compression because of its large size, or by rupture into the surrounding area. Complete excision of the AVM is the treatment of choice, but, because of the size, location, number of vessels involved, and age and condition of the patient, may not be possible. Embolization, in which small Silastic spheres are purposely introduced into the AVM to cause clotting off, is sometimes used to treat these patients.

Assessment of the Patient with an Intracranial Aneurysm

The order of assessment depends partly on the condition of the patient at the time of admission. If the patient is more alert, beginning with a careful neurologic assessment would be appropriate. In any event, the patient should ultimately receive a total body assessment and detailed neurologic assessment; the nurse is usually the one who discovers that re-bleeding has begun, noting changes in the neurological baseline data.

The entire neurologic assessment will not be repeated here. See the chapter on patient assessment and the section on intracranial pressure. Of particular interest in the aneurysm patient are the signs of meningeal irritation: stiff neck, headache, occasionally opisthotonos, positive Kernig's sign, and inability to do the straight leg raising test. These all reflect meningeal irritation from blood in the CSF. In addition, a slight temperature elevation may be due to blood in the CSF.

Photophobia is often present with aneurysm patients; this makes the testing for pupillary light response very uncomfortable.

If the patient is scheduled for surgery, the reader might wish to read the section on assessment of the client with head injury, since it parallels neurosurgery.

Careful and frequent monitoring of blood pressure is important. It may be appropriate to determine some blood pressure limits, above which the physician should be called or emergency measures undertaken. In many patients hypertension is thought to contribute to the rupture of the vessel.

Interventions for Patients with Intracranial Aneurysms

Pre-Surgical Care—The Basal Living Routine

During the pre-surgical period, the efforts of the nurse should be directed toward preventing re-bleed, and preventing complications. The patient regime designed to hopefully prevent re-bleed is based on the desire to keep intracranial pressure down and to keep blood pressure down.

The patient should be placed on bedrest in a private room with limited activity. Some patients cannot tolerate complete restriction of activity, so small concessions may be made such as allowing use of the bedside commode, or permitting the patient to sit in a chair several times per day. These deviations from the usual plan should be allowed only after consultation with the physician. The patient should also be helped to understand the importance of limiting activity. While in bed, the head of the bed can usually be elevated 30-45°. The patient can usually be permitted to feed himself.

Rest should be encouraged. In some patients it may be necessary to use mild sedation, but the decision to do so should be made carefully since sedation may mask the patient's true level of consciousness. In some cases, patients are not permitted to watch television, listen to the radio or read. Such drastic measures often contribute to patient agitation since there is little else to do while confined in bed. Visitors should be limited, but again it is necessary to decide the degree of limitation based on the individual patient's response. Family (and any other visitors) should be instructed about the treatment program and their help encouraged.

Safety is important. Side rails should be up, unless someone is with the patient. It may be necessary to pad the side rails. Use of restraints is contraindicated since restraints usually contribute to agitation as the patient fights to be free. If the patient is agitated, assess him to see why: distended bladder, hunger, confusion?

Preventing constipation and associated straining at stool are important to keep the intracranial pressure and blood pressure down.

A bowel routine which incorporates use of stool softeners and appropriate diet manipulations (prune juice, roughage) is usually helpful. Use of enemas and rectal suppositories should be discouraged since stimulation of the anal area causes a vagal response and can increase blood pressure. Thus, use of rectal thermometers may be contraindicated. (It is necessary to set priorities; in the unconscious patient obtaining a rectal temperature may be less hazardous to the patient than obtaining *no* temperature).

The use of special diets partly depends on the patient's condition. If the patient is alert, a regular diet may be appropriate; if the patient is hypertensive a sodium restricted diet may be needed. Many physicians do not want patients to receive extremely hot or extremely cold beverages, so only room temperature food would be allowed. Coffee, tea and other stimulating beverages are usually restricted or forbidden. The water at the bedside should not contain ice. In the patient who is not alert, a nasogastric tube can be used for feeding. The tube feeding should not be given while ice cold, but, of course, should not be allowed to stand at room temperature for a long period.

Intake, output, specific gravity, weight, and presence of occult blood (guaiac) in stools should be monitored.

If the patient is unconscious, eye care should be done every four hours. This includes cleaning around the eyes and instilling artificial tears. If the eyes remain open it may be necessary to tape them shut. If photophobia is present in the alert patient, keeping the room dark will be more comfortable for him.

Steroids are usually employed to reduce cerebral edema. Careful observation of the patient for side effects of steroids is appropriate.

Aminocaproic acid (Amicar) has been used in recent years to promote clot formation. This drug is a systemic antifibrinolytic which acts by preventing fibrinolysis (clot dissolution) from occuring. Known side effects or untoward effects include nausea, cramping, diarrhea, dizziness, and headache. Too rapid intravenous administration can result in bradycardia, arrhythmias and hypotension.

In both the pre- and postoperative periods, nursing care should include: skin care, frequent positioning, *passive* range of motion exercises, regular assessment of respiratory status and use of measures to prevent respiratory problems. For further enumeration of appropriate nursing measures see the sections on intracranial pressure, and interventions for the patient who has had a head injury.

Finally, the need to provide emotional support to the patient and family cannot be overemphasized. The sudden nature of the ruptured aneurysm is difficult to accept, and the period of waiting before surgery is anxiety-producing. The patient and family need to know what is being done to them or asked of them at each step along the way. Consultation with Social Service and the Chaplain may be helpful.

Etiology of TIA and Stroke

A stroke, or cerebrovascular accident (CVA), can actually have several causes. A cerebral thrombosis is a blood clot that forms somewhere in the cerebral circulation and blocks the circulation distal to that point. An embolism is the blockage of a vessel by a foreign substance: a clot, air, fat, or plaques. Hemorrhage occurs from rupture of a vessel.

A transient ischemic attack (TIA) is a temporary stroke-like situation in which the neurologic deficit or signs are present for only seconds or hours, but which usually disappear. A stroke-in-evolution describes the situation of worsening neurologic signs. A completed stroke describes a static neurologic conditon.[43]

Pathophysiology of TIA and Stroke

Any time the blood supply to an area is interrupted, there is an alteration in the oxygen supply and metabolism to that area. If the interruption continues, ischemia will develop. Ultimately, tissue anoxia results in infarction, that is, necrosis following the loss of blood supply. Once the artery has been blocked by thrombosis or embolus, a series of steps occur: local vasodilation, stasis of blood behind the blockage, edema and necrosis.

In hemorrhage, the blood destroys or displaces large amounts of tissue. Intracerebral hemorrhages can occur anywhere within the cranial cavity, and often do occur deep in the center of the brain or brainstem. As many as 80% of hypertensive intracerebral hemorrhages are fatal.[34]

There is a known stroke-prone profile. Predisposing factors include history of TIA or stroke, hypertension, cardiac abnormalities (e.g., old M.I., left ventricular hypertrophy), clinical evidence of atherosclerosis, (e.g., angina pectoris, arterial bruits), diabetes mellitus, and elevated blood lipids. Cigarette smoking, gout, and other factors may also be implicated.

In the majority of patients, the CVA or TIA is of sudden onset, and reaches maximum intensity within a few hours. In the United States about 70% of strokes are due to atherothrombosis, 20% to hemorrhages of various types and 10% to embolism. Embolism is more common in younger patients, hemorrhage more common in blacks.[34]

It is usually not possible to determine the cause of the stroke at the time the patient is admitted. Presenting signs and symptoms may include headache, dizziness, mental confusion, focal neurologic signs such as hemiplegia, aphasia, visual field deficits, changes in vital signs, convulsions, even coma, with death following quickly. The prognosis cannot be predicted with much accuracy at the time of admission. In non-fatal cases, it may be months until the permanent neurologic problems can be defined with certainty. The course of illness varies with the patient's condition, the course of the stroke, the age, etc.

The course of treatment varies with the nature and severity of the stroke, patient age, history, and variety of factors. Medical management for stroke and TIA will be discussed, followed by surgical.

For both TIA and stroke, initial treatment with adrenocorticosteroids, specifically dexamethasone (Decadron), may be helpful in controlling edema and thus improving symptoms. If the TIA has cleared with residual neurologic deficit the physician may wish to forego the steroids.

Anticoagulants can be of particular help to patients with TIA, arterial emboli associated with valvular heart disease, or a predisposition to venous thrombi. They are contraindicated in patients in whom intracranial hemorrhage may have occured. Anticoagulants should be used with caution in the hypertensive. Finally, the anticoagulants will not cure present symptoms, but may prevent progression of the stroke or TIA.

Antihypertensive therapy may be started in patients with an extremely high blood pressure. The goal is to reduce the blood pressure very slowly and in a controlled fashion, as a sudden reduction can alter vessel resistance and flow factors, and precipitate additional strokes or emboli.

In acute cases a variety of intracranial pressure reducing agents may be of help for emergency treatment: urea, mannitol or glycerol.

Surgery for the patient with a completed stroke is usually not indicated unless the presence of a hematoma is suspected. The location of the hemorrhage and hematoma will influence the decision about surgery since clots deep within the brain usually cannot be removed with much success.

For the patient with TIA, it may be possible to remove the thrombus or reconstruct stenosed or occluded arteries. Endarterectomy is the removal of the intima of the artery along with whatever is obstructing it, usually thrombus or plaque. In many cases, surgery will be withheld until the patient stabilizes after his TIA.

Diagnostic measures used with TIA and stroke patients vary depending on suspected cause of neurologic dysfunction, age of the patient, acuity of symptoms, and so on. These procedures include lumbar puncture, CAT or other scans, arteriogram, and echoencephalogram.

Complications of TIA and Stroke

In some ways, any permanent neurologic deficit that results from a stroke may be regarded as a complication. Certainly, if a TIA is a forerunner of stroke, then that stroke could be regarded as a complication.

In the seriously ill stroke patient, that is, with major severe neurologic deficits, any complication associated with immobility and bedrest can occur, particularly in the absence of preventive care: pneumonia, infection, decubitus formation and contractures.

Assessment of the Stroke and TIA Patient

Initially, the nurse needs to ascertain the degree of respiratory function and assure a patent airway. The stroke patient may present almost moribund, and maintenance of respiratory function is of prime importance.

The next major step in assessment of the stroke patient is to do a complete neurologic exam to determine the baseline state of the patient. This assessment should include evaluation of higher functions such as orientation, appropriateness of response, memory, and so on. Speech problems (aphasias) are common with stroke and often make assessment difficult. It may be possible to gather information from the patient's family. Even though the patient may not be able to speak coherently to the nurse, he may still understand the nurse. The patient should be reassured, if possible, and still included in the discussion as much as possible.

Visual field defects are common in stroke. Careful assessment of visual field problems will alleviate later difficulties that may arise in trying to approach the patient or ask him to do activities on a side where he cannot see.

Classically, loss of motor function accompanies stroke. Certainly, this is not true in every case, but a careful assessment of motor function and position sense should be done. The patient who still retains some motor function may complain of paresthesias.

At the time the patient is admitted with a stroke or TIA, it is not always possible to determine if it is a TIA, a stroke in evolution, or a completed stroke. For that reason, careful recording of baseline information is important for documenting any later changes.

Interventions for Patients with TIA and Stroke

In perhaps no other situation, except spinal cord injury, does nursing care make the ultimate difference in prognosis for rehabilitation. From the time of admission the nurse should be observing for changes, preventing complications, and preparing for discharge to the rehabilitative situation.

Refer to the care of the spinal cord injured for a discussion of respiratory management, skin care, positioning, and other preventive measures. The patient with dense hemiparesis is similar to the spinal cord injured patient who suffered a partial transection of the cord: instead of the lower portion of the body being paralyzed, it is one side or one extremity. Consider the following in addition to reviewing the section on spinal cord injury.

If the patient has a visual field defect it is important to approach him from the side that he can see. Thus, it is often helpful to choose a bed in which the functional vision is on the side that all people entering the room must face. The same concern about functional vision should carry over to all activities: place food trays, water pitchers, call bells, etc., where the patient·can see them.

Meal times may be a source of embarrassment and frustration to the stroke patient who may have lost use of his dominant arm, or who has facial weakness, making eating and swallowing difficult.

There is no easy way to solve these problems, but careful assessment and planning to discover how to best position the patient during meals, what foods are easier for him to chew or swallow, where in the mouth to put food or straws, etc., will make meals less upsetting. Of course, reassuring the patient and providing privacy are important.

Aphasias can be very difficult to work with. Patience is essential. It is also helpful to use hand movements to demonstrate/illustrate what is being said, speak slowly using simple words, and repeat as needed. If all else fails, at least communicate concern through gentle touch and occasional hand holding, if appropriate.

MENINGITIS

Etiology and Pathophysiology

Meningitis, or inflammation and infection of the meninges, can be caused by a variety of microorganisms. The severity of any one case of meningitis depends on such variables as the organism(s) involved, the speed of diagnosis, and the presence of other neurologic problems.

In the intensive care setting, meningitis may be the primary diagnosis, or it may be secondary to contamination from a head injury, an infected shunt, or contamination during lumbar puncture.

Signs and symptoms may include chills, headache, temperature elevation, nausea and vomiting, stiff neck, irritability, confusion, stupor, coma, and seizures. The individual appears acutely ill. A few of the more common types of meningitis will be briefly discussed.

Meningococcal meningitis: The causative agent (Neisseria meningitidis) may enter through the nasopharynx or the blood stream; it can often be cultured from the blood before the symptoms of meningitis appear. Cases may be fulminant. Mortality rate is low in treated cases, as is the incidence of complications and sequalae.

Pneumococcal meningitis (Diplococcus pneumoniae) is usually a complication of otitis media, mastoiditis, sinusitis, skull fractures, upper respiratory infections and lung infections.[34] Mortality still approaches 30%. The best prognosis is in cases following skull fracture or with no known site of infection; the poorest prognosis is for meningitis following pneumonia, empyema, lung abscess or a persistent endocarditis.

Staphylococcal meningitis is relatively infrequent, but may follow subdural or epidural abscesses and neurosurgical procedures.

Streptococcal meningitis is also infrequent and usually follows nasal sinus infection.

Meningitis caused by *Hemophilus influenzae* accounts for 18% of all cases of meningitis.[34] It is usually secondary to acute sinusitis, otitis media and skull fracture; in infants it is usually primary. Mortality in treated adults is less than 5%, but sequelae are not uncommon.

Tuberculous meningitis is always secondary to tuberculosis elsewhere in the body. This form of meningitis is characterized by a more prolonged course and a higher mortality rate. Prognosis is influenced by age of the patient and the speed with which treatment is instituted. Major and minor sequelae occur in as many as 24% of patients, including deafness, seizures, blindness, hemiplegia, paraplegia, and in children, decreases in IQ.

Fungal meningitis: The occurrence of fungal meningitis has increased in recent years due to several factors: new antimicrobial agents and their more frequent use have destroyed normal flora, paving the way for fungal overgrowth; use of corticosteroids has increased the "incidence of infections with fungi of low pathogenicity to man,"[34] and contributed to the severity of infection with more pathogenic organisms; immunosuppression in treatment of patients with organ transplants, Hodgkin's disease and leukemia predisposes to systemic infection with fungi.

Diagnosis of fungal meningitis is difficult, and treatment, at best, is unsatisfactory. Amphotericin B has been used with some success in recent years, but treatment lasts for weeks, there are many side effects to the drug, and death is not uncommon.

Sarcoidosis is a generalized disease which resembles tuberculosis in many respects. Nervous system involvement is most often seen in cranial nerves, but peripheral nerve involvement and meningitis are not uncommon. No specific therapy is known, but the disease may have a benign course with spontaneous recovery. Death may result from increased intracranial pressure.

Complications and Sequelae

Complications and sequelae from meningitis vary and depend on the severity of the patient's illness, the causative organism, age, speed of diagnosis and treatment, effectiveness of treatment, and general patient condition.

Complications include increased intracranial pressure, and appearance of worsening neurologic signs. Adhesions and scar tissue formation may prevent complete recovery. Death can ensue in many cases.

Sequelae can include cranial nerve palsies, hemiplegia, quadriplegia, blindness, deafness and decreases in IQ.

Assessment

Any alteration in a patient's level of neurologic function or level of consciousness should be thoroughly investigated. Assessment for meningitis would include a careful neurologic examination, especially of level of consciousness.

An increase in temperature may be present. If there is access to the cerebrospinal fluid it should be inspected for cloudiness or changes in character. Specimens of CSF for culture should be sent.

A stiff neck, that is, inability to touch the chin to the chest, may indicate meningeal irritation. In the case of meningitis, this irritation is caused by infection and inflammation.

There may be a positive Kernig's sign: reflex contraction and pain in the calf muscles when an attempt is made to extend the leg after flexing the thigh.

Observation for signs of increased intracranial pressure is essential.

Interventions

The nurse will be working in conjunction with the physician in an attempt to confirm diagnosis. Measures to prevent and treat increased intracranial pressure may be employed.

Adequate hydration should be maintained; the patient should receive about 3,000-4,000 cc. per 24 hours. Alterations in electrolytes are not uncommon, so blood work should be done and evaluated regularly.

Many antibiotics and, in the case of fungal infection, Amphotericin B, will usually have to be given intravenously. In high doses all of these drugs have associated side effects, including neurologic signs and symptoms and blood dyscrasias. Therefore, systemic neurologic examination of the patient should be done regularly. Remember, too, that Amphotericin B loses potency when exposed to sunlight; usually the IV bottle can be covered with a dark paper or plastic bag to decrease contact with light.

Careful emotional support of the patient and family is important. While it is true that the majority of patients do recover from meningitis without long-term problems, the nurse should not be falsely optimistic.

REFERENCES

1. Alexander MM, Brown MS: Physical examination. Performing the neurological examination. Part 17. *Nursing '76* 6:38-42, June, 1976; Part 18. *Nursing '76* 6:50-55, July, 1976.
2. Anthony CP, Kolthoff, NJ:*Textbook of Anatomy and Physiology.* 9th Ed. C.V. Mosby, St. Louis, Mo., 1975.
3. Bordeaux MP: The intensive-care unit and observation of the patient acutely ill with neurologic disease. *Heart & Lung* 2:884-887, 1973.
4. Beland IL, Passos JY: *Clinical Nursing. Pathophysiological and Psychosocial Approaches.* 3rd Ed. Macmillan Publishing, New York, 1975.
5. Berkovsky D: Physiological effects of closed head injury. *Journal of Neurosurgical Nursing* 4:125-139, Dec., 1972.
6. Bouvette JM: Preoperative and postoperative care of patients with cerebral aneurysms. *Nursing Clinics of North America* 9:655-666, 1974.
7. Breunig KA: After the blowup . . . How to care for the patient with a ruptured cerebral aneurysm. *Nursing '76* 6:37-45, Dec., 1976.
8. Burrell ZL, Burrell LO: *Critical Care.* 3rd Ed. C.V. Mosby, St. Louis, Mo., 1977.
9. Calvin RP: Continuous ventricular or lumbar subarachnoid drainage of cerebrospinal fluid. *Journal of Neurosurgical Nursing* 9:12-14, March, 1977.
10. Carini E, Owens G: *Neurological and Neurosurgical Nursing.* 6th Ed. C.V. Mosby, St. Louis, Mo., 1974.
11. Chusid JG; *Correlative Neuroanatomy and Functional Neurology.* 16th Ed. Lange Medical Publications, Los Altos, Calif., 1976.
12. Confirmation and cure of acute subdural hematoma. *Nursing '72,* 2:15-16, Feb., 1972.

13. Cooper CR: Anticonvulsant drugs and the epileptic's dilemma. *Nursing '76* **6**:44-50, Jan., 1976.

14. Erickson R: Cranial check: a basic neurological assessment. *Nursing '74* **4**:67-68, Aug., 1974.

15. Feustel D: Autonomic hyperreflexia. *American Journal of Nursing* **7**:228-230, 1976.

16. Frankel HL: A symposium on spinal injuries from the national spinal injuries centre, Stoke Mandeville Hospital: traumatic paraplegia. *Nursing Mirror* **141**:47-52, Nov. 6, 1975.

17. Guyton AC: *Textbook of Medical Physiology.* 5th Ed. W.B. Saunders, Philadelphia, Pa., 1976.

18. Hanlon K: Description and uses of intracranial pressure monitoring. *Heart & Lung* **5**:277-282, 1976.

19. Hinkhouse A: Craniocerebral trauma. *American Journal of Nursing* **73**:1719-1722, 1973.

20. Hoffman JJ: Arterial blood gas analysis as a basic criterion for the management of the neurosurgical patient. *Journal of Neurosurgical Nursing* **9**:29-33, March, 1977.

21. Jacobs GB: The treatment of intracranial aneurysms. *Journal of Neurosurgical Nursing* **8**:149-154, Dec., 1976.

22. Jimm LR: Nursing assessment of patients for increased intracranial pressure. *Journal of Neurosurgical Nursing* **6**:27-38, July, 1974.

23. Johnson M, et al.: The subarachnoid screw. *American Journal of Nursing* **77**:448-450, 1977.

24. Jones AJ: Nursing implications in the administration of urea. *Journal of Neurosurgical Nursing* **7**:37-41, July, 1975.

25. Kealy SL: Respiratory care in Guillain-Barré syndrome. *American Journal of Nursing* **77**:58-60, 1977.

26. Kinney AB, Blount M: Systems approach to myasthenia gravis. *Nursing Clinics of North America* **6**:435-453, 1971.

27. Lindh K, Rickerson G: Spinal cord injury: you can make a difference. *Nursing '74* **4**:41-45, Feb., 1974.

28. Mack EW, Dawson WN, Jr.: Injury to the spine and spinal cord. *Hospital Medicine* **12**:23-25+, July, 1976.

29. Maddox M: Subarachnoid hemorrhage. *American Journal of Nursing* **74**:2199-2201, 1974.

30. Mauss MK, Mitchell PH: Increased intracranial pressure: an update. *Heart & Lung* **5**:919-926, 1976.

31. Mazzola R, Jacobs GB: Social and psychological implications of paraplegia. *Journal of Neurosurgical Nursing* **5**:63-68, Dec., 1973.

32. McGuckin M: Microbiological studies. Tips for assisting with cultures of CSF and other body fluids. Part 5. *Nursing '76* **6**:17-18, April, 1976.

33. Metzer L, et al.: *Concepts and Practices of Intensive Care for Nurse Specialists.* 2nd Ed. Charles Press Publishers, Bowie, Md., 1976.

34. Merritt HH: *A Textbook of Neurology.* 5th Ed. Lea and Febiger, Philadelphia, Pa., 1973.

35. Michner F: Patient assessment: neurological examination. Programmed Instruction. *American Journal of Nursing* Part I. **75**:P.I. 1-24, Sept., 1975; Part II. **75**:P.I. 1-24, Nov., 1975; Part III. **76**:P.I. 1-25, April, 1976 (Reflexes).

36. Mitchell PH, Mauss N: Intracranial pressure: fact and fancy. *Nursing '76* **6**:53-57, June, 1976.

37. *Myasthenia gravis. A manual for the nurse.* Free, from the Myasthenia Gravis Foundation, Inc., 230 Park Ave., New York, New York 10007.

38. Nikas DL, Konkoly R: Nursing responsibilities in arterial and intracranial pressure monitoring. *Journal of Neurosurgical Nursing* **7**:116, 122, Dec., 1975.

39. Nursing grand rounds. Caring for the totally dependent patient. Some traps, some guidelines. *Nursing '76* **6**:38-43, July, 1976.

40. Odachowski S: Cerebrospinal fluid acid-base balance: importance in neurosurgical nursing. *Journal of Neurosurgical Nursing* **6**:117-121, Dec., 1974.

41. Parsons C: Respiratory changes in head injury. *American Journal of Nursing* **71**:2187-2191, 1971.

42. Reid M: The berry aneurysm patient: the surgical management—from hemorrhage to follow-up. *Journal of Neurosurgical Nursing* **6**:78-84, Dec., 1974.

43. Riehl J, Chambers J: Better salvage for the stroke patient. *Nursing '76* **6**:24-31, July, 1976.

44. Rudy E: Early omens of cerebral disaster. *Nursing '77* **7**:58-60+, Feb., 1977.

45. Sawitzke S, Teter A: Arteriovenous malformations of the brain. General review including role of embolization. *Journal of Neurosurgical Nursing* **8**:132-143, Dec., 1976.

46. Sodaro E: Guillain-Barre: the syndrome, patient care and some findings. *Journal of Neurosurgical Nursing* **6**:97-108, Dec., 1974.

47. Stackhouse J: Myasthenia gravis. *American Journal of Nursing* **73**:1544-1547, 1973.

48. Stephens GJ, et al.: A delicate balance: managing chronic airway obstruction in a neurosurgical patient. *American Journal of Nursing* **75**:1492-1497, 1975.

49. Swift N: Head injury. Essentials of excellent care. *Nursing '74* **4**:26-33, Sept., 1974.

50. Tindall GT, et al.: Current methods for monitoring patients with head injury. *Clinical Neurosurgery* **19**:98-120, 1972.

51. Vincent PJ, et al.: Treatment of patients with spinal cord injuries. *Canadian Nurse* **71**:26-30, Aug., 1975.
52. Wiley L: The stigma of epilepsy. *Nursing '74* **4**:36-45, Jan., 1974.
53. Williams A: Classification and diagnosis of epilepsy. *Nursing Clinics of North America* **9**:747-760, 1974.
54. Youmans JR: *Neurological Surgery.* W.B. Saunders, Philadelphia, Pa., 1973.

CHAPTER 6

Care of the Patient with Gastrointestinal Problems

by Susan M. Daum, RN and
Barbara J. Daly, RN, MSN

INTRODUCTION

The gastrointestinal system includes those organs and structures involved in the intake and passage of food, the breakdown and metabolism of foodstuffs, and the elimination of solid waste products. This chapter will deal with those disorders which commonly result in critical illness requiring intensive medical and nursing care.

For convenience of discussion, the major organs of the gastrointestinal (GI) system can be thought of as belonging either to the alimentary canal or to the accessory metabolic system. The alimentary canal is essentially a nine meter tube whose major function is to propel the food and begin the breakdown of nutrients into usable form. The accessory metabolic system provides the enzymes and other substances necessary for the further breakdown, uptake, utilization, and storage of essential nutrients.

The alimentary canal consists of the structures of the oropharynx (mouth, teeth, salivary glands, palate, tongue), epiglottis, esophagus, stomach, large and small intestine, rectum, and anus. The accessory organ system includes the liver, gallbladder, and pancreas (Figure 6-1).

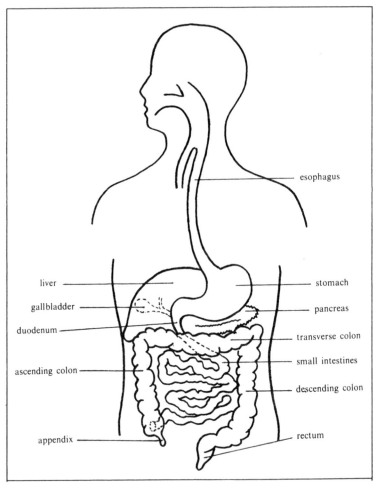

Figure 6-1. Organs of the digestive system.

Under normal conditions, food is taken into the mouth, chewed and lubricated, and formed into a bolus. The bolus of food is passed into the esophagus by swallowing. It is then conveyed down the esophagus through peristalsis, and into the stomach, where further breakdown occurs. Peristalsis continues to slowly move food through the large intestine; here bile, pancreatic enzymes, and intestinal secretions complete the breakdown of carbohydrates, fats, and proteins. Absorption of water and essential nutrients occurs prior to passage of feces into the rectum.

Although adequate intake and metabolism of food stuffs is certainly essential for life, disorders of or interferences with normal digestive processes do not usually, in themselves, constitute a critical illness. Certain diseases of the digestive system may, however, progress to the point where other life support systems, such as the circulatory system, are involved or may have sequelae, such as infection, which become life-threatening. The structures which are most commonly involved in these critical states are the esophagus, stomach, bowel, gallbladder, liver, and pancreas.

The following sections will first briefly describe the normal anatomy and physiology of these six organs, then discuss those associated conditions with which the intensive care nurse will deal. Disorders will be grouped under three headings which represent the aspect of the illness which entails critical management—bleeding, infection, and severe metabolic disturbance. Nursing interventions applicable to each of these situations will then be discussed.

ANATOMY AND PHYSIOLOGY

Esophagus

The esophagus serves two functions in man: lubrication of food and passage of food into the stomach. When food is swallowed, the presence of the bolus in the rear of the mouth stimulates pressure receptors which activate the swallowing center in the medulla, via afferent nerves. The swallowing center coordinates the activity of the pharynx, larynx, and esophagus. As food reaches the pharynx, the glottis closes, the epiglottis folds over it, and the bolus enters the esophagus.

The esophagus is a tube-like structure, 22-25 cm. in length, 1.25-2.5 cm. in diameter. The upper third of the esophagus is composed of skeletal muscle, arranged longitudinally and circularly; the lower two-thirds are composed of smooth muscle. The lining is made up of a collagen and elastic network with mucus secreting cells. Innervation is through both sympathetic and parasympathetic fibers, and afferent fibers carry sensation from the esophagus.

When relaxed, the esophagus is closed. As a bolus of food reaches the pharynx, the swallowing center initiates the opening of the hypopharyngeal sphincter, the entrance into the esophagus, by contraction of the skeletal muscles. After the bolus has passed, the muscles relax and the sphincter closes.

Once in the esophagus, the bolus is propelled by peristaltic waves. The peristaltic wave is a "sequential activation of its (the esophagus) muscles by efferent firing in a pattern . . .,"[13] and begins just below the junction of the pharynx and esophagus. The contraction reaches the lower end of the esophagus about nine seconds after it has begun. If food remains in the esophagus, thus distending it, a secondary peristaltic wave is initiated to force the bolus into the stomach. Consistency of the bolus and position of the person affects the rate at which food passes through the esophagus. When flat or upright, water reaches the stomach one second after swallowing; semi-solid masses usually pass into the stomach within five to six seconds. Peristalsis normally decreases with old age.

The last 4 cm. of the esophagus is referred to as the gastroesophageal sphincter, and the last 2 cm. is sometimes termed the vestibule. This sphincter normally remains tonically contracted when empty, thus preventing the reflux of food from the stomach. As the peristaltic wave begins, the gastroesophageal sphincter relaxes to let food pass into the cardia of the stomach, and then contracts again.

Reflux is also prevented by the constriction imposed by the diaphragm, through which the last portion of the esophagus passes. It is the higher pressure existing in the esophagus that actually prevents food from re-entering the esophagus from the stomach, and several mechanisms operate to maintain this pressure. Because the lower portion of the esophagus is below the diaphragm, abdominal distention, which raises gastric pressure, also raises esophageal pressure. Even distention of the stomach with food does not elevate stomach pressure above that of the esophagus. With gastric distention, the hormone gastrin is released; gastrin causes an increase in pressure in the lower esophagus, thus preserving the pressure gradient necessary to prevent reflux.

Abnormalities of the esophageal musculature or gastroesophageal sphincter and severe increases in abdominal pressure will result in reflux. This is a common occurrence in pregnancy. If the gastric contents have a pH below 4, a burning sensation, often termed "heartburn" will result. In addition to pH, the esophagus is sensitive to distention and abnormal contractions or spasms.

Stomach

The stomach can be likened to a balloon in that when empty it has a volume of approximately 50 ml. but when fully expanded it may hold up to a liter. In relation to the rest of the gastrointestinal tract, the stomach lies between the esophagus and the small intestine. The cardiac sphincter is at the proximal end of the stomach and allows the passage of food from the esophagus into the stomach; the pyloric sphincter lies at the distal end of the stomach where it joins the duodenum and prevents backflow of intestinal contents. These two areas, the cardiac and pyloric sphincters, are the only locations where the stomach is fixed and provide important landmarks when x-ray examination of the stomach is performed.

The stomach has four areas: the cardia, which is the upper portion surrounding the cardiac sphincter; the fundus, which rises above the cardia and to the side of it; the body, which is the major portion, lying below the fundus; and the antrum, which is the narrowed portion extending from the pyloric sphincter (Figure 6-2).

The stomach has two curvatures. The lesser curvature is the inferior, concave portion, extending from the cardia to the pylorus. The greater curvature extends from the cardiac orifice, bends up and backwards around the fundus, and ends at the pylorus (see Figure 6-2).

The muscle layers of the stomach are responsible for emptying the stomach of its contents. The walls have two layers of smooth muscle. The longitudinal layer, when contracted, pushes food forward throughout the gastrointestinal tract. The internal circular layer is responsible for a squeezing type motion that causes food to mix and subdivide into smaller pieces. The combined action of these two muscle layers causes peristalsis. This peristaltic wave continues throughout the gastrointestinal tract, but is strongest as food enters the antrum. The muscle layers are therefore thickest at this point, where food and gastric secretions become mixed to the greatest degree.

Peristaltic movements of the stomach can be affected by the emotional state of the individual. Depression and fear cause decreased motility and anger and aggression increase motility. However, it is important to note that gastric emptying is mainly controlled by the chemical composition and amount of chyme in the duodenum and not the volume of contents in the stomach.

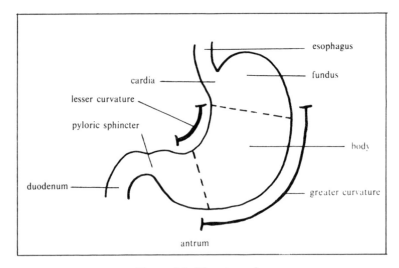

Figure 6-2. The stomach.

There are three other layers of the stomach wall, in addition to the muscle layer. The serous outer layer is called the visceral peritoneum; it extends from the lower portion of the stomach as a double fold, referred to as the omentum, and covers the intestines. This serous layer allows fluid to be filtered into the peritoneal space.

The submucosa lies between the muscular layer and the mucosa. This layer permits the movement of the mucosa with peristaltic action.

The surface epithelium of the last layer, the gastric mucosa, is often divided into the body and the pyloric areas. The body area is pierced by numerous glands which are responsible for the secretory functions of the stomach. The body glands, or fundic glands, contain mucus neck cells which secrete mucus, parietal cells which secrete HC1 and water, and the chief cells which are responsible for both mucus and pepsinogen production.

The pyloric glands, which lie near the pylorus, secrete primarily mucus and a small amount of pepsinogen. It is also felt that gastrin is produced and released by the pyloric glands.[13] When gastrin is released from the mucosa it passes through the liver and then into the general circulation, where it reaches the mucosa and may stimulate acid secretion in the stomach.

Neuromuscular innervation

Motor function of the gastrointestinal tract is due to smooth muscle innervation. The only exception is at the pharyngeal-esophageal junction, as mentioned, and at the anus. Smooth muscle cells have no characteristic resting length and therefore maintain some degree of tension throughout life. Smooth muscle contraction and gland secretion in the gastrointestinal tract are regulated by both nerves and hormones.

Extrinsic nervous innervation of the stomach is divided into sympathetic and parasympathetic branches of the autonomic system, both of which carry afferent and efferent fibers. The chief function of sympathetic fibers is to inhibit contraction of smooth muscle and, to some extent, the secretion of mucus. Sympathetic innervation comes from the greater splanchnic nerves and the celiac ganglia. Afferent fibers at the 6th to 10th thoracic spinal segments are responsible for visceral gastric pain, which may be stimulated by muscle contraction, distention, or inflammation. This visceral pain causes referred pain in the epigastrium.

Parasympathetic innervation of afferent and efferent nerves is accomplished by the vagus nerve. The anterior vagus, which is a continuation of the left vagus supplying the esophagus, also supplies the liver and the gallbladder, and the right vagus innervates the posterior surface of the stomach. When stimulated, the vagus causes increased secretion of acid and pepsinogen.

The gastrointestinal tract has two major nerve plexuses in its walls. The myenteric plexus is found between the longitudinal and circular layers of the smooth muscle. The submucosal nerve plexus is located in the submucosa itself. These two plexi are found throughout the gastrointestinal tract. In both, the axons branch profusely. This means that a stimulation at any one point may lead to activity at any other point in the GI tract.

Small Intestine

The small intestine is a tube approximately 350 cm. long and 2.5-3 cm. in diameter, leading from the stomach to the large intestine. It is further divided into three segments: the duodenum, which is approximately 20 cm., the jejunum, which is approximately 90 cm., and the ileum, about 240 cm. long.

The mucosa of the intestine is highly folded and contains finger-like projections called the villi. The villi are composed of microvilli which, along with the folded mucosa, increase the total surface area of the small intestine many times, thereby enabling a large amount of absorption to take place. It has been estimated that the small intestine has a total surface area of 2,000 square feet,[2] equivalent to the area of a singles tennis court.[59]

The surface of the small intestine is protected by mucous glands, called Brunner's glands. These are particularly located in the duodenum, where a high concentration of pancreatic juices are emptied. The main function of these glands is to prevent the duodenal wall from being digested by pancreatic and other enzymes. Secretion from these glands is increased by tactile or vagal stimuli and by intestinal hormones. Sympathetic stimulation inhibits the action of Brunner's glands, which then leaves the duodenum unprotected; this may help to explain why 50% of peptic ulcers occur in this area of the GI tract.

Mucus is also secreted over the entire surface of the intestinal mucosa by goblet cells in the epithelial layer. The secretion of mucus here is due to chemical or tactile stimulation of the mucosa by chyme.

Motility of the bowel is due to the activity of the circular and longitudinal muscle layers. The circular muscle layer movement, which is referred to as the segmenting contractions, are ring-like local contractions which occur at a rate of 11 contractions per minute in the proximal small intestine and at a rate of 8 contractions per minute in the distal small intestine. These contractions are regular and rhythmic, causing the intestinal contents to subdivide into segments and mix. This also exposes larger areas of the mucosa, which facilitates absorption and digestion. Peristaltic movement is responsible for the distal movement of intestinal chyme, but these waves are much weaker than in the stomach.

The longitudinal muscle layers are responsible for a pendular motion. This motion, together with segmentation, causes a back and forth motion of the chyme. The total effect is that of moving the chyme toward the large intestine and further mixing the intestinal contents.

In the last portion of the ileum, just as it joins the large intestine, is a sphincter, the ileocecal valve. This valve is usually closed, but when ileal contractions increase after a meal, the sphincter relaxes and allows food to enter the large intestine. This is referred to as the gastroileal reflex and is initiated by excitation of receptors in the stomach, mediated by nerve fibers to the intestinal muscle.

The entire surface of the small intestine is covered with crypts of Lieberkuhn. It is believed that these crypts have epithelial cells which form up to 2,000 ml. of fluid per day. It is the circulation of this fluid from the crypts to the villi that provides the watery fluid through which substances are absorbed.

The secretions of the small intestine have almost no enzymes except enterokinase, which activates trypsin, and a small amount of amylase. However, the epithelial cells of the mucosa have large quantities of digestive enzymes which digest food as it is absorbed through the intestinal epithelium.

Large Intestine

The large intestine or colon is approximately 150 cm. in length and 2.5-8.5 cm. in diameter. It leads from the ileocecal valve to the anus and constitutes the last portion of the GI tract. The colon is not folded as is the small intestine, but has three relatively straight segments, the ascending, transverse, and descending colon. Below the junction of the small and large intestine is a blind pouch which is termed the cecum. The small finger-like projection at the end of the cecum is the appendix; the function of the appendix is unknown. The final portion of the descending colon is an S-shaped structure, the sigmoid colon, which empties into the rectum.

Like the small intestine, the colon is composed of longitudinal and circular smooth muscle; however, in humans this is incomplete. The walls of the colon are composed of haustra, which are small sacs that form as the circular smooth muscle contracts. Circular muscle contraction also causes a slow segmentation motion.

Once material from the small intestine has entered the colon, it usually remains there for 18-24 hours. Marked increases in motility occur at varying times during the day, usually after meals. This is known as the mass movement, during which large segments of the ascending and transverse colon contract at the same time to propel fecal material a third to three-fourths of the length of the colon within a few seconds. There may also be some peristaltic movement in the descending colon which aids in moving the fecal material into the rectum. The degree of distention of the rectal walls by fecal material, rather than any specific amount of feces, produces the normal stimulus for defecation and initiates the defecation reflex.

Within the mucosa of the large intestine are crypts of Lieberkuhn, similar to those in the small intestine. Instead of epithelial cells secreting enzymes, though, the large intestine has mucus secreting goblet cells. This represents the only significant secretion of the large intestine. Mucus aids in protecting the intestinal wall from erosion (mucus is alkaline, with a pH of about 8), provides a medium in which fecal material is held together, and protects the wall of the bowel from bacterial activity.

Absorption in the colon takes place primarily in the proximal portion; most of the available water and electrolytes are absorbed here, leaving 100 to 200 ml. out of about 2,000 ml.) to be excreted in the feces. The distal portion of the colon then functions mainly as a storage place for fecal material until defecation takes place.

Bacterial activity is significant in the large intestine. Both aerobic and anaerobic bacteria reside in the colon, including Escherichia coli, Pseudomonas aeruginosa, Clostridium perfringens, Bacteroides, and fungi such as Candida albicans. Bacteria aid in the formation of vitamin K, B_{12}, thiamine, riboflavin, and various gases. Vitamin K formation is probably most important since ingested foods do not usually have an adequate amount of vitamin K to maintain normal blood coagulation.

The feces are usually three-fourths water and one-fourth solid material, of which 30% is dead bacteria. The brown color of the feces is due to bilirubin derivatives, stercobilin and urobilin.

Pancreas

The human pancreas is an elongated retroperitoneal gland approximately 12.5 to 17.5 cm. long. It is subdivided into three parts: head, body, and tail. The head lies within the loop formed by the duodenum and is often attached to it. The head of the pancreas and the duodenum share the same blood supply (which makes total pancreatectomy a difficult procedure to perform). The body, which constitutes the major portion of the gland, extends horizontally across the abdomen and behind the stomach. Much of the pancreas is hidden by the stomach and the transverse colon; because of this, tumors or injuries to the pancreas are easily overlooked. The tail, which is at the level of the first and second lumbar vertebrae, almost touches the spleen. Because of the relative fixed position of the pancreas and its close association with the vertebral column, it is prone to injury by blunt trauma.

The pancreas is a mixed gland, the largest portion of which is exocrine; less than 1% functions as an endocrine gland. The exocrine or digestive portion of the pancreas is responsible for secreting digestive enzymes, water, and electrolytes into the duodenum. The pancreas is composed of lobes, which in turn are made up of many small alveoli lined with secretory cells. A group of these cells is termed an acinus. The lobes are marked by loose connective tissue septae, which contain nutrient blood vessels, nerves, and lymphatic channels. The acini cells, which are responsible for pancreatic exocrine secretion, have a thin membrane on one side and a duct on the other. The lobes themselves also have small ducts which empty into the duct of Wirsung, which is the largest pancreatic duct, extending the entire length of the pancreas. The duct of Wirsung joins with the common bile duct from the gallbladder to form the ampulla of Vater, which then empties into the duodenum. (This arrangement of ducts varies among individuals, however.) (Figure 6-3.)

Pancreatic secretions include water, bicarbonate, the enzymes trypsin, chymotrypsin, carboxypeptidase, amylase, and lipase, and RNA and DNA. The presence of HCl, glutamic acid, and proteolytic by-products in the duodenum stimulates the release of secretin from the duodenal mucosa; secretin in turn stimulates the release of pancreatic juice rich in bicarbonate, which then is able to neutralize the acidic chyme. Pancreozymin, another duodenal hormone, stimulates pancreatic secretion rich in enzymes and low in bicarbonate. Pancreozymin is stimulated by peptides, amino acids, and fatty acids.

Increased vagal stimulation also causes an increase in pancreatic juice rich in enzymes; as much as 700 units of amylase can be produced in this fashion. Vagal stimulation may be the result of the sight or smell of food or anticipation of eating.

The endocrine function of the pancreas comes from the small spherical islets of Langerhans. These islets have no ductal system; they are scattered throughout the pancreas. Their products are released directly into the circulation.

Three distinct types of endocrine cells have been identified: alpha, beta, and delta. The alpha cells produce glucagon. Glucagon is a hyperglycemic stimulating hormone which acts by inducing the

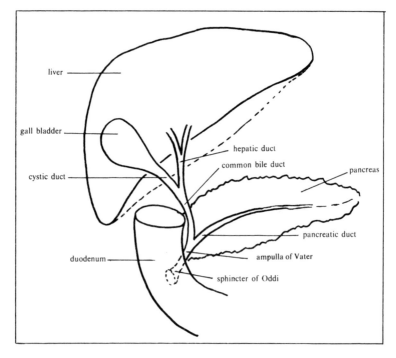

Figure 6-3. Bile and pancreatic ducts.

breakdown of liver glycogen, resulting in a release of glucose into the circulation. Glucagon also inhibits gastric acid secretion, inhibits gastric and intestinal motility, and stimulates the flow of bile. Beta cells produce insulin. Insulin production by these cells of the islets is stimulated by alterations in the concentration of serum glucose. The exact function and significance of the delta cells are not known.

Arterial blood supply to the pancreas is from the celiac and superior mesenteric arteries, which branch along the connective tissue septae and ducts. The venous supply draining the pancreas accompanies the arteries and empties into the splenic and portal veins. Blood supply is rich, and hemorrhage remains the major cause of death in injuries involving the pancreas.[49]

Liver

The liver is the largest organ in the body, weighing between 1200 and 1600 grams. The liver lies in the right side of the upper abdomen; the upper surface conforms to the undersurface of the diaphragm and the inferior surface rests on the viscera of the upper abdomen. The liver is held in position primarily by intra-abdominal pressure, assisted by support from the thoracic cage. Under normal conditions the liver cannot be palpated on physical exam. Most of the liver is covered by the peritoneum with the exception of a small area of the posterior aspect.

The liver has four lobes, which are further divided into lobules. The basic functional unit of the liver is the lobule. Each of the 50,000 to 100,000 separate lobules is constructed around a central vein that empties first into the hepatic veins, then into the vena cava. The lobules are composed of many hepatic cellular templates which are further divided into thick cells containing small bile canaliculi between them. These empty into terminal bile ducts which originate in the septae between adjacent liver lobules.

The portal venules, receiving blood from the portal veins, are also located in the septae; thus,' hepatic cells are continually exposed to portal venous blood which has drained from other abdominal veins. This blood supply transverses the liver and eventually empties into hepatic veins, which then return blood to the heart via the vena cava. Oxygenated blood is supplied by the hepatic artery; arterioles empty directly into hepatic sinusoids found between hepatic plates. The liver also has a rich lymphatic supply, which forms a network surrounding the lobule.

Venous sinusoids are lined by two types of cells, endothelial and Kupffer cells. Endothelial cells have large pores with a space beneath, the space of Disse, which allows plasma to move freely. The Kupffer cells are capable of phagocytosis of bacterial or foreign matter and of aged erythrocytes.

Vascular

One of the most important functions of the liver is the providing of a blood reservoir. Approximately 1400 cc. of blood reaches the liver per minute. Of this, 1000 cc. comes from the portal vein and 400 cc. comes from the hepatic artery. Normal pressure in the hepatic vein, emptying the liver, is 0 mm. Hg. Portal vein pressure is usually 9 mm. Hg; thus, there normally exists no resistance to blood flow from the portal venous system to the systemic venous system. In disease states, the portal pressure may rise to 20 or 40 mm. Hg. Portal hypertension then causes the formation of collateral circulatory channels and a reflected increase in pressure in the veins leading to the portal system. Cirrhosis, in which normal liver tissue is replaced by dense fibrous bands, is the most common condition causing a rise in pressure due to blocked exit pathways from the sinusoids to central lobular venules.

With this rich blood supply, the liver normally contains as much as 200-400 cc. of blood. When there is increased pressure in the vascular system the veins draining the liver will cause blood to be "dammed" in the sinusoids, and up to an additional liter of blood can be stored. In cases of blood loss, with decreases in systemic venous pressure, a large percent of the blood in the sinusoids is released into the systemic circulation in order to replace volume.

Hepatic congestion is primarily due to cardiac failure. When central venous pressure remains consistently elevated to 10-15 mm. Hg, stretching of the sinusoids occurs. This results in stasis of blood and can eventually be associated with necrosis of hepatic cells.

Lymph and ascites

The large pores in the sinusoids create a permeability which allows a large quantity of lymph to be formed with a high protein content. About 1/2 to 1/3 of all of the lymph in the body is formed in the liver, with a protein concentration of about 6 gram %. When there is an increase in hepatic venous pressure, the formation and flow of lymph increases, which then causes a transudation of fluid from the surface of the liver into the peritoneal cavity. The exact reason for this increased lymph flow in cirrhosis is unknown.

Another major factor involved in ascites formation is hypoalbuminemia. Albumin is normally synthesized in the liver. When hepatic disease interferes with albumin formation, a decrease in serum osmotic pressure occurs which then facilitates the loss of large amounts of serous fluid from the liver. As more protein is lost in this manner, osmotic pressure drops further, and the ascites worsens. Sodium and water retention, related to abnormal renal function, and portal hypertension are the other factors usually associated with ascites.

Reticuloendothelial system

The Kupffer cells lining the sinusoids are responsible for filtering the blood passing through the liver. Portal blood coming from other abdominal organs contains a large number of bacteria, including colonic bacilli, which are then removed before passing out of the sinusoids.

Detoxification also occurs in the liver. A variety of mechanisms are involved in this function, including oxidation and conjugation by enzymes.

Secretion

Bile is secreted by the liver but stored and concentrated in the gallbladder. Hepatic cells constantly form small amounts of bile which are secreted into bile canaliculi, leading to terminal ducts and eventually reaching the hepatic and common bile ducts. Bile is then emptied either into the duodenum or directed into the gallbladder. Approximately 800 to 1000 cc. of bile is secreted per day, but the gallbladder can store only 40-70 cc. Electrolytes and water are reabsorbed by the gallbladder mucosa so bile constituents such as bile salts, cholesterol, and bilirubin are up to four times more concentrated in the gallbladder.

Bile salts

Approximately 0.5 Gm. of bile salts are produced per day. The precursor is cholesterol which is supplied by the diet or synthesized in the liver during fat metabolism. Bile salts exert a detergent action in the intestine; they emulsify fat particles, reducing surface tension and allowing the breakdown of globules into smaller particles. Bile salts also aid in the absorption of fatty acids, monoglycerides, cholesterol, and lipids from the intestinal tract. Without bile salts, up to 40% of dietary lipid is lost in the stool and metabolic deficiencies result. When fats are not absorbed, fat soluble vitamin absorption is also impaired. Vitamins A, D, and E can be stored in other parts of the body, but vitamin K cannot. When bile secretion ceases, vitamin K deficiency develops within a few days. This may lead to an impairment in the formation of several blood coagulation factors such as prothrombin, which is normally synthesized in the liver with vitamin K.

Usually 94% of bile salts are reabsorbed by the intestinal mucosa in the distal ileum. They are returned to the liver by portal blood and then absorbed by hepatic cells, thus conserving the majority of salts. A small amount is lost in the feces.

Bilirubin excretion

Bilirubin is the major endproduct of hemoglobin decomposition and bile pigment metabolism. Bilirubin is converted to urobilinogen after it has been secreted into the bowel. After conversion, most of it is excreted in the stool, and a small amount is reabsorbed and excreted into bile and urine.

The normal concentration of bilirubin is 0.5 mg. per 100 cc. of plasma; when the concentration reaches 1.5 mg., jaundice, a yellow tint of body tissues, occurs. Jaundice may be caused by the increased destruction of RBCs, by an obstruction of the bile ducts, or by damage to liver cells and destruction of ducts. When bilirubin cannot be excreted via the gastrointestinal tract, it is reabsorbed into blood, producing jaundice.

Glucose regulation

The liver is responsible for storage of glycogen, conversion of galactose to glucose, and gluconeogenesis. Hypoglycemia stimulates the conversion of amino acids to usable glucose, and hyperglycemia stimulates the liver to remove excess glucose and store it as glycogen.

Fat metabolism

Fat metabolism can occur in almost any body cell but certain aspects occur more rapidly in the liver. The hepatic cell is capable of high rates of oxidation of fatty acids, formation of lipoproteins, and conversion of large quantities of carbohydrates and proteins to fat.

Protein metabolism

In the liver, deamination of amino acids occurs before the amino acids can be used for energy or converted to fats or carbohydrates. An especially important aspect of this function relates to the metabolism of ammonia, which is produced from deamination of amino acids in the liver and through bacterial activity in the bowel. Under normal conditions ammonia is converted to urea, which can then be excreted by the kidneys. In liver disease this process is impaired, leading to the accumulation of ammonia and resultant central nervous system disturbance.

Gallbladder

The gallbladder is a pear-shaped organ usually located on the underside of the right lobe of the liver, although its position can vary greatly. The gallbladder is usually 7 to 10 cm. long and 2-3 cm. wide, and can hold approximately 30 to 70 cc. of fluid. It is divided into the fundus or tip, which extends from the anterior edge of the liver, the corpus or body, called Hartmann's pouch, and a narrow neck which leads into the cystic duct. The hepatic duct has two branches coming from the liver, 2-4 cm. long, which join to form one large hepatic duct. The cystic duct then joins this hepatic duct to form the common bile duct, which descends 8-15 cm. into the duodenum at the ampulla of Vater (see Figure 6-3). This is surrounded by the sphincter of Oddi which is responsible for the control of bile secretion into the intestine.

Arterial blood supply to the cystic and hepatic ducts comes from the hepatic artery. Venous drainage of the gallbladder is accomplished by the cystic vein.

Gallbladder tissue consists mainly of mucosa of columnar epithelium, muscularis, subserosa, and serosa. Mucous glands are found only in the neck. When the gallbladder becomes inflamed, it is usually this area which is most affected. The bile ducts also contain mucous glands.

The most common problem faced by a surgeon in treating gallbladder disease is the great variability of the biliary system. Variations in number, location, and structure of the ducts is common and requires careful surgical technique. The most common abnormality is the existence of one or more accessory hepatic ducts which enter the gallbladder directly from the liver. A duct overlooked in the performance of a cholecystectomy can result in leakage of bile into the peritoneal cavity, then making re-operation and drainage of the gallbladder bed a necessity. Abnormalities of the gallbladder itself are rare, but include absence of the gallbladder, duplication, and the "floating" gallbladder, which is suspended from the liver by peritoneal mesentery.

The main function of the gallbladder is the collection, concentration, and storage of bile until it is needed for digestion. As described in the preceding section, up to 1000 cc. of bile per day is formed by the liver. After delivery of the bile to the gallbladder, the bile is concentrated through the constant absorption of water and electrolytes.

During digestion, bile empties from both the gallbladder into the duodenum and from the liver into the gallbladder as the sphincter of Oddi is opened and relaxed. Fat or protein, as it enters the duodenum, triggers the release of the hormone cholecystokinin-pancreozymin (CCK-PCZ) from the duodenal and jejunal mucosa.

This is transported in the bloodstream to the gallbladder and stimulates it to contract, which then forces bile to flow into the duodenum. Mild vagal stimulation also causes contraction of the gallbladder and relaxation of the sphincter of Oddi; strong stimulation, however, causes constriction of the sphincter.

Between meals the sphincter of Oddi remains closed. As pressure builds within the closed duct system, bile is forced to flow from the liver into the gallbladder for storage and concentration until needed.

CHEMICAL PHASE OF DIGESTION

Having briefly described the anatomy and physiology of the major organs of the gastrointestinal tract, a summary of the chemical or enzyme phase of digestion can be made. The organs of the gastrointestinal system are responsible for the synthesis of many digestive enzymes. These enzymes are specific in their action in that those that act on carbohydrates cannot act on proteins, those that act on proteins cannot act on fats, etc. Enzymes have traditionally been known by the suffix -ase. For example, enzymes that break down carbohydrates are called carbohydrases and those breaking down lipids are called lipases. In addition, they are named according to the part of the digestive system from which they originate, as shown in Figure 6-4. Because of the specificity of the enzyme system, if the organ source of an enzyme is damaged, other enzymes cannot take over that function.

Although chemical digestion begins in the mouth through the action of salivary amylase, the first major activity takes place in the stomach with secretion of gastric juice rich in HCl and pepsinogen. Hydrochloric acid, produced by the parietal cells, converts the inactive pepsinogen to the active form of pepsin. Pepsin, produced by the chief cells, is a protein splitting enzyme which also helps destroy bacteria entering with food and increase mineral solubility.

Several factors stimulate the secretion of gastric juice. Eating causes 3 ml/minute of juices to be secreted, and even the sight, smell, and taste of food can lead to increased secretion. Distention results in continued secretion. Thus acid and enzyme concentration is usually increased during the first few hours after eating, decreasing in the following hours until the next meal. Patients with gastrointestinal disease are often prescribed diets high in fats and carbohydrates, which provide little gastric stimulation, and are en-

Source of Enzyme Secretion	Site of Enzyme Action	Name of Enzymes and the Substances They Act On			
		Starches	Sugars	Fats	Proteins
salivary glands	mouth	salivary amylase (Ptyalin)			
stomach	stomach			gastric lipase	gastric protease (pepsin)
pancreas	small intestine	pancreatic amylase		pancreatic lipase	pancreatic proteases
wall of small intestines	small intestine		sucrase maltase lactase		intestinal proteases

Figure 6-4. Digestive enzymes (from: Wilson ED, et al.: Principles of Nutrition. John Wiley and Sons, Inc., New York, 1975, p. 105. Used with permission.)

couraged to avoid alcohol, caffeine, and high protein meals, which are all strong stimulants.

As food leaves the stomach and enters the duodenum it is in a semi-liquid form referred to as chyme. In this phase of digestion intestinal juices, pancreatic juice, and bile are added to the chyme and complete the breakdown of fats, carbohydrates and proteins. It is in the duodenum where the majority of carbohydrate digestion takes place. Pancreatic amylase converts starch to the disaccharide maltose, and small intestine enzymes eventually break the disaccharides into simple sugars, glucose, fructose, and galactose, for absorption.

The digestion of fat also occurs primarily in the small intestine through the actions of bile and pancreatic lipase. Bile salts begin the process of fat digestion by emulsifying fat globules, lowering the surface tension so that each globule may be broken into smaller, more easily digested droplets. Pancreatic lipase can then hydrolize these droplets into glycerols, fatty acids, and glycerides which are absorbable.

Protein digestion, like fat and carbohydrate digestion, begins in the stomach, through the action of pepsin, but the majority of enzyme activity takes place in the small intestine. The pancreas secretes several precursors or inactive proteases which are converted to active enzymatic form in the intestine: trypsinogen is converted to trypsin, chymotrypsinogen to chymotrypsin, and procarboxypolypeptidase to carboxypeptidase. The active forms of these enzymes break down the links of polypeptide chains, producing smaller units of polypeptides. The final conversion of these polypeptides into amino acids occurs through the action of the enzymes aminopolypeptidase and dipeptidase in intestinal secretions. It is these enzymes, primarily from the pancreas, which are capable of fat and protein breakdown that are so destructive to body tissue when fistula formation occurs in disease.

As described earlier, little enzyme action occurs once the end products of digestion have moved into the large intestine. Here the most significant activity consists of water and sodium absorption and bacterial activity. It should be noted, however, that disease states which interfere with these processes, leading to excessive water loss or disturbance of normal colon flora, can easily lead to severe electrolyte disturbances or vitamin deficiencies which have serious consequences if not corrected.

PATHOPHYSIOLOGY AND INTERVENTION

Introduction

As mentioned earlier, disease or malfunction of the gastrointestinal tract does not, in and of itself, mandate intensive medical or nursing care. However, all disease states which involve the gastrointestinal system have the potential of precipitating infection, bleeding, or severe metabolic disturbances, and it is these sequelae which then necessitate intensive care.

Infection is most commonly associated with abdominal surgery, particularly when performed for bowel obstruction or ruptured viscus. The two disease entities which cause bleeding severe enough to constitute a critical illness are ulcer disease and esophageal varices. Conditions producing life-threatening metabolic disturbances include liver disease, particularly cirrhosis and hepatic encephalopathy, pancreatitis and prolonged vomiting and diarrhea. It is readily apparent that all of these diseases have elements of all complications; for example, the patient with a bowel obstruction may present in the Intensive Care Unit with metabolic alkalosis following severe vomiting, may develop peritonitis following surgery, and could begin bleeding from a suture line. However, each disorder will be reviewed under the heading which represents the sequela or complication most often accompanying it. Relevant medical and nursing interventions will then be discussed.

Causes of Infection

Infection of the abdominal cavity may occur following rupture of any of the viscera, or may be a complication of any abdominal surgery. It is a frequent cause of admission to the Intensive Care Unit. Although localized infection of a viscera or fistula tract may occur, this section will focus on peritonitis.

Peritonitis may be defined as any inflammation of the peritoneum and may be caused either by bacterial contamination or irritation from any foreign substance. However, it is the number and nature of bacterial invasions which determine the severity and mortality.[53] Mortality rate from peritonitis averages about 7%,[28] and it is the most common cause of death following abdominal surgery.[22] Bowel obstruction, the second most common disorder requiring emergency abdominal surgery,[58] and diverticular disease, which is present in 40% of all patients by age 70,[46] will be discussed as common precursors of peritonitis.

Bowel obstruction

Obstruction is said to occur whenever there is lack of movement of intestinal contents due either to functional or mechanical obstruction. Functional obstruction, or paralytic ileus, may be a temporary and normal postoperative phenomenon, or may result from spinal cord damage, peritonitis, metabolic disturbance (e.g., hypokalemia), or bowel ischemia. Mechanical obstruction may be caused by adhesions from previous surgery, by obstruction of the lumen of the bowel by tumor, inflammatory processes, diverticulitis, intussusception, gallstones, or by extrinsic compression resulting from neoplasm, hernia, or volvulus. Prompt surgical intervention is usually indicated once mechanical obstruction has been diagnosed.

Signs and symptoms present with bowel obstruction include pain or abdominal cramps, vomiting, constipation, and abdominal distention. Bowel sounds usually include peristaltic rushes, or high-pitched tinkling sounds; absence of sound occurs with functional ileus. The nature of the vomiting and the degree of distention depend on the location of the obstruction. Colon obstruction is not usually associated with vomiting because the ileocecal valve prevents regurgitation. This disorder usually causes the most pronounced distention, however, as fluids and gases cannot be expelled and rapidly accumulate. Ileal obstruction causes regurgitation of brownish liquid that may have a fecal odor resulting from advanced digestion of foodstuffs and bacterial activity. Distention will accompany this obstruction because the vomiting only partially decompresses the bowel. Jejunal obstruction is associated with the greatest amount of vomiting, of a thin greenish liquid, and the least amount of distention.

Diagnosis of obstruction is confirmed by x-ray. Plain abdominal films may reveal distended loops of bowel, or barium enemas may be used to pinpoint the location and cause of obstruction.

When obstruction occurs, several physiological processes begin. Distention diminishes absorption in the bowel while increasing gastric and intestinal secretions. It may also compromise arteriolar supply and lead to edema. There is often an increase in cell permeability secondary to edema or ischemia, and plasma proteins exude into the peritoneal cavity. The most severe initial result of these combined processes is dehydration. If prolonged vomiting has accompanied the obstruction, the patient may also be alkalotic, with hypochloremia and hypokalemia.

A bowel obstruction necessitates immediate treatment. If the obstruction is not relieved, bowel necrosis, rupture, and sepsis will occur, in addition to hypovolemic shock. Initial treatment consists of decompression of the stomach by means of a nasogastric tube and fluid and electrolyte replacement. Once these measures have been instituted, the decision concerning corrective measures can be made. If the obstruction is partial and thought to be temporary, as is the case with adhesions or post-radiation enteritis, a Miller-Abbott tube may be used to decompress the bowel. This drainage tube has a bag at the tip of the tube which contains three to ten cc. of mercury; the weight of the mercury assists in the movement of the tube through the intestines.

If surgery is deemed necessary, several alternative procedures may be chosen, depending on the type and location of the obstruction. When possible, mechanical causes of obstruction, such as adhesions, are removed without entering the bowel. More often it is necessary to make some repair of the colon itself. This may involve only a cecostomy, in which an opening is made in the cecum and a drainage tube temporarily placed, a temporary colostomy, or a permanent colostomy.

The most common temporary procedures are double barrel colostomy and loop colostomy. These temporary procedures are performed when it is thought possible to eventually restore bowel continuity. With the double barrel colostomy, the colon is divided and the two ends externalized out through separate skin openings. The proximal end will then drain fecal material and the distal end, called a mucous fistula, may drain a minimal amount of blood and mucus. The two ends of the bowel are anastomosed 4 to 6 months after the original operation. In the loop colostomy, the bowel is brought to the surface of the skin and held in place with a glass rod inserted under the loop of colon. After the skin sutures underneath the loop have begun to heal, in two to three days, an opening is made in the bowel, usually by cautery. The bowel is then later anastomosed; this procedure is somewhat easier and simpler to perform than a double barrel colostomy.

Permanent colostomy is most often performed for cancer. When the colostomy is intended to be permanent, only one stoma is created. This distal end of the bowel or rectum is then resected and sutured (Figure 6-5).

Diverticulitis

Diverticular disease is the most common disorder of the colon in Western countries.[45] The term diverticula refers to an outpouching of a segment of the mucous membrane of the bowel through the circular muscle layer. Diverticulosis is used to indicate the presence of several diverticulae. Diverticulitis is the inflammatory condition which may or may not complicate diverticulosis.

Diverticulae are found most often in the sigmoid colon, and, as

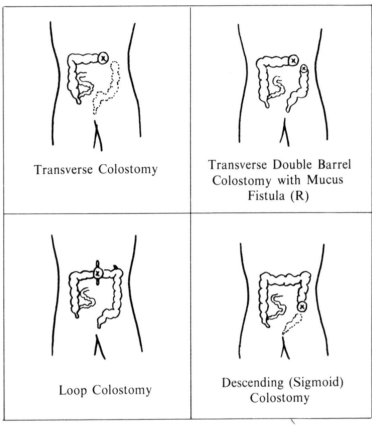

Transverse Colostomy

Transverse Double Barrel
Colostomy with Mucus
Fistula (R)

Loop Colostomy

Descending (Sigmoid)
Colostomy

Figure 6-5. Colostomy procedures.

mentioned earlier, are present with increasing frequency with aging, occuring in one out of every three patients by age 60.[39] The etiology of this disease is thought to be related to changes in the muscular wall and mucous membrane induced by dietary factors. It has been noted that diverticulosis does not occur in very underdeveloped countries, such as Africa, but the incidence increases as industrialization and economic advancement occur. This societal change is associated with a change in diet from one that includes a high fiber content to one that includes processed foods with low fiber content. The low fiber content results in a fecal mass which moves sluggishly through the bowel, allowing more time for water absorption and producing a firmer stool.

This change in diet then leads to two anatomical alterations. First, the presence of more viscous stools in the colon requires higher pressures in order to move the stool; these higher pressures, which are produced during the segmental contractions of the colon, then lead to muscular thickening and outpouching through the mucosa. The mucous membrane itself is also often found to have proliferated into excessive folds. An inherent weakness of the muscle wall is the third factor which is thought to have an etiologic role in the development of diverticulosis.

The majority of patients with diverticulosis experience no symptoms, or only recurrent mild constipation. Others will have more difficulty with distention, pain, and diarrhea. Diverticulitis is thought to occur when fecal accumulation and high intralumen pressures cause perforation or, at the least, mucosal abrasion. At this point the symptoms occurring are related to the inflammatory process and extent of involvement. The inflammation may be confined to the immediate pericolic tissues; in this case a low-grade fever, leukocytosis, and hyperactivity of the bowel may be present. If perforation has occurred, and peritoneal irritation occurs, diffuse, rebound tenderness is usually present. Signs of sepsis, the most common sequela of diverticulitis, will then ensue. Obstruction also frequently occurs as a result of the edema associated with this process.

Surgical treatment is indicated when recurrent attacks of diverticulitis occur, when abscess formation is present, or, of course, when frank peritonitis secondary to a communicating or open perforation is present. A temporary colostomy is the procedure of choice, including resection of the diseased segment if possible.

Peritonitis

Having provided a brief background of two conditions which are common precursors of intra-abdominal infection, the discussion will now focus on peritonitis itself and intervention.

Once peritoneal inflammation has occurred, regardless of cause, several processes will be initiated by the body as defense against the insult. First, the peritoneum will exude large amounts of a plasma-like fluid. Second, paralytic ileus usually occurs in response to the irritation. The loss of fluid from the peritoneum itself and associated with the ileus may total as much as 5 liters per day.[28] Thirdly, there is usually an associated increase in adrenocortical hormone secretion if the process is severe. (See chapters 8 and 9 for a more detailed description of endocrine response to stress and shock).

Classical peritoneal signs include abdominal pain on coughing, rebound tenderness, and tenderness to percussion over the area of peritonitis. There will be rigidity of muscles overlying this area, or over the entire abdomen. When ileus is present, bowel sounds are absent and abdominal distention present. Leukocytosis and electrolyte imbalances are prominent. Respiratory impairment may be present if the process is diffuse.

Primary peritonitis refers to the process which occurs spontaneously, not associated with trauma, ruptured viscus, or surgery. It may be due to cirrhosis, bacterial invasion via Fallopian tubes in young females, or nephrosis. Treatment consists of fluid replacement and antibiotic therapy; surgery is not indicated.

Secondary peritonitis is by far more common, and is most often related to perforated viscus, abdominal trauma, or abdominal surgery, particularly of the lower GI tract. Surgical intervention is usually indicated to repair the source of infection or irritation (e.g., ruptured appendix or anastomotic leak), drain abscesses, and remove debris from the peritoneal cavity. The particular procedure performed depends on the primary disorder, but regardless of procedure, other aspects of treatment necessitated most often include:

1. antibiotic therapy
2. decompression of the gastrointestinal tract
3. fluid and electrolyte replacement
4. respiratory support
5. restoration or maintenance of nutritional balance

Assessment

As with any illness, specific intervention measures are based upon accurate assessment. Abdominal assessment of the critically ill, which was not included in the first chapter on Physical Assessment, will be briefly described before discussing aspects of treatment of the patient with peritonitis.

The abdomen may be divided into either 4 quadrants or into 9 regions. Figure 6-6 illustrates this and Table 6-1 lists structures

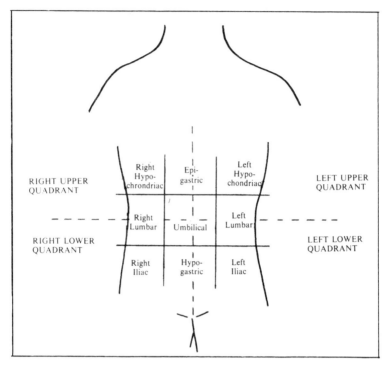

Figure 6-6. Abdominal quadrants and regions.

found in each. The names of the quadrants or regions are used in describing physical findings.

The first aspect of assessment is inspection. With the critically ill patient the nurse should be particularly alert for signs of dehydration, such as poor skin turgor and dry mucous membranes. All wounds and stomas should be carefully inspected; if drainage is present, the amount, color, consistency, and odor may yield important clues as to source. Skin condition surrounding the drainage site is also noted. Abdominal girth should be measured at the umbilicus; if a large bulky dressing is in place, measure during dressing changes when the wound can be lightly covered with one layer of gauze. Marks should always be made on the skin with a pen to insure that subsequent measurements will be made at the same location.

Any abnormal findings should be carefully recorded. Spider nevi, or angioma, reddened, spider-like blood vessels, indicate liver

TABLE 6-1

Organs Located in Abdominal Quadrants[22]

Quadrant	Organ
Right upper	liver gallbladder head of pancreas top of right kidney and right adrenal pyloric sphincter of stomach start of duodenum bowel: transverse colon and possibly loops of small bowel
Left upper	left tip of liver spleen stomach pancreas top of left kidney and left adrenal bowel: transverse colon and possibly loops of small bowel
Right lower	remainder of right kidney appendix bladder and ureter ascending colon and loops of small bowel uterus and ovary
Left lower	remainder of left kidney bladder and ureter descending colon and loops of small bowel uterus and ovary

disease, as does thick, glistening skin which is produced with ascites. Grey-Turner's sign, a discoloration around the flanks, or Cullen's sign, a bluish color of the umbilicus, may indicate either intra-abdominal hemorrhage or peritonitis. Observation of the contour of the abdomen may reveal ascites.

Auscultation should be performed before palpation, to avoid inducing reflex peristalsis. Auscultation is performed by placing the diaphragm of the stethoscope lightly on the upper abdomen, then moving to all four quadrants. Table 6-2 lists possible findings on auscultation.

Palpation will assist in determining the degree of abdominal distention. The abdomen should be fairly firm in individuals of muscular build, but it should be possible to palpate as deep as 3 to 4 inches if the patient can relax his muscles. Rigidity, tautness, and involuntary guarding are indications of underlying pathology. The

TABLE 6-2

Abdominal Sounds

Sound	Interpretation
1. Gurgling, swishing, or tingling, from 5 to 30 sounds per minute	Normal bowel sounds
2. High pitched, long, intense rushes or tinkling	Hypermotility; often heard with mechanical bowel obstruction; accompanied by pain
3. Borborygmi: waves of loud gurgling or tinkling noises	Indicates abdominal contents are being squeezed through narrowed opening, as with partial obstruction; accompanied by cramping
4. Absence of bowel sounds	Functional obstruction, paralytic ileus
5. Bruit in midabdomen or epigastrium	Abdominal aortic aneurysm; pulsatile mass is often palpable

liver itself is not usually palpable, although the edge can be felt with deep palpation by pressing the fingers down along the right costal margin. If the edge of the liver can be felt below this, liver enlargement is present and the number of centimeters it is palpable below the costal margin should be recorded. The spleen, on the left side, should not be palpable.

Antibiotic therapy

Antibiotic therapy may be administered by two routes in treating peritonitis: systemically or locally (intra-abdominally). Systemic, intravenous antibiotic administration is essential, but if the patient's condition permits, may be withheld until culture reports yield positive identification of pathogens. Without specific identification of the bacterial contaminant, adequate therapy is difficult to insure. In the absence of culture reports, the most common recommendations include combinations of penicillin, clindamycin, gentamicin, ampicillin and chloramphenicol.[28,40,53] The nurse administering these antibiotics must of course be alert for sensitivity and anaphylactoid reactions, in addition to being knowledgable concerning toxic effects, such as renal damage with gentamicin and bone marrow depression with chloramphenicol.

Thought regarding the use of peritoneal lavage remains divided. Some feel that the technique of irrigating the peritoneal cavity with large amounts of fluid and antibiotics spreads contamination, that systemic antibiotics are well distributed to the peritoneum and local administration not necessary. Others believe that irrigation reduces the number of bacteria in the peritoneal cavity and also washes out foreign material, thus contributing to a decreased mortality rate.[28,53] Lavage is usually continuous and carried out via either several sumps or peritoneal dialysis catheters placed into upper and lower quadrants, two for instillation of fluid and two for drainage. The solution itself may be dialysate solution, saline, or a balanced salt solution.

In administering intraperitoneal lavage the nurse is concerned primarily with two aspects: maintenance of the irrigation system and prevention of complications related to the procedure. Although with continuous rapid infusions overall fluid balance is difficult to regulate, the nurse must be able to estimate positive or negative balances. If a large amount of debris such as blood or feces is present, drainage catheters may become clogged and must be cleared in order to prevent fluid accumulation. The potential for large fluid shifts across the peritoneum also exists, just as occurs with peritoneal dialysis. Measurement of drainage is often difficult because of leakage of fluid around sump drains and through incisions: if accurate measurements cannot be made, the patient should be weighed twice daily.

Respiratory impairment may result if large amounts of fluid are retained in the abdominal cavity and inhibit diaphragmatic excursion. The patient having peritoneal lavage should be kept in semi-Fowler's position in order to minimize this risk. Some also believe that keeping the head of the bed slightly elevated also reduces the risk of pleural effusion associated with sub-diaphragmatic or sub-phrenic abscesses. These effusions are thought to occur through the passage of fluid into the pleural cavity from the peritoneal cavity either via the lymphatics or through unrecognized openings in the diaphragm.[49]

Skin care is difficult whenever there is a communication between skin and peritoneal cavity. As mentioned previously, the stomach, small intestine, and particularly the pancreas are rich sources of enzymes all capable of damaging the skin. Irrigation does dilute these enzymes and lessen their effect on skin surfaces, but it also makes it very difficult to keep the skin dry and clean. Use of such protective material as Karaya or Stomadhesive is essential, and real ingenuity is required in designing and applying drainage bags which will keep the leaking irrigant away from the skin.

Decompression of the GI tract

Decompression through the use of a nasogastric or intestinal tube is utilized in order to relieve fluid accumulation and prevent recurrent distention. Levine tubes and Salem sump tubes are used for gastric aspiration, and Miller-Abbott and Cantor tubes for bowel aspiration. The Levine, Salem, and Miller-Abbott, the most commonly used, are shown in Figures 6-7 and 6-8.

In order to insert a nasogastric tube, the first step is to explain the procedure to the patient and obtain his consent and cooperation. Next, determine the length of tubing necessary to reach the stomach by measuring the distance from the nose to the earlobe plus the distance from the nose to the tip of the sternum, and mark the tube accordingly. Position the patient in a high-Fowler's position with head straight or neck flexed very slightly forward; having the neck hyperextended makes entry into the trachea more likely, especially with an unconscious patient.

The first two or three inches of the tube should be lubricated with a water-soluble jelly prior to insertion. With very flexible tubes, such as red-rubber feeding tubes or small Levine tubes, it may also be helpful to immerse the tube in ice for a few minutes in order to stiffen it.

Insert the tube gently through one nostril. If obstruction is met, try the other side. After two or three inches of insertion, have the patient take small sips of water through a straw. This will facilitate passage into the esophagus. It ususaly causes less discomfort if the patient can continue to swallow several times as the tube is advanced. There is *no reason* to rush this procedure and the patient should be allowed to stop and rest a moment if he wishes.

Once inserted the pre-determined distance, the position of the tube should be verified. This can be done by aspirating, which should yield gastric material, by injecting 30 cc. of air through the tube and listening with a stethoscope over the stomach for the sound of the air passage, or by immersing the end of the tube under water and looking for the presence of bubbling, which would indicate entry into the respiratory tree.

When position has been determined, the tube should be taped in place, with a *minimum* amount of tape. Excessive tape succeeds

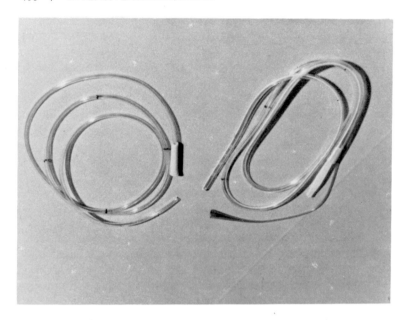

Figure 6-7. Levine (R) and salem sump (L) tubes.

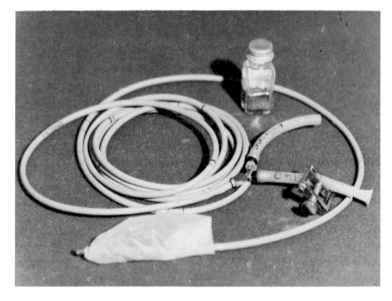

Figure 6-8. Miller-Abbott tube.

only in making the patient uncomfortable; it does not keep the tube in place if it is handled carelessly or if the patient is uncooperative or disoriented and wishes to remove the tube. The tube should be taped in the position which it naturally assumes; it should not be pulled to one side or taped to the forehead. Both of these maneuvers create pressure on the nostril and lead to skin breakdown. Pinning the tube to the patient's gown will prevent traction on it as the patient moves about in bed.

Maintenance of a functioning nasogastric drainage and irrigation system is the nurse's responsibility. General principles and guidelines include the following:

1. Saline is used as irrigant in order to avoid electrolyte depletion.
2. Whenever anything other than saline is instilled via the tube, such as antacids, the tube should be flushed afterward with saline in order to avoid clogging the lumen.
3. In choosing nasogastric tubes, keep in mind: the Levine tube is smaller and less irritating, but the Salem tube, with air vent, is less likely to pull at the gastric mucosa and cause damage. The Salem, having a larger lumen, is also less likely to become clogged.
4. In assessing patency of a Salem sump tube, it should always be possible to hear or feel air being pulled through the air vent. If the air vent has become plugged, it can be irrigated by injecting air or saline through it.
5. The NG tube, if functioning, should always drain at least 50 cc. per 8-hour shift. If there is no drainage whatever, the tube is not functioning. Similarly, if there is a sudden marked decrease in drainage from one shift to another, the system should be checked.
6. If there is reason to suspect that the NG tube is not draining properly, but patency has been assured by irrigation, the tube should be repositioned.
7. If the patient has had gastric or esophageal surgery, the tube *should not* be repositioned without checking with the physician. It is possible, in the early postoperative period, to disrupt suture lines by frequent tube manipulation.

Level of suction used with nasogastric tubes varies, but generally low intermittent suction (-30 mm. Hg) is used with Levine tubes, which have no air vent to keep the tip away from the stomach wall. Salem sump tubes function best at a constant setting of −60 to −80 mm. Hg suction, or intermittent suction of 80-120 mm. Hg.

Although NG tubes may seem commonplace in the intensive care setting, the consequences of inattention to the system can be disastrous to the patient. Distention of the stomach after gastric surgery places tension on suture lines, prolongs ileus, and may result in vomiting and aspiration when level of consciousness is depressed.

Long gastrointestinal tubes, such as the double lumen Miller-Abbott tube, are used for bowel decompression. The insertion procedure is the same as for short nasogastric tubes. After the tube has reached the stomach, the balloon at the end of the tube is inflated with 3-10 cc. of mercury which assists in passage through the intestines. The tube is left untaped so that it can advance freely with peristalsis. The physician may also order that the tube be advanced or inserted an additional one or two inches every few hours. The tube may be irrigated frequently to maintain patency, but it is often not possible to aspirate the irrigant back because of the location of the tube in the bowel.

Fluid and electrolyte balance

As has been mentioned, vascular fluid loss in peritonitis can be extensive. Sequestration of fluid in the peritoneal cavity also follows major abdominal surgery and is often referred to as "third space loss." Consequently the patient may exhibit signs of hypovolemia and shock despite constant administration of intravenous fluids at standard rates. This "third space" accumulation of fluid may persist for several days, then slowly be reabsorbed into the vascular system, complicating assessment of fluid balance. The most reliable measures of adequate fluid replacement are a urine output of 30-60 cc./hr., stable hematocrit, and vital signs, including central venous pressure, within the normal range. Pulmonary capillary wedge pressure readings will yield a more sensitive index of cardiac function and fluid status in the very complex patient or in high-risk patients.

The potential for disturbance in fluid balance is readily appreciated in reviewing the following facts. The gastrointestinal tract normally secretes 8000 cc. of fluid per day, including saliva, gastric juice, bile, pancreatic and intestinal juices.[22] All but 200-300 cc. of this is reabsorbed by the time feces are eliminated. Thus, any disease or treatment interfering with normal reabsorption can easily lead to fluid imbalances of several thousand ccs. per day.

Maintenance of normal electrolyte levels can be quite difficult in the peritonitis patient. Depending upon the underlying disease condition and length of time it has persisted, as well as certain treatment modalities, almost any electrolyte may be depleted or accumulated. The following considerations relative to electrolyte balance should be kept in mind.

Acid-base abnormalities are common occurrences. Prolonged vomiting most often leads to metabolic alkalosis because of the loss of hydrogen ions in gastric acids, and prolonged diarrhea usually results in metabolic acidosis because of the loss of bicarbonate ions from intestinal juices. Most significant in knowing which abnormality to expect is knowledge of the specific location of electrolyte loss. For example, if the patient has an upper bowel obstruction and vomits bowel contents, acidosis rather than alkalosis may occur. Similarly, nasogastric suction will result in alkalosis while Miller-Abbott drainage leads to acidosis. Slow, shallow respirations, indicating the respiratory response to alkalosis, or rapid, deep respirations, (Kussmaul) which compensate for metabolic acidosis, may be the nurse's first indication of acid-base status in the absence of arterial blood gas results.

Loss of sodium ions often accompanies loss of fluid from any part of the GI tract. All gastrointestinal fluid contains large quantities of sodium, particularly bile and intestinal juice, and the nurse should be alert for signs and symptoms of hyponatremia. These include apprehension, abdominal cramping, and, in severe cases, convulsions.

Potassium imbalances may have life-threatening consequences. Hypokalemia is common when vomiting or diarrhea have been persistent, and also accompanies prolonged nasogastric suction. Parenteral potassium supplements must be provided whenever the patient is NPO. Sixty mEq/day is an average replacement dosage, but this amount varies considerably depending on renal status, use of blood infusions, amount of tissue necrosis, degree of catabolism, acid-base status, and many other variables. Consequently, the nurse caring for the patient with any gastrointestinal disorder must have as a priority the monitoring of potassium levels. Weakness, tremors, diminished reflexes, and paralytic ileus are common manifestations of hypokalemia; ECG changes (peaked T waves, widened QRS, flattened P waves) are predominant in hyperkalemia.

Calcium is the third electrolyte which is often altered in GI disease. Calcium is less soluble in alkaline solutions and can be precipitated by certain digestive enzymes, thus removing it from serum. Hypocalcemia is evidenced by hyperreflexia, muscle cramps, tingling of fingers and toes. Chvostek's sign, a spasm or numbness of the facial muscle elicited by tapping the hollow of the cheek an inch in front of the ear, is a simple bedside test to confirm suspicions of hypocalcemia.

Respiratory support

Respiratory complications in the patient with peritonitis are common and are related to several factors. Prolonged anesthesia time and postoperative hypoventilation and secretion accumulation lead to atelectasis in patients undergoing abdominal surgery. Upper abdominal procedures are particularly associated with restricted breathing patterns postoperatively because of pain, and these patients, *more than any others,* should receive intensive pulmonary care, including adequate pain medication. A new fever in the first 24 postoperative hours should alert the nurse to pulmonary complications.

Restriction in diaphragmatic excursion is a second factor leading to pulmonary complications. Abdominal distention limits the extent to which deep breathing can be performed; elevating the head of the bed will reduce the extent to which abdominal contents impinge upon respiratory movement of the thorax and make coughing and deep breathing easier.

The third factor, mentioned earlier, is the frequent occurrence of pleural effusion associated with infectious processes below the diaphragm. Diminished or absent breath sounds in lower lobes or posteriorly, deteriorating blood gases, and increasing respiratory rate and pulse may be the first clinical signs; chest x-ray will confirm the presence of effusion, which may then require thoracentesis or placement of a chest tube.

Maintenance of nutrition

The treatment of gastrointestinal disease and peritonitis frequently includes resting that segment of the GI tract involved, or carefully regulating the initial introduction of food. Tube feedings, either via nasogastric tube or a tube inserted through a stab wound into another segment of the GI tract, e.g., jejunostomy tube, are used to provide nutrition when possible. Parenteral hyperalimentation, the alternative to tube feedings, has several complications, particularly sepsis, and is used only when the stomach and bowel must be kept empty for a period of time.

Tube feedings of various formulas are commercially available or can be blenderized to provide specific amounts of nutrients by the hospital's dietary department. Consultation with the dietician is essential in planning feedings which best meet the patient's need. Regardless of specific formula of feeding, however, some general guidelines should be followed.

Feedings that are prepared in the hospital should be refrigerated until needed, as should commercial mixes once opened. However, the solution should be warmed prior to administration to the patient. Very cold feedings may cause diarrhea.

Another cause of diarrhea is overly rapid administration of feedings. When feedings are initiated, small volumes should be given, e.g., 100 cc. over not less than one hour, and the residual volume left in the stomach at one, two, and three hour intervals checked in order to assess the tolerance to the feeding. The amount of each feeding can then be gradually increased and/or the interval between feedings decreased. The length of time of administration should not be shortened. If diarrhea persists, a very slow continuous infusion of the feeding may be necessary.

The most common cause of diarrhea associated with tube feedings is an intolerance to the concentration of the feeding. Solutions with a high osmolality may retard water absorption in the bowel and result in diarrhea. Giving half-strength feedings will resolve this problem.

A recent study of tube fed patients has pointed out that the most common fluid and electrolyte problems associated with this form of nutrition are states of dehydration and hyponatremia.[33] Consequently, the nurse administering tube feedings should be alert for complaints of thirst, dryness of mucous membrances, abdominal cramping, and hypotension.

Bleeding

Bleeding from any site in the GI tract—stomach, small intestine, large bowel, due to any cause—ulcer disease, diverticulae, trauma, may progress to hemorrhage and threaten the survival of the individual. Gastrointestinal bleeding is an unfortunately common problem, ranking second only to cardiovascular disease as a reason for emergency hospitalization. It is also associated with a mortality rate ranging from 5 to 30%; if the bleeding reaches massive proportions, the mortality rate reaches as high as 50%.[50] Although bleeding may originate at any point, such as pancreas or biliary system, representative conditions that will be discussed are gastritis, peptic ulcer disease, and esophageal varices.

Gastritis and ulcer disease

Gastritis is usually defined as an inflammation of the gastric mucosa, but the etiology may include several different factors. It may exist in an acute or chronic form. In acute gastritis the gastric mucosa is reddened, inflamed, edematous, and has areas covered by exudate and mucus. Erosive areas may be present which cause bleeding; this is usually self-limited, though, and most often is not massive in nature.

Acute gastritis may occur asymptomatically, eventuating in the patient presenting in the emergency room with upper GI bleeding and no history of previous difficulty. Acute alcoholism and/or the use of medications such as salicylates are the precipitating causes in most cases. In other instances the patient may experience anorexia, fever, vomiting, or epigastric pain of varying duration. Hospitalized patients may develop acute gastritis related to the stress of illness or intensive care. Uremia, food and heavy metal poisoning may also precipitate this condition.

Diagnosis can accurately be made by gastroscopy. Treatment consists of blood replacement, ice water lavage, and large doses of anticholinergic medications. Bleeding which has not been controlled within twelve hours is usually an indication for surgical intervention in the form of vagotomy, pyloroplasty, or gastrectomy.

Chronic gastritis is a more progressive condition. The exact cause is unknown, although it is frequently associated with other disease entities, such as rheumatoid arthritis, ulcerative colitis, chronic renal disease, and chronic infection. In this form of gastritis the mucosa initially becomes thickened, but as the disease progresses the walls and lining of the stomach become thin and atrophy. The mucosa of the body, the acid producing area, is primarily involved.

Chronic gastritis is most often asymptomatic, but vague complaints such as anorexia, vomiting after meals, or epigastric burning may be present. In severe cases, decreased acid secretion (achlorhydria) from the body of the stomach may lead to poor iron absorption. When this intrinsic factor is missing, vitamin B_{12} absorption is affected and pernicious anemia results.

Gastric ulceration may also occur because of a decrease in the resistance of the mucosa, despite the decreased acid secretion. There are few characteristic findings on x-ray or gastroscopy, and gastric biopsy is necessary to confirm atrophy of the mucosa and rule out carcinoma. Treatment is conservative and often includes diet modification, antacids, and vitamin B_{12} replacement.

Antral gastritis is the third kind of gastritis which may bring the patient to the ICU. In this disorder there is pitting and reddening of the antral mucosa, with chronic inflammation and fibrosis. Antral gastritis has been associated with duodenal ulceration because the chronic exposure of the antral mucosa to intestinal contents causes irritation and hyperplasia of the parietal cells, thus leading to excessive gastrin release.

Gastritis is often a precursor to peptic ulcer disease because of the changes in the mucosal wall. A peptic ulcer is a circular break in the mucosal wall of the stomach due to contact with gastric juices such as hydrochloric acid and pepsin. The break usually extends beyond the epithelium. Peptic ulcers may occur in any part of the gastrointestinal tract but are usually found in the lower end of the esophagus, in the stomach, or in the duodenum.

Gastric ulceration may occur in any part of the stomach. It is often associated with normal or even decreased acid production, but some acid and pepsin are necessary for ulcer production. The etiology is believed to be related to an imbalance in those factors which protect the gastric mucosa and those that potentiate damage. An increased permeability of the mucosal barrier to hydrogen ions allows a back diffusion of hydrogen, which in turn causes mucosal cells to release histamine. There is resultant vasodilation, capillary stasis, and hemorrhage.[5] This back diffusion also causes a decrease in acid secretion and leads to changes in the mucosal resistance to other substances. Other factors believed to have an etiologic role in ulcer development include a greater than normal regurgitation of duodenal contents into the stomach due to abnormal pyloric function, increased vagal activity, hypersecretion of gastric acid, and an enhanced sensitivity of the mucosa to gastric juices. Certain drugs may also lead to increased mucosal susceptibility—aspirin, cortico-steroids, and vasopressors, in addition to alcohol, are associated with mucosal damage. Smoking and environmental-emotional factors are other etiologic agents.

Gastric ulcers occur more frequently in men than women and increase in incidence with age. Pain associated with the ulcer is located to the left of the epigastrium, is not relieved by food ingestion, and may occur a short time after eating. Other symptoms include nausea, vomiting, a feeling of abdominal distention, and, in some cases, progressive weight loss.

When the patient's history and physical exam are suggestive of a gastric ulcer, further diagnostic tests must be employed to differentiate this diagnosis from gastric cancer or duodenal ulcer. Upper GI x-rays may reveal a sharply defined crater with mucous folds leading to the base of the ulcer, whereas a malignant lesion is more often flat, irregularly shaped, with rolled margins. Gastroscopy is by far the most helpful tool and improves diagnostic accuracy as much as 75%.[25] Cytologic examination and gastric analysis are used to rule out the presence of carcinoma.

Ulcers that are deep and consist of chronic lesions, usually involving the first portion of the duodenum, are known as duodenal ulcers.[37] Duodenal ulceration is most commonly due to excessive hydrochloric acid and pepsin secretion. Hydrochloric acid may be secreted in excess of 12 mEq/hour,[25] and may be related to parietal cell hyperplasia, increased vagal stimulation, increased pyloric regurgitation, and antral gastritis.

Assuming that an excess of hydrochloric acid and pepsin are responsible for duodenal ulcer formation, there are a multitude of mediating factors thought to influence the development of the ulcer crater. Men are affected more often than women, in a 7 or 8:1 ratio,[37] particularly when employed in a high-tension occupation. There is no exact proof of the effect of high stress jobs, but the emotional tension is thought to increase gastric secretion or reduce mucosal resistance.[25] Certain other disease entities, such as liver disease, and emphysema, are associated with a higher incidence of ulcer formation. As with gastric ulcer, drugs such as steroids and aspirin, alcohol, caffeine, and cigarette smoking are all thought to contribute to pathogenicity.

Individuals with duodenal ulcers may complain of epigastric pain or burning located in the mid-epigastrium, but more frequently the complaint is of pressure, muscle spasm, or the occasional feeling of hunger. Pain occurs when the stomach is empty, often awakening the patient at night. Duodenal ulcer pain is probably caused by the unbuffered gastric acid bathing the ulcer and is quickly relieved by ingesting food or antacids.

Definitive diagnosis depends upon x-ray studies, duodenoscopy, gastric analysis, and serum gastrin levels, all interpreted in light of accurate history and physical examination. Gastric analysis is performed to determine if the patient has increased or decreased gastric secretion, increased secretion being associated most often with duodenal ulcers and decreased secretion with gastric ulcers. Serum gastrin levels are also used to rule out hypogastrinemic states, which are indicative of other types of peptic ulcer disease. Like gastroscopy, duodenoscopy significantly increases the accuracy of diagnosis.

Varices

Portal hypertension, caused by any form of fibrotic liver disease, is associated with the development of varices. Portal hypertension is said to occur when there is a sustained elevation in portal vein pressure above the normal 6-12 cm. H_2O,[25] and may be the result of intra- or extrahepatic obstruction to blood flow. The increase in portal pressure may exceed 400-500 cm. H_2O pressure in severe instances.

The portal vein, which supplies most of the blood to the liver, is formed by the junction of the superior mesenteric vein and splenic vein. The coronary vein, which drains the lesser curvature of the stomach and the lower portion of the esophagus, joins this plexus prior to entering the liver (Figure 6-9). Consequently, with obstruction to flow, pressure will elevate throughout this venous system.

When portal pressure rises, collateral circulation develops as a compensatory mechanism. Collateral vessels may arise in the esophagus, abdomen, stomach, intestines, and vagina, but those in the esophagus are of the greatest clinical significance. Varices are characteristically dilated, tortuous vessels with little elastic tissue; consequently they are fragile, with low distensibility and bleed readily. These esophageal vessels are located in the submucosa and have no valves to regulate flow. They are subject to wide changes in pressure and rupture may be caused by the Valsalva maneuver, as occurs with coughing or sneezing, by regurgitation of food or acid secre-

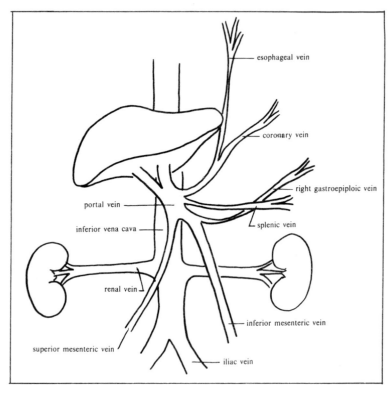

Figure 6-9. Portal venous circulation.

tions from the stomach, or simply from gradually increasing portal pressure.

Individuals with bleeding esophageal varices commonly present with complaints of hematemesis and melena; bleeding may be extensive enough to cause shock. Physical exam that reveals abdominal collateral vessels, ascites, and splenomegaly indicates portal hypertension. This diagnosis may be confirmed by liver function tests, liver biopsy, and x-ray studies; esophagoscopy and gastroscopy are used to definitively locate the site of bleeding. Celiac and mesenteric artery angiography may also be used to diagnose varices.

Intervention

Peptic ulcer disease in general may be medically treated in a variety of ways. However, belief in the adage "no acid, no ulcer" underlies almost all interventions.[56] Treatment usually includes antacids, tranquilizers, anticholinergics, dietary restrictions, and a prescription for physiological and emotional rest, all designed to reduce and neutralize acid secretion. If medical management is not successful in halting the progression of the disease, pyloric obstruction, perforation, and hemorrhage may occur. Hemorrhage due to upper GI bleeding and esophageal varices will be discussed.

The patient with active GI bleeding usually seeks treatment because of hematemesis and/or rectal bleeding. Hematemesis, the vomiting of blood, is almost always followed in time by melena, the passage of bloody stools. Hematemesis occurs most commonly with gastric ulcers, whereas melena is more common in duodenal ulceration, although both may be present in either condition.

The color of the vomitus and stools yields some diagnostic information. When blood has been exposed to gastric acids the bright red color of hemoglobin is changed to brown, giving it a "coffee ground" appearance. Bacterial action on stools containing blood causes the feces to become black and shiny, or "tarry." Medications such as iron or bismuth compounds may also cause black stools, but they are not shiny and are not guaiac positive. Melena may occur with as little as 50-100 cc. of blood in the intestines. Decreased bacterial action, or increased motility as is caused by the cathartic effect of blood in the bowel, will result in maroon colored stools. Bright red bleeding from the rectum indicates a lower GI bleed, as opposed to the stomach or duodenum as bleeding sites.

History and a physical may be difficult to obtain when the patient presents in shock, but are essential to determine any previous history of gastrointestinal disease or surgery, and to obtain a drug history. The patient and/or family should be questioned about the recent use of salicylates and alcohol, the most common causes of hemorrhagic gastritis, as well as anticoagulants and over-the-counter drugs, many of which contain aspirin.

If the patient is actively bleeding and in critical condition, diagnostic tests to determine the exact site of bleeding are not done until bleeding has been controlled. Large clots in the stomach often obscure GI x-rays and barium studies make later endoscopy difficult. Even if a lesion is demonstrated on x-ray, this does not definitively establish it as the actual bleeding site. Consequently, endoscopy is the first procedure to be performed when the patient's condition stabilizes.

The degree of shock exhibited by a patient may help to estimate the amount of blood that has been lost. Mild hypotension, in which systolic blood pressure is 90 mm. Hg or above and pulse rate 110 or below indicates a blood loss of 25% or less; moderate shock, in which blood pressure ranges 70-90 systolic and pulse 110-130, reflects a blood loss of 25-40%; and severe shock with systolic pressure below 70 and pulse greater than 130 indicates severe blood loss which may precipitate cardiovascular collapse.[60] Moderate blood loss, e.g., 2-3 units, over a period of several weeks may not cause any signs or symptoms other than weakness, fatigue, and pallor; however, a sudden loss of 2-3 units will cause definite signs of hypovolemia, with syncope and hypotension.

When the patient is admitted to the Intensive Care Unit, close monitoring of all parameters and careful nursing observation is necessary. Oxygen therapy and cardiac monitoring are indicated because low hemoglobin levels may cause tissue hypoxia. Arrhythmias are not uncommon and there is a reported 1-2% incidence of acute myocardial infarction in patients with gastrointestinal bleeding.[60]

Hemoglobin and hematocrit levels should be obtained immediately. These initial values will often not reflect actual blood loss because it may require several hours for body fluids to be redistributed following a sudden loss in blood volume, but the initial levels are needed for comparison with later samples. A four percent drop in hematocrit usually indicates a loss of one unit of blood.

Sodium, potassium, and BUN levels also should be frequently measured. Vomiting and the decompression of the stomach by NG suction, as well as saline irrigations, all may alter sodium levels. Potassium may be lost through vomiting and diarrhea and may accumulate when large amounts of stored blood are given. The BUN may rise 24-48 hours after the initial bleed because of the absorption of blood from the GI tract and conversion into urea. If blood ammonia levels rise it may be necessary to give enemas in order to clear the intestines of old blood.

The importance of emotional support to the patient and family during the crisis of a GI bleed cannot be overemphasized. The suddenness of the episode and the many procedures to which the patient is initially subjected are very frightening. Explanation of everything that is done, such as insertion of IV or CVP lines, should not be overlooked in the haste to accomplish tasks.

When blood replacement has begun, the nurse must be alert for signs of transfusion reactions, such as fever, chills, urticaria, and hematuria. All blood must be double-checked by two persons. Patients such as GI bleeders who are likely to receive multiple transfusions should always have micropore blood filters used on every unit, in addition to the standard mesh screen blood administration sets, in order to filter debris from stored blood and prevent later pulmonary complications.

A large nasogastric tube is usually inserted for iced lavage. A large diameter tube is chosen in order to allow aspiration of blood clots and prevent clogging, even though it is more uncomfortable for the patient. Iced lavage (gastric cooling) will decrease gastric blood flow, and thus bleeding, by up to 50%,[50] in addition to removing blood and clots. There is some disagreement as to whether saline or water is the better irrigant. Some believe that the use of saline may contribute to hypernatremia, particularly in cirrhotic patients, while iced water irrigation may lead to hyponatremia. The procedure involves cooling one or two liters of solution with ice, then instilling the cold solution, 100-300 cc. at a time. It is allowed to drain out by gravity or by the use of low suction. Manual aspiration may be necessary to clear the tube of clots, but this should be done gently to avoid further trauma. The procedure is continued until the returns are clear or lightly pink tinged.

Nursing measures necessary during iced lavage include frequent checking of temperature for hypothermia, providing blankets to keep the patient warm, and monitoring for complications. Aspirations, cardiac arrest secondary to MI, and respiratory arrest secondary to systemic hypothermia have occurred with the use of gastric cooling.[24]

When hematemesis is due to gastric and/or esophageal varices, a Blakemore-Sengstaken tube is used. This tube consists of 3 lumens, one for inflation of an esophageal balloon, one for inflation of a gastric balloon, and one for aspiration of gastric contents (Figure 6-10). It can be used to provide gastric and esophageal tamponade, and to differentiate between the esophagus and stomach as the site of bleeding.

Before inserting the Blakemore, the balloons should be tested by inflating them under water. The lumens should be clearly marked according to the balloon or port to which each leads. This tube is usually inserted through the nose, although it can be inserted through the mouth, and should be chilled in order to make it stiffer

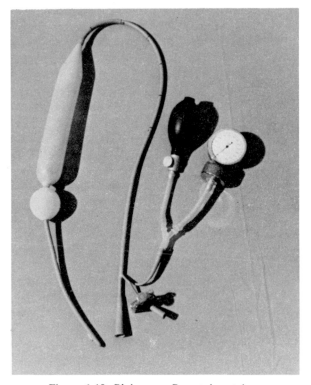

Figure 6-10. Blakemore-Sengstaken tube.

prior to use. Vomiting may occur during insertion, and the appropriate suction equipment should be ready. It is uncomfortable for the patient and the procedure should be thoroughly explained prior to beginning.

The tube is inserted to its full length (40 cm.) and 50-100 cc. of air used to inflate the gastric balloon. The position of the tube should be verified by x-ray. When certain of the location, the gastric balloon can then be fully inflated with an additional 100-200 cc. of air. It is then pulled back to rest firmly against the cardio-esophageal junction, and traction used to keep it in place; the balloon thus effectively seals off the esophagus from the stomach. Foam rubber should be used to protect the nares from the pressure created by traction on the tube. Some hospitals use a helmet type of device which allows a designated amount of traction, e.g., one-half

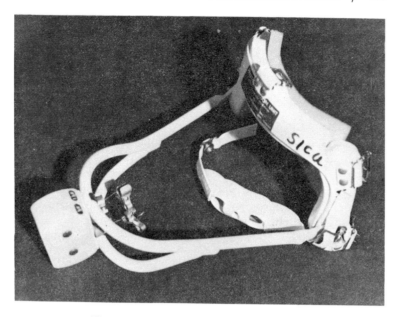

Figure 6-11. Blakemore-Sengstaken helmet.

pound, to be applied in addition to securing the tube (Figure 6-11).

If blood is not aspirated from the gastric lumen, esophageal varices must be the cause of bleeding. The esophageal balloon can be inflated with air to provide tamponade and stop bleeding. The amount of air used is not as significant as is the amount of pressure exerted. A manometer should be connected to the esophageal balloon lumen; the pressure should not exceed 40 mm. Hg. Esophageal tamponade will arrest bleeding from varices, at least initially, in 50-80% of cases.[50] It may in some instances be necessary to insert an additional NG tube into the esophagus to drain accumulated blood.

Safety measures to be employed when the Blakemore-Sengstaken tube is used begin with the use of double clamps on the balloon lumens to prevent the leakage of air. Neither the esophageal or gastric balloons should be left continually inflated for more than 24 hours in order to prevent necrosis of the mucosa. Scissors should be kept at the bedside at all times; if the gastric balloon should break, the traction will pull the tube up into the nasopharynx, thus obstructing the airway. In this situation both lumens should be cut and the tube immediately removed.

In conjunction with all of these measures, antacids will frequently be used. The three antacids most often chosen are magnesium hydroxide, aluminum hydroxide, and calcium hydroxide. All of these chemically neutralize acid. Magnesium hydroxide has laxative properties while aluminum hydroxide is constipating. Because of this they are often given together in alternating hourly doses. Calcium hydroxide is somewhat constipating and may also cause alkalosis and hypercalcemia in a minority of patients.

If bleeding persists, intra-arterial vasopressors may be used. The intra-arterial route is preferred over intravenous because smaller amounts can be used and will act locally, thus minimizing side effects. Epinephrine in combination with propranolol has been used in the past, but the effect of epinephrine stops as soon as the infusion stops, making it less advantageous. Vasopressin is the drug of choice today, at a dose of 0.2 units per minute. Infusion of vasopressin via the superior mesenteric artery successfully controls bleeding associated with both ulcers and portal hypertension. Unlike epinephrine, it acts primarily at distal vessels, has prolonged action, and few side effects. The use of vasopressin is particularly important when surgery is contraindicated because of sepsis, renal failure, or other superimposed disease states.

Side effects which have been seen with vasopressin use include hypertension, bradycardia, arrhythmias, and reduced cardiac output. Although these are infrequent, they do dictate close monitoring by the nurse.

Surgery is indicated if these medical interventions have not succeeded in stopping bleeding. In the case of duodenal ulcer, if there has been a loss of more than six units of blood or if bleeding episodes have been repeated, surgery is also usually desirable. Surgery is the eventual treatment of choice for gastric ulcers, even when bleeding is controlled. Indications for surgery for esophageal varices will be discussed at a later point.

Surgical intervention

Many surgical procedures may be performed for treatment of gastric or duodenal ulcers. In general all procedures are designed to reduce the capacity of the stomach to produce acid and/or to remove diseased tissue. Some of the more common surgical approaches are listed on pp. 423-424 (Figure 6-12).

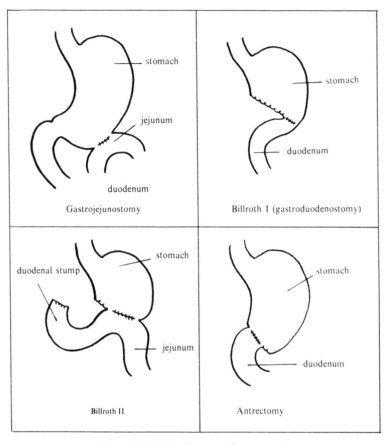

Figure 6-12. Gastric resection procedures.

1. *Plication:* this is the simple over-sewing of an ulcerated area, sometimes including the use of a patch of omentum to cover the ulcer. It is a much less extensive procedure than gastric resection.

2. *Vagotomy:* division of vagus nerve branch to the stomach. This is usually performed in conjunction with gastric resection and is done in order to reduce stimulation, thus decreasing the volume of HCl secretion and slowing the emptying of the stomach.

3. *Pyloroplasty:* pyloric sphincter is enlarged in order to establish a

larger outflow tract. This is done to allow better emptying in a stomach made hypotonic by vagotomy.

4. *Gastrojejunostomy:* the jejunum is brought up and sutured to the greater curvature of the stomach, thus providing a second outlet for gastric contents. This procedure is associated with a higher rate of ulcer recurrence and is performed less often than others.

5. *Billroth I:* partial gastrectomy is done, removing the distal one-half to two-thirds of the stomach; this is also termed gastro-duodenostomy, referring to the anastomosis of the remaining portion of the stomach to the duodenum.

6. *Billroth II:* removal of lower one-half to two-thirds of stomach (partial or subtotal gastrectomy) and anastomosis of remaining stomach to jejunum (gastrojejunostomy or gastroenterostomy). The duodenal stump is sutured closed.

7. *Hemigastrectomy:* this term refers to the removal of one-half of the stomach and may include the resection of the first portion of the duodenum.

8. *Antrectomy:* the entire antrum is removed, thus eliminating the source of gastrin. Hemigastrectomy or antrectomy may be performed for duodenal ulceration in order to stop the bathing of the ulcer by stomach acid, thus allowing the ulcer to heal.

9. *Total gastrectomy:* removal of the entire stomach and anastomosis of the esophagus to the jejunum. This procedure is not used often because of the high mortality rate (10-20%), but may be indicated for recurrent ulcers, cancer of the stomach, or Zollinger-Ellison syndrome (gastric hypersecretion, multiple peptic ulcers, and gastrin producing pancreatic tumor).

Postoperative care of the patient who has undergone gastric resection includes those nursing interventions common to the care of any individual after a major surgery. That is, careful monitoring of fluid and electrolyte balance, pulmonary status, and renal function are all appropriate. In addition, patients who have had any of the above procedures are subject to rebleeding and hemorrhage from suture lines or anastomoses.

Leaking from the duodenal stump is associated with gastro-jejunostomy. Peritonitis, either chemical or bacterial, is a major complication which requires immediate treatment. Impaired nutritional status, the dumping syndrome, diarrhea, gastric stasis, and pyloric obstruction are sequelae which may develop in the later postoperative period.

Surgical intervention for portal hypertension: The many consequences of liver disease have been discussed earlier. The existence of varices caused by portal hypertension are perhaps the greatest threat; of all individuals with cirrhosis, as many as one-third will die from bleeding due to ruptured varices.[19] At this time, the most common method of intervention is surgical decompression via shunt procedures.

Portasystemic shunts were first attempted in the early 1900s, but the technique was not perfected until 1945.[4] Whipple and associates, in performing the first operations, demonstrated that by anastomosing the portal vein to the vena cava, end to side, a marked decrease in portal pressure could be achieved, thus reducing the risk of bleeding from a varix. Since that time, several modifications in the procedure have been made. To be successful, the shunt must meet the following criteria:

1. portal pressure is reduced and varices decompressed;
2. hepatic blood supply remains adequate;
3. blood flow to other areas is not compromised;
4. the shunt has a high probability of remaining patent.

The most often chosen shunt procedures (portacaval, splenorenal, and mesocaval) are shown in Figure 6-13. Table 6-3 summarizes characteristics of each of these. Other less commonly used shunts include the portacaval with synthetic graft, portorenal, and distal splenorenal.

The decision to operate depends upon several factors. In general, it is thought best not to operate during the first few days of an acute bleeding episode; however, with improvements in surgical technique and medical management, this is less significant than it used to be. Surgery may be indicated in order to stop active bleeding after 24-48 hours of medical treatment, providing the patient is not in shock and has adequate cardiac and renal function. Age and related medical conditions, such as heart disease, affect the mortality rate of this procedure as they do any surgical intervention. The most significant factor in determining survival is hepatic function at the time of operation.[4]

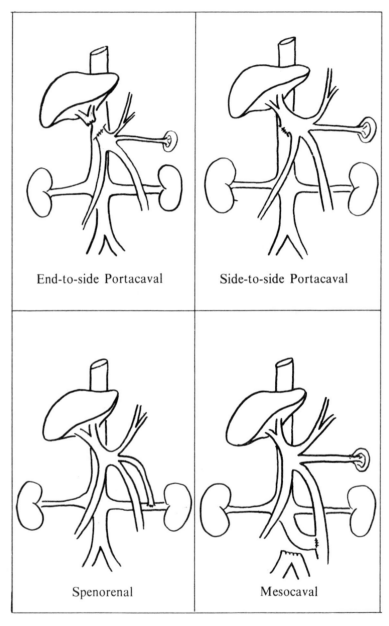

End-to-side Portacaval

Side-to-side Portacaval

Spenorenal

Mesocaval

Figure 6-13. Porta-Systemic shunts.

TABLE 6-3

Porta-Systemic Shunts and Their Characteristics[2,4,19,29]

Shunt	Operative Procedure	Characteristics
End-to-side Portacaval	Ligation of portal vein prior to entry into liver; anastomosis of distal end to side of inferior vena cava	Technically easy Achieves incomplete decompression of hepatic sinusoids because of persistent blockage of outflow tracts Less effective than side-to-side anastomosis or mesocaval shunt in eliminating ascites Lowest 5-10 year survival rate High incidence of postoperative encephalopathy
Side-to-side Portacaval	Anastomosis of side of portal vein to side of inferior vena cava	Somewhat more difficult than end-to-side shunt Achieves more complete decompression of hepatic sinusoids because blood in liver can flow retrograde through portal vein to vena cava More effective than end-to-side or splenorenal shunts in eliminating ascites Higher 5-10 year survival rate than end-to-side; slightly lower than splenorenal High incidence of postoperative encephalopathy
Splenorenal	Splenic vein anastomosed to renal vein. The anastomosis may be side-to-side or end-to-side, which is done in conjunction with splenectomy	More difficult than end-to-side portacaval Less effective decompression than end-to-side or side-to-side portacaval shunts Less effective than end-to-side or mesocaval shunts in eliminating ascites Highest 5-10 year survival rate

(Continued)

TABLE 6-3 *(Continued)*

Porta-Systemic Shunts and Their Characteristics[2,4,19,29]

Shunt	Operative Procedure	Characteristics
		Lower incidence of postoperative encephalopathy than end-to-side or side-to-side portacaval
		High incidence of postoperative bleeding
		High incidence of shunt thrombosis due to smaller diameter of vessels
Mesocaval	Inferior vena cava is divided and end is anastomosed to side of superior mesenteric vein. May also be done by using a prosthetic graft between the vena cava and mesenteric vein	Achieves decompression equivalent to end-to-side portacaval shunt
		As effective or better than end-to-side portacaval in eliminating ascites
		Particularly useful when there is portal hypertension due to extra-hepatic occlusion of portal vein
		High incidence of postoperative encephalopathy
		Greatest problem is severe edema of lower extremities due to interrupted venous return; may be used more in younger patients because of this
		Use of graft prevents edema, but is associated with a high incidence of thrombosis

Scoring or classification systems have been devised in order to evaluate prospective shunt candidates. These systems differ somewhat from one another, but usually include the following criteria in determining desirability of operation:

1. serum bilirubin below 2.0 mg./100 ml.
2. serum albumin above 3.5 mg./100 ml.
3. ascites absent
4. nutritional status adequate
5. hepatic encephalopathy absent

The degree to which the individual deviates from these criteria determines the risk of surgery.[2]

Postoperative care of the patient who has undergone a portasystemic shunt begins with an appreciation of the magnitude of the procedure. The patient who has undergone a shunt requires all usual postoperative measures but is particularly at risk of developing fluid and electrolyte problems. The preoperative existence of ascites, the dissection of lymphatics during surgery, and the reallocation of a major portion of cardiac output all predispose the individual to fluid disequilibrium. Sodium, potassium, and glucose levels are often abnormal in patients with liver disease and must be monitored closely. Abdominal girth should be measured every 8 hours, and the patient must be weighed daily.

Temporary impairments in liver function usually occur after shunts and mild hepatic encephalopathy is not uncommon. The use of anesthesia, sedatives, and reabsorption of blood may be partially responsible for the reported 19% incidence of this postoperative syndrome.[19,2] Appropriate safety measures must be taken to protect the confused patient, and family members often need support and reassuring explanations concerning this syndrome.

Bleeding is of particular concern after surgery. The shunt patient is prone to this complication because of the interference in prothrombin production. Vitamin K is given and prothrombin and partial thromboplastin times are monitored. The increased risk of bleeding dictates measures such as padded side rails, assessment of all drainage for the presence of blood, use of small gauge needles and catheters, and restrictions in the number of venous and arterial punctures. Antacids are frequently given to reduce the risk of gastric and duodenal ulceration.

If the patient is able to eat, a diet similar to that ordered for the individual with chronic liver disease is usually chosen. Sodium may be restricted to 1-2 Gram and protein content kept below 100 Gm. Caloric intake should be at least 3000 per day.

Other surgical procedures currently being evaluated for treatment of portal hypertension include ligation of varices, devascularization of the esophagus and stomach, and construction of prosthetic shunts. All of these have been performed, but at this time the available data do not support their use in most patients.[4]

In summary, portasystemic shunts are the most effective means of treating bleeding varices. This intervention is also advantageous in that in most cases it reduces or eliminates chronic ascites. However, the shunt procedures do carry a significant hospital mortality rate, ranging from 6 to 23%.[4] It should also be remembered that this operation does not cure the underlying disease. The fact that only 50% of patients survive more than five years after a shunt has been performed is an undeniable indication for early diagnosis and prevention of those conditions which lead to portal hypertension.

Causes of Severe Metabolic Abnormalities

Two final conditions with which the intensive care staff must be prepared to deal with are hepatic encephalopathy and acute pancreatitis. Both of these diseases have underlying pathologies which exist in a chronic form, but both can be exacerbated and interfere with homeostatic mechanisms to the extent that the patient's condition becomes critical.

Hepatic encephalopathy

Because of the variety of functions performed by the liver, damage to this organ, regardless of cause, has numerous manifestations. Nutritional deficiencies result from the inability to metabolize vitamins, regulate glucose levels, and deaminate amino acids for metabolic processes. Blood coagulation defects occur. Jaundice is often present when bilirubin breakdown is impaired. Water and electrolyte disturbances occur secondary to reduced plasma protein levels and altered hormonal secretions. Abnormalities of the central and peripheral nervous systems are caused by the accumulation of toxic products that the damaged liver could not degrade or detoxify. Bleeding, which was discussed in the previous section, and

CNS disturbances are the sequelae which most often necessitate admission to the Intensive Care Unit.

Hepatic encephalopathy is the term used to describe the syndrome of cerebral dysfunction caused by liver disease. It has also been termed hepatic coma and nitrogenous encephalopathy. The pathogenesis of coma is not completely understood. However, it is generally accepted that the accumulation of ammonia, due to the failure of the liver to reconvert ammonia to non-toxic glutamine for storage and later conversion to urea, inhibits cerebral energy metabolism.[21] It is also thought that the damaged liver may be unable to produce substances needed for cerebral function.[20]

Causes of the underlying liver disease are quite varied. Cirrhosis, related to excessive alcohol intake; viral hepatitis or chronic biliary disease; and drug or chemical injury, are some of the most common. Once disease is present, several factors may precipitate coma, including azotemia, use of sedatives, tranquilizers, and analgesics, gastrointestinal hemorrhage, hypokalemic alkalosis, and excessive protein intake.

The contribution of all of these factors is explained by the following mechanisms. The substances implicated in hepatic coma are produced in the body by the metabolism of protein, the conversion of urea to ammonia in the intestine by bacteria, or may result from the breakdown and absorption of free blood from the gut. The shunting of blood around the liver that characteristically occurs with portal hypertension then prevents the detoxification of ammonia which reaches the cerebral circulation. Thus excessive dietary intake of nitrogenous substances or the presence of GI bleeding can both lead to azotemia. It is not clear if the use of CNS depressant drugs merely over-sedate an already susceptible brain or if these drugs induce encephalopathy in some other way.[21] When alkalosis occurs, either because of the direct loss of hydrogen ions or loss secondary to the depletion of potassium ions as with diuretic therapy, the entry of ammonia into cells is facilitated. Constipation also promotes the increased uptake of ammonia from the intestine.

Signs and symptoms of hepatic encephalopathy progress from mild mental impairment, lethargy, and irritability, to slurred speech, ataxia, and deepening coma. Asterixis, a tremor of the hand elicited by extending the wrist upward, and coarse tremors of the face and arms, are present in the early stages. Fetor hepaticus describes the sweet, musty odor of the breath sometimes present due to the abnormal metabolism of sulfur compounds. Hyperreflexia and hyperventilation proceed to loss of deep tendon reflexes and stertorous respirations. The progression of the coma is related to the underlying disease; when caused by acute fulminant liver failure, without previous chronic liver disease, coma occurs more rapidly and is more often fatal.

Objective data used in the assessment of encephalopathy includes blood ammonia levels, CSF glutamine levels, and EEG pattern. Serum ammonia levels, normally 100 mgm./100 ml., vary among individuals in hepatic disease, and a baseline level should be established early during hospitalization. CSF glutamine is usually elevated to 35 mg./100 ml. in encephalopathy. Other tests of liver function, such as bilirubin, protein, and enzyme studies, do not correlate with degree of coma. Clotting studies, however, should be done to monitor the associated risk of bleeding.

Intervention is aimed at eliminating or reducing those factors which contribute to the accumulation of ammonia. Because the primary source of ammonia is the intestine, efforts are directed at reducing intestinal absorption. The diet, first, is modified to reduce protein intake. In acute progressive disease, the protein content may be restricted to 0-20 Gm. protein/day. Provision of adequate calories is essential, however, to prevent the catabolism of body protein.

Bowel sterilization in order to deplete bacterial flora which produce ureases, the enzymes which convert urea to ammonia, is the second aspect of reducing intestinal uptake of ammonia. This is usually accomplished by administering nonabsorbable antibiotics such as neomycin or kanamycin in enemas. More recently lactulose, a synthetic disaccharide, has been used either in addition to neomycin, or in place of it in patients with renal contraindications to neomycin. Lactulose acts as a cathartic, thus reducing the length of time for absorption of bowel contents, and also causes a reduction in colon pH. The acidification of bowel contents further reduces ammonia absorption.

Nursing assessment of the patient in hepatic coma is extremely important. Because there are no direct laboratory tests available to gauge progression or improvement of clinical status, determination of the effects of treatment is dependent upon frequent, accurate assessment. Neurological checks should be done every four hours, following a consistent format. In addition, the nurse must be alert for the development of other sequelae to the disease which may, in themselves, increase the threat to survival or worsen the coma.

Gastrointestinal bleeding is a major complication. As mentioned, blood in the GI tract is a rich source of ammonia. GI bleeding is a common associated disorder both because of the frequent history of alcoholism and gastritis and because of the inability of the diseased liver to produce clotting factors. Nasogastric drainage, emesis, and stools should be routinely checked for the presence of occult blood. Vitamin K is often administered to correct the deficiency caused by reduced bacterial production.

The diarrhea produced by antibiotic or lactulose enemas also may lead to fluid, electrolyte, and pH abnormalities. As mentioned, hypokalemia and alkalosis precipitate coma, and frequent arterial blood gas and electrolyte determinations should be done. Daily weights are essential, particularly in view of the hypoproteinemia, ascites, and edema that usually accompanies liver disease. The use of steroids in the treatment of active chronic hepatitis may further complicate fluid and electrolyte balance in promoting sodium and water retention.

More extreme forms of treatment that are currently being evaluated include exchange transfusions, which are thought to both eliminate toxic substances and perhaps supply unknown substances necessary for brain metabolism, and use of artificial livers, which has not yet been technically perfected. L-dopa therapy is currently under investigation as a possible means to alter amino acid synthesis, which may be a pathogenic factor in coma. Manipulation of plasma amino acids by the infusion of various commercial solutions of essential and non-essential amino acids is also being evaluated.

The exact cause of death in hepatic coma is not known. Cerebral edema, morphologic changes in the cerebral cortex, and demyelination of the cerebrospinal tracts has been found at autopsy in very fulminant cases, but the significance of these changes in terms of identifying the central causative mechanism has not yet been determined.[21]

Pancreatitis

This disorder is considered under the heading of metabolic abnormalities because the effects of pancreatitis usually include a major interference in the normal metabolism of foodstuffs. In addition, pancreatitis has been linked to a metabolic abnormality, hyperlipidemia.

Pancreatitis, as the term suggests, is an inflammatory state that may exist as a chronic or acute condition. Several etiologic agents have been identified in addition to hyperlipidemia; some of the more common causative factors are listed in Table 6-4.

TABLE 6-4

Etiologic Agents in Acute Pancreatitis
1. ALCOHOLISM
2. ABDOMINAL ORGAN DISEASE   a) Biliary tract obstruction or inflammation   b) Duodenal ulcer   c) Duodenal diverticulum   d) Regional enteritis
3. TRAUMA   a) Operative   b) Direct, external (e.g., auto accident)
4. DRUGS   a) Thiazide diuretics   b) Adrenocorticosteroids
5. METABOLIC   a) Hyperlipoproteinemia   b) Hyperparathyroidism
6. INFECTION   a) Mumps   b) Scarlet fever

Regardless of the exact precipitating factor or cause, it is thought that the central mechanism in pancreatitis is autodigestion of the organ by pancreatic enzymes released as a result of inflammation. This leads to edema and eventual necrosis and hemorrhage. Chemical peritonitis results from the release of activated pancreatic enzymes into the abdominal cavity.

These local effects are serious in themselves, but more profound systemic alterations may bring the patient to the Intensive Care Unit. The damaged pancreas also releases kinins (such as bradykinin) which are powerful vasodilators. The presence of these kinins, combined with the loss of circulating volume which may accompany the peritoneal inflammation, can result in hypotension, which may progress to shock and even subsequent dealth.

Hyperglycemia may also be present if the beta cells of the pancreas have been damaged. However, even when present, this is not usually the aspect of the disease which is most threatening to the patient.

Clinical manifestations of pancreatitis classically include hypotension, pain, elevated serum amylase, and nausea and vomiting. The pain is characteristically quite intense, occurring in the mid-epigastric or periumbilical area, made worse by lying supine and lessened somewhat by sitting with knees flexed and drawn up. This severe pain is probably caused by peritoneal irritation, spasm or stretching of the pancreatic duct, or stretching of the pancreatic capsule.

Amylase is the enzyme most commonly and most quickly elevated, usually exceeding 200-400 Somogyi units within several hours of the onset of the episode; the elevation may reach 2000 units before stabilizing. The level of amylase usually begins to fall within 72 hours, although urinary amylase may not return to normal for 3-7 days. Serum lipase elevations usually occur more slowly but parallel amylase elevations; similarly, the level falls more slowly and thus may be more helpful in late diagnoses.

Peritoneal involvement in the inflammatory process gives rise to a number of signs and symptoms. Nausea and vomiting usually occur and may be accompanied by distention; these reflect paralytic ileus. Ascites may be present due to the effusion of protein and fluid into the abdominal cavity with increased peritoneal permeability. In addition, the patient may exhibit generalized abdominal tenderness and rigidity with the epigastric pain.

Intervention is primarily medical, supportive, and aimed at facilitating the healing process and preventing complications. Analgesic administration is usually one of the first measures ordered. Meperidine is the drug of choice, since opiates may cause spasm of the sphincter of Oddi and worsen pain, in addition to leading to false elevations of amylase and lipase. Frequent administration of pain medication will be required throughout the most acute phase of the disease. Severe pain can contribute to hypotension and tachycardia, and analgesia should not be withheld even when the patient's blood pressure is decreased.

Efforts are directed at reducing pancreatic secretion. Nasogastric suction is used to keep the stomach empty and prevent duodenal stimulation of pancreatic enzymes. It is important to understand that the rationale for the use of the NG tube is not merely for treatment of ileus in order to appreciate the necessity of maintaining patency of the drainage system. High doses of anticholinergics may be ordered to further reduce pancreatic stimulation, but opinion varies concerning the usefulness of the measure.[15]

Insulin is usually administered both to correct existing hyperglycemia and to prevent additional stress on the pancreas. Hyperglycemia in the initial phase may reflect the shock state more than actual islet cell damage and consequently, may be quite transient. A continuous intravenous infusion or frequent small subcutaneous doses of regular insulin are used, rather than large doses of long-acting insulin.

Antibiotics are often administered for prophylaxis. Tissue that has been destroyed by free pancreatic enzymes provides an excellent medium for bacterial growth and secondary infection is a common complication of acute pancreatitis.

Other therapeutic measures employed are related to specific complications which may develop. As mentioned, fluid and electrolyte disturbances may continue to be a serious problem; dehydration and metabolic acidosis, from loss of bicarbonate, are the two most common imbalances.[54] Hyperkalemia may result from severe tissue destruction. Hypocalcemia develops when peritoneal fat is hydrolyzed by enzymes and combines with serum calcium, precipitating into an insoluble soap.

As with liver disease, gastrointestinal bleeding may occur, related either to the associated alcoholic gastritis or diminished clotting ability. Prothrombin level may be abnormally low due to interference with vitamin K synthesis in the bowel or from the destructive action of pancreatic proteolytic enzymes on clotting factors in the blood.

Respiratory distress occurs in as many as 20% of patients during an acute attack.[25] Daily chest x-rays and arterial blood gas determinations should be an integral part of the monitoring of these individuals and the nurse must be alert to the more subtle signs of increasing respiratory impairment, such as increased respiratory effort and respiratory rate, and changes in behavior and breath sounds.

Surgical intervention is usually not employed because of the high mortality rate, unless more conservative measures have failed to halt the progression of the disease and tissue destruction becomes extensive. Surgery is more often used when there has been a penetrating abdominal wound which involves the pancreas or when pancreatic cancer has been diagnosed. The preferred procedure for pancreatic cancer is the Whipple operation, which involves the resection of the head and portions of the body of the pancreas in addition to the duodenum, the end of the common bile duct, and a portion of the stomach. The jejunum is then anastomosed to the remaining pancreas and stomach. When there has been disruption of the pancreas by trauma, a Roux-en-Y pancreaticojejunostomy may be performed; this involves anastomosis of the severed ends of the pancreas into a loop of jejunum and is also used to provide open pancreatic ductal drainage when stricture of the ducts is causing recurrent pain in chronic pancreatitis. Simpler procedures involve the insertion of sump tubes for drainage of the pancreatic bed, performed in addition to gastrostomy for keeping the stomach and duodenum empty and jejunostomy for feeding.

The most serious complication of pancreatic surgery is hemorrhage. This event is made likely because of the difficulty in adequately visualizing the pancreas and all of the closely approximated blood vessels, the aorta, vena cava, superior mesenteric artery and veins, and splenic vessels. Strictures of other organs, such as the duodenum, may follow extensive reconstructions, or anastomotic leaks may develop. Exocrine and endocrine replacement therapy is also necessary following pancreatectomy, and may lead to complications after the patient has recovered from surgery.

REFERENCES

1. Alexander MM, Brown MS: Physical examination; Part 13: Examining the abdomen. *Nursing '76* **6**:65-70, January, 1976.
2. Altshuler A, Hilden D: The patient with portal hypertension. *Nursing Clinics of North America* **12**:317-330, 1977.
3. Bachrach WH: Advice on antacids. *Peptic Ulcer.* Medcom, Inc., Fort Washington, Pa., 1971.
4. Bengmark S: Surgical management of portal hypertension. *Clinics in Gastroenterology* **4**:395-419, 1975.
5. Bermar PM, Kirsner JB: The gastric ulcer. *Peptic Ulcer.* Medcom, Inc., Fort Washington, Pa., 1971, pp. 54-59.
6. Botsford TW, Wilson RE: *The Acute Abdomen.* 2nd Ed. W.B. Saunders, Philadelphia, Pa., 1977.
7. Bouchard R, Owens NF: *Nursing Care of the Cancer Patient.* 2nd Ed. C.V. Mosby, St. Louis, Mo., 1972.
8. Boyer CA, Oehlberg SM: Interpretation and clinical relevance of

liver function tests. *Nursing Clinics of North America* **12**:275-290, 1977.

9. Brunner LS, Suddarth DS: *The Lippincott Manual of Nursing Practice.* J.B. Lippincott, Philadelphia, Pa., 1974.

10. Burrell ZL, Burrell LO: *Critical Care.* 3rd Ed. C.V. Mosby, St. Louis, Mo., 1977.

11. Clearfield HR, et al.: Control of bleeding varices. *Emergency Medicine* **7**:62-71, April, 1975.

12. Colcock BP: Diverticular disease: proven surgical management. *Clinics in Gastroenterology* **4**(No. 1):99-119, 1975.

13. Davenport HW: *Physiology of the Digestive Tract.* 3rd Ed. Year Book Medical Publishers Inc., Chicago, Ill., 1971.

14. Dineen P, Brown T: A guide to the diagnosis of intra-abdominal abscesses. *Hospital Medicine,* February, 1976.

15. Dinoso VP, et al.: The acute abdomen. *Emergency Medicine* **7**:209-214, 1975.

16. Donovan MI, Pierce SG: *Cancer Care Nursing.* Appleton-Century-Crofts, New York, 1976.

17. Durham N: Looking out for complications of abdominal surgery. *Nursing '75* **5**:24-31, February, 1975.

18. Eisenberg MM: Vagotomy and Pyloroplasty for Treatment of Duodenal Ulcer. In Najarian JS, Delany JB (Eds.): *Surgery of the Gastrointestinal Tract.* Intercontinental Medical Book Corp., New York, 1974.

19. Ellis PD: Portal hypertension and bleeding esophageal and gastric varices: a surgical approach to treatment. *Heart and Lung* **6**:791-798, 1977.

20. Felsher BF: Hepatic Encephalopathy. In Zschoche DA (Ed.): *Mosby's Comprehensive Review of Critical Care.* C.V. Mosby, St. Louis, Mo., 1976, pp. 513-519.

21. Fischer JE, Baldessarini RJ: Pathogenesis and Therapy of Hepatic Coma. In Popper H, Schaffner F (Eds.): *Progress in Liver Disease,* Vol. 5. Grune and Stratton, New York, 1976, pp. 363-397.

22. Given BA, Simmons SJ: *Gastroenterology in Clinical Nursing.* 2nd Ed. C.V. Mosby, St. Louis, Mo., 1975.

23. Goligher JC: The Surgical Treatment of Peptic Ulcer. In Najarian JS, Delaney JB (Eds.): *Surgery of the Gastrointestinal Tract.* Intercontinental Medical Book Corp., New York, 1974.

24. Goodale RL: Use of Endoscopy and Gastric Cooling for Massive Upper GI Hemorrhage. In Najarian JS, Delaney JB (Eds.): *Surgery of the Gastrointestinal Tract.* Intercontinental Medical Book Corp., New York, 1974.

25. Greenberger NJ, Winship DH: *Gastrointestinal Disorders: A Patho-*

physiologic Approach. Year Book Medical Publishers, Inc., Chicago, Ill., 1976.

26. Gutowski F: Ostomy procedure: nursing care before and after. *American Journal of Nursing* **72**:262-267, 1972.

27. Guyton AC: *Textbook of Medical Physiology.* 5th Ed. W.B. Saunders, Philadelphia, Pa., 1976.

28. Holliday RL: Peritonitis—old and new thoughts. *Heart and Lung* **4**:456-460, 1975.

29. Horovitz JH, Luterman A: Postoperative monitoring following critical trauma. *Heart and Lung* **4**:269-79, 1975.

30. Hughes LE: Complications of diverticular disease: inflammation, obstruction and bleeding. *Clinics in Gastroenterology* **4**(No. 1):147-163, 1975.

31. Jarvis CM: Perfecting physical assessment: part 3. *Nursing '77* **7**:44-53, July, 1977.

32. Katz D: What is gastritis and what is not? *Peptic Ulcer.* Medcom, Inc., Fort Washington, Pa., 1971, pp. 34-39.

33. Kubo W, et al.: Fluid and electrolyte problems of tube-fed patients. *American Journal of Nursing* **76**:912-916, 1976.

34. Literte JW: Nursing care of patients with intestinal obstruction. *American Journal of Nursing* **77**:1003-1006, 1977.

35. McConnell EA: All about gastrointestinal intubation. *Nursing '75* **5**:31-37, September, 1975.

36. McConnell EA: Ensuring safer stomach suctioning with the salem sump tube. *Nursing '77* **7**:54-61, September, 1977.

37. Menguy R: The duodenal ulcer. *Peptic Ulcer.* Medcom, Inc., Fort Washington, Pa., 1971, pp. 60-74.

38. Menguy R: An Approach to the Clinical Management of Diffuse Gastric Mucosal Bleeding. In Najarian JS, Delaney JB (Eds.): *Surgery of the Gastrointestinal Tract.* Intercontinental Medical Book Corp., New York, 1974.

39. Morson BC: Pathology of diverticular disease of the colon. *Clinics in Gastroenterology* **4**(No. 1):37-51, 1975.

40. Munster AM: Sepsis following gastrointestinal surgery: some recent considerations. *Heart and Lung* **3**:615-619, 1974.

41. Naish JM, Read AE: *Basic Gastroenterology.* 2nd Ed. Year Book Medical Publishers, Inc., Chicago, Ill., 1974.

42. Najarian JS, Sutherland DE: Intra-Arterial Vasopressors for Control of Gastrointestinal Bleeding. In Najarian JS, Delaney JB (Eds.): *Surgery of the Gastrointestinal Tract.* Intercontinental Medical Book Corp., New York, 1974.

43. O'Brien KA: Cross circulation for hepatic coma. *American Journal of Nursing* **77**:1459-1462, 1977.

44. Ostrow JD: The disintegrating liver. *Emergency Medicine* **7**:87-94, 1975.

45. Painter NS: Diverticular Disease of the Colon and Dietary Fiber. In Clearfield HR, Dinaro VP (Eds.): *Gastrointestinal Emergencies.* Grune and Stratton, New York, 1976.

46. Painter NS, Burkitt DP: Diverticular disease of the colon, a 20th century problem. *Clinics in Gastroenterology* **4**(No. 1):3-19, 1975.

47. Pierce L: Anatomy and physiology of the liver in relation to clinical assessment. *Nursing Clinics of North America* **12**:259-274, 1977.

48. Rickert RR: Pathology of gastritis and peptic ulcer. *Peptic Ulcer.* Medcom, Inc., Fort Washington, Pa., 1971, pp. 22-26.

49. Sabiston, DC, (Ed.): *Davis-Christopher Textbook of Surgery.* 10th Ed., W.B. Saunders, Philadelphia, Pa., 1972.

50. Severance SR: Gastrointestinal Bleeding. In Zschoche DA (Ed.): *Mosby's Comprehensive Review of Critical Care.* C.V. Mosby, St. Louis, Mo., 1976, pp. 520-535.

51. Shaninpour N: The adult patient with bleeding esophageal varices. *Nursing Clinics of North America* **12**:331-344, 1977.

52. Sherlock S: Primary Biliary Cirrhosis. In Schaffner F, Popper H (Eds.): *Progress in Liver Disease,* Vol. 5. Grune and Stratton, New York, 1976, pp. 550-575.

53. Simmons RL, Uranga VM: The Peritoneum and Peritonitis. In Najarian JS, Delaney JP (Eds.): *Surgery of the Gastrointestinal Tract.* Intercontinental Medical Book Corp., New York, 1974, pp. 575-583.

54. Simmons S, Given B: Acute pancreatitis. *American Journal of Nursing* **71**:934-939, 1971.

55. Spiro HM: On the disorder called ulcer. *Peptic Ulcer.* Medcom, Inc., Fort Washington, Pa., 1971, pp. 8-13.

56. Spiro HM: The management of peptic ulcer disease. *Peptic Ulcer.* Medcom, Inc., Fort Washington, Pa., 1971.

57. Spiro HM: *Clinical Gastroenterology.* 2nd Ed. Macmillan Publishing, New York, 1977.

58. Stahlgren LH, Morris NW: Intestinal obstruction. *American Journal of Nursing* **77**:999-1002, 1977.

59. Vander AJ, et al.: *Human Physiology—The Mechanisms of Body Function.* McGraw-Hill, New York, 1970.

60. Wiley L, (Ed.): The G.I. Bleeder. *Nursing '75* **5**:49-54, September, 1975.

CHAPTER 7

Death and Dying in Intensive Care Units

by Benita C. Martocchio, RN, PhD

DEATH AND DYING IN AMERICAN SOCIETY

Death, a ubiquitous and inevitable occurrence, is a part of life. Although a naturally occurring phenomenon, the contemporary American views dying as an "abnormal" event,[7] a catastrophe.[18] Death and dying have been described as taboo topics.[10]

There are many speculations on the reasons why death has become an unspeakable and dreaded event to be avoided at all costs. It may be that death reminds us of our "finiteness",[18] or perhaps it is its unpredictable quality. Death strikes indifferently, old or young, rich or poor, high status or low, good or bad. No one is exempt. Perhaps it makes us all too aware of our vulnerability in spite of our technological advances.[15] We pride ourselves on our ability to fly to the moon, to cure once incurable ills, to delay dying. We can postpone but we cannot eliminate death.[5]

There are those who would say that it is difficult to accept death because few Americans witness death.[7,15] In our modern technological society, dying is something that is done in hospitals or in other institutions. Children are exposed to violence and violent deaths on television; however, they are protected from people who are dying or who have died. One can only speculate on the lasting fears these practices engender.

However, witnessing death in itself neither leads to its acceptance, nor helps us to know what to say, what to do, how to act, or

441

how to be helpful. In fact, some physicians and nurses who do witness death exhibit the same avoidance tactics as lay people when interacting with dying patients and their families.[13,19] This finding is not so surprising if we recognize that nurses and physicians, no less than lay people, reflect the attitudes of society. It has been, and in most instances is, the purpose of hospitals and of health care practioners to heal, to cure, to restore, to rehabilitate, and to return the individual to living a life of quality.

THE DILEMMA: DEATH ON ICU

Intensive Care Units epitomize the charge of cure, and restoration of health. They are geared to waging war with death. They were designed to care for people who face the threat of dying due to some acute temporary crisis. They are staffed by a cadre of highly skilled personnel and are equipped with an array of complex, life-sustaining equipment.

Nowhere is the issue of life versus death placed in sharper focus. Although other divisions house patients with a high probability of dying, Intensive Care Units are unique. Their patients are considered to be salvageable and able to return to some quality of life, *if* they can be maintained through the period of acute crisis. The staff is expected to and does make every effort to sustain life during these periods of crisis. This effort includes the use of all available technologies and extreme personnel effort. It is undergirded by the belief that it is possible to accomplish the task.[2] Conflict is inherent in the situation. There is to be battle; the enemy is death and the staff cannot always win. Further complicating the situation is the fact that the same technologies and equipment used to sustain lives and to win the battle with death also give rise to many moral, ethical, and psychological issues related to life (What constitutes living? Who shall be kept alive?) and related to death (What is the definition of death?).

A central issue concerns the quality of human life. We have become so adept at maintaining life in the desperately ill that we are now faced with the question of when are we prolonging dying rather than prolonging life. This basic question leads to other no less difficult questions: what constitutes extraordinary means; under what conditions do ordinary means become extraordinary; who decides when to discontinue the use of equipment, such as respirators (an act which may or may not eventuate in death); and what constitutes euthanasia.

Another major issue is economic: the age-old problem of supply and demand. There are many seriously ill people but there is a limited supply of intensive care facilities and personnel. Moreover, the financial and emotional costs of care are astronomical.

Tension rises as decisions must be made to continue treatment, discontinue treatment, and/or discharge patients in order to accommodate other patients. Recall that it is the task of the ICU to provide the *best* chance of survival for those with acute, temporary, life-threatening problems. Patients for whom death is certain or for whom the return to life with some quality is improbable do not fit this criteria. However, they may still be housed on ICU. This situation raises additional problems and conflicts that are not solved by transferring the patient to another service. These problems are provoked by issues related to dying and death and constitute the crux of this chapter.

There is a growing belief in society today that dying and death should *not* be taboo subjects. There is an increase in literature which emphasizes the benefits of discussing dying and death and of perceiving dying as an integral part of living not as a deplorable event to be avoided at all costs. Some consumers are demanding that dying and death no longer be hidden behind closed doors. There is a movement to recognize that dying persons have rights, as do living patients. These rights have been identified and in some cases, written.[4,6] One of these rights is to know they are seriously ill and that they may die. Having this knowledge they are able to have some control over what happens to them, to participate in decisions about their care, and complete unfinished business. They are entitled to do this in an atmosphere of hopefulness. They have the right to die in peace and dignity surrounded by loved ones, unencumbered by tubes, machine, and strangers (however highly skilled). They have the right to privacy. They are entitled to be cared for by caring, sensitive, knowledgeable people who attempt to understand their needs and the needs of their significant others, including family and friends.

The concern that patients be allowed to die with dignity has led to the development and use of the living will.[9] The living will is a document which is directed to the person's family, lawyer, clergyman, or any individual who may become responsible for the individual's health, welfare, or affairs. This includes any medical facility in whose care the person may be. It requests that under conditions when (1) the individual can no longer take part in decisions of his/her own future, and (2) there is no reasonable expectation for recovery, the individual be allowed to die and not be kept alive by artificial or "heroic measures." It further requests that medication be administered to alleviate suffering even though it may hasten the moment of death.

At the present time, living wills are not legally enforceable in all states. In addition, there are many questions related to the conditions under which the wills can, or should be, honored. However, the important factor, for purposes of this chapter, is that the wills may compound the conflicts and decision-making dilemmas which already exist in the setting. Whether or not the wills are *legally* binding does not negate the fact that wills usually are perceived as *morally* binding. It is not unusual for ICU staff and family members to express feelings of anger, guilt, and anguish when extraordinary or artificial means are instituted or continued to maintain life when death is seen as inevitable. These feelings are intensified when a will, either inadvertently or intentionally, is not honored.

Although legal enforcement of these wills may be held in question, the law is clear on one point: mentally competent people may refuse treatment, and no doctor who complies with the request will be guilty of murder.[4,5] However, how many of the patients dying on ICU are mentally alert?

Thus far we have explored some of the characteristics of our contemporary society which contribute to making death on ICUs more difficult than in other environments. Let us now turn to the ICU itself and examine those factors which contribute to some of the dilemmas associated with caring for the dying patients and their families.

Intensive Care Units: Structure And Atmosphere

Intensive Care Units are structurally designed for a specific purpose: to maintain life through acute but temporary life-threatening episodes. Accurate monitoring and continuous observation are essential to this charge. Consequently, the units generally are open wards which provide high visibility of patients, but result in a lack of privacy, one of the rights of dying people and their families. In other ICU situations, patients are placed in small rooms or cubicles, which may provide more privacy, but may also preclude visitors because of the more limited space. Thus, the dying person is more likely to be alone or surrounded by highly skilled, well-intentioned strangers, rather than family and friends.

What about the atmosphere of ICUs? Think about your first working day on ICU. What was happening? What did it sound like? What were the doctors and nurses doing? What were the patients like? What were they doing? What did you think they expected of you? Now, think again, what did you see as your primary charge . . . to help save lives or to care for dying people and their families?

Except to those well-initiated to ICUs, they are very awesome places. There is a feeling of tension in the air, the kind of tension that accompanies readiness for the unexpected. The tension and strangeness are reinforced by the sounds of respirators and monitors, and by personnel, usually in strange garb, busily going about their work. There are ominous signs on the door prohibiting entrance to all but a select group. Visitors are relegated to special waiting rooms. Generally, they are allowed to enter the ICU only at specified times. Even at these times, they must request permission to enter, usually through use of some kind of telephone or intra-office communications system. In most places, permission to enter is given by a secretary or clerk of some type. Visitors enter, spend a few minutes with the person they come to see, exchange a nod or a few amenities with the staff, and return to the waiting room until the next permitted visiting period. In the waiting room, visitors share their hopes, fears, criticisms, anxieties, and misconceptions.

Thus, an aura of mystique prevails and is maintained. It is important to address this atmosphere, because it is the mystical aura in conjunction with the primary purpose of the ICU which adds to the difficulties of dying or caring for the dying on ICU. The very atmosphere is conducive to distancing the patient from family, friends, and staff. The family members are reassured that they are not needed. In fact, they are made to feel that they are in the way. In some institutions, there is a restriction that allows only two designated family members to visit. These designated people are expected to report back to any other concerned individuals.

In most instances, patients' care is dependent on the use of complicated machinery and equipment. This use of machinery is another factor which reduces the chances for human contact, especially since it may represent the last hope of maintaining life.

Dr. Avery Weisman describes the ICU patient as occupying a kind of "sacred space." "It seems required that visitors put on a special face before entering, walk softly, speak in hushed and respectful tones, be ever so careful about what is said and done . . ."[28] However it is not just the family who "puts on a special face." The same observations can be made of the conscious patients and the members of the staff. This putting on of a "special face" may influence how people interact and how aware they are of the reality of the situation.

Awareness And Interactions

Glaser and Strauss[13] have described the influence of the degree of awareness of the realities of the situation possessed by each person involved in the dying process on interactions. They described four levels, which range from closed awareness, in which the patient did not recognize his impending death, although others had this information, to open awareness, where both the patient and those around him acknowledge that he is dying.

The levels of "suspected awareness" and "mutual pretense" are most pertinent to this discussion. The suspicious patient will engage in attempts to validate his suspicion that death is inevitable. This situation may resemble a contest with the patient attempting "to reveal" and the others (family or staff) trying "to conceal" the facts.

Once the patient has confirmed his suspicions a new game is to act as normal as possible. The rules of this game are very stringent, conforming, and restrictive. To achieve the goal, topics of conversation are restricted, length of conversations may decrease, or conversations may be avoided entirely by avoiding the patient. Facial expressions are controlled, as are emotions. Multiple tactics for avoiding the patient and/or his family are called into play. Although Glaser and Strauss focused upon the dying person, a similar process can be observed between the family member and the doctors and nurses.

The achievement of "open awareness," especially in an Intensive Care Unit, will not in and of itself, serve as a panacea for the solution of problems nor for making difficult decisions. It may or may not lead to mutually acceptable solutions to identified problems regarding the patient and his care.

Dying is a lonely process, for the patient, for the family, and for the health care provider. Each individual in the situation reacts to the imminence of death in his or her own way. In addition, everyone has his or her own idea of how the patient should die, of what constitutes a "good" death. The differences in reactions, coupled with divergent views of what constitutes an appropriate way to die, and who is ultimately responsible for making decisions regarding treatments, can and usually does lead to an atmosphere of conflict and high tension. Although the conflicts and tensions may be acted upon, the causes are rarely if ever addressed directly. As a consequence, individuals feel more alone and further alienated from each other.

At the same time that dying is lonely, it is also a shared situation. People may feel lonely but they do not die alone in the sense that they die in relationships with other people—family, friends, health care providers. Thus, dying persons influence, and are influenced by those around them.

Each care provider must cope with dying just as each dying person and his or her family are also dealing with it. There are probably as many ways of coping with dying as there are people and stages of life. Our perceptions toward life, as toward death are shaped by our past experiences, by our stage in the life cycle, and by the prevailing attitudes in our society.

ATTITUDES TOWARD DEATH AND DYING

Although there are no pure attitudinal types, there are four identifiable prevailing attitudes toward death in our society today. These are the attitudes of: denial of death, defiance of death, desire for death, and acceptance of death.

Denial Of Death

Denial of death is frequently seen in hospitals. It is manifested by avoidance of the subject and, in some instances, avoidance of the dying person. For those who hold this attitude, discussion of dying, especially with the dying person, is taboo. As a result, health care practitioners and others who encourage honest discussion of dying with the patients and their family members may well be seen as inhumane by those with this attitude. These individuals justify their stance by expressing the belief that they are "protecting" the patient. The question must be raised, who is being protected? They may be protecting themselves from the anxieties that are provoked by their feelings toward death and toward their own finiteness. For whatever reason, vigorous denial of death is generally more prevalent among physicians than others in our society.[11] Such denial on the part of physicians can contribute to conflicts in decision making and also can contribute to difficulties in reaching agreement regarding the approach to patients, their care and treatment. The problem is compounded because society has relegated decisions related to the care of dying patients to the physician. Doctors, by virtue of the emphasis upon cure provided by their education, are not well prepared to care for dying people; yet, they are reluctant to formally acknowledge their lack of expertise in this area. Although nurses are more vocal in expressing how the dying patient should be cared for, they are reluctant to assume the responsibility which accompanies this role for which they may be better prepared. The result is that no mutual agreement is reached as to the course of action to be taken. Thus, when the physician withdraws from the situation, the family and the nursing staff are left in a quandary as to what to do. This problem is intensified in the ICU where it is all too easy for the physician to make rounds once or twice a day and walk away. That is not the case for nurses. Nurses, in contrast to any other health care practitioners or members of clergy, spend their entire daily energies in working with the patient. In addition, it is nurses who must face families, and respond to, or evade, their forthright, and sometimes desperate questions. The situation is further complicated by other physicians, who would be equally evasive under the same circumstances, but who are pressing for ICU space for their own patients and are criticizing colleagues for not facing the inevitable. Unfortunately, in this struggle for ICU space, physicians express their views to nurses rather than to fellow physicians.

When it becomes clear that the patient has no chance for recovery, and a physician evades responsibility for making any explicit decision regarding treatment, the continuation of intensive care becomes a mockery of the physical and emotional efforts of the nurses. The result is deterioration of morale.[23] Decreased morale may lead to increased difficulty in approaching the patient's family members, especially if the latter are not directly informed of the futility of continued intensive efforts.

Transfer of the patient to another service, based upon an inability to face a difficult situation, is not a solution. It is a precursor to no less difficult problems. It not only has negative consequences in terms of the morale of the staff of the receiving service, but it also leaves the ICU staff with feelings of guilt and lack of closure, especially if they disagreed with the decision. Of greater importance, the transfer may be accurately interpreted as abandonment of the patient.

Defiance Of Death

The second attitude, death defiance, is a part of the Judeo-Christian heritage. It is exemplified in instances where people have fought for causes or ideologies in spite of the fact that they might die in the attempt. This attitude is reflected in the battle for life against death that is waged on ICU, not only·by the patient, but dramatically by the professional staff. However, while the professional staff takes on the cause, that of saving people's lives, their own lives are not in jeopardy. It is the patient who dies; nevertheless, the staff lives with the sense of a battle lost. In addition, they are reminded of their own finiteness and the inevitability of death.

Desire For Death

Although it is not generally considered acceptable to express our desire to die or our desire for others to die, the death desiring attitude is quite common in our society. There are many circumstances which give rise to the desire to die. Some seek relief from the miseries of life—pain, disability, uncertainty, and loneliness. Others seek reunion with loved ones in some other place. Still others may look forward to death as the last phase in the fulfillment of life.

Patients express their desire to die in many ways. The expression of the desire to die in many instances confirms that death is seen as inevitable. This recognition leads to observable patterns of adaptation to the recognition. The following patterns of adaptation were identified in a study of hospitalized dying people.[17] One pattern is *relief from uncertainty*. It is characterized by searching for some kind of closure, some answer to the question "will I live or will I die," by dealing with fate or the supernatural. The following are examples of how people expressed their wish for life or for death as an end to the anguish generated by uncertainty. Notice the underlying hope in addition to the "live while you live and die and be done with it" attitude. "It is up to God, I've been through enough, now it's up to God." "It's just up and down, up and down, I just wish that one way or another it would end."

Another pattern is the desire for *escape*. It is characterized by (1) resignation and (2) escape from loneliness and despair. One person expressed it by saying, "I have nothing left to live for. I pray I die. I pray to God I die before I get put away in some home or other." Another said, "Dying is just another experience. I'm not afraid of dying. It can't be worse than lying here day after day, all alone with only nurses who care. No family, even my friends don't come any more."

The families of dying patients, as well as the staff members, may desire the death of the patient. The reasons vary. They may wish to see the end of human suffering. Perhaps, there is the desire for relief from personal or financial responsibilities, or the burden of care, or the uncertainties of the situation.

Two overt patterns were manifested by family members. They openly expressed their desire that patients die by (1) granting them *permission to die* or by (2) *the invitation to die*. Either approach is not as shocking as it may at first appear.

Granting *permission to die* generally occurs in situations where there is an illness of short duration culminating rapidly in death, e.g. accidents. Initially, the family members encourage the patient "to try," "you will get better if you just try." However, as the patient's condition becomes worse, and as family members begin to recognize that death is inevitable, their focus changes to one of sanctioning dying. For example, the following comments were made to a fifteen-year-old patient in a surgical Intensive Care Unit. The boy was dying of septic shock following emergency surgery. "It's okay, we know you won't be apart from us, you pray for us when you get up there. It's okay, son, I'm getting old myself and I'll be coming to join you, so you won't be alone."

One woman granted her husband permission to die by telling him what a good husband he had always been and by acknowledging how hard he had tried. "You were a good husband, you always took good care of us. You tried, there's nothing more you can do. We understand."

The overt *invitation to die* occurs under situations where all known treatments have been tried, the patient has made a concerted effort to get well and yet there is still unrelenting symptomatology. In addition, it usually occurs in situations where there have been close family relationships and where patients were actively involved in decisions regarding their care through at least the latter stages of their illnesses. The invitation is usually directly made by a family member; however, the responsibility may be given to someone else, such as a member of the clergy.

The following example is included to demonstrate that neither the tone nor the intent of the *invitation to die* is one of abandonment. Jeff was a twenty-eight-year-old man dying of cancer. He had had multiple surgeries, radiation therapy, and chemotherapy. It was his eighth admission to the Intensive Care Unit. One day his mother turned to her son, washed his face, stroked his forehead and spoke to him as though he were an overtired, obstreperous, but much loved child who needed a nap. She simply and directly stated: "Jeff, Jeff darling, why don't you just die."

It is important to understand that the desire for death is not a deplorable, inhuman, uncaring attitude. More importantly, the behaviors or patterns of adapting such as overtly expressing the wish that someone die, granting permission to die, or overtly inviting someone to die are not horrendous or abnormal. Neither is it abnormal or horrendous to identify a dying person as a source of anger, frustration, or resentment. It should be expected that someone's death may at the same time, be a welcomed relief and a terrible loss.

The last form of adaptation reflects this dilemma. This pattern is seen in interactions between family members and staff. It occurs in situations where patients are no longer able to communicate in some meaningful way, either verbally or nonverbally; and where death is inevitable. Essentially, the patients are seen as *non-persons*. Under these circumstances, common in the Intensive Care Unit, patients are no longer perceived as living people. Because they are unable to interact or respond in any meaningful way, they are perceived as dead, socially at least. However, they are biologically alive and therein lies the dilemma. Under these circumstances, family members may well turn to the nurse or other staff members, expressing their distress. The following statement reflects the dilemma for the family member. It is also an example of how family members may express their frustration.

"I've done my crying now. I just want him peaceful. He can't do anything. He can't be anything, he can't even talk anymore. When you can't talk, you are not a person. What are you people doing anyway? Can't you do something to end all this?"

Acceptance Of Death

The last attitude to be discussed is the death-accepting attitude. It is this attitude which places death as a normal, natural, and integral part of living. Resignation to and acceptance of our limited existence has been defined as the central task for achieving maturity.[1] With this acceptance, death becomes the conclusion of life's plan. But, as Schneidman[20] points out, this is a rather romantic view which makes early or accidental death an unnatural event. Thus, the attitude of death acceptance, like open awareness, is not a magical solution to the dilemmas surrounding the dying process.

What is there to be gleaned by the nurse from this brief categorization of attitudes toward death in our society? First, there are no pure attitudes toward death. There are combinations of attitudes, which differ between and among people, and in the same person under varying situations and during different stages of life. Second, we are moving, or at least advocating, that we move from a death denying to a death integrating society. However, it is incorrect to think in terms of a scale with death denial being most negative and death acceptance as most positive. It is equally inappropriate for us to have some imaginary grading system for ourselves and for those around us based upon our or their abilities or lack of abilities to interact in an open fashion with any one patient or any one family. It is more important to understand that there is no one well-defined way to die or to act toward the dying just as there is no one well-defined way to live or act toward the living.

We all harbor feelings of love-hate quality. They are intrinsic to all our relationships. Unless we recognize and accept that caring for people who are expected to die just as caring for people who are expected to live, evokes feelings of anger, frustration, and despair, as well as feelings of compassion and love, we will neither be able to cope effectively ourselves nor be able to assist the patient and his family to cope effectively.

To cope effectively does not mean that we will all cope in the same way. Working with dying patients, especially in the face of failure of our modern life saving devices, evokes intense personal feelings. Although we may all experience these intense feelings, there is no assurance that they are the same feelings, or that we will or need to act them out in the same way.

There is no recipe for caring for the dying patient in the Intensive Care Unit or elsewhere. We are just beginning to accumulate knowledge about how people die and how people act and react to dying, to death and to those who are dying.

The identification of this body of knowledge can offer us some guidelines, for there are universal concerns related to the process of dying. In addition, there are general principles which can be gleaned from identifying the common problems of dying. These principles can be beneficial for patients, family members and health care practitioners if the individual, the personal, and the unique characteristics within the common problems are not only recognized, but considered, and if a stereotyped approach to the care of dying is avoided.

PHASES AND PATTERNS OF DYING

Phases Of Dying

Pertinent to this discussion is the question raised by E. Mansell in his book, *The Experience of Dying*.[20] He asks "Are there stages or phases of dying"? The question is raised in reaction to the many people who adopted Kubler-Ross's stages of dying as an inevitable process. As you may recall, Elizabeth Kubler-Ross[14] organized her observations about the dying process around a series of stages.

She described a series of psychological reactions to dying. This series began with initial shock and numbness, followed by denial and isolation, anger, bargaining and depression. Individuals who successfully moved through these stages achieved a stage of acceptance and lived in hope. It is improbable that Kubler-Ross ever intended that these stages be interpreted as some concretized process, as hard facts of reality. Nonetheless, many people latch on to these stages as though they are facts. As a consequence, patients are expected to conform and to pass through these stages. They are expected to "die in the right way" and the "right way" is not only to pass through these stages but to do so in sequence and in an observable fashion. The misapplication of these stages has consequences for practitioner and patient alike. Patients who do not pass through these stages are chastised by the staff. They are seen as deviant, and in many instances forced into this "scientific" way of dying. Practitioners are no longer allowed to respond to patients as individuals with unique responses to dying. They question why the patients are not passing through the appropriate stages in the expected sequence. They also question their own abilities as practitioners because they can not assist or force patients to conform to the "scientific" way of dying.

In recent years, there are many who question the stages of dying concept. Weisman[27] describes the idea of staging psychosocial episodes as orderly but artificial. He suggests that there is no well-recognized succession of emotional responses that are typical of people throughout their process of dying. Neither Shibles,[22] nor Schulz and Aderman[21] offer support for the concept. Shibles found that the stages are too narrow and fixed. They do not adequately account for the thought, images, perceptual and motor abilities of the dying person. Schulz and Aderman observed that patients adopted a pattern of behavior which persisted until death occurred. Pattison[16] found no evidence to support stages of dying. In agreement with Weisman,[27] he suggests that it may be clinically useful to conceptualize the dying process in terms of phases. He divides the period of living-dying into three clinical phases: (1) the acute crisis phase; (2) the chronic living-dying phase; and (3) the terminal phase.

The acute crisis phase occurs when patients are confronted with the crisis of knowledge of death. During this crisis, there is an increasing anxiety that will reach a peak of tolerance. Since no one can continue to function at this level of anxiety, psychological mechanisms are called upon to reduce the anxiety. Patients may become immobilized, express disbelief, or exhibit the anger, denial, and bargaining behaviors described by Kubler-Ross.[14]

During the crisis period, the person is faced with an unsolvable problem. Death is inevitable and there is no way to stop it. The individual is faced with dying, a new experience, with no prior experience to rely upon. Whether old or young, there is a major threat to life goals. Unresolved problems from the past such as dependency, passivity, and identity, among others, may be evoked. Thus, during this phase, the person may not only be faced with dying but with unresolved problems and conflicts from the past.

At this time, nursing care can be directed toward the reduction of anxiety. This is accomplished by focusing upon reality issues—

those factors or things which are actually occurring. Given our interest, support and guidance, the dying persons can learn to face death as an unknown and apply their energies to dealing with living even as they know they are dying. Pattison describes this period of living even when knowingly dying, as the chronic living-dying phase. During this phase, dying people face many fears: fears of the unknown, of loneliness, of sorrow, of loss of family and friends, of suffering, of loss of identity. However, if not deprived of human contact, they can learn to endure the inevitable degrees of separation without loneliness. They can face the loss of friends, relatives, and former activities if they can actively mourn their loss in a situation where grief is defined and accepted, and where others accept the loss. Dying people can tolerate the loss of self-control if they can exercise some control where feasible, and if the loss of self-control is not perceived as a shameful experience by themselves or by others. Pain can be tolerated if the dying person can see the source and its meaning so that it is not transformed into suffering. In essence, dying people can maintain their dignity and self respect if they can place their lives in perspective within their own personal history, family and human tradition. Once this latter task is accomplished, the person can enter the terminal phase, where it is possible to give up one's battling with life, and where an acceptable regression and withdrawal occurs.

Pattison's conceptualization of phases of dying should be used as a frame of reference, as one way of looking at the dying process. One phase may or may not lead to the next. There may be situations where a phase may be repeated, or even skipped. Death may be so sudden there is no time to enter a second or third phase; or perhaps there is recovery followed by another period of crisis.

Patterns of Dying

In the Martocchio study of hospitalized dying people,[17] four general patterns of dying were identified. These are: (1) Peaks and Valleys; (2) Descending Plateaus; (3) Downward Slopes; and (4) Gradual Slants. Recognition of different patterns of dying, each with its own inherent problems, offers additional understanding of the situation of people and their families. These are schematically diagramed in Table 7-1.

The *"Peaks and Valleys"* pattern of dying is characterized by

TABLE 7-1

Patterns of Dying

PEAKS AND VALLEYS   DESCENDING PLATEAUS

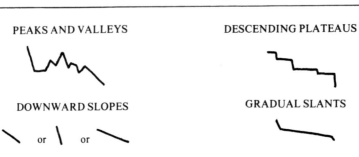

DOWNWARD SLOPES   GRADUAL SLANTS

periods of crisis (exacerbation) and periods of quiescence (remissions). This pattern can be conceptualized as a series of erratic peaks and valleys, with the peaks representing remissions (periods of greater health) and the valleys representing times of crisis (exacerbations).

Both the heights of the peaks and the depths of the valleys are indeterminate, as is the length of time spent at any one point. However, there is an overriding downward slope. The peaks become less high and the valleys not necessarily lower but lasting longer periods of time.

It is a pattern of dying frought with uncertainty and false hopes. Patients and their families talk about the "hopeful highs" and "the terrible and depressing lows." Health care practitioners are also distressed. It is difficult to know whether to prepare the person for living or for dying. Most likely the answer is to prepare for living even while preparing for dying; in other words, address dying as an integral part of living.

Descending Plateaus is another pattern of dying. This is a pattern of progressive degeneration plateauing an unpredictable number of times and for varying periods of time. These individuals experience a major crisis, recover from the crisis, but do not return to their former level of health or functional ability. They continue on a relatively stable course until another crisis intervenes. This pattern can be depicted as a series of steps; the depths and the duration of the plateaus may vary. This pattern entails continuous adjustment to greater debilitation, or continuous rehabilitation with no certainty regarding the future.

The third pattern is the continuous *downward slope*. In this pattern there is a persistent, consistent, easily discernable downward slope. The degree of the slope represents the acuity of illness and the length of the slope represents the length of the illness.

Generally, these individuals are essentially healthy, and then experience a major crisis. They have shorter periods of illness before death than those dying in the other patterns. There is little time to prepare. Interactions are intense, and there is an observable increase in tension. This pattern is frequently seen on Intensive Care Units. There is a dramatic concerted effort to stop the downhill course. The focus is upon the patient, who is probably unconscious. In the supreme effort to save the patient, the family is all but forgotten. In most instances they are relegated to the visiting room where they wait until the end, usually without information regarding their family member.

The last pattern, *gradual slant* is depicted by an almost continuous low ebb of life, gradually, and sometimes almost imperceptibly, leading to actual death. Generally, these individuals experience a major debilitating bodily insult. This pattern may be long or short in terms of duration of time preceding actual death.

This pattern creates many dilemmas when it continues for long periods of time. It is under these circumstances that questions are raised regarding definitions of death, what actions constitute extraordinary means, where the person should be cared for and by whom. For instance, is the person alive when there is a beating heart, but a non-functioning brain? Should the use of respirators be discontinued although "living" would probably cease without them? Are modern technologies prolonging life or death?

These models and conceptualizations offer us a frame of reference from which to better understand the situation of and surrounding dying people. Such understandings can be used as guides in caring for dying people and for assisting their families. However, the primary task is to respond to *each* individual's actual dying experience. To respond to each individual's actual dying experience entails identifying the crisis and related stress at a specific time and responding to it and the emotions generated by it. It entails responding to where people are in their living as well as in their dying. The task, that of responding to each individual's actual dying experience, precludes forcing any person to conform to our pre-conceived notions of what dying should entail.

REFLECTIONS ON SOME FREQUENTLY ASKED QUESTIONS

There are some questions which are frequently raised by nurses when caring for dying patients and their families. For some questions there are no answers. For others there are many responses, but no one best answer. I shall reflect on some of these questions and suggest that the responses be used as a springboard for your own reflections.

One frequently asked question is, how detached should the nurse be when caring for the dying patient? Stated differently, is it accep-table or "professional" to become "emotionally involved"? In gen-eral, the goal for the professional is to achieve a state of "detached concern."[17] This state includes understanding the dying person while maintaining objectivity.

We have all been exposed to the notion that to understand dying in others we must deal with dying in ourselves. Yet, we cannot rec-ognize the thought of our own deaths for long periods,[1] if at all.[12] Weisman[26] states that caring for dying people evokes many uni-versal fears—fears of extinction, abandonment, disfigurement, and of loss of self-esteem. We could not care for patients long if we were to consistently and directly face our own finiteness. It is necessary to appropriately repress our own death anxieties if we are to care for patients. Appropriate repression[16] is the capacity to call forth an awareness of our death anxiety, to feel comfortable about our own mortality, and to allow our more fundemental concerns to lie out of our conscious sight most of the time. It is rather like looking at the sun indirectly.

Perhaps detached concern can be better understood if we look at two extremes of behavior: complete detachment and overinvolve-ment. Complete detachment is gaining emotional distance through professionalization or intellectualization. For these individuals, death is made an impersonal, external problem. It is an object to be studied, to be treated. There is an appropriate plan for treatment, and there is an appropriate way to die.

The other extreme is overinvolvement or overidentification. In these situations, the health care provider becomes overinvolved in the life and death of the dying person. In many instances, these practitioners use the situation to work through past guilts, to rework their prior death experiences or to restore or build their own self-esteem.

In contrast, detached concern is the practice of maintaining objectivity even while personalizing the approach. The essential aspects include demonstrating understanding and revealing concern.

Another frequently asked question is, what should the nurse say if a family member asks if a patient is dying? For this, and other similar questions, the key lies in focusing upon the reality of the situation. Before responding, it is essential to find out if the question should be interpreted at face value. What is the person really asking? Remember, family members are aware of the seriousness of the situation by virtue of the fact that their family member is a patient on an Intensive Care Unit. Helpful answers are those which help the family member grasp the reality of the situation. They are usually brief factual answers which are informative and/or clarify misconceptions. In addition, they are conversational, in the sense that the family member is listened to, responded to, and time is taken to express understanding of their worry and concerns.

Above all, the answers should be honest but not unthinking and unfeeling. In many instances, a verbal reply is not wanted nor expected. Sometimes non-verbal behaviors such as eye-to-eye contact, a nod, a touch or gently escorting the visitor to the bedside and staying with the visitor is all that is necessary. Other times a short response such as "it must be so difficult for you to wait and wonder" will suffice. On other occasions, more specific answers are needed. For example, you might say, "your wife will get better if we can get her kidneys to work again." It is important that the response is geared to the intent of the question and to the patient's actual condition at the time the question is asked.

If you do not know the family member, or know when he/she last visited the patient, it is important to find out what his/her frame of reference is. A very different response may be appropriate if the visitor is seeing the patient for the first time than if the person has observed a decline in the patient's condition.

It is essential to respond in terms of the reality of the situation at the specific time. Listen, identify the stressors, and then respond to the emotional responses and to the questions that are generated by the situation. Respond simply, honestly and in a caring and concerned fashion using the family members' cues and the reality of the situation as a guide.

A closely related and important question frequently raised is what if the family does not recognize, or does not accept that the patient will not recover and most probably will die; what, then, is the nurse's role? This is a question which cannot be answered directly without some preceding discussion. First, we make assumptions based upon verbal and non-verbal responses we observe. Then we attempt to act on those assumptions. However, our assumptions are not always correct. We may misinterpret the behaviors; thus, at times our interventions are not only inappropriate, they are dysfunctional for the family, the patient, and ourselves.

Let us explore this further. First, as in the preceding question, it is important to identify the *realities* in the situation as *perceived by the family.* To what are they responding? What have they been told? What kind of explanations have they been given? How many double messages have they received? How many different and incongruent explanations have they received? In other words, what is their actual information base? What is the situation as they perceive it? Second, what are other factors to consider in understanding and interpreting a behavioral response? There are some general factors which serve as guides in understanding behavioral responses. First, most behavior is an effort to achieve or to maintain one's equilibrium. Second, the responses of individuals are determined by how they perceive the situation, the symptoms, the treatments, and more importantly, by their general patterns of response to life and life's crises.

Individuals, family members and others bring to the situation all they are or have been. Every person's behavior is comprised of his history or past experiences, his culture, his personality, and his past and present environment. All these factors influence how the person perceives the situation and develops styles of coping. Coping styles may alleviate, or they may increase stress. In addition, the person's response will be influenced by his/her interpretation of the reality of the situation. It is helpful to identify the factors influencing the response, but it is not the role of the nurse to attempt to change the basic life patterns of a person. It is the role of the nurse *to support and to guide people as they move toward a way of life that accommodates the illness, the treatment, or lack of treatment for however long that accommodation is necessary.* The success of this endeavor can be evaluated in terms of the ability of the person and his family to live *comfortably* or *resignedly* with the real situation.

This process of adaptation begins when the person and the family learn either by diagnosis or by change in condition that life is threatened.[3,8] For the patient in ICU, it may have preceded admission. Initially there is a response of disbelief, especially if the person appeared to be recovering and then experienced another crisis.

Family members may overtly express disbelief. They may even deny that death is a possibility. Denial is not a negative and inappropriate response. It is a protective device. Moreover, denial or acceptance of death is not an either/or proposition. Most likely there are degrees of acceptance and denial occurring continuously and simultaneously. Therefore to eliminate denial and to achieve acceptance is not a justifiable goal.

Expressions of denial and anger are appropriate and necessary parts of the process of adaptation. The nurse can help by allowing the patient and family to express how they feel and by assisting them to clarify their own feelings. This is not the time to directly confront them with the cold facts of reality. It is a time to establish yourself as a person who understands and accepts their feelings but is aware of the facts. It is a time to ask how you can help. It is a time to demonstrate to the family that you are a person who can be depended upon to deal with the reality they are not yet ready to face. It is a time for listening, for expressing warmth and understanding while maintaining the stance of the professional. Stay with the patient and family; give competent procedural care; let your actions indicate the reality of the situation.

As the inevitability of death becomes more apparent, there may be expressions of anger, guilt and greater dependency. Feelings of helplessness evoke feelings of anger, frustration and guilt in us all. Listen to the expressions of anger and guilt and recognize them for what they are. Lengthy explanations and arguments about the competence of the care lead to more anger and defensiveness. In general, address needs as they arise. Accept but do not probe for expressions of feelings. Remember that if a person's life pattern was to avoid or ignore problems, it is not the time, the place, nor the nurse's role to change it. It *is* the nurse's role to recognize and to capitalize upon behaviors which assist the patient and his family in adjusting to the reality of the situation. This includes recognizing her/his own behavior and that of other health professionals.

We all influence each others behavior even as our own behavior is being influenced. Nurses and physicians, no less than patients and family members are continually adapting and changing as they interact with each other. Although it is necessary for health professionals to remain objective and realistic, this stance does not preclude the need to be humanistic. For most, the overwhelming desire is to be treated humanly, and with respect.

REFERENCES

1. Becker E: *The Denial of Death*. Free Press, Riverside, New Jersey, 1973.
2. Caughill RE: Coping with Death in Acute Care Units. In Caughill RE (Ed.): *The Dying Patient: A Supportive Approach*. Little, Brown, and Company, Boston, Mass., 1976, pp.95-124.
3. Crate MA: Nursing functions in adaptation to chronic illness. *American Journal of Nursing* 65:72-76, 1965.
4. Curtin L: *The Mask of Euthanasia*. 2nd Ed. N.C.F.L., Inc., Cincinnati, Ohio, 1976.
5. Dempsy D: *The Way We Die: An Investigation of Death and Dying in America Today*. McGraw-Hill, New York, 1977, p.107.
6. Donovan ML, Pierce SG:*Cancer Care Nursing*. Appleton-Century-Crofts, New York, 1976, pp.19-33.
7. Dumont R, Foss D: *The American View of Death: Acceptance of Denial?* Schenkman, Cambridge, Massachusetts, 1972, p.2.
8. Engel G: Grief and grieving. *American Journal of Nursing*. 64:93-98, 1964.
9. Euthanasia Educational Council, 250 W 57th Street, New York, New York, 10019
10. Feifel H: Death. In Faberow NL (Ed.): *Taboo Topics*. Atherton Press, New York, 1963, pp. 8-12.
11. Feifel H: The functions of attitudes toward death in *Death and Dying: Attitudes of Patient and Doctor*. Group for Advancement of Psychiatry, New York, 1965.
12. Freud S: Thoughts for the times on war and death. *Collected Papers*. Vol.4, Hogarth, London, 1915.
13. Glaser BG, Strauss AL: *Awareness of Dying*. Aldine, Chicago, 1965.
14. Kubler-Ross E: *On Death and Dying*. Macmillan Publishing, New York, 1969.
15. Kubler-Ross E: *Death: The Final Stage of Growth*. Prentice-Hall, Englewood Cliffs, New Jersey, 1975, p.5.

16. Mansell PE: *The Experience of Dying.* Prentice-Hall, Englewood Cliffs, New Jersey, 1977.
17. Martocchio BC: *The Social Processes Surrounding The Dying Patient.* (Doctoral dissertation, Case Western Reserve University, 1975). *Dissertation Abstracts International, 1976, 37,* 1239A. University Microfilms No. 76-16, 055.
18. McClelland DC: The Harlequin Complex. In White R (Ed.): *The Study of Lives.* Atherton Press, New York, 1963, p. 95.
19. Quint J: *The Nurse and the Dying Patient.* Macmillan Publishing, New York, 1967.
20. Schneidman ES: On the deromantization of death. *American Journal of Psychotherapy* **25**:4-17, 1971.
21. Schulz R, Alderman D: Clinical research and the stages of dying. *Omega* **5**:137-143, 1974.
22. Shibbles W: *Death: An Interdisciplinary Analysis.* Language Press, Whitewater, Wisconsin, 1974.
23. Skillman JJ: Ethical dilemmas in the care of the critically ill. *Lancet* **2**:7881, 634-637, 1974.
24. Tiedt E: The psychodynamics process of the oncological experience. *Nursing Forum* **14**:264-277, 1975.
25. Wahl CW: The fear of death. In Fulton RL (Ed.): *Death and Identity.* John Wiley and Sons, New York, 1965, p.57.
26. Weisman AD: Misgivings and misconceptions in the psychiatric care of the terminal patient. *Psychiatry* **33**:67-81, 1970.
27. Weisman AD: *The Realization of Death.* Aronson, New York, 1974.
28. Weisman AD, Kastenbaum R: The psychological autopsy. *Community Mental Health Journal, Monograph Series,* No. 4, 1968, p. 47.

CHAPTER 8

Special Problems in Critical Care: Trauma

by Martha L. Allen, RN, MSN

INTRODUCTION

The nurse working in the critical care setting deals daily with patients who have highly complex health problems that require extensive, in-depth understanding of the human organism in every aspect of its functioning. Among the most complex and challenging cases the nurse may encounter in the critical care setting is the patient who has suffered a single or multiple life-threatening trauma. The major objective of this chapter is to expand the nurse's depth of understanding and skills in caring for these acutely ill patients.

Clinically, trauma is often perceived as an intense injury of varying magnitude to the body. Such injuries are frequently thought of in terms of fractures, lacerations, or wounds, and are usually associated with accident victims. However, the term trauma encompasses a wide range of insults to the body, from one or a combination of external noxious forces, such as thermal, chemical, deceleration, missile or impact.[22] When viewed within this context, any insult from an external noxious force is a trauma; therefore, surgical incisions and minor sunburns, although not often perceived as "accidents," fall within the classification of trauma.

The term trauma encompasses a wide variety of insults of varying magnitude and intensity. Because of this intricacy, it is essential that the nurse caring for the trauma patient have a *basic* understanding of the significance of different types and varying degrees of trauma.

Basically, there are three major categorizations of trauma. They are: wounds (contusions, incisions, lacerations, punctures), crushing injuries, and burns. Within each of these broad categorizations, each specific degree of trauma is determined by a variety of factors and clinical findings. Among these are the characteristics of the external force causing the injury, the type of injury it inflicts, the parts of the body affected, and the extent of functional impairment as well as the degree of contamination of the injured area(s).

The type of trauma the patient has suffered, the area(s) of the body it affects, and the extent of the insult it inflicts on normal body functioning, all help to determine the acuity of the injury (Table 8-1) as well as the long-term physiological consequences for the patient in every phase of the illness experience. However, no system of classification exists that is able to accurately predict the response of any individual patient to trauma. A bullet wound in one patient may initially affect only one organ system, while in a second patient, a deep third degree burn initially has a broader systemic effect; the final outcome, however, may be clinically similar for both patients. The complex and often interacting responses of the body may have a "snowballing" effect that leads to involvement of many or all tissues and organs throughout the body.[24] Thus, not only the specific injury itself, but also the magnitude of the response to injury contribute to the eventual patient outcome.

The types of trauma encountered in the critical care setting are usually profound and involve multiple, severe injuries affecting any or all bodily functions. The efficiency of the body's response as well as the care the patient receives to support vital functions and aid in healing may determine whether and to what extent the patient will recover from the trauma. The following pages of this chapter will consider the physiological reactions and pathological sequelae that arise as a result of trauma and the nurse's responsibilities in dealing with these responses in caring for the trauma patient.

PHYSIOLOGICAL RESPONSES
AND PATHOLOGICAL SEQUELAE

Physiological Responses to Trauma

From the onset of the acute traumatic event, observable physiological manifestations occur which reflect an automatic response by the body to the external, noxious insult. These responses occur at every level from the individual cell up to and including complete organ systems. The responses of the organism are directed toward healing of the injury and restoration of steady, optimal functioning of the body. These responses occur both *locally* and *systemically* and may be either rapid or slow depending upon: (1) the nature of the trauma inflicted; (2) the type and extent of the injury which has occurred; and (3) the adequacy of the response or the degree to which the response meets the body's needs.[23]

The body's response to trauma has three major characteristics: (1) the responses occur in a continuous, on-going fashion with definable phases; (2) there is involvement of both neurological and endocrine mediated mechanisms; and (3) there is a major alteration in metabolic systems and pathways. The clinical manifestations of trauma will be discussed in terms of these three characteristics.

The sequential phases which occur in the event of acute trauma of a life-threatening nature include the alarm phase (flight/fright), followed by the resistance phase, in which there is mobilization and activation of all available resources to cope with the trauma. The third phase is one of exhaustion of resources and an inability to sustain life without support from external sources, and is often seen in acute trauma with shock secondary to burns or multiple injuries.[23] Both neuro-hormonal and metabolic mechanisms are involved throughout all three phases, and are active both locally and systemically. All of these phases are likely to be seen in Intensive Care Units. With adequate care and support, the patient then progresses into what may be termed recovery or convalescent phases.

The first or acute phase has the most observable effects and is, in a sense, the most crucial to the patient's survival. The three major occurrences of this initial phase are the release of amino acids and electrolytes into the extracellular fluid, maintenance of extracellular fluid volume and the conversion of body fat to carbohydrate to provide an adequate, long-term source of energy for the body.

Through these mechanisms, the body is able to support the circulatory system, essential for immediate survival. It is also able to alter normal body metabolism which relies on dietary intake of carbohydrate and other essential foodstuffs for energy to an effective starvation-like state of metabolism in which body fat is used as the primary resource for metabolism.

The key elements which maintain the integrity of the

TABLE 8-1
Injury Description*

Injury Category Severity Code	General	Head and Neck	Chest	Abdominal	Extremities
No injury 0	None	None	None	None	None
Minor 1	Minor lacerations, contusions and abrasions. All 1°, small 2° and 3° burns.	Cerebral injury without loss of consciousness. "Whiplash" without vertebral damage. Ocular abrasions and contusions.	Minor chest wall contusions, abrasions.	Muscle contusions; seat belt abrasion.	Minor sprains and fractures, and/or dislocation of digits.
Moderate 2	Extensive contusions, abrasions; large lacerations; avulsions (<3" diameter) 10-20% 2° or 3° burns.	Cerebral injury with <15 minutes unconsciousness; no amnesia. Undisplaced skull or facial bone fractures. Eye lacerations, retinal detachment. "Whiplash" with vertebral injury.	Simple rib or sternal fractures. Major contusions of chest wall without hemo- or pneumothorax, or respiratory embarrassment.	Major contusion of abdominal wall without intra-abdominal injury	Compound fractures of digits or nose. Undisplaced long bone or pelvic fractures. Major joint sprains.

(Continued)

TABLE 8-1 (Continued)
Injury Description*

Injury Category Severity Code	General	Head and Neck	Chest	Abdominal	Extremities
Severe 3 (not life-threatening)	Extensive contusions or abrasions; large lacerations or avulsions (>3" diameter). 20-30% 2° or 3° burns.	Cerebral injury with unconsciousness >15 minutes without severe neurologic signs; <3 hours post-traumatic amnesia. Displaced closed skull fractures without signs of intracranial injury. Loss of eye, or avulsion of optic nerve. Facial bone fractures, displaced or without antral or orbital involvement. Cervical spine fracture without cord damage.	Multiple rib fracture without respiratory embarrassment. Simple hemo- or pneumothorax. Rupture of diaphragm. Moderate pulmonary contusion.	Contusion of abdominal organs. Extraperitoneal bladder rupture. Retroperitoneal hemorrhage. Avulsion of ureter. Laceration of urethra. Thoracic or lumbar spine fractures without neurologic involvement.	Displaced simple long bone fractures, and/or multiple hand and foot fractures. Single open long bone fractures. Pelvic fractures with displacement. Dislocation of major joints. Lacerations of major nerves or vessels of extremities.

Severe 4 (life-threatening, survival probable)	Severe lacerations and/or avulsions with dangerous hemorrhage. 30-50% 2° or 3° burns.	Cerebral injury with or without skull fracture, with unconsciousness of >15 minutes with definite abnormal neurologic signs; post-traumatic amnesia 3-12 hours. Compound skull fracture.	Open chest wounds; flail chest; pneumomediastinum; myocardial contusion and pericardial injuries without circulatory embarrassment.	Minor lacerations of intra-abdominal viscera including kidney, spleen and tail of pancreas. Intraperitoneal bladder rupture. Avulsion of genitals. Dorsal and/or lumbar spine fractures with paraplegia.	Multiple closed long bone fractures. Amputation of limbs.
Critical 5 (survival uncertain)	Over 50% 2° or 3° burns.	Cerebral injury with unconsciousness of >24 hours; post-traumatic amnesia >12 hours; intracranial hemorrhage; signs of increased intracranial pressure Cervical spine injury with quadriplegia. Major airway obstruction.	Chest injuries with major respiratory embarrassment (laceration of trachea, hemomediastinum, etc.) Aortic laceration. Myocardial rupture or contusion with circulatory embarrassment.	Rupture, avulsion, or severe laceration of abdominal vessels or organs, except kidney, spleen or ureter.	Multiple open limb fractures.

*From: Ballinger WF, et al: *The Management of Trauma.* W.B. Saunders Co., Philadelphia, Pa., 1973, p. 27. Used with permission.

circulatory system are the neuro-hormonal responses, which will be discussed in the next section in more detail. Increased secretion of epinephrine and norepinephrine in appropriate concentrations and proportions permits redistribution of vascular fluids to essential areas of the body while minimizing the adverse effects of diminished circulation to other areas. The secretion of ADH by the neurohypophysis and aldosterone from the adrenal cortex, in response to ACTH, also facilitate circulation through the conservation of water and sodium chloride.

In terms of the metabolic response, the acute phase is characterized by evidence of increased gluconeogenesis and a diabetogenic-like hyperglycemic state. There are concurrent increases in glucose, urea, and creatinine levels in the urine.

Local responses to trauma are also significant in the alarm or initial phase. These responses are activated at the site of injury (i.e., the location of tissue destruction, blood loss, or site of infection). These local responses mediated through the actions of the autonomic and endocrine systems begin immediate healing. The degree to which wound healing will be accomplished will depend to a great extent on oxygenation of the wounded area and amount of contamination accompanying the injury.[21]

To maximize oxygenation and minimize infection of the wound due to contamination in the acute phase, there is localized dilatation of blood vessels to aid circulation through the area. This increased vascularity in the wound area is accompanied by alterations in the vascular cell wall membranes; such alterations lead to an outpouring of plasma and migration of leukocytes and macrophages into the interstitial spaces of the wound.

The initial reactions in the acute phase set the stage for the classic inflammatory process to occur. Damaged and necrotic tissue is broken down and removed by substances which neutralize toxins, aid in phagocytosis and absorb necrotic material.[22]

In the next ("the collagen," "productive" or "fibroblastic") stage of local healing there is a proliferation of collagen which walls off the area, prevents the spread of infection and aids healing by a progressive increase in the stability of the wound. The collagen content reaches its maximum in 10 to 12 days after the initial injury.

The final stage is characterized by maturation of the collagen into a weave that appears clinically as dark red-pink granulation tissue. This final phase of the healing process occurs over 6 weeks or more.[2,16]

The Neurohormonal Response System

The application of any external stress, such as trauma, triggers a generalized neurohormonal response by the autonomic and endocrine systems that prepares the body to defend itself against an actual or perceived threat to homeostasis. The responses are defensive adaptations which attempt to restore or maintain the normal mechanisms regulating circulatory, metabolic and other processes essential to the maintenance of life and the normal functioning of the human organism in its environment. Sensory input due to trauma results in stimulation of the hypothalamus in the central nervous system and leads to activation of neurohormonal responses which maintain the internal environment of the organisms (Figure 8-1). The magnitude of the chemical, metabolic, and neurological changes which develop and the clinical symptoms which accompany them are determined by the intensity of the trauma and the body's ability to respond to it.

The autonomic system is actually comprised of two interacting divisions, the parasympathetic and sympathetic systems, which innervate the same organs in response to different stimuli from within the internal and external environments (Table 8-2). This interaction allows for a wide range of variations within the environments without adverse effects on the normal functioning of the body.

The parasympathetic system exerts its effect on one organ without disturbing the other organs which it innervates. Generally, its responsibility lies in the domain of internal "housekeeping." That is, it responds to the on-going vegetative (digestion, defecation, urination) or feed-breed activity adjustments during normal daily functioning of the body.

The sympathetic division of the autonomic nervous system, quite unlike the parasympathetic division, acts as the body's first line of defense against stress. When the body is inflicted with any trauma, this division exerts effects which result in simultaneous changes in all organs it innervates. The behavioral responses to stress (fight or flight) have very specific purposes, such as increasing heart rate and blood pressure in the face of blood loss.[27]

When an individual is subjected to a massive trauma, the initiating stimuli which lead to activation of the systemic responses are multiple. Fear, pain, and disruption of regulatory organ functioning all play a part in activating the sympathetic system to

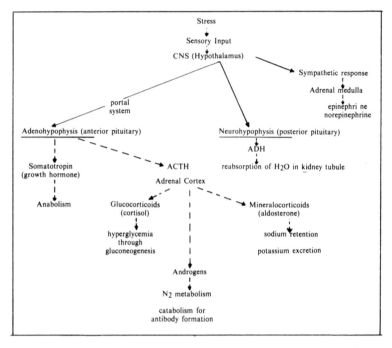

Figure 8-1. Neuro-endocrine response to injury (From the Course Syllabus in Medical-Surgical Nursing, *Frances Payne Bolton* School of Nursing, Case Western Reserve University, Cleveland, Ohio).

defend against the insult and maintain the functional integrity of the body. No stimuli, however, have a greater influence on activation of the system than volume loss or alterations in the blood pH. Acute reductions of total blood volume, which may involve hemorrhage externally or into tissues or hollow viscera such as the abdominal cavity, plasma loss through areas of increased capillary permeability (burns, peritonitis, hypoxic tissue, large areas of damaged tissue), and acute extracellular volume deficiencies all precipitate intense stimulation of the receptor sites of the sympathetic division.

The most obvious result of sympathetic stimulation is secretion of catecholamines (epinephrine and norepinephrine) by the adrenal medulla. The clinical manifestations of sympathetic catecholamine activation are profound skin pallor, tachycardia, sweating, and the absence of cutaneous motor reflexes. Other significant clinical manifestations include the following:

TABLE 8-2

Selected Actions Resulting from Activation of the Sympathetic and Parasympathetic Divisions of the Autonomic Nervous System

Site of Effector Cells	Activation of Sympathetic Division (Thoracolumbar) Tends To:	Activation of Para-Sympathetic Division (Craniosacral) Tends To:
Heart	Increase rate and output	Decrease rate and output
Coronary arteries	Dilate	Dilate
Blood vessels in nose, salivary glands, and pharynx	Constrict	Dilate
Cutaneous vessels	Constrict	
Bronchi	Dilate	Constrict
Gastrointestinal motility and secretion	Decrease peristalsis and muscle tone; constrict sphincters	Increase; relax sphincters
Glycogenolysis by the liver	Increase	
Glands	Decrease secretion	Increase secretion
Sweat glands	Increase (some authorities classify this as parasympathetic function)	
Pupil of eye	Dilate	Constrict
Ciliary muscles	Lessen tone, eyes accommodate to see at a distance	Contract ciliary muscle, eyes accommodate to see near objects
Mental activity	Increase	

1. stimulation of cardiac contractility
2. reduction of venous capacity through venoconstriction
3. increased vasoconstriction in selective areas
4. favoring of transcapillary movement of fluid into the blood (hemodilution)
5. post-traumatic activation of the intrinsic coagulation system and fibrinolysis
6. mobilization of carbohydrate stores and acute hyperglycemia and lactic acidosis

7. lypolysis and mobilization of fatty acids to the blood from blood stores
8. decreased salivation and a fall in gastric acid-peptic secretions
9. decreased motility of the gastrointestinal tract.[24]

The sympathetic responses which occur with major life-threatening situations such as blood loss or alterations in blood pH are directed toward providing adequate perfusion and effective metabolism in areas of the body which are essential to life, such as the brain, heart and lungs. Tissue perfusion and metabolic activity are compromised in all other areas except these and the areas directly affected by the trauma in order to preserve the life of the organism.

Although the autonomic nervous system is essential to the preservation of a patient's life after sustaining an acute trauma, its effects alone will not suffice. The responses of the autonomic system must occur in intricate coordination with those of the endocrine system if the patient is to survive the initial insult and recover from his injuries. Stimuli such as decreased vascular volume, altered fluid and electrolyte balance, and tissue injury lead to activation of the hypothalamus by the central nervous system after acute trauma and precipitate activation of other organs of the endocrine system (see Figure 8-1).

Antidiuretic hormone (ADH) secretion is evoked by stimuli originating in the hypothalamus and traveling via the neurohypophysis or posterior pituitary gland. The afferent stimuli arise from volume receptors in the wall of the left atrium responding to volume depletion which would arise; for example, with hemorrhage following acute trauma. The secretion of ADH causes water, sodium, and chloride retention by the distal renal tubules. This leads to reduced urine formation, which then helps to re-establish a proper relationship between vascular blood volume and increased vascular capacity.

Aldosterone, a major mineralocorticoid, is secreted by the adrenal cortex in response to the corticotrophic hormone (ACTH) and more specifically in response to plasma angiotensin, a precursor of renin, a hormone produced in the juxtaglomerular cells of the renal cortex. Renin production is stimulated in hemorrhagic states when blood pressure falls and circulation to renal cells diminishes or when sodium concentration in the distal tubules declines.[26] Reabsorption of sodium chloride and water from the renal tubules and excretion of potassium in response to aldosterone secretion help to maintain the composition of the extracellular spaces after trauma, when dehydration and hyperkalemia are potentially lethal events.[5] In summary then, ADH and the mineralocorticoid aldosterone together support the circulatory system and maintain electrolyte balance, particularly in the extracellular spaces of the body.

The glucocorticoids of the endocrine system act in every phase of trauma, from its acute onset through convalescence. A number of glucocorticoids (steroid hormones) are also secreted in response to corticotrophin (ACTH) stimulation and activation of the adrenal cortex. The glucocorticoids influence carbohydrate and nitrogen metabolism and suppress ACTH secretion by the anterior pituitary by negative feedback.

Cortisol, one of the major hormones secreted by the adrenal cortex in response to ACTH production, facilitates gluconeogenesis, the process by which glucose is synthesized from protein. This alternate form of glucose production has significant complications in the immediate fasting stages associated with acute trauma. This method of glucose production helps sustain an adequate level of blood glucose, the chief substrate for energy metabolism by the brain. Cortisol also facilitates mobilization and degradation of protein from skeletal muscle, possibly providing essential amino acids for protein synthesis by the liver or by injured tissues during repair. Other significant actions of cortisol in addition to hepatic gluconeogenesis and suppression of protein synthesis in muscle are: (1) stimulation of protein synthesis in the liver; (2) lytic action on lymphocytes and eosinophils; (3) antiallergic and anti-inflammatory actions; (4) influences on the distribution of water across all cell membranes; (5) increased mobilization and utilization of fat; and (6) an influence on cells and synapses of the central nervous system (observed clinically with recovery by improved mood, appetite and weight gain).[24,26,5]

Growth hormone (somatotrophin) production also rises after trauma but its exact mechanism of action varies in the child and the adult. It is known to stimulate anabolism in young animals and pharmacologically can produce positive balances in nitrogen, phosphorus, calcium, potassium and sodium. In the injured adult it may act as a diabetogenic agent. After moderate trauma, insulin plasma levels rise and may remain elevated for several days but the rise appears to be insufficient to counter the insulin antagonizing effects of both growth hormone and the glucocorticoids. This antagonistic action is thought to be an abnormal response by growth hormone to changes in carbohydrate metabolism that occur after trauma and the prolonged starvation state which may accompany profound trauma.[24,26]

Metabolic Response

The primary objectives of the metabolic response are to maintain the stability of the organism, to repair damaged tissue, and to restore the body to its normal composition and activity. Protein, carbohydrate, and fat metabolism are all involved in this response.

Protein Metabolism

Gluconeogenesis, or the formation of glucose from non-carbohydrate sources, is largely confined to the liver. Amino acids derived from proteolysis are the new primary source of glucose by this means, although glycerol from fat is also contributory. It is now believed that this process of glucose formation after injury provides essential carbohydrate intermediates for the purpose of synthesis, including the synthesis of glucose for subsequent oxidation by tissues such as the brain, which cannot utilize fat for fuel.[11]

The process of gluconeogenesis is usually fully activated within 24-36 hours after any significant trauma; at this time increased concentrations of urea and creatinine are usually noted in the urine. The activation of this process appears to be related to the changes which occur with the neurohormonal response to injury. The glucocorticoids also play a permissive role in the gluconeogenic process.[10,18] As mentioned, cortisol facilitates this process in the liver, where glucogenic amino acids (e.g., alanine) are converted into glucose.[26]

Although gluconeogenesis results in the synthesis of protein intermediates needed for glucose production for vital organs, it may contribute in an adverse manner to the ultimate survival of the organism. Gluconeogenesis from protein sources taps a large caloric reserve found largely in lean, peripheral tissue, primarily muscle mass. The extent to which gluconeogenesis has an ultimate detrimental effect on the organism's survival will be dependent upon the type and severity of the trauma, the age, sex, and size of the patient and previous nutritional status.[11] If a patient loses one-third to one-half of the lean tissue (muscle) mass by gluconeogenesis, profound cachexia will develop. This loss of muscle mass affects not only the ability of the patient to perform simple tasks such as eating and ambulating, but also impedes the patient's ability to breathe normally. Because of the catabolism of protein in the respiratory muscles, the patient's ventilation may become impaired. Impaired ventilation may lead to the development of sepsis in the vulnerable lower respiratory tract as well as respiratory failure. Therefore, female patients who are elderly, thin, or debilitated and are subjected to a major, life-threatening trauma of a sustained nature are more susceptible to such complications as respiratory failure than their young, well nourished, male counterparts with a similar trauma.[5]

The pre-traumatic characteristics of the patient such as age and sex may determine to a significant extent whether the patient will develop such complications as respiratory failure secondary to lean tissue loss, but the one variable which must always be considered is the trauma itself. The nature and the extent of the trauma determines, to a great extent, the energy requirements of the body after injury. They, in turn, will determine the amount of body tissue required for fuel and, to some extent, the caloric contribution of lean tissue protein for energy demands. It has been demonstrated that there is a significant increase in resting metabolic expenditure with severe traumas such as multiple fractures (25%) and major burns (50-100%).[19] The clinical significance of this change lies in its persistence over days or weeks. This patient becomes increasingly vulnerable to any mechanism producing shock, because in the face of increased demand for oxygen to the tissues, there is superimposed a decreased transport of oxygen.[11] In this situation, a young male patient who has suffered a major burn may succumb to a respiratory infection because of an inability to meet oxygen demands while an older, more debilitated patient may survive a similar infection if his trauma is less extensive in nature.

Another relevant aspect of the gluconeogenic process and protein catabolism is the relationship to the starvation state. Although glucogenesis and a negative nitrogen balance occur after trauma in the absence of starvation, the starvation state frequently accompanies trauma of an acute nature. Starvation contributes to the alteration of normal metabolism in which protein initially provides glucose for intermediary metabolism and fat ultimately becomes the body's main source of glucose in the absence of dietary sources.[26,17]

It should be emphasized at this point that no single factor alone is responsible for the negative nitrogen balance which occurs after trauma or the clinical manifestations which accompany it. The negative nitrogen state is a reflection of a degree of catabolic imbalance, tissue injury and breakdown, decreased oral intake, and immobilization. Clinical manifestations which persist under these conditions are: weight loss, anorexia, lethargy, tissue breakdown, and impaired healing as well as impaired ventilation and electrolyte imbalance, with associated loss of phosphorus, calcium, potassium, magnesium, and sulphur.[26,5,24,9,13]

One final aspect of altered protein metabolism is that of a marked decrease in serum albumin following trauma. The decrease occurs in spite of the fact that there is a significant increase in the synthesis of all fractions of plasma proteins after trauma.[4] Part of this decrease may be due to the sequestering of albumin at the site of the injury as well as a reduction in the half-life of albumin.[2] Although it is not clearly understood why the reduction in albumin occurs, the very fact that such a reduction does occur has clinical significance. Albumin is largely responsible for the colloidal osmotic pressure of plasma and is essential to the maintenance of vascular volume. When it is sequestered at the site of an injury, whether the injury is at a joint or in the abdominal cavity, its colloidal osmotic properties will result in the accumulation of fluid at the site of the injury. Such accumulations are observed locally as edematous, swollen areas. On the other hand, a significant lack of serum albumin could result in decreased vascular volume and serum osmotic pressure, with signs of generalized edema, decreased urinary output, hypotension, and tachycardia. Such changes may lead to the development of hypovolemic shock.[25,27,5]

Carbohydrate Metabolism

The characteristic rise in blood sugar to a hyperglycemic state after trauma is, in part, felt to be related to gluconeogenesis and the subsequent increase in glucose production. However, this process is unlikely to contribute significantly to the dramatic rise in the blood sugar level which occurs within hours after major, severe trauma.[24]

Normally the blood glucose represents a balance between rate of input and rate of removal. The endocrine system regulates this fine balance largely by altering the secretion of insulin according to the body's needs for both immediate energy and reserve stores of protein and fat. Figure 8-2 indicates the normal major metabolic pathways of the major foodstuffs in the absorptive phase.

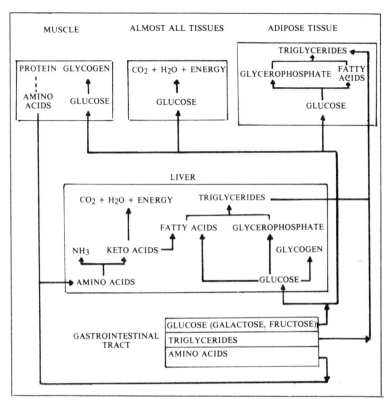

Figure 8-2. Major metabolic pathways of the absorptive phase (From: AJ Vander, et al: *Human Physiology: The Mechanics of Body Function.* 2nd Ed. McGraw-Hill Publishing Co., 1975, p. 407. Used with permission).

Insulin is the chief anabolic hormone. Its secretion in response to increased blood sugar levels in the absorptive phase promotes glycolysis (the breakdown of glucose to pyruvic acid or lactic acid), glycogen synthesis, fatty acid and glyceride synthesis, and protein synthesis.[26] Although there is an increase in insulin secretion after major trauma that corresponds with a rise in the blood sugar levels, the normal response becomes altered to favor catabolic rather than anabolic reactions. Opposing roles in intermediary metabolism appear to arise between insulin on the one hand and the catabolic hormones (adrenalin, cortisol and diabetogenic [growth] hormone) on the other hand.[2,11] Adrenalin probably plays the major opposing role in this response in that it depletes carbohydrate stores and promotes hyperglycemia and lipolysis.[25,26,28] Cortisol, in direct contrast to insulin, supresses glycolysis and stimulates gluconeogenesis and protein breakdown for gluconeogenic purposes. The diabetogenic hormone not only promotes glycogenolysis but inhibits the utilization of glucose by tissues, again in exact contrast to insulin.[24]

Accompanying these changes in carbohydrate metabolism are clinical signs of a hyperosmolarity of body fluids with transient osmotic diuresis, and metabolic acidosis due to increased production of lactic acid, and, to a lesser degree, pyruvic acid. These clinical changes parallel the rise in blood sugar. However, severe lactic acidosis is most commonly noted in severe cases of trauma which are accompanied by shock.[2,24,11] The extreme rise in lactic acid in the presence of shock reflects an alteration in the lactic/pyruvic ratio with lactic acid levels far in excess of pyruvic acid. Such a clinical change is indicative of general tissue hypoxia secondary to poor tissue perfusion, a state in which the body is forced to convert to an anaerobic form of metabolism (Figure 8-3). If shock is allowed to prevail after trauma, hypoglycemia rather than hyperglycemia will develop due to tissue hypoxia and the prevailing lactic acidosis.

Fat Metabolism

Glycogen stored in liver and muscle tissue can be rapidly mobilized to supply energy for a sudden burst of stress such as that occurring with trauma. This anaerobic source of glucose is, however, limited in its usefulness. When glucose is produced in this manner, it becomes incompletely oxidized to lactate, which has limited energy value. In addition, conversion of glycogen to glucose can provide only twelve hours of basal caloric need without further ingestion of basic foodstuffs. Consequently, the glucose needs of the body cannot be met after trauma by this source.[28] The patient must first rely on gluconeogenesis from protein for glucose and ultimately on the large reserve stores of fat.

Fat is the body's most effective, potential source of fuel and serves as a ready source of abundant calories.[7] Just as the catecholamines and cortisol are responsible for mobilization of carbohydrate stores in protein and carbohydrate metabolism after trauma, so too are they responsible for the mobilization of glucose from fat. These hormones either cause or aid in increased triglyceride break-

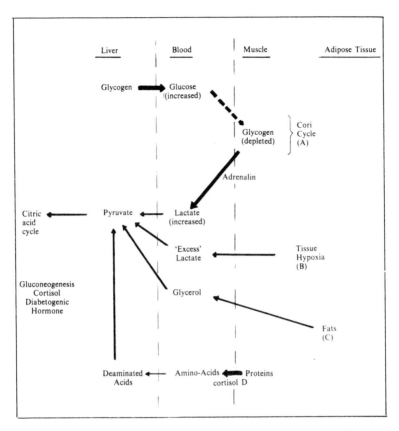

Figure 8-3. Diagrammatic representation of altered carbodydrate metabolism occurring after injury (with heavy arrows indicating probably impaired activity) (From: S Sevitt: *Reaction to Injury and Burns.* J.B. Lippincott, 1977, p. 123. Used with permission).

down, increased concentration of free fatty acids, glycerol and ketone bodies in the blood, accumulation of lipid in the liver, and increased oxidation of fatty acids.[24,25,28] Rises have been noted clinically in triglyceride levels within hours after trauma and in cholesterol and phospholipid levels as well.[24]

Although these changes are noted within hours after trauma, most changes that occur in fat metabolism appear to be closely related to the catabolic, starvation state which follows severe, extensive trauma. Any clinician who has cared for the acutely ill trauma patient is familiar with the trauma-associated catabolic effects of injury and starvation. These patients classically appear cachexic with the muscle wasting of severe illness, poor wound healing, increased susceptibility to skin breakdown, weakened respiratory muscles, inadequate clearing of secretions, and pneumonia.[25]

A starvation state will develop within 24 hours without food. In this state, the patient's body will revert almost entirely to fat as the primary source of fuel for the body, including the brain. Without this source of fuel, the brain alone could deplete one-third of the total protein stores in a healthy person after only three weeks of fasting. These same protein stores would be depleted at an astounding rate in the face of total body needs in an injured patient.[25]

The presence of this catabolic starvation state leads to the breakdown of fats to keto-acids to be used instead of glucose in order to spare nitrogen, and thus, protein.[7] The brain, as well as the rest of the body, will adapt to this ketotic state; as long as the stores of fatty acids in adipose tissue are adequate, the patient can survive, and life threatening protein loss may be minimized. In fact, with prolonged starvation, ketoacidosis, which is usually an abnormal state, becomes essential. A moderate, compensated form of this metabolic acidosis will exist with total bicarbonate concentrations as low as 17 to 18 mEq. per liter.[25]

It must be pointed out that even while the acutely ill trauma patient is receiving glucose infusions, he/she may still exist in a catabolic-starvation state. One of the greatest problems in the care of the acute trauma patient, for several reasons, is nutrition. In the acute phase, the catabolic hormones (especially the catecholamines) inhibit normal digestion of complex foods due to their direct action on the gastrointestinal tract. Therefore, oral feedings are prohibited.

Secondly, trauma creates a set of unique problems because of altered utilization of glucose. Intravenous infusion of glucose will not significantly alter protein catabolism. Increased insulin resistance is so marked that even increased concentrations of exogenous glucose cannot be effectively utilized by the body.[7] The excessive secretion of the catabolic hormones not only increases insulin resistance, but also causes cellular redistribution of sodium, potassium, and water, thus leading to hyperglycemia, hyponatremia, and sodium retention and excessive excretion of potassium and nitrogen in the cell. To effectively counterbalance the catabolic hormones, the acutely ill patient may be given large concentrations of glucose supplemented with potassium and insulin,which is administered either as continuous infusion or subcutaneously in divided doses determined by the blood sugar level.[24] Given effectively, such therapy may aid in reversing the effects of the catabolic hormones and result in a general improvement in the clinical status of the patient. The patient's blood pressure and pulse may stabilize and he may appear more alert, active, and involved with his environment. Metabolic and electrolyte parameters will improve. Laboratory and clinical data will reflect an increased secretion of sodium and water from the cell, and a rise in plasma sodium level, a decrease in potassium and nitrogen excretion and a restoration of vascular volume.[24]

The changes in fat metabolism, as well as those in protein and carbohydrate metabolism, serve to meet the body's need for maximal energy output over a sustained period of time. Although they are essential to the preservation of life, they are not without adverse consequences for the patient.

Pathological Sequelae

The neurohormonal responses of the acute phase of trauma, in addition to creating the previously described hazards to the patient, may cause other complications as well. These complications arise because of limitations in the body's homeostatic adaptation and defense mechanisms. Among these may be:

1. necrosis of tissue and increased heart load following prolonged vasoconstriction and decreased tissue perfusion.
2. degeneration or renal tubular necrosis with possible renal failure following renal vasospasm
3. increased internal body temperature causing increased metabolism with vasoconstriction of the skin to prevent heat loss
4. diminished lung perfusion with CO_2 retention and a hyperventilatory response to blood loss following the fall in cardiac output and redistribution of the systemic circulation
5. decreased oxygen-carrying capacity of blood due to decreased hemoglobin concentration
6. severe hypertension secondary to prolonged and excessive secretion of adrenalin

7. altered homeostasis between coagulation and fibrinolysis, leading to the appearance of disseminated intravascular coagulation.[24,2,5]

Another pathological sequela which should always be considered after trauma with fracturing of bone is pulmonary fat embolism. Pulmonary fat embolism usually occurs within 24 hours after the trauma and represents a potentially lethal event for the patient. Such emboli are thought to arise from the release of fat droplets into the circulation from the marrow of long bone.

Because of the persistent threat of pulmonary fat embolism, any patient who has suffered a fracture should not be subjected to unnecessary handling which may increase the possibility of such a complication. They should also be observed closely for such signs and symptoms as mild apprehension or agitation, altered consciousness, shortness of breath accompanied by pallor, cyanosis and tachycardia, and most specifically, petechial hemorrhages of the chest and conjunctiva. This last sign is a classic occurrence in the presence of pulmonary fat embolism.[12]

NURSING CARE OF THE TRAUMA PATIENT

In order to prevent or deal with the pathological sequelae which may develop after an individual has been subjected to trauma, it is essential that nursing care be organized into an effective plan of action which reflects insight and understanding of all of the trauma patient's problems, both existing and potential. The need for such a plan cannot be overemphasized. The trauma patient requires intense monitoring and highly skilled, coordinated care if he is to survive and potentially lethal or crippling complications are to be prevented. For example, a young healthy seventeen-year-old male who suffered a fractured leg and pelvis and internal hemorrhage after an auto accident developed acute renal failure only 24 hours after the accident. Although the initial injury would not be considered as acute as a severe multiple trauma involving vital organ systems, the threat to full recovery is equal. A comprehensive understanding of the pathophysiology of trauma is essential. Excessive blood loss, with hypotension and the super-imposed effects of the cholinergic drugs, predisposes the trauma patient to acute renal failure. An awareness of the potential for this complication as well as an understanding of the signs and symptoms of acute renal failure can contribute significantly to the institution of nursing measures which may help prevent or minimize the effects of such a complication.

As noted previously, comprehensive care must be instituted immediately in the acute phase of trauma and must reflect the nurse's awareness of the multiple potential problems which the trauma patient may develop. The key note should always be to anticipate potential problems and prevent their development. This means monitoring of all physiological parameters with continuous ongoing systematic assessment. The importance of continuous assessment will be illustrated in the following pages utilizing a case study of an acutely ill multiple trauma patient. The objective of the discussion of this patient's care is to illustrate the problems, needs and nursing care requirements of the trauma patient in each stage of the illness experience. Because the ICU nurse is most often involved in providing care during the acute period, the emphasis in the discussion will be on this phase. The later phases of recovery will be summarized, however, in order to illustrate the necessity for early planning of measures to assist the patient with all aspects of his/her illness.

PATIENT CARE STUDY

Phase I—The Acute Phase

Mrs. Smith was a 45-year-old black woman, a divorcee, and mother of three children, ranging from 2 to 26 years of age. She had been employed in several types of manual jobs, including domestic and factory work. At the time of her accident, she had been unemployed and had received welfare assistance for almost eight months.

Mrs. Smith was the victim of a hit-and-run accident. Prior to her accident, she had been in relatively good health with the exceptions of slight obesity and mild hypertension. After the accident she was taken to the emergency room of a large medical center where she was diagnosed as having the following injuries: a small right subdural hematoma, concussion, cephalohematoma, multiple lacerations of the face and hips, ruptured bladder, contusion of the right lung, large contusion of the right hip, and multiple fractures (right clavical, right scapula, sacrum, lumbar vertebrae 3 and 4, subcapital fracture of the right femur, bilateral fractures of the inferior and superior pubic rami, compound trimalleolar fractures of the right ankle, and compound bimalleolar fractures of the left ankle). While in the emergency room, Mrs. Smith had a grand mal seizure and was noted to be in hypovolemic shock.

Question: In light of the data presented and knowledge of the pathophysiology of trauma, what might be the anticipated clinical findings on a patient such as this? Also, what immediate problems and needs of such a patient would be expected?

Discussion: In response to the first question, the presenting diagnoses alone should suggest that the patient's condition would be critical. It should also be expected that the patient's basic homeostatic balance would be grossly altered and that all physiological parameters would be in a constant state of fluctuation due to both the multiple severe injuries and the body's attempt to defend against these massive insults. The patient's prior physical status was relatively normal; however, her chances of surviving the acute trauma could have been affected by the fact that she was a middle-aged, overweight, slightly hypertensive female.

Because of the complex nature of Mrs. Smith's injuries, it would be unwise to attempt to consider her clinical findings only in terms of her specific injuries. Doing so in the critical care setting often leads to an overwhelming intellectual exercise or isolation of specific problems without consideration of their relationship to other problems. A systematic, methodical approach is essential. Make a mental assessment of the patient clinically, from head to toe and system by system. As this is done, it should become easier to assess the clinical findings and predict the effects of a single injury in one system on the functioning of any other system.

General

First, visualize the general appearance of the patient, given the available data. One would expect a great deal of swelling and bruising of the head and right side of the body from the description of the injuries. Because the patient was in hypovolemic shock, one would also expect that the patient would appear pale and that the skin would be cool and diaphoretic. In fact, Mrs. Smith had such excessive swelling of the face and head that normal features were distorted. There was a 4-6 cm. hematoma on the forehead with blackening of both eyes. Swelling and extensive bruising were also noted from the midchest, progressing up the right shoulder and arm and down to the right aspect of the thorax along the border of the diaphragm. There was also extensive edema in all extremities with a large contusion encompassing the entire right hip. The bed sheets were soaked from the patient's profuse diaphoresis.

Neurological

The severe trauma to the head along with hypoxia and severe metabolic disturbances which accompany hypovolemic shock probably contributed to the seizure the patient had in the emergency room. Such insults to the nervous system would significantly alter normal neurological functioning. One would expect that the patient would be at least somnolent, or more probably comatose. Normal reflexes might also be altered. In fact, the patient was in a deep coma and responsive only to deep pain. Other neurological findings included equally light reactive pupils, intact dolls' eyes, and spontaneous movement of the upper and lower extremities.

Respiratory

Again, if one evaluates the clinical findings of the respiratory system, the expectation would be that the lung contusion and hypovolemic shock would alter the functioning of this system. Both ventilation and perfusion might be expected to be *drastically* altered. Chest wall instability should also be considered.

Patients such as Mrs. Smith usually present with severe respiratory distress and she was no exception. Her respirations were rapid, shallow and extremely labored with intercostal retracting and nasal flare. There was no paradoxical movement of the chest wall. Hypoxia was severe and the patient had markedly diminished breath sounds on the right side as well as crepitant rales and scattered wheezing throughout. These findings are consistent with a contusion of the right lung. Admission arterial blood gases with a pH of 7.31, pCO_2 of 35, pO_2 of 68, HCO_3- of 18 and a base deficit of -8 on 50% oxygen indicated mixed respiratory and metabolic acidosis with hypoxia. This too should be expected in light of the lung trauma sustained, severe blood loss, and the poor tissue perfusion accompanying such an extensive trauma.

Cardiovascular

In the presence of hypovolemia of an acute nature and severe tissue injury, the cardiovascular system becomes severely taxed. The neurohormonal response should increase stroke volume and vascular perfusion and thus aid oxygenation to both injured tissues and vital organs. If the system is effective in the initial response to the blood loss it will be reflected in a rising diastolic pressure and a relatively normal systolic pressure. However, continued blood loss taxes the normal defenses of the body to the point that intense vasoconstriction and increased cardiac output cannot compensate for the increasing deficit. If it becomes increasingly difficult to hear the Korotkoff sounds, stroke volume is probably falling.[29]

Mrs. Smith remained in hypovolemic shock; this fact suggests that the patient probably was continuing to bleed and circulation to the tissues was inadequate. The presence of metabolic acidosis confirms this. It should, therefore, be anticipated that the combined effects of the neurohormonal response and hemorrhage would be manifested clinically by cyanosis, a rapid pulse, marked lowering of both the systolic and diastolic pressure, distant heart sounds, and faint or absent peripheral pulses.

Mrs. Smith had all of these clinical findings. Her lips and nail beds were slightly dusky. She had a rapid, thready pulse with a rate of 130-150/minute. The heart sounds were distant and difficult to hear. The blood pressure was labile and also difficult to hear. It ranged from 100/60 to 70 mm. systolic by palpation. The patient did continue to have internal bleeding. Initially she received 4 units of blood and this figure eventually increased to a total of 20 units, as her hematocrit continued to fall.

Gastrointestinal

Although the admission diagnosis did not reveal any damage to the gastrointestinal tract, gastric motility could be expected to be severely impaired. As discussed earlier, sympathetic stimulation decreases salivation, diminishes gastric acid and peptic acid secretion and slows the motility of the gastrointestinal tract. Hemorrhaging from the bladder also would be expected to interfere with normal digestion by creating peritoneal irritation, thus altering normal functioning of the gastrointestinal tract.

One of the earliest clinical manifestations of these changes would be the finding of decreased or absent bowel sounds. Gastrointestinal contents pool and a paralytic ileus usually develops, resulting in abdominal distension and, not infrequently, vomiting. In Mrs. Smith's case one might also expect to find blood in the gastrointestinal tract for several reasons. She may have swallowed blood from the trauma to the face and head or from the irritation associated with nasogastric and endotracheal tubes, placed on admission. She might also develop active intra-abdominal bleeding due to physiological stress, trauma, or both. Abdominal tenderness and guarding should also be expected due to the ruptured bladder.

Mrs. Smith did have severe abdominal distension that continued to increase after admission. In addition, there was marked rebound tenderness in the lower abdomen. Bowel sounds were absent and remained so for several days. Nasogastric contents were dark brown and were significantly positive for blood for approximately 48 hours.

Renal

Evaluating expected clinical findings of the renal system would be complicated because the patient was known to have a ruptured bladder. If extensive bleeding existed, urinary output could be altered due to obstruction from clots. One would again anticipate abdominal distension, tenderness, and possible persistent pain due to spasms as the bladder attempts to contract and expel clots. Urinary output would be grossly bloody if the rupture were significant. It would not be possible to determine urine volume or urine electrolytes in the presence of active bleeding, and kidney function, i.e., urine formation, would be difficult to evaluate at this time. She had a tight, distended abdomen. When the lower abdomen was palpated, she responded with grimacing and mild agitation. There was continuous expulsion of clots both around and through the Foley catheter that was inserted on admission. The bleeding did not clear with continuous irrigation; rather, it increased until surgical intervention the following day.

Musculoskeletal

Anticipating the clinical findings of the musculoskeletal system would also be difficult. The patient had spontaneous movement of all extremities on admission to the emergency room. However, with the extent of the fractures sustained, Mrs. Smith would undergo surgery for stabilization and casting prior to admission to the Intensive Care Unit. As a result of the continued progression of the inflammatory process and surgical manipulation, swelling, bleeding in the tissues and joints, and limited tissue perfusion would alter the clinical findings.

Following this line of thinking, one would expect to find diminished sensation, tone and mobility, especially in the lower extremities. This should be true because of injury to the system, altered neurological status, and limitation of movement due to casting and traction.

Mrs. Smith lacked both sensation to pain and spontaneous movement in the right leg and had diminished sensation in the left leg. The response to painful stimulus in the upper extremities was equal, with withdrawal to painful stimuli. Tone was also diminished although spontaneous movement was noted occasionally in the left hand and arm. The deficits in Ms. Smith's lower extremities persisted for several weeks. Her mobility was limited for a month due to her pelvic fractures and muscle tone diminished extensively in all extremities.

Question: Given the available data, now consider the patient's problems and needs. What nursing interventions would be necessary to meet the patient's needs and to help resolve her problems? The nursing plan of care should reflect insight into not only existing problems but also problems that may evolve.

The nature of Mrs. Smith's injuries precipitated numerous, complex, interrelated health problems. Because of the number and the magnitude of the problems which evolved after her admission, future discussion will be limited to three major problem areas: the neurological, respiratory, and gastrointestinal systems.

Discussion—*Neurological:* Mrs. Smith's problem in this area may be defined as an altered state of consciousness. On admission, she presented in a deep coma and was responsive only to deep painful stimuli. The problem could have been due to the small right subdural hematoma, the concussion, the severe hypoxia and metabolic disarrangement that evolved secondary to hypovolemia and trauma, or the combination of all these variables. Although all of these variables certainly contributed to the patient's altered state of consciousness, hypoxia appears, in retrospect, to have contributed most significantly to the problem. As the patient's tissue oxygenation improved, so too did her level of consciousness. This examplifies the importance of evaluating all clinical findings in light of the patient's total injury rather than in isolation.

At the time of admission, one should not exclude any variables which could have contributory effects on the problem. The basic objectives of care should be to: (1) maintain and support normal body functioning for the patient; (2) to identify and eliminate the cause of the problem; and (3) to prevent complications which delay or prevent full recovery from the trauma.

All nursing interventions should be directed toward meeting the clinical objectives from the outset of the patient's admission to the intensive care setting. It goes without saying that improving the patient's ventilation and perfusion would be essential to improvement of her neurological status. Vital signs, neurological signs, arterial blood gases, and blood electrolytes should all be monitored frequently in an effort to find the source of the problem and to prevent the development of further neurological complications.

A flow sheet should be kept with vital signs and neurological signs monitored every hour, half-hour or more frequently if necessary. Such documentation reflects the relationship among changes in all monitored physiological parameters. Many Intensive Care Units utilize additional flow sheet check lists for neurological assessment. Such sheets provide an exact, continuous means of reporting objective observations and become an important source of documented clinical change. These sheets may include data such as: neurological response to sensations such as pain, touch, and voice; the presence or absence of normal reflexes; the presence and degree of purposeful movement and nonpurposeful movement; types of posturing; response to commands (e.g., consistently, occasionally, never); orientation to the environment; and a description of seizure activity.

It is important to document not only serial observations on a patient such as Mrs. Smith, but to be cognizant of the significance of changes in parameters. For example, a fixed dilated pupil in the presence of a slowing pulse, widening pulse pressure and constantly fluctuating temperature may indicate increased intracranical pressure. Such changes must always be reported immediately when observed. If the intracranial pressure is rising and is not reduced within 15 to 60 minutes, irreversible brain damage or death may ensue.[20]

This type of patient should also be observed for bleeding from the ears and nose and for ocular hemorrhage. Bleeding from such areas is indicative of further intracranial hemorrhage. Drainage of clear fluid from the nose (rhinorrhea) may be due to leakage of cerebrospinal fluid from a fracture through the cribriform plate and should, therefore, be reported without delay.[15]

A temperature elevation cannot be overlooked in a patient with a head injury. An elevated temperature increases cerebral irritation and may precipitate seizure activity. If an elevation occurs, the physician should be notified and medication ordered to prevent further rising. Remember, however, that the trauma patient is also susceptible to the development of stress ulcers. Therefore, medication such as aspirin should be avoided. If medication alone does not alter the rise, hypothermia should be instituted. The goal should be to maintain the patient's temperature at or near normal (37°C or 98.6°F).

The unconscious trauma patient is unable to regulate and control most aspects of normal body functioning. It thus becomes the nurse's responsibility to meet all basic ongoing needs such as bathing, oral hygiene, and activity to maintain muscle tone. Attention to the basic nursing arts is essential in the care of the acute trauma patient. Negligence in this basic area of nursing may contribute to the development of life-threatening infections and debilitating tissue breakdown.

For patients such as Mrs. Smith, nursing care which will maintain normal body functioning must be consistent and complete. Mrs. Smith received complete baths daily and skin lubrication with lotion. During the bath and during position changes the skin was checked for pressure areas and developing abrasions.

The patient's nails were kept cleaned and trimmed to prevent scratching and contamination of open wounds. Rings were also removed to prevent the patient from lacerating herself. Mrs. Smith's hair was washed weekly and combed and braided each shift to prevent matting and diminish circulation to the scalp, especially the back of the head.

Protective eye care was also instituted to prevent corneal damage. This care included sterile saline irrigations every four hours, application of eye lubricants, and the use of a protective eye shield. This was instituted because, while unconscious, Mrs. Smith's eyes remained open and edematous. Her cornea became dried and inflamed. When corneal irritation occurs in patients such as this, taping and eye patches should be avoided. These often do not effectively close the eyes and may cause further damage due to their abrasive nature.

Feminine hygiene can also become a persistent problem with trauma patients such as Mrs. Smith. Perineal care should be done daily or more frequently if necessary. Such patients often develop vaginal fungal infections after long-term antibiotic therapy. These infections arise due to alterations in the normal flora of the vagina. The presence of a foul-smelling, cheesy vaginal discharge should alert the nurse to the presence of such an infection. Treatment should then include vaginal irrigations on a daily basis and the use of antifungal vaginal suppositories.

Although Mrs. Smith's mobility was limited by her injuries and the casting and traction, safety measures were necessary to prevent further injury due to seizures or unconscious movement. Her siderails were kept up and padded. She was checked for dentures and a loose tooth was pulled to prevent airway obstruction. An oral airway was inserted along with an oral endotracheal tube to prevent the patient from biting her tongue and to assure adequate ventilation. Intravenous infusion sites were secured and daily sterile cleansing and dressing changes were done of all indwelling catheter sites to prevent injury and infection.

Because the unconscious patient is unable to respond to excessive changes in heat or cold, all external sources effecting significant temperature change should be used with discretion. External sources of heat and cold (e.g., heating pads, heat lamps, hypothermia blankets) were used with caution in order to avoid injury to the skin. Also, all casts and dressings were checked each shift to insure adequate circulation and prevent the development of pressure areas and lacerations. Restraints were used only when absolutely necessary and were checked frequently each shift and padded extensively when used.

Positioning and exercise posed a severe nursing problem in Mrs. Smith's unconscious state. Ideally, nursing care in such a patient should include turning and positioning every two hours or more frequently. Passive range of motion exercises, performed hourly, should also be a routine procedure. However, Mrs. Smith's fractured pelvis and legs made such procedures impossible.

Mrs. Smith was placed immediately on an alternating air mattress to decrease the risk of tissue ischemia and prevent decubitus ulcer formation. When the traction was released on the left leg, passive range of motion exercises were then done hourly. Leg positioning was maintained and checked frequently. Because of the weight of the cast and the patient's unconscious state, her left leg became increasingly rotated in an external abducted position and had to be constantly supported with pillows. Foot drop was prevented by the cast, but some degree of contracture became unavoidable for the same reason.

An individually designed and molded brace was made to support Mrs. Smith's left wrist and hand. Such molds should be used with the unconscious patient to prevent wrist drop and forward drop of the thumb. The brace was removed every four hours from the hand, and exercises of the wrist and fingers done to prevent contractures and maintain muscle tone.

Moving the unconscious patient requires adequate support of the head and extremities because of the patient's inability to support himself. To prevent falling or dislocation of a limb, adequate help should be available. Mrs. Smith was moved only when necessary to check her skin and to change her linen. This was done once a shift. Other movement was avoided to prevent embolism and further injury to her pelvic and leg fractures.

When Mrs. Smith was moved, seven people were required. The patient was lifted as a single unit. While being held off the bed, her sheets were changed by pulling the sheet through from the top to the bottom of the bed. While being held, the patient's back, buttocks, legs, and arms were checked for pressure areas and the skin massaged with lotion. This procedure prevented the development of pressure areas and decubitus ulceration.

Maintaining adequate nutrition and elimination also exist as potential problems in the unconscious, acutely ill, trauma patient. Mrs. Smith developed a severe problem due to malnutrition. This problem will be discussed at an appropriate point later in the chapter as will her problem with elimination. It is noted here only to emphasize the effect of alteration of one system on the normal functioning of other systems.

Another point which too often is overlooked in caring for the comatose patient in the Intensive Care Unit is that hearing is the last sensory response a patient loses. Dialogue regarding the patient's condition should never be carried on at the patient's bedside. Every effort should be made to communicate with the patient whether the patient responds to the verbal stimulus or not. The family should also interact with the patient on a consistent basis. Often patients will begin to respond to their families before responding to members of the staff.

Families also require support to deal with the stress of an acutely ill family member. In acute trauma cases such as Mrs. Smith's, the family may be devastated by the patient's appearance and lack of responsiveness. They often, after seeing the patient for the first time, fear the worst. Because of this, families should be prepared for what they will see. It should be explained that the swelling, bruising and distortion of normal appearance are temporary. Families also need honest, clear appraisals of the patient's condition on a consistent basis. They benefit from having their questions answered simply, in terms they can understand. Families may ask the same question repeatedly, and repeatedly need to hear the same answer. This is often because the devastating shock of the situation hinders internalization of the responses being given to their questions. Such support can contribute greatly in minimizing stress for the patient's family during the acute phase of the patient's illness.

Respiratory

It may be recalled that on admission to the hospital, Mrs. Smith presented with severe respiratory distress with marked hypoxia and a metabolic acidosis. Initially, the problem was defined as respiratory insufficiency due to hypovolemic shock, a contusion of the right lung, and severe metabolic disturbance. The problem did not resolve with initial treatment and within twenty-four hours profound respiratory failure secondary to adult respiratory distress syndrome developed.

Adult respiratory distress syndrome, or shock lung, as it is commonly defined, is a frequently occurring phenomenon after acute trauma or any acute insult to the body. The syndrome was first clearly defined during the Second World War by Brewer as the "post-traumatic wet lung syndrome."[6] It has been classically described clinically by diffuse haziness of the lungs (the wet snow storm) on x-ray, with diffuse rales and rhonchi, and hypoxia. When shock lung occurs, there is a loss of compliance due to exudated plasma, and an interference with surfactant function.[8] Until the advent of contemporary treatment such as the volume respirator and hemodynamic monitoring, the patient with respiratory failure due to shock lung often died.

In Mrs. Smith's case, profound respiratory failure posed the greatest consistent threat to her life during the acute phase of her illness. Her symptoms were classic in nature. The patient had, by x-ray, a massive, hazy infiltrative process in the right lung with increasing infiltrates in the left lung. Without supportive mechanical ventilation her respirations were grossly inadequate. Her breath sounds were almost inaudible with fine rales and rhonchi throughout and tight wheezing in the upper lobes on expiration. Even with the assistance of the MA-1 respirator at 20 cm. of PEEP, the patient was hypoxic with a partially compensated metabolic acidosis (pH = 7.36; CO_2 = 29; PO_2 = 56; HCO_3^- = 18.5; Base deficit = -8), probably evolving as a result of several predisposing factors. As in the case of the patient's other problems, the evolution of this problem was due, in part, to alterations in the functioning of other systems and the body as a whole. The most significant predisposing factors to the respiratory failure were the contusion of the right lung, hypovolemic shock, and generalized trauma. Pulmonary damage probably occurred during the initial hypotensive episode when there was diminished perfusion in the lungs. This slowing of blood flow may have allowed stasis and clotting in the pulmonary vessels. Polymorphonuclear leukocytes could then, according to present theory, accumulate and release lysosomes which damage or destroy the lung cells.[21]

When such injury occurs, the cells of the lungs and other vital organs do not receive adequate oxygenation and damage to the cells may result. This plus the accumulation of metabolites due to inadequate perfusion and exchange further damages cells and cell membranes. In addition to these factors, the patient's lung tissue could also have been damaged by the metabolites and other toxic materials accumulated when receiving massive blood transfusions. Thus, these predisposing factors plus the impaired lung function from the contusion probably precipitated the shock lung process and the subsequent respiratory failure.

The main objectives of care for the trauma patient with acute respiratory failure should be: (1) support the patient's respiratory system (i.e., appropriate use of mechanical ventilation); (2) institute necessary measures to improve the patient's ventilation and perfusion; (3) prevent complications which may further impair respiratory functioning; (4) eliminate causes of the problem; and (5) provide emotional support for the patient during a period of intense crisis.

Patients such as Mrs. Smith require detailed observation and assessment of all physiological parameters. This is as important in the area of respiratory failure as it was in the area of altered neurological functioning. Documentation of the rate, depth and quality of ventilation should be noted on an hourly basis. It is essential that the nurse also be aware of the significance of changes in the patient's respiratory status. For example, the sudden absence of breath sounds in the left lung field may be due to alterations in the placement of an endotracheal tube. It could, however, also be due to a pneumothorax caused by rupturing of an alveolus with high positive end expiratory pressures (PEEP) used with mechanical ventilation.

Care of a patient such as Mrs. Smith also requires in-depth understanding of respiratory physiology and the use of mechanical ventilation. In such cases, the patient will always require supportive ventilation with a volume respiratory and the use of PEEP. Although such equipment has provided a life-saving means of supporting a patient's respiratory system, it is not without its hazards. Artificial ventilation cannot replace normal, physiological ventilation. The warm, moist environment in the ventilation system is conducive to rapid proliferation of any bacteria in the machine or patient. The patient may also become increasingly dependent on artificial ventilation both physically and emotionally.

Endotrachial tubes provide a patent airway and an easy means for clearing excessive secretions. However, they are also irritating and uncomfortable for patients and may cause severe tracheal damage. Finally, they significantly impair normal communication, and may create frustration and despair for the patient. The nurse caring for an intubated patient should be fully aware of both the benefits and hazards of using respiratory equipment and take appropriate interventions to prevent complications associated not only with the disease but with its treatment.

Mrs. Smith's respiratory failure was accompanied by cardiovascular compromise; continuous monitoring of blood pressure, heart rate and rhythm, central venous pressure, pulmonary artery pressure, cardiac output, urine output and serial blood gases and electrolytes was required. The reader is directed to the chapters on the care of the critically ill patient with respiratory and cardiac disorders for further study of the intricate relationship of these parameters.

Nutrition

Mrs. Smith had a persistent problem with respiratory insufficiency throughout the acute phase of her illness. She developed pneumonia during the first week of her illness and this persisted for several weeks. In part, the problem of malnutrition with negative nitrogen balance contributed to the persistence of this problem. As was noted earlier, protein wasting of skeletal muscle tissue of the thorax may result in diminished muscle strength for breathing. This loss of muscle strength further impedes an already compromised respiratory system, thus contributing to ineffective ventilation, the accumulation of secretions and atelectasis, and the development of pneumonia. In terms of threatening ultimate survival of the acute trauma patient, the problem of severe malnutrition has no equal.

It may be recalled that shortly after a major trauma is inflicted on the body, normal metabolism is altered. The cholinergic responses to trauma act to impede the normal, ongoing vegetative processes of the body. Activity in the gastrointestinal tract is reduced to a minimum and the patient presents clinically with diminished or absent bowel sounds, anorexia, and possible vomiting. As long as the stress of trauma exists, these clinical findings will persist.

The neurohormonal response to trauma and the gastrointestinal disturbances which accompany it alter normal metabolism with first protein and later fat becoming the primary source of fuel for essential cellular activities. The trauma patient's situation is different, however, from other types of malnutrition. This patient's metabolism is unique because of the presence of insulin resistance. The problems, therefore, become two-fold. First the patient lacks both the means and desire to take in normal nutrients and secondly, his body is forced to rely on increasingly limited sources of endogenous nutrients.

Although such alterations in digestion and metabolism are essential for initial survival of the patient, they create severe potentially lethal problems the longer they exist. Pneumonia is an example of only one of the many potential problems which may arise as a result of this malnutrition state.

Mrs. Smith exhibited many of the classical signs and symptoms of a patient with such alterations in digestion and metabolism due to trauma. At various times during the acute phase of trauma the patient had many of the commonly observed electrolyte disturbances noted after trauma. Initially, she had a severe metabolic acidosis. This state persisted in a compensated form for 3-4 days. At one point her bicarbonate level dropped as low as 19. She also developed hyponatremia and mild hypokalemia, both of which were effectively treated with potassium supplements, intravenous infusions, and meticulous monitoring of both blood and urine electrolytes and intake and output. Mrs. Smith also had hyperglycemia on admission with a blood sugar of 320. As expected, this hyperglycemic state persisted for approximately 48 hours.

The most significant indicators of Mrs. Smith's poor nutritional status and negative nitrogen balance were manifested clinically as she progressed towards the end of the acute phase of the trauma. Initially, the problem was compounded by the fact that the patient was also unconscious and intubated. Her weight dropped from 128.9 kg. on admission to 118 kg. after one week of hospitalization. As time passed, her appearance became more cachexic and muscle wasting was marked.

Although Mrs. Smith was awake, alert, and extubated within two weeks after her admission, her nutritional status continued to be a problem throughout her hospitalization. Initially, she could not eat because of a persistent paralytic ileus. A nasogastric tube had to be reinserted on at least two different occasions. It was finally left in place for two weeks after resolution of the paralytic ileus because of the patient's severe anorexia. During this time, the patient demonstrated little interest in either eating or her environment. She complained of feeling weak and tired. Soon thereafter she developed ulcerations on her lips and upper palate and refused almost all foods offered her.

In the case of patients such as Mrs. Smith, the question becomes, how can the pattern be reversed? The more the patient's body is forced to rely upon endogenous stores for nutrition, the greater will be the chances that complications will evolve. Therefore, in caring for a patient such as this, the objectives of nursing care should be focused on: (1) providing adequate external sources of nutrition for the patient; (2) preventing potential complications of malnutrition; and (3) providing the patient with emotional support during this most trying period.

During the acute phase, the patient must receive parenteral nutrition to survive because the energy requirements needed to deal with multiple acute injuries exceed available endogenous resources. Hyperalimentation infusions, a combined solution of hypertonic glucose plus amino acids and polypeptides, are given intravenously to promote anabolism and achieve tissue synthesis.

Hyperalimentation has provided an invaluable means of meeting the critically ill trauma patient's nutritional needs. It does, however, create the potential for life-threatening problems. Infection has become the primary complication from this form of therapy. The infusion of this complex glucose solution into a major vein (usually the subclavian) provides a perfect medium for bacterial growth. This can occur through contamination of the catheter on insertion, seeding from blood-borne bacteria, or contamination of the fluid. To prevent this complication, meticulous aseptic technique should be used in every aspect of care. In Mrs. Smith's case, this complication was avoided. The solution was prepared under sterile conditions in a laminar flow room, by the pharmacy. No additional drugs were added to the solution on the division. The indwelling subclavian line was also inserted under strict sterile conditions in the operating room. Cultures of the puncture wound and intravenous tubing were done every other day and the infusion site was changed within two weeks.

The use of aseptic technique in the insertion and care of hyperalimentation lines cannot be overemphasized. Although techniques may vary from hospital to hospital, it is strongly recommended that the nurse change the dressing every 48 hours, and that she gown, glove, and mask while doing the procedure. The skin should be thoroughly cleaned with an antiseptic solution such as povidone-iodine solution and an antibiotic ointment applied at the insertion site. A sterile dressing should then be applied securely to prevent air and moisture contamination. The date of insertion of the catheter should be noted and the date of the dressing change written on the dressing to insure a consistent schedule of dressing changes.

A second complication of hyperalimentation infusion is acute hyperglycemia due to rapid infusion of the solution. Because this may precipitate acidosis, regulation of the infusion must be exact.

Many institutions now use infusion pumps to administer such solutions. Whether the infusion is regulated manually or by pump, the rate of infusion should be checked on an hourly basis to prevent an excessive rapid infusion and subsequent hyperglycemia, acidosis, and a hyperosmolar state from occurring.

Patients who have such lines inserted should also be monitored for respiratory complications. Accidental perforation of the pleura may occur when the catheter is inserted, allowing fluid to enter the chest cavity and a pneumothorax to develop.

Air in the infusion line always presents a potential threat. Air may be sucked into the vena cava during a tubing change because of the volume and pressure changes in the thoracic cavity which occur with breathing. To prevent a large bolus of air from entering, the patient should either be placed in a slight Trendelenberg position when the tubing is opened or the patient should be asked to perform the Valsalva maneuver, which will increase intrathoracic pressure.[20]

It is important to note that although parenteral alimentation is an effective means of providing temporary nutritional supplements for acutely ill patients, its effectiveness in long-term therapy is limited. Too often patients develop sepsis even with the use of aseptic technique or have to have the insertion site changed so frequently that finding adequate new sites becomes impossible. In such cases, reversing the catabolic state becomes extremely difficult. The patient becomes increasingly vulnerable to the complications of malnutrition and may succumb to a complication such as pneumonia or sepsis if protein loss becomes excessive.

Mrs. Smith could not eat because of the ulcerations in her mouth, anorexia, and persistent difficulties with diminished gastrointestinal motility. She did not, however, succumb to the complications of malnutrition, primarily for two reasons. First, the catabolic process was slowed by the institution of parenteral alimentation first and then by tube feedings. Significant in the success of these measures is the fact that they were instituted early, very soon after her admission.

Before parenteral alimentation was discontinued, tube feedings were begun on a gradual basis. Because of Mrs. Smith's diminished gastrointestinal motility, feedings were given in small volumes (50 cc.) every two hours. Nasogastric aspiration was done before each feeding to ascertain the residual left from the previous feeding. This provided a means of determining how well the patient's digestive system was functioning. If the residuals remained minimal (10-15 cc.), the volume of feeding was gradually increased until the maximum tolerable volume could be given. Exact documentation was kept of the patient's dietary intake, her tolerance of tube feedings, bowel elimination patterns (e.g., the number of stools each shift, their color and consistency) and bowel sounds.

Mrs. Smith's problem with gastrointestinal motility also created chronic difficulties with elimination. Extended bed rest due to pelvic fractures further contributed to these difficulties. She lost bowel control and had alternate bouts of constipation and diarrhea. To deal with this problem, the patient was given mild cathartics every other day and was placed on a bedpan at regularly scheduled intervals to prevent incontinence.

Such attempts to regulate bowel elimination were instituted for two reasons: (1) to prevent skin irritation and tissue breakdown; and (2) to avoid the incontinence which the patient found extremely distressing. The patient perceived this loss of bowel control as humiliating and "something only babies have." A great deal of time was also devoted to allowing the patient to verbalize these feelings and helping her to understand that she was not, in fact, losing permanent control of all body functions.

Other complications which the patient developed as a result of malnutrition and immobility were muscle wasting with decreased muscle tone and a tendency to become exhausted with minimal activity. For example, the patient had a great deal of difficulty holding a fork or cup long enough to complete a meal. She would become so exhausted during meals that she would fall asleep while holding a hot cup of coffee.

To maintain as much muscle tone as possible, passive range of motion exercises were instituted. When the patient became fully alert, the physical therapist set up a schedule of exercises for the patient, such as squeezing a hard rubber ball with her hands hourly to restore muscle tone in her upper extremities. The patient was also given one new task to master each week, such as combing her hair, and encouraged to become involved in her own care. Initially, her first responsibility was to wash her own face; as she gained strength, other minor aspects of her own care were encouraged. Because exhaustion readily overwhelmed her, rest periods of at least 45 minutes were provided between each procedure (e.g., eating, bathing, changing of the bed, and exercises).

Mrs. Smith also developed hemolytic anemia as a result of her trauma. The anemia could have become an even greater problem because of inadequate intake of foods high in iron. To prevent this and other vitamin deficiencies, the patient was given iron three times daily as well as other vitamin supplements, such as folic and ascorbic acid. Again, the evolution of this problem, secondary to blood loss and malnutrition, could have precipitated complications in a multitude of other areas such as increased strain on the lungs and heart due to the decreased oxygen carrying capacity of the blood, or skin breakdown due to decreased oxygenation of tissues. The ulcerations she developed in her mouth probably were due to both the anemia and vitamin E deficiency.

Mrs. Smith never developed a serious problem with tissue breakdown during her entire hospitalization. She had a high potential for this, not only because of her malnutrition but also because of her extremely limited mobility, her neurological problems, and her anemia. This complication was avoided because of the nursing interventions noted previously. Mrs. Smith did, however, develop a chronic problem with poor wound healing. Malnutrition and the negative nitrogen balance which evolved contributed to this problem.

Protein deficiency may interfere with the assembly of amino acid chains and the formation of collagen which is essential to wound healing.[16] Severe and prolonged catabolism will contribute to protein loss and, thus, poor wound healing. Wounds which do not heal then become prime media for bacterial growth and infections. Often this sequence of events becomes the Achilles heel for the acutely ill trauma patient and ultimately leads to death.

Mrs. Smith's problem with malnutrition and slow wound healing delayed her recovery from the trauma significantly. Because of this delay in healing and subsequent wound infection, the patient underwent surgery on three occasions for drainage and debridement of wound infections in the fracture sites of both ankles and her right hip. The nursing care of a patient such as Mrs. Smith who has slow healing wounds should be directed toward minimizing the possibility of, or the extent of infection and preventing further loss of function.

The care of a wound should be done using the same aseptic technique one would use in any sterile procedure. If the wound is open and draining, as was Mrs. Smith's, sterile gloves used to remove the old dressing should not be used to apply the new dressing. The wound should be assessed daily for signs of necrosis, purulent drainage, and impaired circulation to the affected part. Dry skin is more resistant to infection than moist skin; thus, the wound should be kept dry and clean at all times.

If the wounds are casted, as Mrs. Smith's ankles were, close attention should be paid to assessment of the extremities and the casting each shift. Documentation should clearly describe changes in the color, warmth, smell, sensation and movement in the casted extremities. Often the first indications that a patient has developed an infection under a cast are the evidence of a foul odor and the patient's persistent complaint of pain in a specific area that is casted. The skin under cast edges should also be checked for abraded areas and padded to prevent ulceration and infection.

Nothing is more discouraging for the trauma patient than chronic complications and wounds which never seem to heal. Mrs. Smith was terrified of dressing and cast changes. She faced them with dread because they caused increased pain and she lived with pain constantly. To minimize the pain, she was always medicated an hour before her dressings were changed. Each step of the procedure was explained to her before it was done to eliminate unexpected changes and sensations which would increase her stress. Her discouragement with her slow progress was never fully overcome; however, the depression it created was significantly altered through consistent reinforcement of realistic goals. She was encouraged to think in terms of the immediate future and our objectives for her recovery in that period rather than focusing on the distant, vague future. When this was accomplished, Mrs. Smith became more optimistic and involved in her care.

RECOVERY PHASES

Phase II—The "Turning Point" Phase of Trauma

A great deal of the previously described aspects of the problem of malnutrition evolved during the second phase of Mrs. Smith's trauma. This phase usually begins on the fourth to seventh day after the trauma, but Mrs. Smith did not reach the turning point in her illness until approximately two-and-a-half weeks after sustaining the trauma. If and when a patient reaches this or other stages of recovery from trauma will depend upon the influences of the variables described at the outset of this chapter (e.g., age, sex, nature and extent of injuries, and state of health prior to the injury). This second phase is characterized by decreased catabolism of tissue and decreased nitrogen excretion, acquisition of tensile strength by the wound, increased appetite, and a spontaneous increase in activity as well as an increased involvement with the environment.

Mrs. Smith did not completely manifest all of the classical characteristics of this phase. Although her total blood protein levels increased from 4.9 mg. to a normal level of 7.6 mg., suggesting a decrease in the rate of catabolism, other clinical findings indicated that she was still in a catabolic state. Her weight continued to decline to 98 kg. three weeks after admission. Urine urea nitrogen excretion also remained elevated (normally 5-13, Mrs. Smith's was 800). Also her SGOT, LDH and CPK blood enzyme levels, which normally rise with muscle tissue injury, rose consistently for over two weeks after the initial injury. The patient's wounds also did not show the normal improvement expected during this period. Although she did begin to take solid foods orally, her dietary intake remained marginal.

The most marked improvement for Mrs. Smith during this period came in the areas of increased activity and interest in the environment. Mrs. Smith began to gain strength and expressed increasing desire to do things independently. She now asked frequently about her children and parents and waited anxiously each day for visits from them.

The progress the patient made during this second phase of her illness also precipitated a commonly observed state of frustration and depression noted among acute trauma patients during this time. As Mrs. Smith began to feel better and more aware of her environment, she also became acutely aware of how sick she really had been. When she realized this and then saw how she looked in a mirror she became depressed and angry. Because she felt better, she wanted to *be* better and look better. At one point she went through a grave crisis due to alteration of her body image and what she perceived as a loss of sexuality due to her injuries. As she put it, "they keep telling me I should be happy. It's a miracle that I'm even alive. Well, if I had died I wouldn't have to know anything. I wouldn't look this way or feel any pain. Now I can't take care of my kids. I'm no use to anyone anymore. It would have been better if I had died."

Shortly after this dialogue, her physicians told her that it would be some time before she could again have sexual relations because of her fractured pelvis. Mrs. Smith did not clearly understand but was afraid to discuss the subject with either her mother or her physicians. She thought she would never be "normal" again.

Although some of this patient's perceptions were not totally accurate, they were very real concerns. Her fears about her family's welfare were very real concerns and should always be considered when a patient requires long-term hospitalization. The younger children needed to be cared for, fed, and supervised. Bills needed to be paid and the patient had no source of income to pay for her medical expenses. She constantly worried about these real problems of daily living. When the nursing staff became aware of her concerns, they contacted the social service department. The social worker was able to coordinate the services of several local and state agencies. As a result, the patient's family received the assistance they needed during her hospitalization and the patient's concerns were alleviated.

Dealing with a patient's concerns regarding body image required insight and sensitivity on the part of the nurse. The patient will often provide clues that he is concerned about this. If, however, the nurse lacks a sensitive awareness of the meaning of these clues, the patient's problem may never receive attention. Initially Mrs. Smith could not express her concerns openly. She would be talkative and cheerful one minute, and sullen, withdrawn, and angry the next. The nurses spent a considerable amount of time simply sitting and talking with the patient. During these times, an effort was made to enter the patient's room not just to perform tasks or procedures, but also just to talk, in order to direct the focus of the interactions to her psychological needs and her concerns.

Once a stable, involved relationship was developed with Mrs. Smith, it became possible for her to more freely discuss her feelings. After this point, the nursing staff was able to help the patient put her concerns into a more realistic perspective. It was found that the patient's knowledge of her sexual anatomy was limited. Teaching was then instituted to help her understand how her injuries were temporarily expected to impair normal sexual activity. The patient's physicians were also consulted and asked to sit and discuss with her again the nature of her injuries and how long it would be before healing would occur. She was also offered psychological counseling but she felt that as long as she could "talk with my nurse" she did not need further help. Finally, as was noted previously, her energies were directed toward more immediate, obviously attainable goals so she could realistically perceive the extent of her progress.

The coordinated teamwork which went into Mrs. Smith's care helped a great deal to diminish the psychosocial problems she encountered particularly while hospitalized in the acute care facility. As the patient was entering the third or anabolic phase of trauma, she was transferred to an extended care rehabilitation hospital where she convalesced from her injuries for several months.

Phase III—The Anabolic Phase

Had it been possible to continue to follow the progress of Mrs. Smith, one would expect that her negative nitrogen balance would resolve and there would be renewed reconstruction of lean tissues. Her appetite would continue to improve and her increased dietary intake should lead to weight gain and increased strength. The emotional frustrations of "slow progress" could pose even greater stress for the patient during this period because of her boredom with confinement and her desire to be active and involved.

Localized wound healing should accelerate at this point as long as dietary intake improves. Normally, this phase might begin within 7-10 days after the trauma, but, again, progression would be affected by several variables. Mrs. Smith's progression to this phase did not occur until almost one month after her trauma.

Phase IV—The Convalescence Phase

This phase occurs for weeks or months after the trauma. It is characterized by a return to full body weight and function, restoration of fat deposits, return of normal dietary intake, full restoration of lean body tissue, and culmination of localized healing at the site of the injuries.

Fully two years after Mrs. Smith's accident, she continued to have residual effects from her accident, including a severe limp and chronic bladder problems. Although this patient did not fully recover from her injuries, she did survive what could have easily been an irreversible traumatic insult to her body.

This case presentation demonstrates why thorough, coordinated treatment of the critically ill trauma patient is essential. The survival of patients such as Mrs. Smith can only occur in a critical care setting where nursing care is based upon a comprehensive understanding of the pathology of trauma and the problems and needs evolving as a result of it.

REFERENCES

1. Bailey H: *The Emergency Surgery.* 9th Ed. Williams and Wilkins Company, Baltimore, Md., 1972.
2. Ballinger WF, et al.: *The Management of Trauma.* 2nd Ed. W.B. Saunders, Philadelphia, Pa., 1973.
3. Beland IL: *Clinical Nursing: Pathophysiology and Psychosocial Approaches.* 2nd Ed. Macmillan Publishing, New York, 1975.
4. Birke G, et al.: Albumin catabolism in burns and following surgical procedures. *Acta Chir Scandaniva* **118**:353, 1959-60.
5. Boyd RJ, et al.: *Trauma Management.* Year Book Medical Publishers, Inc., Chicago, Ill., 1974.
6. Brewer LA, et al.: The "wet lung" in war casualties. *Annals of Surgery* **123**:343, 1946.
7. Cahill GF: Body fuels and metabolism. *Bulletin of the American College of Surgery* **20**:12, 1970.
8. Cook WA: Shock lung: etiology, prevention, and treatment. *Heart and Lung* **3**:933, 1974.
9. Deitrick JE, et al.: Effects of immobilization upon various metabolic and physiologic functions in normal man. *American Journal of Medicine* **4**:3, 1948.
10. Dudley HA, et al.: The permissive role of adrenal cortical hormones after injury in man. *Metabolism* **8**:895, 1959.
11. Duke JH, et al.: Carbohydrate and Nitrogen Metabolism After Injury. In Knight J, Porter R (Eds.): *Energy Metabolism in Trauma.* J. and A. Churchill, London, 1970, pp. 103-126.
12. Ferguson J, et al.: Multiple fractures. *Nursing '74* **11**:26, 32, 1974.
13. Fleck A, Munro HN: Protein metabolism after injury. *Metabolism* **12**:783, 1963.
14. Frohlich ED: *Pathophysiology: Altered Regulatory Mechanisms in Disease.* J.B. Lippincott, Philadelphia, Pa., 1972.
15. Gardner B, Shatan GW (Eds.): *Quick Reference to Surgical Emergencies.* J.B. Lippincott, Philadelphia, Pa., 1974.
16. Heughan C, Hunt TK: Some aspects of wound healing research: a review. *The Canadian Journal of Surgery* **18**:118, 125, 1975.
17. Holden WD, et al.: The effect of nutrition on nitrogen metabolism in the surgical patient. *Annals of Surgery* **146**:563, 1957.

18. Johnston IDA: The role of the endocrine glands in the metabolic response to operations. *British Journal of Surgery* **54**:438, 1967.

19. Kinney JM: The effect of injury on metabolism. *British Journal of Surgery* **54**:435, 1967.

20. Luckman J, Sorensen KC: *Medical-Surgical Nursing: A Psychophysiological Approach.* W.B. Saunders, Philadelphia, Pa., 1974.

21. National Institute of Health: The status in trauma and the critically injured. *A Report by the Surgery Training Committee of the National Institute of General Medical Sciences.* Washington, D.C., 1970.

22. Peacock E, et al.: *Wound Repair.* 2nd Ed. W.B. Saunders, Philadelphia, Pa., 1976.

23. Selye H: The stress syndrome. *American Journal of Nursing* **65**:98, 1965.

24. Sevitt S: *Reactions to Injury and Burns and Their Clinical Importance.* J.B. Lippincott, Philadelphia, Pa., 1974.

25. Skillman JJ, Ed.: *Intensive Care.* Little, Brown, and Company, Boston, Mass., 1975.

26. Tepperman J: *Metabolic and Endocrine Physiology.* 3rd Ed. Year Book Medical Publishers, Inc., Chicago, Ill., 1974.

27. Vander AJ, et al.: *Human Physiology: The Mechanisms of Body Function.* McGraw-Hill, New York, 1970.

28. Walt AJ, Wilson RF: *Management of Trauma; Pitfalls and Practice.* Lea and Febiger, Philadelphia, Pa., 1975.

29. Wilson RF: Shock: Its Definition, Classification, Diagnosis, Pathophysiology, Monitoring, and Treatment. In Wilson RF (Ed.): *Principles and Techniques of Critical Care.* Upjohn Company, Philadelphia, Pa., 1976.

CHAPTER 9

Special Problems in Critical Care: Septic Shock

by Helen A. Schaag, RN, MSN

INTRODUCTION

Septic shock is a frequent and serious problem despite the advances in the management of critically ill patients. When septic shock occurs the mortality rate approaches 60 to 80%.[26] Because of the high mortality rate of septic shock one of the goals in the care of critically ill patients is the prevention of the occurrence of sepsis and septic shock. Once it occurs, the goal is to bring the sepsis and septic shock under control while maintaining "normal" body functions.

To assist in achieving these goals, the nurse must have an understanding of the etiology of sepsis and septic shock, the associated pathophysiological and hemodynamic changes, and the medical and nursing management of sepsis and septic shock. Although complete understanding does not exist in all of these areas, a review of current knowledge is presented in this chapter. A case study of a patient with septic shock is incorporated following the discussion.

The nursing process provides the framework for nursing management. Outcome criteria focusing on priority problems provides the basis for the evaluation of effectiveness of management. Questions related to septic shock and the case study are presented at points throughout the chapter. These questions are intended to assist the clinician or student to critically evaluate the clinical data, taking into account the multiple system involvement, plan nursing care for the total patient, and apply the concepts to the nursing care environments.

One of the areas that cause confusion in the understanding of septic shock is the use of multiple terms without clear definitions. Table 9-1 provides commonly used words and their definitions.

Predisposing Factors

From the preceding definitions it is apparent that before sepsis and septic shock can occur, a pathogenic organism must invade the bloodstream. Several predisposing factors play a role in the increased frequency of sepsis.

1. Antibiotic therapy has been indiscriminately used at times.
2. Nosocomial infections occur more frequently.
3. The number of compromised hosts has increased as advances in medical technology keeps more patients alive.
4. Invasive procedures are more frequently used for diagnosis, monitoring, and treatment.

Laboratory techniques which isolate and identify organisms are also more sophisticated and reliable, thus increasing the frequency of detection.

The last three factors will be discussed in more detail.

Nosocomial Infections

Nosocomial infections occur in approximately 5% of all patients admitted to general hospitals.[33] Typically, common sites for nosocomial infections involve the urinary tract, the respiratory tract, surgical wounds, subcutaneous tissue and skin or septic thrombophlebitis and bacteremia. Two-thirds of all patients who develop sepsis do so after being hospitalized 1 to 2 weeks and following specific manipulative events such as surgery, catheterization, and intravenous therapy.[43]

Compromised Host

A higher incidence of nosocomial infections occurs in persons whose "normal" defense mechanisms are deficient in some manner. Interference with defense mechanisms can be due to pathological or iatrogenic states that interfere directly or indirectly with cellular or

TABLE 9-1

Common Terms and Definitions

Bacteremia:	the presence of viable bacteria in the bloodstream.
Compromised Host:	any individual who has an increased susceptibility to infections. The increased susceptibility can be due to a wide variety of reasons.
Endotoxemia:	the presence of specific parts of the cell wall of gram-negative bacteria in the bloodstream.
Nosocomial Infection:	infection acquired in the hospital.
Sepsis:	the presence of various pus-forming and other pathogenic organisms or their toxins in the bloodstream or tissues.
Septic:	related to or caused by sepsis.
Septicemia:	condition with metabolic and hemodynamic changes due to the presence of microorganism, their toxins, or other fractions in the bloodstream or tissues.
Septic Shock:	a syndrome resulting from the presence of a pathogenic organism and/or its toxic products in the bloodstream. It is characterized by circulatory maldistribution, inadequate tissue perfusion and oxygenation, and inadequate cellular metabolism.

humoral immunity. Table 9-2 lists some commonly occurring pathological and iatrogenic states that will be seen in hospitalized patients. The major immunological defect, common infective organisms, and types of infections are identified.

This table provides a list of specific types of patients who should be considered as compromised host. When giving nursing care to any of these patients, their high risk for infection must be kept in mind, and nursing actions designed to decrease their chance of infections must be incorporated into their care. This can lead to an elimination or reduction of nosocomial infections. Other patients who should be considered as compromised hosts are those patients who are malnourished; those patients undergoing oral, GI, and/or GU procedures; those patients with urinary stasis, urinary obstruction, prostatism, or prostatitis; and those patients who have an

TABLE 9-2

Pathological and Iatrogenic States in the Compromised Host*

Conditions	Immunological Defect	Infective Organisms	Types of Infections
Leukemia, Aplastic anemia, agranulocytosis	Neutropenia, monocytopenia	Staphylococcus aureus, E. coli, Klebsiella, Pseudomonas, Candida, Pneumocystis, Aspergillus	Pneumonia, bacteremia, ulcers and abscesses of oropharynx, anus, and skin
Chronic granulomatous disease	Decreased bactericidal activity	Staph. aureus, E. coli, Serratia, Salmonella	Lymphadenitis, abscesses in lung, liver, and bone
Hodgkin's disease—lymphoma	Lymphocytopenia, reduced delayed hypersensitivity, decreased chemotaxis	M. tuberculosis, E. coli, Listeria, Salmonella, Candida, Cryptococcus, herpes zoster, herpes simplex, cytomegalovirus	Pneumonia, hepatitis, bacteremia
Agammaglobulinemia, dysgammaglobulinemias, intestinal lymphangiectasia, multiple myeloma, chronic lymphocytic leukemia, splenectomized pt.	Decreased opsonization	Strep. pneumoniae, H. influenza, rubella, Giardia lamblia	Sinusitis, pneumonia, and bacteremia
Complement deficiencies: C3, C5	Decreased chemotaxis and opsonization	Staph. aureus, Proteus, Pseudomonas	Otitis, sinusitis, pneumonia, septicemia
Burns	Tissue necrosis, loss of epithelial barrier, lymphocytopenia	Strep. pyogenes, Staph. aureus, gram-negative enteric bacilli, particularly Pseudomonas, Candida, herpes simplex	Cellulitis, bacteremia, pneumonia
Diabetes	Reduced neurovascular supply, decreased leukocyte chemotaxis and bactericidal activity	Staph. aureus, Candida, gram-negative enteric bacilli, M. tuberculosis, Mucoraceae	Cellulitis, urinary tract infection, and bacteremia

(Continued)

TABLE 9-2 (Continued)
Pathological and Iatrogenic States in the Compromised Host*

Conditions	Immunological Defect	Infective Organisms	Types of Infections
Hemolytic disease	Reduced monocyte-macrophage function (RES clearance)	Salmonella, Bartonella, Strep. pneumoniae	Bacteremia, pneumonia, osteomyelitis, meningitis
Uremia	Lymphocytopenia, impaired delayed hypersensitivity, decreased chemotaxis	E. coli, Klebsiella, Staph. aureus, Pseudomonas	Urinary tract infection, pneumonia, bacteremia
Cystic fibrosis	Bronchial obstruction by hyperviscous mucus	Staph. aureus, Pseudomonas	Bronchitis, pneumonia
Glucocorticosteroids	Decreased cellular immunity, decreased chemotaxis	Staph. aureus, gram-negative enteric bacilli, Candida, Toxoplasma, herpes zoster, herpes simplex, Pneumocystis	Cellulitis, bacteremia, pneumonia
Cytotoxic drugs	Neutropenia, monocytopenia, lymphopenia, loss of mucosal barriers	Gram-negative enteric bacilli, Candida, Pseudomonas	Bacteremia
Antibiotics	Colonization by resistant bacteria	Staph. aureus, resistant gram-negative bacilli, especially Pseudomonas, Serratia, Mima-Herellea	Superinfections
Prosthetic devices	Foreign body	Staph. aureus, gram-negative enteric bacilli, Candida	Abscesses, bacteremia

*Adapted from : Petersdorf RG, Dale, DC. In Thorn GW, et al, Ed.: *Harrison's Principles of Internal Medicine*, 8th Ed. McGraw-Hill, New York, 1977, p. 766. Used with permission.

unmanageable disease process. Also, the very young and the very old should always be considered to be compromised hosts, regardless of their disease state.

Invasive Procedures

Almost every hospitalized patient will have some type of invasive procedure. Intravenous therapy, intraurethral catheterization, endotracheal intubation, and various other instrumentations and surgical interventions are just a few of the invasive procedures that are done with hospitalized patients. These procedures cannot be eliminated, but utilization of stringent sterile techniques when carrying out the procedures and daily meticulous care of urethral catheters and intravenous and intra-arterial catheters will prevent infections in some of these patients.

The intravenous catheter is so frequently used that its potential as an etiological agent in sepsis in hospitalized patients may be overlooked. Approximately 1 out of every 4 hospitalized patients receives intravenous therapy.[33] Of those patients receiving IV fluids for more than 48 hours, as many as 57% having plastic intravenous catheters have had positive cultures from their catheter tips and 0 to 12% having metal needles have had positive cultures from their needle tips.[16]

When the site of an intravenous or intra-arterial catheter becomes inflamed and infected, the patient typically complains of tenderness or pain near the insertion site or proximal to this. The vague complaints could indicate thrombosis but the discomfort increases as phlebitis, thrombophlebitis, or cellulitis develops. Objective assessment of the infused extremity reveals signs of inflammation and a palpable or cord-like vein around the insertion site. Once phlebitis or cellulitis develops, the intravenous catheter must be removed to prevent further infection. To minimize the infection potential of intravenous and intra-arterial catheters, it is recommended that insertion sites be changed at least every 72 hours,[16] intravenous tubings and bottles be changed every 24 hours, and inspection and dressing changes around the insertion site be completed every 24 hours.[21] In addition, strict attention to aseptic technique is essential when using pressure transducers for monitoring. There are multiple opportunities for the introduction of contaminants into the blood stream, from the catheter and catheter site to the delivery system. Therefore, it is essential that all health team members follow stringent sterile techniques during the preparation of the skin, the changing of bottles and tubings, the addition of medications, the adjustment of air filters, and the daily inspection and cleansing of the insertion site.

QUESTIONS

1. In your institution or unit, how frequently is intravenous therapy used?
2. How long are intravenous catheters commonly left in place on any one patient in your unit?
3. Does your health institution have a policy or procedure regarding care of intravenous insertion sites, tubing, fluids, etc?
4. Has your health institution ever studied the rate of infections from intravenous therapy?
5. Do you know how frequently infections from intravenous therapy occur in your health institution?
6. Would an intravenous therapy team or an intravenous additive program assist the health team at your institution to reduce the present or potential incidence of infections from intravenous therapy?

Preventive Management and Monitoring

The following parameters should be monitored on a routine basis on any patient with a compromised host status. The frequency for monitoring may need to be increased if invasive procedures are done.

The earliest signs of septic shock result from a decrease in blood flow to specific organs. Observe the patient's sensorium level. Sometimes disorientation, restlessness, or a change in the patient's usual behavior will be the first sign of infection. Also, observe the skin temperature and degree of moisture for early signs of vasoconstriction. Typically, the skin will be warm and dry at this stage. In addition, various degrees of oliguria may be seen.

Monitor the blood pressure, pulse, respiration, and temperature every four hours or more, as indicated. Usually, the pulse and respiratory rate will increase when infection occurs. The blood pressure may fall but this could vary. Also, one would anticipate a low grade to moderate temperature elevation. In some situations, rectal temperatures present unnecessary risks for precipitating infections. Insertion of the temperature probe into the rectum has the potential for irritating or scraping the mucosa, and bacterial flora in the rectum can enter the bloodstream.

It is important to monitor the serial white blood cell count. Generally, if the WBC count falls below 1500/cu. mm., various degrees of protective isolation should be initiated as a protective measure for the patient. A protective isolation routine can be set up in any institution. The use of protective isolation *does not* negate the need for careful handwashing between patients and before caring for the patient, and care in not assigning infectious personnel to care for the patient. Protective isolation procedures can be initiated at the nurse's discretion.

Although there are classical changes to expect in the parameters mentioned, some patients do not show typical signs and symptoms when infected. The important concepts in picking up early subtle changes are to monitor all parameters carefully and to continually assess and compare the patient's present condition to base line state.

QUESTIONS

1. What is the procedure for protective isolation in your health institution?
2. What parameters would you monitor to detect early signs and symptoms of infection?

Although nurses in Intensive Care Units usually care for septic shock patients, all nurses in health institutions need to be able to identify compromised host patients in their setting. Many patients develop sepsis while on a general division and are transferred to the ICU only after the development of sepsis.

QUESTIONS

1. What specific patients in your work area would you categorize as being compromised hosts?
2. What potential etiological events routinely occur with these patients?
3. Do nurses in your institution independently initiate any monitoring or interventions to decrease the risk of infections?

If the patient has an infection, determine if the infection is in close proximity to a mucous membrane which has been or will be subjected to surgery, trauma, or other invasive procedures. This assessment will determine the degree of risk. Mucous membranes are highly vascular and have an abundance of gram-positive and gram-negative bacteria. A bacterial invasion into this prime medium could precipitate a massive bacteremia.

The focus of controlling infections should begin with prevention or reduction of their incidence. If your institution has an active infection control committee or an infection control nurse, surveillance of infection rates may be done. By surveying over an extended period of time, patterns of infections, their causative organism, and routes of transmission may become apparent. The identification of these patterns can be utilized in identifying measures to decrease the infection incidence. In addition, surveillance can be used to pick up increased incidence of infections over the normal expectations. If no established means of surveillance exists, nurses can institute surveillance for infection control. Table 9-3 is an example of a data collection tool which can be used in infection surveillance.

Infective Organisms

Once a patient has an infection, the patient has the potential for developing septic shock. Any organism (gram-positive or gram-negative bacteria, fungi, viruses, or rickettsiae) can precipitate septic shock. However, the most common organism is the gram-negative bacteria. There may be many reasons for this, but one very important reason is the fact that antibiotic therapy is more effective against gram-positive organisms than gram-negative organisms; thus, gram-negative bacteria proliferate while gram-positive bacteria are being eliminated.[26] Approximately 50% of all patients with gram-negative septicemia and 5% of all patients with gram-positive septicemia develop septic shock.[50]

Table 9-4 lists common organisms found in blood cultures over a two-year period in one institution. The incidence and Gram stain reaction for each organism are indicated.

Exotoxins and Endotoxins

Important in the development of the hemodynamic and meta-

TABLE 9-3

Surveillance Form For Infection Control

BACTERIA	JAN	FEB	MAR	APR	MAY	JUN	JUL	AUG	SEP	OCT	NOV	DEC
E. coli												
Blood												
Urine												
Staph. aureus												
Blood												
Wound												
Sputum												
Staph. epidermidis												
Blood												
Wound												
Propionibacterium sp.												
Blood												
Wound												
Proteus mirabilis (indole negative)												
Blood												
Urine												
Proteus sp.												
Blood												
Urine												

(Continued)

TABLE 9-3 (Continued)
Surveillance Form For Infection Control

BACTERIA	JAN	FEB	MAR	APR	MAY	JUN	JUL	AUG	SEP	OCT	NOV	DEC
Pseudomonas sp.												
Blood												
Urine												
Sputum												
Klebsiella sp.												
Blood												
Urine												
Sputum												
Enterobacter sp.												
Blood												
Urine												
Bacteroides sp.												
Blood												
Urine												
Sputum												
Enterococcus												
Blood												
Urine												
Other												

TABLE 9-4

**Incidence of Bacteria in Blood Cultures and Their
Gram-Stain Reaction***

Organism	No.	Gram-Negative	Gram-Positive	Other
Staphylococcus aureus	141		X	
Staphyloccus epidermidis	133		X	
Micrococcus sp.	4		X	
Sarcinia sp.	3		X	
Peptococcus sp.	10		X	
Streptococcus pyogenes Group A	8		X	
Streptococcus pyogenes Group B	17		X	
Streptococcus pyogenes Group D:			X	
Enterococci	31		X	
Not enterococci	2		X	
Streptococcus-nonhemolytic, not Group A, B or D	12		X	
Streptococcus (viridans group)	30		X	
Streptococcus pneumoniae	68		X	
Peptostreptococcus sp.	10		X	
Propionibacterium sp.	73		X	
Eubacterium lentum	3		X	
Clostridium perfringens	3		X	
Clostridium felsineum	1		X	
Clostridium paraputrificum	1		X	
Clostridium ramosum	2		X	
Listeria monocytogenes	4		X	
Bacillus sp.	12		X	
Corynebacterium	24		X	
Yeast	19			X
Escherichia coli	194	X		
Salmonella typhi	3	X		
Citrobacter diversus	3	X		
Citrobacter freundii	1	X		
Klebsiella pneumoniae	71	X		
Enterobacter aerogenes	1	X		
Enterobacter cloacae	22	X		
Serratia marcescens	10	X		
Serratia liquefaciens	2	X		
Proteus mirabilis	27	X		
Proteus morganii	1	X		
Yersinia enterocolitica	3	X		
Acinetobacter calcoaceticus	1	X		
Acinetobacter Iwoffi	2	X		
Moraxella sp.	1	X		

TABLE 9-4 (Continued)

Organism	No.	Gram-Negative	Gram-Positive	Other
Pseudomonas aeruginosa	55	X		
Pseudomonas maltophilia	1	X		
Haemophilus influenzae	3	X		
Eikenella corrodens	2	X		
Neisseria gonorrhoeae	3	X		
Veillenella sp.	7	X		
Bacteroides fragilis	40	X		
Bacteroides oralis	4	X		
Bacteroides melaninogenicus	2	X		
Bacteroides corroden	2	X		
Fusobacterium sp.	4	X		

*Microbiology Laboratory, Huntzel Hospital, blood culture results Sept. 1, 1973 to Aug. 31, 1975. There were 10,966 blood cultures (aerobic bottle and anaerobic bottle = 1 culture: 1,077 positive/10,966 cultures = 9.8% positive. (From: Brown WJ: A classification of microorganisms frequently causing sepsis. *Heart and Lung* 5(3): 403, 1976. Used with permission.)

bolic changes that occur in septicemia and septic shock are not only the effects of the organisms themselves, but also the effects of toxins released by the organisms. Both gram-positive and gram-negative bacteria can produce toxins.

Toxins are classified as exotoxins or endotoxins. A summary of the characteristics of exotoxins and endotoxins is presented in Table 9-5. Exotoxins are protein in nature, are produced within the interior of the gram-positive bacteria cell, and can diffuse through the bacterial cell wall. Some exotoxins diffuse very easily while others do not leave the bacterial cell until the cell is destroyed. Endotoxins are lipopolysaccharide in nature; gram-negative bacteria release their endotoxins from the cell only when the cell is destroyed. Most exotoxins are produced by gram-positive organisms; endotoxins are produced only by gram-negative organisms.

Exotoxins and endotoxins differ in several other ways. Exotoxins are much more potent than endotoxins. Exotoxins are easily denatured with heat, whereas endotoxins are relatively heat stable. Exotoxins seem to exert their pathological effect directly on specific tissues and cells, whereas endotoxins are inert unless they com-

TABLE 9-5

Characteristics of Toxins

Features	Exotoxins	Endotoxins
Type of bacteria	Gram-positive	Gram-negative
Chemical nature	Protein	Lipopolysaccharide
Location of toxin	Within bacteria cell (toxins diffuse through bacteria cell wall)	Within cell wall of bacteria (toxins released* with disruption of bacterial cell)
Body reaction to toxins	Specific (toxins have specific affinity to specific tissues)	Nonspecific (local reaction to systemic reaction and septic shock)
Potency	Usually greater than endotoxins	Usually lesser than exotoxins
Stability	Unstable (denatured with heat, light)	Stable
Conversion to toxoid	Yes	No

bine with one or more elements in the blood. These elements are believed to be antibodies and complement.

The combination of endotoxin, antibodies, and complement produce anaphylatoxin. The anaphylatoxin is the "vehicle" that precipitates the pathological effects.

Fungi, Viruses, and Rickettsiae

The incidence of these organisms causing septicemia and septic shock is low. Their individual infectious processes may be localized or disseminated. However, invasion of any of these organisms into the body further compromises the patient, makes the patient more susceptible to other infectious diseases, and makes management and prevention of any infectious process more difficult.

PATHOPHYSIOLOGICAL CHANGES

There are a wide variety of signs and symptoms associated with septicemia and septic shock. The signs and symptoms vary with the stage of shock. Table 9-6 compares early and late signs and symp-

TABLE 9-6

Signs and Symptoms of Early and Late Shock

Parameters	Early	Late
BP	Mildly decreased	Markedly hypotensive to inaudible
P	Mildy tachycardic	Markedly tachycardic, peripherally weak and thready
R	Increased	Increased
Skin	Usually warm and dry but may be cool and clammy	Usually cold and moist but may be warm and dry
Mental status	Restless, periods of confusion and disorientation	Markedly disoriented to unconscious
Renal	Output normal to mildly decreased	Output markedly decreased to oliguric
CVP	Normal to elevated	Variable
Pulmonary artery pressure/pulmonary wedge pressure	Normal to increased	Increased
Cardiac output	Normal to increased	Decreased
Acid-base balance	Respiratory alkalosis	Metabolic acidosis and respiratory acidosis
Respirations breath sounds	Clear	Congested
PO_2	Normal	Decreased
PCO_2	Normal to decreased	Increased
Serum K^+	Mildly decreased	Mildly increased

toms of septic shock. Numerous unanswered questions still exist regarding the exact mechanism by which the bacteria and/or the toxins produce all the signs and symptoms seen in septic shock. Some patients with septic shock may display many of these signs and symptoms, while other septic patients may only exhibit a few signs and symptoms of early and late shock. The time span between the early and late signs and symptoms is highly variable and unpredictable. In the next section the major changes that occur in various body systems will be discussed. The analysis of these changes will include a description of some of the signs and symptoms associated with septic shock.

Hemodynamic Changes

In man, there are two types of hemodynamic situations that occur in different stages of septic shock. Early in septic shock, a hyperdynamic state exists where there is increased cardiac output, decreased peripheral resistance, and slowed circulation time. The patient is warm and dry. The "warm flushed state" is due to generalized vasodilation and pooling of blood in capillary beds, shunting of blood around capillary beds through arteriovenous shunts, and redistribution of the circulation with shunting of blood to the inflamed or infected area. The cause of these circulatory changes is probably the release of vasoactive substances such as histamine and kinins from body cells that were injured by the exotoxins or endotoxins, and the antibody-complement combination.

The circulatory changes and decreased peripheral resistance causes an immediate stimulation of the sympathetic adrenal medullary mechanism. Stimulation of this mechanism causes the heart rate to increase. In some patients, the cardiovascular system can respond to a degree sufficient to maintain the blood pressure and the "warm" shock picture exists.

This state is followed by a hypodynamic state in which peripheral vascular resistance increases, the cardiac output decreases, and the patient becomes cold, clammy, and eventually cyanotic. The cause of the movement of the patient from the hyperdynamic state to the hypodynamic state is unknown.

It is speculated that cardiac failure occurs and makes it impossible for the heart to maintain cardiac output in the presence of massive vasodilation. Also, the shunting of blood to the inflamed area may become sequestered within the area and decrease vascular volume. Cardiac failure and/or the sequestration of fluid causes cardiac output to decrease. This change activates the sympathetic adrenal medullary mechanism causing increased heart rate and massive arteriole and venule vasoconstriction. This should increase the blood pressure, but in septic shock these compensatory mechanisms are inadequate.

Metabolic Changes

Cellular metabolism is radically altered during septic shock. It must be remembered that even in the hyperdynamic state cellular metabolism is altered. Even though adequate blood flow may be getting to the capillary beds, the cells seem to be unable to utilize the oxygen, glucose, and electrolytes. It is hypothesized that the toxic products interfere with oxidative phosphorylation[26,50] or interfere with diffusion of these elements across the cell membrane.

Normal metabolism

In a typical cell, the cytoplasm contains enzymes for the anaerobic glycolytic cycle, and the mitochondria contain enzymes for the aerobic citric acid cycle. Sugar enters the cell and is catabolized anaerobically to pyruvate. In the absence of oxygen, pyruvate is converted to lactic acid and can leave the cell. In the presence of oxygen, pyruvate is converted to acetyl coenzyme A (acetyl CoA), enters the Krebs cycle, and is catabolized to CO_2, H_2O, and energy.

The energy formed in anaerobic and aerobic metabolism is held in the cell as adenosinetriphosphatase (ATP). ATP is the major fuel utilized for cellular function. The importance of oxygen in producing greater amounts of energy can easily be seen from the fact that in the absence of oxygen, only 2 molecules of ATP are produced from each molecule of glucose. Under aerobic conditions, 38 molecules of ATP can be formed from each molecule of glucose.

The reaction in which pyruvic acid is converted to acetyl CoA, which then enters the Krebs cycle, is critical in the metabolism of glucose because it is an irreversible reaction. In contrast, the anaerobic reaction between glucose and pyruvic acid can be reversed. This reversible process permits any of the anaerobic intermediates to synthesize glucose, but because of the irreversibility of pyruvic acid to acetyl CoA, acetyl CoA cannot be used to synthesize glucose.

The breakdown and synthesis of neutral fats is similar to the metabolism of glucose because of the formation of intermediates common to both pathways. The breakdown of neutral fats produces fatty acids and glycerol. Glycerol enters the anaerobic glycolytic pathway and continues into the Krebs cycle. Fatty acids are broken down to acetyl CoA and enter the Krebs cycle at that point. As previously mentioned, the reaction leading to the formation of acetyl CoA from pyruvic acid is irreversible and thus acetyl CoA derived from fatty acids cannot be used to synthesize glucose. Glucose can provide the acetyl CoA required for fatty acid synthesis and can readily be converted into fatty acids. When acetyl CoA is unable to enter the Krebs cycle, acetyl CoA can be formed into ketone bodies in the liver.

Proteins are formed from 20 different amino acids and have different chemical structures and pathways for their synthesis and degradation. Unlike carbohydrates and lipids, amino acids contain nitrogen. Once nitrogen is removed, the remainder of the molecule can enter the Krebs cycle to be broken down or can be converted to glucose. There are several ways of removing nitrogen from amino acids: (1) amino acids may be deaminated in a reaction with H_2O to form a keto acid and ammonia; or, (2) amino acids may transfer their amino group to a keto acid forming a new amino acid and a new keto acid. The keto acids can enter the Krebs cycle at the appropriate steps.

The various metabolic processes for glucose, fat, and protein metabolism proceed at various rates and in various directions. There are two factors that directly determine the reaction rates: (1) the concentration of various substrates present in the cell; and (2) the activity of the cell's enzymes. The availability of substrates within cells is dependent on cell membrane permeability and transport systems.

Metabolism in septic shock

During stress, catabolic states, and in the absence of adequate oxygen, various changes in metabolic pathways occur. Normally, glucose is the major source of energy but in catabolic states or in the absence of oxygen when metabolism cannot proceed as usual, other sources of energy may be used.

Septic shock is a catabolic state characterized by inadequate cellular perfusion. With the presence of these two states, the source of energy will be drastically changed. In shock states, cellular metabolism is essentially anaerobic because of the lack of oxygen. The Krebs cycle is virtually shut down. Glucose is only anaerobically metabolized and produces only 2 ATPs per glucose molecule and large amounts of lactic acid. The lack of energy production from glucose metabolism leads to rapid breakdown of glycogen.

When glycogen stores are limited, the body normally compensates by breaking down fats and proteins. Proteins are used to produce new sugars by the process of gluconeogenesis. In catabolic states, skeletal muscle is the principal source of protein for gluconeogenesis. However, in septic shock, the proteins broken down for gluconeogenesis are not utilized in that manner. Animals in septic shock do not have the ability to carry out gluconeo-genesis.[37] Studies in man with shock due to sepsis indicate similar findings.[42]

Since there is an inefficient utilization of glucose in sepsis, rapid depletion of glycogen occurs. With the inability to carry out gluconeogenesis, energy requirements of the body must be met by fat catabolism. The fat catabolism does not proceed by the normal pathway. The acetyl-CoA from fat breakdown cannot proceed through the Krebs cycle because of a lack of oxygen. Energy requirements are met by ketogenesis. The danger of increased ketogenesis is the likelihood of developing ketoacidosis. Ketones are formed more rapidly than they can be oxidized and the ketones overflow into the blood.

One of the major effects of this altered metabolism is metabolic acidosis. The metabolic acidosis is due to increased production of lactic acid from anaerobic glucose metabolism, aminoaciduria from increased protein breakdown, and ketosis from incomplete fat breakdown. Phosphatases are also increased, probably because they are not utilized in bonding to ATP molecules. The serum pH thus drops below normal due to the increased amount of anaerobic acid metabolism. Lactic acid levels must be determined to adequately monitor the patient in septic shock.

Another major effect of altered metabolism is deficient amounts of ATP production. Deficient ATP production causes profound alterations in cellular membrane function. A very large portion of the body's total energy expenditure (ATP utilization) is at the cellular membrane level to maintain the sodium-potassium pump.[38] When deficient amounts of ATP are available, major dysfunctions in the membranes occur, such as efflux of potassium from the cell and the influx of sodium and water into the cell. This results in intracellular edema. Intracellular edema is a common sign in shock states and further interferes with or blocks other cellular metabolic reactions and activities.

Endocrine Changes

Multiple endocrine changes occur in the presence of septic shock. Hormones are released in an effort to compensate for the altered hemodynamic and metabolic state. The release of most hormones is mediated by the hypothalamus. The hypothalamus receives input directly or indirectly from all parts of the brain.[30] The stimulation of the medulla by the hemodynamic changes can be directly or indirectly transmitted to the hypothalamus, and the hypothalamus then mediates the release of appropriate hormones.

The hormones that play the biggest role in the compensatory responses are adrenocorticotropic hormone (ACTH), glucocorticoids, mineralocorticoids (aldosterone), growth hormone (GH), antidiuretic hormone (ADH), glucagon, and insulin. The effects of each of these hormones will be briefly described. The reader should consult the identified texts for more information.[30,49]

Increased secretion of ACTH occurs in the presence of physical and psychological stressors and in the presence of endotoxins in the blood.[2] ACTH· stimulates the release of adrenal cortex hormones, particularly the ketosteroids and glucocorticoids. Some mineralocorticoids (aldosterone) may be released in response to increased ACTH, but the major stimulus for the release of aldosterone is due to the renin angiotensin system. This is discussed in a later section. The role of ketosteroids in septic shock is uncertain. The major effects of ACTH and glucocorticoids are:

1. insulin antagonism, thus making more glucose available for brain metabolism.
2. promotion of glycogenolysis and gluconeogenesis.
3. promotion of protein and fat catabolism.
4. retention of sodium and H_2O.
5. accentuation of vasopressor effects of norepinephrine.

Growth hormone production is stimulated by physical and psychological stressors such as trauma, prolonged fasting, acute febrile conditions, and shock. Growth hormone reinforces the insulin antagonism effect of glucocorticoids by inhibiting the uptake and oxidation of glucose by many tissues in the body. Likewise, GH reinforces the fat mobilizing effects of other hormones by increasing adipose tissue triglyceride breakdown.

The posterior pituitary hormone, ADH, is increased in stress states such as pain and decreased arterial pressure. This hormone acts on the distal tubule cells of the kidney and leads to the active reabsorption of water and thus increases the vascular volume.

Aldosterone, a hormone produced by the adrenal cortex, is also released in stress states such as septic shock. In the kidneys, cells in the juxtaglomerular apparatus monitor the blood level of sodium and the vascular volume. A decrease in serum sodium or vascular volume stimulates these cells to release renin. Renin acts on a serum protein, angiotensinogen, converting it to angiotensin. Angiotensin directly stimulates the adrenal cortex to release aldosterone. Aldosterone acts on the renal tubule cells and enhances the reabsorption of sodium and water. This effect will help to increase vascular volume. The hypoperfusion to the renal tubules, occurring in septic shock, because of pooling or vasoconstriction would stimulate this response.

Glucagon and insulin, both secreted by the pancreas, are affected in shock states. In septic shock, insulin action is decreased and glucagon production is increased. The increased need for glucose in catabolic states stimulates glucagon release. The increased levels of epinephrine and norepinephrine resulting from sympathetic-adrenal medullary stimulation decrease insulin secretion. The resultant effect of these endocrine changes are hyperglycemia due to gluconeogenesis, glycogenolysis, and the inability of some cells to utilize glucose without insulin.

The overall effect of all of these changes is an increase in vascular volume and increase in nutrients for cell metabolism. As with other compensatory responses, the effect may not always be beneficial. The increased sodium and water reabsorption by the kidneys in response to ADH and aldosterone, may overtax a stressed heart and will increase the chance of renal shutdown. Prolonged production of the other hormones can lead to hyperglycemia and severe protein depletion.

Renal Changes

Although some capillary beds may be dilated, others are constricted as the body responds to septic shock. The maldistribution of blood flow within critical organs is unpredictable and difficult to directly measure. It has been shown that in humans, the kidney is one of the primary organs affected by septic shock. Renal damage is due to the shunting of blood flow away from the kidney.

The degree of kidney function reflects the adequacy of its tissue perfusion and extent of tissue anoxia. Kidney function can be evaluated by urine output volume/time, osmolarity ratio, urinary sodium concentration, serum creatinine, and BUN. These parameters should be monitored on a continual basis. It must be remembered that any patient with septic shock is a candidate for acute tubular necrosis and ARF. (See Chapter 4 for details of the pathophysiology of renal failure.) Shunting of blood flow in the kidney results in tubular ischemia and tubular damage.

Hematological Changes

Various hematological changes can occur in septic shock. Changes in RBC, WBC, and platelets as well as other clotting factors may result. Typically, the patient with septic shock will have a leukocytosis because of the presence of infection prior to septicemia and septic shock. A predominate neutrophilic granulocytic picture usually results.[53] The mature neutrophilic granulocytes, polymorphonuclear leukocytes (PMNs), are the body's first defense in fighting an infection. Neutrophils are drawn to the site of infection by a process called chemotaxis and proceed with their phagocytic activity at that location.

In some instances, when the onset of septicemia and septic shock is rapid, a reduction in white blood cells may be seen due to a reduction in neutrophils. The acute infection and toxic reaction causes a depression of the bone marrow. In addition, patients with leukemia or those receiving chemotherapy may not show leukocytosis.

Anemia is a common finding with acute and chronic infections. The anemia, which is probably due to bone marrow depression from the overwhelming infection, usually stabilizes rather than continues. In addition, septicemia may precipitate various degrees of intravascular erythrocyte destruction.

Platelets and other clotting factors can be altered tremendously in septic shock. Platelet levels may be decreased as a result of the bone marrow depression which occurs in acute infection or because of the occurrence of disseminated intravascular coagulation (DIC).

The primary pathophysiology of DIC involves a response to an underlying disease that initiates a generalized activation of the normal clotting mechanism. Endotoxins are known to initiate fibrinolytic activity and activate the Hageman factor.[27] In addition, because of pooling and sluggish flow, platelet aggregation can occur. Once started, the inappropriate and extensive clotting process proceeds at an accelerated rate. The inappropriate clotting depletes available clotting factors and platelets. When the blood coagulating factors become depleted, hemorrhage becomes the major problem. See Chapter 10 for more information on DIC.

Respiratory Changes

Numerous respiratory changes occur in patients with septicemia. Early in septic shock hyperventilation and respiratory alkalosis occurs. The hyperventilation is initiated because with the early hemodynamic and metabolic changes hydrogen ions will increase and diffuse from the blood to the cerebrospinal fluid and stimulate the receptors in the fourth ventricle. At first the hyperventilation is compensatory and helps to keep a "normal pH". The early hemodynamic and metabolic changes may be corrected but because of the delay in the blood-brain equilibrium the hyperventilation persists and respiratory alkalosis results.

Later in septic shock the patient will develop hypoxemia, hypercapnia, and respiratory acidosis as a result of atelectasis, pulmonary edema with ventilation/perfusion mismatching, increased arteriovenous shunting, and/or the development of "Acute Respiratory Distress Syndrome". Any or all of the latter problems may occur and the development of one problem may lead to another pathological condition. The processes initiating the pathological states are not always known but one initiating event may be decreased pulmonary compliance.

Normal inflation of the lungs requires a certain amount of pressure to overcome the elastic forces of the lung and thorax and to overcome the resistance to flow of gas occurring through the respiratory airways. Surfactant, a phospholipid secreted by Type II alveolar cells, is a major factor that determines the degree of lung compliance and regulates surface tension. Surfactant must be continually replaced. Pulmonary edema and passage of plasma and fibrinogen into the interstitial space can destroy surfactant and cause decreased pulmonary compliance and collapse of alveoli leading to atelectasis, increased arteriovenous shunting, and/or "ARDS".

Atelectasis may also result from the lack of deep breathing and sighing. Long-term shallow breathing usually results in plugging of the alveoli with mucus. Pulmonary edema can result from overhydration, left ventricular failure, and/or the increased capillary permeability and movement of colloids into the interstitial space.

Refer to Chapter 3 for further information on respiratory pathophysiology.

MANAGEMENT

The discussion of management of patients with septicemia and septic shock will focus around the presentation of a case study. The case study will utilize the assessment tools from Chapter 1 in obtaining and presenting the patient data. The patient will be initially assessed at admission; at that time the priority patient care objectives and the appropriate nursing action will be presented. The health status of the patient will be reassessed, and the altered status of the patient will be reflected in his care objectives and nursing actions when septic shock develops.

At the time of admission, the initial data collected by the nurse provides the essential baseline data for nursing management. There are many formats available which facilitate the collection of data. Chapter 1 discusses assessment techniques and approaches for collecting data on all body systems. The guidelines in Chapter 1 may be beneficial in designing a complete and realistic assessment tool for your nursing unit. This assessment tool should be appropriate for use at admission and throughout the hospital course. Once the assessment tool has been developed, a flow sheet to record the serial data should be constructed.

The recording of laboratory data is essential but becomes more meaningful when the serial data are recorded on a standardized flow sheet. Identify the laboratory parameters within urine, blood components, and blood chemistry that are appropriate for your nursing staff to monitor. Then formulate a data flow sheet that will reflect the subtle sequential laboratory changes.

Case Study

Mr. S. W., a 51-year-old male Caucasian, has been admitted to your nursing division from the emergency room with a medical diagnosis of fever and hematological changes. On the Problem Oriented Medical Record (POMR), this nursing admission summary has been written.

10/27/77—2 PM—Nursing Admission Summary

S: Mr. S. W., age 51, felt generally well until 6 weeks PTA when he experienced symptoms of an upper respiratory tract infection, non-productive cough, fever, and malaise. He also experienced dyspnea with a 1 to 2 block walk. Three weeks PTA his cough became productive of dark greenish sputum, he experienced epistaxis on several occasions, his throat became sore, and he developed dysphagia. Gradually he became anorexic and frequently vomited. About 1 week PTA, his urine became "dark orange" in color and he frequently became hot and sweaty all over. He denies shaking chills, dysuria, melena, hematemesis, abdominal pain, and easy bruising.

Mr. W. has a positive family history for myocardial infarction, DM, and CVA and a negative family history for cancer. He denies any use of tobacco or alcohol and denies any allergies to foods or drugs.

Significant past medical problems include adult onset diabetes mellitus at age 35, hypertension for many years, and saphenous vein ligation and stripping 5 years PTA. The only medication Mr. W. describes taking is his daily "high blood pressure" pill which his PMD prescribed after his vein surgery. He maintains a 2000-2500 calorie diet at home. He states his usual weight before this illness was about 79 kg. He states he wears glasses only for reading and has no denture plates. He is employed as an electrician. Mr. W. states he is worried about the seriousness of his illness.

O: T 38.5°C (PO), P 100 and regular, R 24, BP 130/80, without postural changes.

Radial, popliteal, and pedal pulses are of good quality and bilaterally equal.

Wt. 74 kg., Ht. 6 ft.

Skin: petechiae over arms and lower extremities; chronic stasis changes to lower extremities; bilateral pitting edema to mid-calves; skin warm and dry to touch, except for bilateral glove and stocking coolness.

Eyes: conjunctiva pale; sclera white.

Nose: small amount of fresh bleeding with clots bilaterally.

Mouth: tonsils bilaterally enlarged with small exudates, and erythematous oral pharyngeal area; many missing teeth; gums infected.

Neck: no bruit and no JVD.

Chest: breath sounds heard in all lobes, bilaterally clear, no rales heard.

Cardiac: PMI 5th ICS, MCL; normal S_1 and S_2 $\overline{s}$ murmurs or gallop.

Abdomen: non-tender, no masses or petechiae; normal bowel sounds; liver 9 cm. span, spleen palpable.

Rectal: stool guaiac +, no gross blood with stool.

Neurological: alert and oriented X 3; comprehends the written and spoken word; walked 10 ft. erect and without limp, swaying, or using any support; moved all extremities, equal strength bilaterally.

Laboratory results:
CBC: Hct 35%, platelets 35,000/cu mm
      WBC 3400/cu mm, 50% cells atypical
Chemistry: Na^+ 130; K^+ 2.4; Cl^- 90; CO_2 25; BUN 23;
         Glucose 160.
Urine: dark orange in color, sp. gravity 1.025, pH 6, RBC 1-2,
      WBC 1-2, sugar/acetone negative
Sputum: mixed gram + and − rods.

ECG: Sinus tachycardia, rate 110 and regular
Chest x-ray: Clear A-P.

A: First admission for this ill-appearing male, not in acute distress.

Patient Problems:
1. Fever
2. Hematological abnormalities
3. High risk for bacteremia and septic shock
4. Electrolyte imbalance

5. Anxious about condition.

P: *Management:* Medical and nursing management of the septic shock patient is individualized and evolves around the underlying pathophysiological condition and the stage in which the shock syndrome becomes apparent. The immediate management is focused towards controlling the infectious process and thus preventing septic shock.

Medical Management:
1. activities as tolerated
2. IV antibiotics
   Gentamicin 120 mg. IV piggyback Stat and Q 8 hr.
   Carbenicillin 5 Gm. IV Q 4 hr.
   Oxacillin 2 Gm. IV Q 4 hr.
3. IVs—5% D/½ NS @ KO rate
4. KCl 40 mEq PO Stat and Q 4 hr.
5. Stat blood, urine, sputum cultures
6. Stat and daily blood and urine studies
7. 2000 calorie diet
8. Folate 1 mg. IV now and then 1 mg. PO daily
9. Tylenol 600 mg. PO Q 4 hr. PRN discomfort

Medical management centers around prescribing the most appropriate medications and treatments. The antibiotic regimen should provide a broad spectrum of coverage for both gram − and gram + organisms until the results of any culture and sensitivity test indicate otherwise. It is not unusual for multiple culture reports to return indicating "no growth." However, the broad spectrum antibiotic coverage should be continued until a full course has been given or until specific antibiotics are indicated by the cultures' sensitivity reports. If after a full course of antibiotic therapy, no particular culture grows an organism, but the patient is still symptomatically septic, the physician will have to evaluate this situation again and may choose to continue the same antibiotics for an extended period or switch antibiotics.

Nursing Management

Nursing management focuses on prevention of septic shock and other problems due to other disease processes. The nursing management includes:

1. early detection of problems due to the underlying disease processes and/or treatment.
2. support of the cardiopulmonary and renal systems.
3. support of psychological status.
4. monitoring for signs and symptoms of the progression of the septicemia state to the septic shock state.
5. modifying activities of daily living as appropriate.

QUESTIONS

1. At this time, what data places Mr. W. into the high risk group for developing septicemia and septic shock?
2. Are there any other physician orders you might expect to see?
3. Are there any other nursing management aspects you would consider at this time?
4. What would be your initial patient objectives and nursing actions for Mr. S. W.?

Discussion: The clinical data which indicates that Mr. S. W. has a high risk for developing septicemia and septic shock is his compromised host status. He is a compromised host because of the leukopenia, abnormal cells, mild anemic state, and the presence of the chronic diseases: diabetes mellitus, hypertension, and gingivitis. In addition, Mr. W.'s history indicates some degree of recent malnourishment.

Patient Objective I

Patient will become afebrile.

Nursing Interventions

1. Vital signs Q 2 hr. or as necessary.
2. No rectal temperatures: indicate whether temperature was orally or axillary.
3. Protective isolation: private room; all people entering patient's room will wear mask, gown, and wash hands prior to care; anyone with a respiratory infection will not enter patient's room; personnel giving direct care also to wear gloves.
4. Administer IV fluids and IV antibiotics per schedule but initiate after STAT cultures obtained.

    a) using sterile technique, apply povidone-iodine ointment to IV infusion site and cover with an occlusive dressing; change Q 24 hr; place time and date when current infusion site was instituted and time and date of last dressing change on tape covering the dressing; change infusion sites at least every 72 hrs.

    b) label all IV bottles, antibiotic containers, and IV tubings with time and date; all bottles and tubings to be changed Q 24 hr. and indicate time and dates when changed.

5. Administer Tylenol 600 mg. PO Q 4hr. PRN discomfort.
6. Oral care with saline mouth gargle TID and brush teeth with soft bristle brush and toothpaste BID; saline gargles for comfort.
7. Record observations and notify physician immediately when PO temperature < 37°C or > 39°C.

Patient Objective II

Patient will not have any uncontrolled bleeding.

Nursing Interventions
1. No IM medications.
2. Hold all venous puncture sites at least 5 minutes and hold all arterial puncture sites at least 10 minutes.
3. Guaiac all stools and any emesis.
4. Observe for any gross evidence of blood in urine and sputum.
5. Observe for any progression in petechiae or evidence of bruising.
6. Shave patient with an electric razor.
7. Record observations and notify physician immediately when any new evidence of bleeding occurs.
8. Remove clutter from room.
9. Assess patient's ability to be up independently; if unstable patient should be up only with assistance; check patient's postural vital signs when getting up.

Patient Objective III

Patient will not develop any undetected signs and symptoms of septic shock. That is:

A) His systolic BP will not be less than 90 mm. Hg and heart rate will not be greater than 110 beats/minute (base line data: BP 130/80, P 110/minute).

B) He will remain oriented x 3 (time, place, person).

C) His skin will remain warm and dry (base line data: skin warm and dry to touch except bilateral glove and stocking coolness).

D) His respiratory rate will range between 16 and 26/minute (base line data: respiratory rate 24/minute).

Nursing Interventions

1. Evaluate BP and pulse Q 2 hr. or more frequently as necessary.
2. Record observations and notify physician immediately when systolic BP < 90 or heart rate > 110 beats/minute.
3. Monitor vital signs during any increase in activities.
4. Evaluate behavior, alertness, and orientation Q 4 hr. or more frequently as necessary.
5. Record observations and notify physician immediately when any changes in sensorium occur.
6. Evaluate skin temperature Q 4 hr.
7. Record observations and report any skin temperature changes immediately to physician.
8. Evaluate respiratory rate Q 2 hr. or more frequently as necessary.
9. Auscultate all lung lobes Q 4.hr. (base line data: breath sounds in all lobes, bilaterally clear, no rales heard).
10. Patient to do coughing and deep breathing exercises at least 3 times/hr. while awake.
11. Observe such characteristics of sputum as color, amount, odor, consistency.
12. Ask patient if he experiences any dyspnea at rest or with exercise, orthopnea, etc., Q 4 hr.; monitor respiratory rate with change in activity.
13. Observe for any dependent edema Q 4 hr.
14. Record observations and report any respiratory rate > 26 or < 16/minutes, ausculatory changes, sputum changes, dyspnea, or edema, to physician immediately.

Patient Objective IV

Patient's fluid and electrolyte status will be stable and in balance.

A) His urinary output will approximate his fluid intake, with a minimum output of 500 ml./24 hr.

B) He will eat his 2000 calorie soft endentulous diet every day.

Nursing Interventions

1. Measure intake and output Q 8 hr.
2. Record observation and notify physician if urinary output < 500 ml/24 hr. or if inequality between I & O occurs.
3. Observe and record color, odor, and specific gravity of urine Q 8 hr.
4. Record observation and report any dysuria or complaints of increase in urinary frequency.
5. Record daily weights (base line data = 74 kg.).
6. Observe for dependent edema, orthopnea, increased respiratory rate, shortness of breath, and moist breath sounds, and record data.
7. Give KCl as ordered.
8. Monitor serum K^+ levels.
9. Maintain IV therapy as prescribed.
10. Record amount of food eaten during each meal.
11. Give mouth care prior to eating to enhance appetite.
12. Check patient's food likes and dislikes and consult dietician about nutritional needs.
13. Record any nausea or vomiting.
14. Clinitest and acetest on double voided urine sample at 7-11-4-9.
15. Provide rest periods before meals.
16. Assist patient with meals as necessary.

Patient Objective V

Patient will state he is less anxious.

Nursing Interventions

1. Explain all procedures and tests to patient.

2. Clarify any information patient receives to make sure the interpretation is correct.
3. Allow patient to verbalize his feelings and worries.

Patient Objective VI

Patient will have ADL needs met without increased energy expenditures.

Nursing Interventions

1. The major intervention will be to identify priority activities and eliminate unnecessary activities. If activities are not prioritized and scheduled, adequate rest cannot be provided.
2. Frequent and adequate back, mouth, and perineal care.
3. ROM exercises to lower extremities when not ambulating.
4. Monitoring of bowel and bladder functions and institution of special measures as necessary if patient incontinent.
5. Assist with meals and fluid intake.

QUESTIONS

1. Are there any additional patient objectives you would prescribe at this time?
2. Are there any additional nursing interventions you would prescribe?

Continuation Of Hospital Course: Seven days post-admission, Mr. W. is transferred to the ICU in acute distress. An up-dated assessment provides the following new information.

S: None.

O: Semi-comatose, restless, unable to follow simple commands. BP 60/?, P 120 with occasional PVB's, respirations 32, shallow and labored, breath sounds decreased in lower lobes bilaterally; T 40°C (ax); nasotracheal suction Q hr., with 5-10 ml. rusty-green secretions obtained; skin cold and clammy, generalized hematomas over body, dependent edema in sacrum and extremities; Serum Na^+ 128, K^+ 6.1, Cl^- 78, CO_2 18, BUN 150, Creatinine 8.8; Hct 26, WBC 1500, Platelets 14,000,

PT 12 c/16 pt, PTT 31 c/40 pt; Blood culture results: E. Coli; Urine output 2-5 ml./hr. for past 8 hr. (Foley), rusty in color, sp. gravity 1.030, urine osmolarity < serum osmolarity; clinitest 2 +, acetest moderate; Stool, emesis, and urine positive for occult blood; Blood gasses: pH 7.25; pO_2 60; pCO_2 40.

A: Infected condition has progressed to septic shock state, and the following problems exist:
1. inadequate O_2/CO_2 exchange in lungs and at the cellular level.
2. acute renal failure.
3. metabolic acidosis.
4. hyperkalemia.
5. thrombocytopenia, leukopenia, and anemia.
6. mental changes.

P: **Medical Management**
1. Intubate and place on volume respirator, rate 18, TV 700 ml FiO_2 40% (See Chapter 3 for discussion of care needs of patients on respirators).
2. Lasix 40 mg. IV push STAT.
3. Sodium bicarbonate 2 amps IV push STAT.
4. Solu-Medrol 1 Gm. IV push STAT.
5. IV antibiotics:
   Clindamycin 600 mg. IV STAT and Q 6 hr.
   Gentamicin 60 mg. IV STAT and Q 6 hr.
6. Transfuse with 6 units of platelets today (See Chapter 10 on DIC for discussion of use of platelet transfusions).
7. Hemodialysis today (See Chapter 4 for discussion of hemodialysis and care needs of patients on dialysis).
8. Dopamine infusion to keep systolic BP > 80 mm. Hg but < 140 mm. Hg.
9. Monitor CVP and PWP Q 1 hr. (See Chapter 2 for discussion of Swan-Ganz monitoring).
10. IV infusion rate to be established Q hr. depending on CVP, PWP, urinary output.

QUESTIONS

1. What is the purpose of administering Lasix, sodium bicar-

bonate, Solu-Medrol, antibiotics, platelets, and dopamine?
2. What effects and/or side effects would you anticipate when administering these medications?
3. Using the laboratory data, explain the rationale for instituting hemodialysis at this time?
4. Using the new data identify appropriate patient objectives and nursing interventions for Mr. W. at this time.

The additional data at the time of transfer to the ICU indicates that the septicemic state progressed into septic shock; the signs and symptoms suggest the late stage of shock. At this time the primary nursing and medical objectives and interventions are focused on maintaining body systems and homeostasis. Since the additional data reflect a change in Mr. W's health status, his care objectives and nursing interventions must be revised to incorporate these changes.

P: **Nursing Management:**

Patient Objective VII

Patient's cullular perfusion, cellular oxygenation, and cellular metabolism will return to normal. (Since the ramifications of septic shock and the effectiveness of cellular perfusion, cellular oxygenation, and cellular metabolism are reflected in the functional ability of various organs and systems, the patient objectives and appropriate nursing interventions will be sub-divided according to specific organs and systems).

A) **Cardiac function**
   1. *Objectives*
      (a) systolic BP will be > 80 mm. Hg but < 140 mm. Hg.
      (b) less than 6 PVBs/minute.
      (c) CVP will range between 6 and 15 cm. H_2O.
      (d) PWP will range between 10 and 12 mm. Hg.
      (e) skin will be warm (not hot) and dry, without cyanosis and mottling.
      (d) sensorium will return to pre-septic shock state.
   2. *Interventions*
      (a) ausculatory and/or arterial monitor of BP Q 15 minutes to Q 1 hr. as necessary and record.

(b) dopamine IV gtt at a rate to maintain systolic BP > 80 mm. Hg but < 140 mm. Hg.

(c) continuous ECG monitoring: check 1 minute strip for number of PVBs/minute Q 1 hr. and as necessary.

(d) monitor CVP and PWP Q 1 hr. and record.

(e) observe and evaluate skin temperature, texture, and color Q 1 hr. and record.

(f) observe and evaluate level of consciousness, pupil reaction, orientation potential, ability to move extremities with and without stimuli Q 1 hr. and record.

(g) weigh patient daily and record.

QUESTIONS

1. Are there any additional patient objectives or nursing interventions you would prescribe at this time?

2. What would be the rationale for the physician to order the dopamine drip?

3. Differentiate between the information provided by the PWP and CVP.

Discussion:

Cardiac function: During the latter stages of septic shock, cellular perfusion is decreased because of the decreased circulating volume resulting from the capillary pooling and vasoconstriction due to the compensatory mechanisms. To improve the cardiac function and thus cellular perfusion, intravenous fluid and drug therapy will be instituted.

The administration of intravenous fluids, by increasing the circulating volume, increases cardiac output and helps to maintain blood pressure. To ensure adequate cerebral circulation, an arterial BP of at least 60 mm. Hg must be maintained. To prevent fluid overload but yet maintain adequate BP and circulating volume frequent and careful monitoring of CVP, PWP, BP, intake and output, heart rate, respiratory rate, skin temperature, and sensorium are essential.

Disagreement exists concerning the advantage of administering vasopressors vs. vasodilator agents in the treatment of shock. Vasopressors increase cardiac output by strengthening cardiac contractility and increasing heart rate and raise arterial blood pressure by constricting blood vessels. The additional strain on the myocardium to overcome the existing increased peripheral resistance and generalized vasoconstriction, which further inhibits cellular perfusion, are the major side effects opposing the use of vasopressors in the shock state. A frequently used vasopressor is dopamine. At moderate doses, dopamine produces a dopaminergic response; that is, selective vasodilatation to the renal, mesenteric, cerebral, and coronary arteries. This selective vasodilatation facilitates cellular perfusion to vital organs and thus supports the use of dopamine. Other commonly used vasopressor agents include epinephrine, norepinephrine, and isoproterenol.

Care must be taken to carefully monitor arterial blood pressure and to ensure proper infusion of any of the vasopressor drugs. Arterial blood pressure must be adjusted to maintain adequate tissue perfusion and yet prevent unnecessary myocardial strain. Several of the vasopressor agents are known to cause ischemia, necrosis, and sloughing of tissues when the intravenous solutions infiltrate. If extravasation occurs, stop the infusion, notify the physician, and prepare phentolamine (Regitine), an alpha adrenergic blocking agent that antagonizes the local vasoconstrictive effects. The subcutaneous injection of Regitine could prevent serious tissue damage and necrosis if injected soon after infiltration.

Vasodilators may be preferred in late septic shock to reverse the existing generalized vasoconstriction especially when high filling pressures exist. Two commonly used vasodilator agents are phentolamine (Regitine) and nitroprusside. Careful and frequent monitoring of BP, CVP, PWP, and heart rate are essential to prevent uncontrolled hypotension, tachycardia, and fluid overload.

Therapeutic benefits of large doses of corticosteroids is controversial in the treatment of septic shock. Experimental studies suggest this therapy may prevent loss of arteriolar vasomotor control and increase capillary permeability associated with septic shock. The effects of steriods on tissue oxygenation and oxygen-hemoglobin affinity must be studied. This therapeutic intervention must be carefully evaluated by the physician before institution.

The primary function of nurses in meeting the objectives in Section A will be the institution of prescribed therapy and the monitoring and recording of observations. The results of the monitoring of cardiac function will be the basis for change in fluid and drug therapy. The patient in shock needs an adequate amount of fluid to promote the most effective cellular perfusion, but this must be carefully evaluated, as the patient in septic shock has a high potential for developing cardiac failure and/or pulmonary edema. An accurate assessment of many parameters is necessary to maintain adequate fluid status without overload.

B) **Pulmonary function**
   1. *Objectives*
      (a) breath sounds will be heard in all lobes.
      (b) arterial blood gas (ABG) results will be:
         pH — range between 7.35 and 7.45
         pCO_2 — range between 30 and 50 mm. Hg
         pO_2 — range between 60 and 100 mm. Hg
         O_2 Sat — 90%
      (c) tracheal and main bronchial areas will be free of secretions.
      (d) respirator will operate at the settings prescribed.

   2. *Interventions*
      (a) auscultate breath sounds in all lobes Q 1 hr. and as necessary; record quality.
      (b) monitor serial blood gases; hold arterial puncture sites at least 10 minutes.
      (c) suction tracheal-bronchial areas Q 15 minutes to Q 1 hr. or as necessary; record amount and type of secretions.
      (d) check settings on respirator Q 1 hr. or as necessary according to that prescribed by physician.
      (e) check endotracheal tube cuff pressure Q 2 hr. (if using high volume, low pressure cuff); cuff pressure not to exceed 25 mm. Hg.
      (f) mouth care Q 2 hr. or as necessary; sterile technique for suctioning.
      (g) report to physician immediately any deviations from set goals.

QUESTIONS

1. What would be the rationale for the physician to order intubation and respiratory assistance?

2. Are there any additional patient objectives or nursing interventions you would prescribe at this time?

Discussion

Pulmonary function: Many patients with septic shock will require intubation and the use of respirators to maintain adequate oxygenation. However, very high concentrations of oxygen must be used with caution. It is important to remember that high concentrations of oxygen over extended periods of time can cause toxic effects. The use of a respirator adds many care needs to the patient. The endotracheal intubation adds a new source for the introduction of infective organisms. Sterile technique with suctioning is essential. See Chapter 3 for a discussion of suctioning. The patient may require suctioning every 15 minutes if secretions are copious. The amount and type of secretions obtained must be recorded.

In addition to suctioning, the nurse must make sure that the respirator is set at the settings ordered and the patient's tolerance to these settings observed. If the patient is fighting the respirator, or does not respond as expected, the physician should be notified immediately so that appropriate adjustments can be made. The monitoring of the patient's respiratory function should be done at least every hour and more frequently if the patient's status is changing rapidly or if adjustments are being made in the respirator settings.

The maintenance of a closed system, when using a respirator and endotracheal tube, requires the use of an inflated cuff. The endotracheal tube cuff should be a high volume, low pressure type which minimizes any damage to the capillaries in the trachea. Refer to Chapter 3 for detailed information on the care of patients with endotracheal tubes and respirators.

The nurse must also remember that the use of a respirator may be very frightening to the patient and/or significant others. It is essential that the nurse and physician give thorough and frequent explanation of all activities to the patient and/or significant others. The intubated patient cannot communicate in the usual way and an alternate means for the patient to communicate with the staff and significant others must be developed.

C) Renal function

1. *Objectives*
   (a) urinary output will be > 25 ml/hr.
   (b) specific gravity will range between 1.010 and 1.025.
   (c) urinary osmolarity will be > serum osmolarity.
   (d) serum electrolytes, BUN, and creatinine will return to normal.
   (e) patient will be hemodialyzed as prescribed.

2. *Interventions*
   (a) measure and record urinary output (Foley) Q 1 hr.
   (b) test urine for specific gravity Q 4 hr. and record.
   (c) collect urine for prescribed tests.
   (d) arrange for the collection of prescribed blood tests.
   (e) arrange for hemodialysis as prescribed.

QUESTIONS

1. Describe how the stated objectives or parameters are used as a guide to monitor renal function.
2. Are there any additional patient objectives or nursing interventions you would prescribe at this time?

Discussion

Renal function: Renal perfusion will be decreased by the original insult, normal compensatory mechanisms, and the use of vasopressors. As can be seen, Mr. W. has developed acute renal failure. All patients with septic shock are candidates for acute renal failure. The primary function of the nurse in meeting these objectives is monitoring of the stated parameters. Monitoring should be done on an hourly basis. The patient will have a Foley catheter which facilitates accurate hourly monitoring.

Although the use of a Foley is mandatory for accurate monitoring of urinary output, it also adds another site for introducing contamination. Strict sterile technique in handling the Foley catheter and drainage bag, and in giving perineal care, and obtaining urine specimens without introducing contamination is essential. When the presence of renal failure has been definitively established, the urinary catheter will be removed in order to avoid the added risk of superimposed infection.

QUESTION

Does your institution and/or unit have a routine procedure for care of urethral catheters? Describe the procedure.

The use of hemodialysis may be necessary for the patient during the acute stage of renal failure. Hemodialysis adds many other needs to patient care (see Chapter 4). The frequency of hemodialysis will be based upon the laboratory studies. The presence of severe hyperkalemia, acidosis, and/or increased urea may require more frequent dialysis. The nurse can assist in decreasing the need for dialysis by instituting measures to decrease the patient's catabolic rate. Catabolism increases protein breakdown and production of urea, releases K^+ from the cells, and produces more acid end products.

Catabolism is increased by anxiety. Good explanation of the unit, procedures, and establishment of communication with the patient may help to decrease anxiety and thus catabolism.

The promotion of rest as feasible decreases metabolic needs, and thus decreases catabolism. Every effort should be made to provide rest periods. This is an aspect where nurses can have major input and institute controls on the patient's environment.

The presence of new infection increases catabolism. Mr. W. has many new potential sites for nosocomial infections (endotracheal tube, respirator, urethral catheter, intravenous and intra-arterial catheters). A procedure for care of each of these invasive devices is necessary. Also, because of the status of the patient and the many monitoring devices, the patient may be kept on his back for extended periods of time. This may aggravate the existing circulatory status. The patient has decreased perfusion, edema, and increased catabolism, all of which makes him very prone to decubitus ulcer formation. A decubitus ulcer will increase protein breakdown and thus increase catabolism.

QUESTION

Describe other nursing interventions which would reduce protein breakdown and catabolism.

D) **Metabolic system**
1. *Objectives*
(a) body temperature will range between 36.5 and 37.5°C.
(b) serum pH will range between 7.35 and 7.45.

2. *Interventions*
(a) monitor body temperature Q 2 hr. or as necessary; use hypothermia unit as needed.
(b) give sodium bicarbonate IV as prescribed.
(c) record observations and notify physician immediately when any of these goals and actions are not being met.
(d) continue with nursing interventions 2, 3, and 4 as described on page 550.

E) **Hematological system**

1. *Objectives*
(a) coagulation factors and platelets will return to normal.
(b) CBC factors (RBC, Hct, WBC) will return to normal.
2. *Interventions*
(a) nursing interventions 2, 3, 4, 5, and 7 as described on page 538 need to be continued. Protective isolation procedures, strict handwashing, and the stringent sterile techniques in the care of the endotracheal tube and respiratory system, IV and arterial catheters, Foley and GU system, and other intrusive diagnostic and therapeutic procedures (in order to avoid infecting other patients, reinfecting Mr. W., or spreading organisms from one site to another) are essential.
(b) give blood and blood components as prescribed.

SUMMARY

The management of the septic shock state is extremely difficult not only because of the septicemia itself, but also because of the compounded underlying pathophysiology. In the ICU, nursing management must focus on all organs and systems at all times. The central focus is the maintenance of all body systems and functions.

Management is continually adjusted to meet new needs based on the continual reassessment. The amount and time of intervention must be very individualized. The monitoring and documentation of the interventions by nurses are essential to accurately treat the patient.

Many sophisticated monitoring techniques (arterial catheters, PWP, CVP, etc.) and treatment techniques (ventilatory, hemodynamic assistance, etc.) will be used to support the patient. It must be remembered that while multiple measures are used to support the patient's altered metabolic and hemodynamic status, other interventions directed toward the underlying disease state are also instituted.

The mortality rate for septic shock is still very high and Mr. S.W. did die one week later. The best treatment still centers around the prevention of bacteremia and septicemia and the detection of such states in the very early stages. Consistent sterile technique in all invasive procedures is an absolute must and may be the activitiy that prevents many patients from developing bacteremia, septicemia, and thus septic shock. In patients who are compromised hosts, like Mr. W., consistent sterile technique and strict handwashing may prevent the massive septic shock syndrome.

REFERENCES

1. Abbey JC: Nursing observations of fluid imbalances. *Nursing Clinics of North America* 3:77, 1968.
2. Ando S, et al.: ACTH release in vivo and in vitro: extrapituitary mediation during Esch. coli bacteremia. *Endocrinology* 74:894, 1964.
3. Aspinall MJ: Scoring against nosocomial infections. *American Journal of Nursing* 78(10): 1704-07.
4. Brand L: A practical approach to infection surveillance in the intensive care unit. *Heart and Lung* 5:788, 1976.
5. Brand L, Wilson RF: Shock. In Meltzer LE, et al. (Eds.): *Concepts and Practices of Intensive Care for Nurse Specialists.* Charles Press Publishers, Bowie, Md., 1976.
6. Brooks SM: *Basic Facts of Body Water and Ions.* 3rd Ed. Springer Publishing Co., New York, 1977.
7. Brown WJ: A classification of microorganisms frequently causing sepsis. *Heart and Lung* 5:397, 1976.
8. Brown WJ: The increasing incidence of sepsis and antibiotic resistance. *Heart and Lung* 5:593, 1976.
9. Cohn JN: Monitoring techniques in shock. *American Journal of Cardiology* 26:565, 1970.
10. Cushing R: Pulmonary infection. *Heart and Lung* 5:611, 1976.

11. Davis BD, et al.: *Microbiology*. 2nd Ed. Harper and Row Publishers, New York, 1973.

12. Duff JH: Cardiovascular changes in sepsis. *Heart and Lung* **5**:773, 1976.

13. Dutcher IE, Hardenburg HC Jr.: Water and Electrolyte Imbalances. In Meltzer LE, et al. (Eds.): *Concepts and Practices of Intensive Care for Nurse Specialists*. Charles Press Publishers, Bowie, Md., 1976.

14. Fisher EJ: Antimicrobial therapy: some guidelines. *Heart and Lung* **5**:437, 1976.

15. Fisher EJ: Surveillance and management of hospital-acquired infections. *Heart and Lung* **5**:784, 1976.

16. Goldmann DA, Maki DG: Infection control in total parenteral nutrition. *Journal of the American Medical Association* **223**:1360, 1973.

17. Goldmann DA, et al.: Guidelines for infection control in intravenous therapy. *Annals of Internal Medicine*.**79**:848, 1973.

18. Goodman LS, Gilman A: *The Pharmacological Basis of Therapeutics*. 5th Ed. Macmillan Publishing, New York, 1975.

19. Guyton AC: *Textbook of Medical Physiology*. 5th Ed. W.B. Saunders, Philadelphia, Pa., 1975.

20. Holliday RL: Intra-abdominal sepsis. *Heart and Lung* **5**:781, 1976.

21. Hoshal VL Jr.: Intravenous catheters and infection. *Surgical Clinics of North America* **52**:1407, 1972.

22. Jacobson ED: A physiologic approach to shock. *New England Journal of Medicine* **278**(15):834, 1968.

23. Jahre JN: Medical approach to the hypotensive patient and the patient in shock. *Heart and Lung* **4**:577, 1975.

24. Lauter CB: Opportunistic infections. *Heart and Lung* **5**:601, 1976.

25. Ledgerwood A: Hepatobiliary complications of sepsis. *Heart and Lung* **5**:621, 1976.

26. Lillehei RC, Dietzman DH: Circulatory Collapse and Shock. In Schwartz SI, et al. (Eds.): *Principles of Surgery*. McGraw-Hill, New York, 1974, p. 133.

27. Linton AL: Diagnosis and treatment of infections of the urinary tract. *Heart and Lung* **5**:607, 1976.

28. Mason JW, et al.: Plasma kallikrein and Hageman factor in gram-negative bacteremia. *Annals of Internal Medicine* **73**:545, 1970.

29. Meltzer LE, et al.: *Concepts and Practices of Intensive Care for Nurse Specialist*. Charles Press Publishers, Bowie, Md., 1976.

30. Mountacastle VB: *Medical Physiology*. 13th Ed. C.V. Mosby, St. Louis, Mo., 1974.

31. Murray J, Smallwood J: CVP monitoring. *Nursing '77* **7**(1):42, 1977.

32. Petersdorf RG: Septic Shock. In Thorn GW, et al. (Eds.): *Harrison's Principles of Internal Medicine*. McGraw-Hill, New York, 1977, p. 770.

33. Petersdorf RG, Dale DC: Infections in Compromised Host. In Thorn GW, et al. (Eds.): *Harrison's Principles of Internal Medicine.* McGraw-Hill, New York, 1977, p. 764.

34. Rodman MJ, Smith DW: *Clinical Pharmacology in Nursing.* J.B. Lippincott, Philadelphia, Pa., 1974.

35. Roellig S: Management of patients with contagious illness. *Heart and Lung* **5**:596, 1976.

36. Rosenberg IK: Renal hemodynamic effects of sepsis. *Heart and Lung* **5**:777, 1976.

37. Schuler JJ, et al.: Effect of glucocorticoids on carbohydrate metabolism and survival of endotoxin-shocked monkeys. *Annals of Surgery* **183**:345, 1976.

38. Schumer W: Metabolism during shock and sepsis. *Heart and Lung* **5**:416, 1976.

39. Schumer W: Shock and its effect on the cell. *Journal of the American Medical Association* **205**(4):75, 1968.

40. Schumer W: Steriods in the treatment of clinical septic shock. *Annals of Surgery* **184**:343, 1976.

41. Schumer W, et al.: Endotoxin effect on respiration of rat liver mitochondria. *Journal of Surgical Research* **10**:609, 1970.

42. Schumer W, Nyhus LM: Corticosteriod effect on biochemical parameters of human oligemic shock. *Archives of Surgery* **100**:405, 1970.

43. Shubin H, Weil MH: Touchstones in critical care medicine: an introduction. *Critical Care Medicine* **2**:281, 1974.

44. Sibbald WJ: Bacteremia and endotoxemia: a discussion of their roles in the pathophysiology of gram-negative sepsis. *Heart and Lung* **5**:765, 1976.

45. Silva J: Anaerobic infections. *Heart and Lung* **5**:406, 1976.

46. Sodeman WA Jr, Sodeman WA: *Pathologic Physiology: Mechanisms of Disease.* 5th Ed. W.B. Saunders, Philadelphia, Pa., 1974.

47. Spengler, RF, Greenough III, WB: Hospital costs and mortality attributed to nosocomial bacteremia. *Journal of the American Medical Association,* Nov. 24, 78 **240**(22):2455-8.

48. Taylor CM: When to anticipate septic shock. *Nursing '75* **5**(4):34, 1975.

49. Tepperman J: *Metabolic and Endocrine Physiology.* 3rd Ed. Year Book Medical Publishers, Inc., Chicago, Ill. 1973.

50. Thal AP, et al.: *Shock: A Physiologic Basis for Treatment.* Year Book Medical Publishers, Inc., Chicago, Ill. 1971.

51. Vander AJ, et al.: *Human Physiology: The Mechanisms of Body Function.* 2nd Ed. McGraw-Hill, New York, 1975.

52. Weinstein, RA, et al.: Pressure transducers as a source of bacteremia after open heart surgery. *Chest* **69**(3):338, 1976.

53. Widmann FK: *Goodale's Clinical Interpretation of Laboratory Tests.* 7th Ed. F.A. Davis Co., Philadelphia, Pa., 1973.

54. Williams SR; *Nutrition and Diet Therapy.* 3rd Ed. C.V. Mosby, St. Louis, Mo. 1977.

55. Wilmore DW: Alimentation in injured and septic patients. *Heart and Lung* 5:791, 1976.

56. Wilson JA: Infection control in intravenous therapy. *Heart and Lung* 5:430, 1976.

57. Wilson RF: Endocrine changes in sepsis. *Heart and Lung* 5:411, 1976.

58. Wilson RF: The diagnosis and management of severe sepsis and septic shock. *Heart and Lung* 5:422, 1976.

59. Wilson RF: The diagnosis and treatment of acute respiratory failure in sepsis. *Heart and Lung* 5:614, 1976.

CHAPTER 10

Special Problems in Critical Care: DIC

by Barbara J. Daly, RN, MSN

DISSEMINATED INTRAVASCULAR COAGULATION

Disseminated intravascular coagulation (DIC) is a syndrome complicating the clinical course of many patients in Intensive Care Units. It is a clotting disorder which occurs only secondarily to a variety of initial or primary pathological states. Before discussing DIC itself, a review of the normal mechanisms of hemostasis is necessary.

COAGULATION AND ANTICOAGULATION

Normally there exists in the body a balance between the processes of coagulation and anticoagulation. Without the presence of injury, trauma, or disease, this balance provides both for the fluid state of the blood and the constant availability of clotting factors, should an injury occur.

Clotting factors are those substances in the blood which interact in the coagulation process. These factors have been assigned numbers (Roman numerals) in order to avoid the confusion arising from differences in nomenclature; these are listed in Table 10-1. The coagulation process is an essential part of the body's ability to stop bleeding.

When an injury to a blood vessel occurs, there is an initial, immediate vasoconstriction, which reduces blood flow to the injured area. Following this is platelet aggregation. Contact with the injured

TABLE 10-1

Clotting Factors

Number	Names Frequently Used
I	Fibrinogen
II	Prothrombin
III	Tissue Thromboplastin, Thrombokinase
IV	Calcium
V	Proaccelerin, Labile Factor, Ac-globulin (Ac-G)
VII	Proconvertin, Serum Prothrombin Conversion Accelerator, Auto-prothrombin I, Stable Factor
VIII	Anti-hemophilic Factor (AHF), Anti-hemophilic Globulin (AHG)
IX	Christmas Factor, Plasma Thromboplastin Component (PTC), Auto-prothrombin II
X	Stuart Factor, Stuart-Prower Factor
XI	Plasma Thromboplastin Antecedant (PTA)
XII	Hageman Factor, Contact Factor
XIII	Fibrin Stabilizing Factor, Fibrinase

vessel wall causes platelets to adhere to each other and to the vessel; this change in platelet characteristics is not completely understood, but is thought to be related to the contact of the platelet with the exposed basement membrane of the blood vessel, with collagen fibers, and with epinephrine, norepinephrine, and ADP.[2] The accumulation of platelets forms a plug which partially blocks the injured vessel and limits blood loss.

The last phase of the body's response is the initiation of the clotting process. There are two coagulation systems which can lead to the production of a clot, the intrinsic and the extrinsic systems. The intrinsic system is initiated when Factor XII, the Hageman Factor, contacts an abnormal surface. Anything which changes the normal surface of the blood vessel, such as endotoxemia, heat stroke, or hypotension, can initiate this. The extrinsic system, which is a shorter and more efficient process, is begun by the release of tissue thromboplastin, Factor III, from damaged tissues, such as caused by blunt trauma or lacerations.

In the intrinsic system, the activated form of Factor XII acts as an enzyme to convert Factor XI to an active form, designated XIa. This activated XI then converts IX, in the presence of calcium, to its active form. With calcium and platelets, IXa joins with Factor VIII, and this complex causes the Stuart Factor, Factor X, to assume its active state. After this point, the intrinsic system follows the same pathway as the extrinsic system.

The extrinsic system converts Factor X to its active form through the interaction of tissue thromboplastin (Factor III), calcium, and factor VII. The activated Factor X, Factor V, platelet phospholipids, and calcium then cause the conversion of prothrombin, which is produced by the liver, using vitamin K, to thrombin. Fibrinogen, which is a large protein molecule also formed by the liver, is then cleaved by thrombin, which acts as a proteolytic agent. In this way single chain fibrin monomers are formed. These monomers polymerize with each other, creating fibrin threads which constitute the inner core of the blood clot. Thrombin also acts in a feedback mechanism to stimulate the production of more prothrombin in the liver. After fibrin polymerization, the clot formed is in a gel phase, and the large molecule of fibrin is composed of loose, easily disrupted bonds. Factor XIII acts to stabilize the clot, which becomes a mesh network, adhering to the vessel wall and preventing the passage of blood. The sequence of these events is shown in Figure 10-1.

To summarize, hemostasis is achieved by three mechanisms: blood vessel constriction, platelet aggregation, and clot formation. The clotting process can be initiated by any condition which changes the vessel endothelium or damages tissue. The major steps in the clotting process involve the reactions leading to the activation of prothrombin, the production of thrombin, and the conversion of fibrinogen into the fibrin thread mesh.

Once coagulation has occurred, several opposing mechanisms begin to operate to prevent extension of the clot and then to dissolve it. First, platelet aggregation is limited to the site of injury. This means that the coagulation factors tend to be contained in this area; factors that are present in areas of the bloodstream where flow is not reduced by platelet clumps are diluted, and their concentration cannot rise high enough to cause clotting. The liver removes these factors as they are circulated. The fibrin threads themselves also absorb thrombin and thus limit its stimulation of prothrombin. It is also thought that neutralization systems or anti-factors exist which

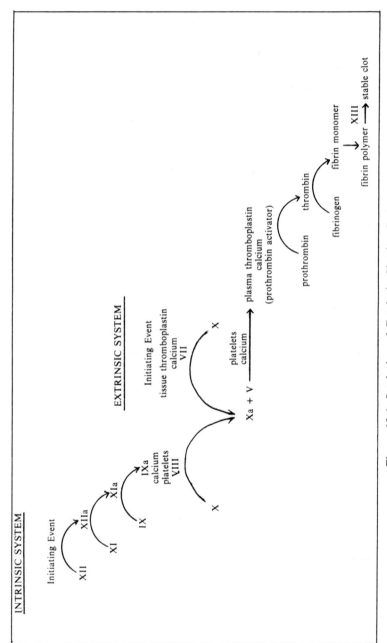

Figure 10-1. Intrinsic and Extrinsic Clotting Systems.

limit and counteract each step in the coagulation process, and that the action of these anti-factors contributes to the fluidity of the blood.[8]

The major control of the clotting process, once it has occurred, is due to the fibrinolytic system. This anticoagulation phase begins with the activation of plasminogen, a proteolytic enzyme, by tissue and bacterial enzymes, and by thrombin. Plasminogen is converted to plasmin, which is incorporated into the clot. Plasmin then dissolves the clot, breaking down the fibrin threads. These pieces of the original fibrin polymer are termed fibrin degradation products (FDP) or fibrin split products (FSP). The anticoagulation process is further assisted by the inactivation of Factors V and VIII by plasmin and the inhibition of thrombin by the FDP.

THE PROCESS OF DIC

The syndrome known as DIC is essentially an imbalance between the coagulation process and anticoagulation process described. Although many terms have been used to describe the phenomenon (defibrination syndrome, consumption coagulopathy, secondary fibrinolysis, intravascular coagulation fibrinolysis), the phrase "disseminated intravascular coagulation" is most appropriate in describing the problem. First, DIC is a *diffuse* process, occurring throughout the body, not localized to any one area. It is a process that occurs wholly *within the bloodstream,* and symptoms are always a result of circulatory impairment. Lastly, although excessive bleeding may be the most significant or first recognized symptom, *coagulation* is the initial event.

As mentioned earlier, DIC is always a secondary, never a primary disease. It occurs as the result or consequence of a generalized activation of the hemostatic processes by some other disorder. Often the primary disease process involves the introduction of a foreign substance into the blood stream, such as endotoxins, snake venom, placental matter from abruptio placentae, which acts as a procoagulant agent. DIC may also be triggered by conditions which predispose to thrombus formation, such as states of hypotension, and direct damage to vascular endothelium. The third way in which DIC may be initiated occurs in diseases or conditions in which large amounts of tissue thromboplastin are released, such as blunt trauma to organs or neoplastic disease. Table 10-2 provides a list of those disorders which frequently are complicated by DIC.

TABLE 10-2

Common Primary Disorders Associated with DIC

Tissue Injury	Neoplastic Disease (carcinoma, leukemia) Extensive Surgery Blunt Trauma
Red Cell Injury	Extracorporeal Circulation Hemolysis (secondary to transfusion incompatibility) Hemolytic Anemia
Foreign Substance	Endotoxemia Snake Venom Abruptio Placentae Amniotic Fluid Embolus
Vascular Changes	Shock, hypotension Direct Trauma Endotoxemia and Viremia
Immune and Antigen- Antibody Responses	Anaphylaxis Systemic Lupus Erythematosus Transfusion Reactions

The primary insult causes the initiation of the coagulation process. Because this occurs not in response to a localized injury, but rather as a generalized response to systemic factors, an overall hypercoagulable state results. The clotting factors involved in coagulation, particularly Factors II, V, VIII, IX, X, XII, and platelets, are thus consumed and their levels fall. This leads to the second phase of DIC, a state of hypocoagulability. Just as coagulation occurred throughout the bloodstream, fibrinolysis takes place in all locations. This then results in the release of excessive fibrin degradation products, which in turn act as antithrombic agents.

The clinical presentation of DIC can be classified as either thrombolic episodes, resulting from the hypercoagulable state, or hemorrhagic episodes, resulting from the hypocoagulable state. Thrombi may occlude the microcirculation of any organ, leading to ischemia and necrosis. Multiple petechiae often appear as a result of these thrombi; in addition to the skin, the brain, pancreas, kidneys, lungs, and adrenals are frequently affected. Bleeding may occur from any site; the gastrointestinal tract, genitourinary tract, and, of course, any wound site are high risk areas.

The diagnosis of DIC is based on several laboratory studies, in addition to the signs and symptoms described. The most common indicators of DIC are: prolonged prothrombin and partial thromboplastin times, decreased platelet and fibrinogen, abnormally high levels of FDP, and the appearance of damaged or fragmented red blood cells.

INTERVENTION

Treatment of DIC must begin with the treatment of the underlying disease. Until the initiating factors are corrected or removed, the imbalance between coagulation and anticoagulation will persist. While therapy for the primary disease is being addressed, there are several measures to interrupt the processes of DIC or control its effects. Most common of these is the administration of heparin. Intravenous heparin, given in doses of 100-150 USP units/kg. body weight every four hours, or 800 U/kg./24 hours as a continuous drip, acts in three places: it inhibits the action of thrombin on fibrinogen, prevents the formation of the prothrombin activator, and increases the absorption of thrombin by fibrin. In these ways, heparin slows the clotting sequence and permits the level of clotting factors to return to normal. There is a certain risk, however, in using heparin with patients who have a major bleeding site which may be activated by the blockage of steps in coagulation.

The second measure available involves the replacement of absent or diminished clotting factors. The availability of these products is sometimes limited, but in acute crisis, platelets, fresh whole blood, and Factor VIII can be administered.

The last therapeutic approach which is helpful includes measures to insure that all other components of the clotting system are present. Vitamin K is often given, in addition to the vitamin B complex, and liver disease is treated as aggressively as possible.

Nursing care of the patient with DIC varies considerably with the extent of the disease and the nature of the underlying disorder. Of absolute priority in the care of these patients is assessment. The identification of thrombic events and determination of specific organ impairment depends upon the observation of the patient's signs and symptoms; early detection is essential in order to institute prompt therapy and minimize the effects of DIC.

Decisions regarding therapeutic measures, such as the administration of platelets, are usually based upon observations of the extent of bleeding. This is the responsibility of the nurse. It is essential that the nurse be able to assess the sources of blood loss, the amount of loss, and, most importantly, the trend in bleeding (progressive increases or decreases). Hourly intake and output, measurement of all drainage, determination of occult blood content in drainage, and weighing of dressings are all necessary measures.

The nursing measures designed to minimize bleeding in patients with any blood dyscrasia, such as hemophilia or leukemia, are all appropriate in caring for the DIC patient. Any kind of trauma to tissues must be avoided; venipunctures and injections are contraindicated. Scabs should be left in place or gradually softened and soaked off to prevent re-bleeding from that site. Tape should not be applied to skin and protective substances such as Karaya gum or Stomadhesive pads can be used around wounds to keep drainage off skin.

The prognosis of the patient whose illness becomes complicated by DIC depends upon the severity of the imbalance between coagulation and anticoagulation, the success of intervention and correction of the imbalance, and the likelihood of recovery from the primary disease. The emotional toll on the patient and family when DIC occurs is quite heavy; DIC represents a second life-threatening event occurring during a crisis state when resources are already stressed. All efforts must be directed toward support of the patient and family's strengths. The following case study exemplifies the challenge and complexity of the care of patients with DIC.

CASE STUDY

Ellen C. was an 18-year-old patient admitted to the hospital with the chief complaint of abdominal pain of 2 weeks' duration. The following are excerpts from the admission history and physical.

Social history

Patient is oldest daughter of middle class parents, both alive and well. Father is an insurance salesman, mother is housewife. Three siblings: 5-year-old brother, 12-year-old sister, 16-year-old sister. Patient lives at home and is currently a freshman at local community college.

Medical history

One previous admission, age 6, for tonsillectomy. Usual childhood diseases—measles at age 8, chicken pox at age 10. No recurrent illnesses.

History of present illness

Patient states she was in good health until two weeks prior to admission. At this time she began to experience intermittent pain, sometimes dull, sometimes of a sharp, stabbing nature, localized over the right lower quadrant. She was taken to private medical doctor, who found nothing abnormal on examination, and she was sent home. In talking with patient's mother at that time, the M.D. suggested that Ellen's symptoms might be a reflection of the stress of upcoming final exams.

Ellen's pain continued, and she returned to her private medical doctor's office, where a repeat examination and CBC were again non-conclusive. When the pain grew worse two days later, Ellen's mother brought her to the Emergency Room (May 11).

Ellen was admitted to the hospital for further observation and diagnosis. When first seen in the Emergency Room, she was in moderate to severe pain, had hypoactive bowel sounds and guarding of the abdomen. By the next day, her abdomen was rigid and she was febrile. On May 12 she was taken to the O.R. and a ruptured Meckel's diverticulum resected. She tolerated the procedure fairly well and was returned to her room from the recovery room in satisfactory condition, with a peripheral IV and abdominal sump and NG tubes in place.

The postoperative course was difficult. By May 15, three days after surgery, Ellen's urine output continued to be low (10-20 cc. per hour) despite adequate hydration, and bowel sounds had not returned. Abdominal cultures taken at the time of surgery had grown enterococcus, coliforms, and clostridium.

By May 17, frank peritonitis was evident. Ellen's respirations had become labored and a chest x-ray revealed bilateral pleural effusions, requiring thoracenteses. At this time petechiae appeared on her chest and abdomen. By that evening, she had become progressively hypotensive, lethargic, and, when respiratory distress again developed, she was transferred to the Intensive Care Unit.

The following note was written by the nurse admitting Ellen:

Admitted via stretcher to SICU from Division 3, 9 PM. Vital signs: 36⁴ 108 48 78/40.

Questionable response to verbal stimuli—responds to pain by groaning and withdrawing. Moves all extremities equally. Pupils small, but react to light. General color grey, with 40% O_2 by mask. Breath sounds audible only in upper lobes, very diminished. Respirations labored, shallow—moaning with each breath. IV in right ankle at 200 cc./hr. NG to intermittent suction, draining brown; Foley to CD., draining dark amber. Petechiae over entire trunk, anterior and posterior. Blood work and chest x-ray done. Left thoracotomy performed; chest tube to water seal drainage, draining bloody purulent material. Right thoracotomy completed. Right paracentesis performed; light brown fecal material obtained. Incision ecchymotic, not well approximated; two new abdominal sumps positioned.

10:30 PM: Tonic seizures noted, upper and lower extremities, lasting 3-5 minutes, including nystagmus. Occurring at 15-20 minute intervals.

10:45 PM: Intubated with 8.0 oral endotracheal tube, placed on MA_1 respirator, 40% O_2, TV = 700 cc.

At 11:30 PM, Ellen was taken back to the operating room for an abdominal exploratory laparotomy. She was given initial does of penicillin, gentamicin, clindamycin, digoxin, and Solu-Medrol. Intravenous fluids included 3 units of whole blood, 2 platelet packs, and Ringer's lactate. In the operating room, it was found that the bowel anastamosis had separated; free air, feces, and bowel content were found in the pelvis. An ileostomy was performed and the patient returned to the SICU, with a CVP line, peripheral IV, arterial line, oral endotracheal tube, NG tube, Miller-Abbott tube, two abdominal sumps, and Foley catheter in place.

Questions

1. Upon her return from the operating room, which parameters should be assessed immediately by the nurse caring for Ellen?

2. After initial assessment, which laboratory studies, in particular, would be of greatest significance to the nurse at this point?

Discussion

In admitting Ellen, assessment of life support systems would certainly take priority. Vital signs should be established immediately, and each parameter then more fully explored. A subnormal temperature would be expected in the first postoperative hour; following exposure in the operating room and use of muscle relaxants, the nurse should expect that the patient's temperature will rise at least one or two degrees. Consequently, if the patient is already febrile, it can be anticipated that some kind of hypothermic agent may soon be necessary, such as a hypothermia blanket.

Heart action should be fully assessed with a cardiac monitor. Even with a patient as young as Ellen, the massive assault of sepsis, hypotension, surgery, and general anesthesia could easily lead to arrythmias. It is much too early at this point to assume that her cardiac function is adequate.

Respiratory rate should be assessed both on and off the respirator. Assuming that anesthesia has worn off or been reversed, respiratory rate and depth may yield clues about acid-base status (i.e., a fast, deep pattern—Kussmaul's respirations—would alert the nurse to the possibility of acidosis).

The blood pressure should be correlated with the skin temperature. For example, is vasoconstriction present and is this a compensatory mechanism contributing to the adequacy of blood pressure, or is the skin warm and dry, indicating a more adequate cardiovascular state?

In view of Ellen's seizure activity, neurological status would also be of added significance. Abdominal girth should be measured as soon as possible, for use in later assessment, and she should be weighed as soon as possible. The color, consistency, and amount of drainage from each tube would be the last of initial observations.

After completing a comprehensive assessment, certain laboratory data will be necessary for the nurse to establish a complete data base. The more information she can gather, the better will be her base; however, there are three which assume priority.

First of these would be arterial blood gas results. The presence of bilateral pleural effusions represents a significant respiratory impairment; this is complicated by having just undergone general anesthesia. Because of altered skin color and questionable neurologic status, it will be difficult to determine appropriateness of ventilator settings without ABG results. The potassium level should be checked immediately, for several reasons. First, the lowered urine output, which persisted ever since Ellen's first surgery, would raise questions about renal function. Although it would not be necessary to establish the extent of kidney impairment at this point, the nurse would need to be alert to cardiac arrythmias, should hyperkalemia be present. The likelihood of hyperkalemia also is increased because Ellen was given three units of stored blood, which contains free potassium from red cell lysis.

The third lab result the nurse should check would be blood glucose level. This would be important in any post-trauma or severely stressed patient (see Chapter 8 for an explanation of the effect of trauma on glucose metabolism), but also significant in Ellen's case because of the frequent occurrence of pancreatic infarctions in DIC.

As the nurse caring for Ellen the next day, May 18, the following data is available.

Laboratory Studies		(Normal Values)	Arterial Blood Gases
Sodium:	148 mEq/1	(135-145)	pH: 7.34
Potassium:	5.2 mEq/1	(3.5-5.0)	pO_2: 57
Chloride:	106 mEq/1	(95-107)	pCO_2: 33
Glucose:	690 mg./dl	(70-110)	HCO_3^-: 17
BUN:	96 mg./dl	(6-23)	
Calcium:	8.1 mg./dl	(9-11)	
Phosphorus:	5.2 mg./dl	(2.5-4.5)	
Creatinine:	6.1 mg./dl	(0.7-1.4)	**Ventilator Settings**
CPK:	7,920 u/l	(0-150)	FiO_2: 40%
SGOT:	245 u/l	(0-32)	TV: 600 cc.
Albumin:	3.1 gm./dl	(3.4-5.0)	Rate: 14
Protein:	5.0 gm./dl	(6.0-7.5)	Peak pressure: 40
Hct:	23	(42-52)	System pressure: 35
WBC:	15,600	(5,000-10,000)	
Platelets:	30,000	(150-350,000)	
Pro. time:	70%	(100%)	
PTT:	control - 41 patient - 48		
FDP:	positive in 1:20 dilution (normally positive in less than 1:5 dilution)		
Fibrin:	510 mg.	(170-410 mg./dl)	

DIC has been diagnosed, and Ellen started on a continuous heparin infusion, of 50,000 U in 250 cc. D_5W, run at 10 cc./hr. She was also given Dilantin, phenobarbital, AquaMephyton, and Chloromycetin on a regular basis, in addition to Digoxin, Solu-medrol, and penicillin, started earlier.

Nurses notes read:

5/18, 10 AM. Vital signs: 38^6 122 18 102/89 CVP = 7

Patient unresponsive to verbal stimuli. Will withdraw to pain. Pupils nonreactive. General color grey; nail beds cyanotic. Skin warm, slightly moist. Oral endo to MA_1; occasionally triggers respirator. TV = 200 cc. off respirator. Suctioning for small amounts of thin yellow material. Breath sounds audible, but moist and diminished in all lobes. Monitor pattern-sinus tachycardia. Having tonic-clonic contraction of extremities every few minutes. NG to intermittent suction, draining greenish-yellow; abdominal sumps to suction, draining small amount purulent brown material, Miller-Abbott tube to suction, no drainage. No drainage from ileostomy. Petechiae evident over trunk and inner upper arms. Incision open entire length, packed with iodoform gauze, edges of wound necrotic. Foley draining 10-15 cc./hr., cloudy urine; specific gravity 1.015. IV intake totals 100 cc./hr. Arterial line patent. Parents in to visit; mother calling Ellen's name, but patient does not respond.
11 AM: ABG on MA_1, 100%: pH 7.36; pO_2 85; pCO_2 34; HCO_3^- 20
MA_1 settings changed to FiO_2 70%, with 5 cm. PEEP
ABG now 7.34; 88; 30; 18

Question 3: Given this data, construct an initial problem list, including both active and potential problems. Specify the data that substantiates each problem.

Discussion

Problem	*Data*
1. Sepsis	Abdominal cultures, following ruptured viscus, grew enteroccus, coliforms, and clostridium. Patient is febrile, with elevated WBC. Purulent drainage from abdominal wound.

2. Respiratory Failure:

a) inadequate airway — Patient has altered level of consciousness and cannot protect airway by cough or gag.

b) ventilatory insufficiency — Tidal volume on spontaneous breathing is only 200 cc.—should be 600 cc. (10 cc./kg body weight). Pleural effusions, secondary to infectious process in abdomen, will reduce lung expansion and compliance. With FiO_2 of 40%, patient was still hypoxic and required use of PEEP to reduce shunt.

Pulmonary infarctions, secondary to DIC, are a possibility.

3. Bleeding Tendency (DIC) — Petechiae indicate wide spread clotting in microcirculation. Thrombocytopenia and the increase in fibrin and fibrin degradation products are all diagnostic of DIC. Shortened prothrombin time and prolonged PTT confirm a clotting disorder.

4. Hyperglycemia — Blood glucose level of 690, secondary to stress and/or pancreatic infarct.

5. Altered Level of Consciousness — Patient is unresponsive, with continuous seizure activity. This may be secondary to brain injury caused by hypotensive episode, hypoxia, infarction associated with DIC, or septic process in brain, although the last is unlikely.

6. Inadequate Renal Function — All laboratory studies are indicative of acute tubular necrosis: elevated potassium, BUN, and creatinine. Specific gravity indicates inability to concentrate urine. Oliguria persists despite adequate fluid.

7. Elevated Liver Enzyme Levels — CPK and SGOT very much elevated. This could be caused by several things, such as myocardial infarction or muscle damage,

but the possibility of liver damage cannot be overruled at this time.

8. Potential Skin Breakdown

Patient is immobile, with open, draining wound, and ileostomy stoma. She is often diaphoretic as temperature rises. DIC will impair circulation to some skin areas.

9. Family in Crisis

Oldest daughter has life-threatening illness, which occurred suddenly, and has worsened over last few days. Mother seems to be looking for some hopeful sign in calling Ellen's name. Patient had been living at home and was presumably still in a somewhat dependent role; parents now have limited ability to do anything for their daughter, even to communicate with her. Siblings have not yet visited.

Question 4: What additional laboratory tests will be helpful in evaluating Ellen's renal function? In relating renal function to cardiac status, of what should the nurse be aware?

Discussion: Urine electrolytes, sodium and potassium should be measured, in addition to urine osmolality. A 24-hour urine collection should be started immediately and creatinine clearance determined. Intake and output should be measured hourly.

In relation to cardiac status, the nurse should be aware of the electrocardiographic indications of hyperkalemia: flattening of the p wave, prolongation of the QRS complex, and peaking of the T wave, in addition to increasing ectopic activity. Achieving a proper digoxin dosage will also be more difficult in light of altered renal excretion and fluctuating potassium levels; digoxin levels should be measured and repeated until the correct dosage is assured.

Question 5: Is it necessary to routinely test spot urines for glucose and acetone in assessing level of hyperglycemia?

Discussion: Assuming that the hyperglycemia persists, the nurse would need to frequently assess blood glucose level. However, before depending upon results of urine spot testing, she would need to determine the renal threshold and the kidney's ability to excrete excess glucose. In acute tubular necrosis, the amount of glucose in the urine is often not a reliable indication of serum glucose, and frequent blood samples must be drawn to assess adequacy of treatment.

Question 6: When first beginning a continuous infusion of heparin, to what change in signs or symptoms should the nurse be alert?

Discussion: The purpose of the heparin treatment is to block certain pathways in the clotting process. Consequently, there may be an initial, transient increase in bleeding. This is especially significant in a patient like Ellen who has a large open wound and numerous other potential bleeding sites, such as chest tubes, arterial lines, and IV lines. It is sometimes not possible to use heparin with a patient who has a fresh surgical wound, and the nurse should be alert to the extent and trend in bleeding.

Question 7: List and discuss nursing interventions related to the problems of respiratory failure and bleeding tendency.

Discussion

Respiratory Failure
a) Turn every one hour; do not use clapping and vibrating because of bruising.
b) Suction when necessary; avoid excessive suctioning and trauma. Instill saline prior to suctioning every four hours to assist in loosening secretions.
c) Tracheal aspirate for culture and sensitivity every other day.
d) Use foam padding or cut 4 x 4s under tapes securing endotracheal tube to prevent irritation and bleeding from corners of mouth.
e) Mouth care every four hours: swab inside of mouth with glycerin to loosen dried secretions; swab with peroxide, then clean with saline. Keep lips moistened with lotion or mouth creme.
f) Measure tidal volume off respirator each shift.
g) Be alert for tension pneumothorax in view of PEEP.

h) Use swivel adaptor on endotracheal tube— respirator connection to prevent pulling and twisting of tube. Especially important because of bleeding tendency and increased likelihood of tracheal damage.

i) Keep head of bed elevated to lower abdominal contents.

Bleeding Tendency

a) Measure *all* blood loss possible.

b) Test all drainage for presence of occult blood, e.g., guaiac test NG drainage, use Lab-stik or other available method for urine testing.

c) Administer all medications intravenously if at all possible— avoid IM injections. If necessary to use IMs, apply pressure to site after injection for 5-10 minutes.

d) Keep all bleeding sites uncovered, in view, at all times—e.g., arterial line, IV line, incision.

e) If seizure activity becomes increased, it may be necessary to protect from injury by placing pillows against side rails.

f) When turning, support extremities under the joints, rather than grasping muscle mass, to avoid bruising.

g) Use gel-pad, foam pad, water mattress, or other protection to prevent bruising over bony prominences.

Ellen's condition did not change drastically in the next week, but she continued on a steady downward course. In addition to the medications already mentioned, she was begun on an insulin infusion of 50 units of regular insulin in 150 cc. D_5W at 30 cc./hr. The dosages of phenobarbital and Dilantin were increased to control seizure activity. A regime of antacids per NG tube was begun to reduce the likelihood of stress ulcer. Her abdominal wound showed no sign of healing. Conjunctival hemorrhage appeared on May 20, and there was slow, but continual oozing of blood from the ileostomy stoma. Two units of fresh whole blood were given every other day.

On May 23, an arterio-venous shunt was inserted and dialysis begun on an every other day schedule. Ellen experienced repeated episodes of hypotension while on dialysis and usually required simultaneous infusions of saline or blood in order to complete each cycle. Urine output continued to average 250-300 cc. per day.

Ellen's respiratory status varied. It was possible by May 21 to achieve adequate oxygenation without PEEP, and tracheal aspirate cultures remained negative. However, on May 22, Ellen had an episode of pulmonary edema, requiring reinstitution of PEEP for 24 hours.

Mrs. C. came to visit her daughter every day, arriving at the first visiting hour, 8 AM, and staying until the last, 8 PM. Mr. C. came after work each day. Mrs. C. frequently stood by Ellen's bed, calling her name, crying, "Wake up, dear, we're here, we're here." At one point she said to Ellen's nurse, "I should have known something was wrong and made her come to the hospital sooner—a mother is supposed to know these things."

The following data sheet summarizes laboratory studies and other parameters.

Blood Work:	5/19	5/22	5/25	5/26
Na	144	147	138	136
K	5.5	5.4	6.8	5.2
Cl	98	70	90	88
CO_2	27	30	26	26
Glu.	380	105	175	70
BUN	150	291	160	105
Ca	7.9	6.3	6.4	6.6
Phos.	3.6	6.6	8.8	7.8
Creat.	4.0	—	6.5	4.7
Protein	5.0	4.0	—	—
CPK	—	10,850	—	—
LDH	345	1,485	—	—
SGOT	195	418	—	—
Hct.	28.4	29.9	38.5	32.0
WBC	13.8	15.5	11.6	7.2
Plat.	18,000	19,000	12,000	11,000
Pro. time:	75%	70%	64%	
PTT control:	41	40	42	
patient:	48	52	56	

Blood Gases:	FiO_2	pH	pCO_2	pO_2	HCO_3
5/20	70% 5 cm. PEEP	7.49	26	175	23
5/25	50%	7.45	28	115	22
5/27	30%	7.46	27	95	22

Tidal volume	5/20	5/25	5/27
off respirator:	300	150	200

Vital Signs:	5/20	5/23	5/26
T	38^2	37^4	38^5
P	100	118	106
R	18	18	24
BP	102/76	110/72	98/70

Given this information, consider the following questions.

Question 8: Was Ellen given two units of fresh whole blood every other day to treat DIC?

Discussion: DIC cannot be treated by administering blood, because the clotting factors are quickly consumed and the underlying imbalance between clotting and lysis of clots persists. However, administering fresh blood will treat the *symptoms* of DIC. Patients with DIC may become anemic if enough sources of significant bleeding are present, as was true of Ellen; the blood then serves merely to replace losses. Also, although no overall improvement can be made, the infusion of active clotting factors can temporarily reduce bleeding tendencies and may be used prophylactically when further surgical intervention is needed such as the insertion of Ellen's arterio-venous shunt.

Question 9: What is the probable explanation for the occurrence of pulmonary edema on May 22?

Discussion: Several factors probably contributed to this development. First, an adequate fluid and electrolyte balance would be difficult to maintain, given renal failure, a damaged gastrointestinal tract, and the many sources of fluid gain and loss. We know that Ellen was receiving 720 cc. of insulin infusion per day (30 cc./hr) and 240 cc. of heparin infusion (10 cc./hr). These alone meant an intake of 660 cc., in addition to the 1,000 cc. (2 units) of whole blood given every other day. Urine output averaged only 250-300 cc. per day; so, even assuming other sources of fluid loss, Ellen would inevitably have been in a positive fluid balance before dialysis was begun. The hypoproteinemia complicated this situation by reducing serum osmotic pressure, and, in a sense, making it "easier" for fluid to leak into the interstitium. The positive pressure provided by PEEP was sufficient to prevent this, but when this was no longer used, pulmonary edema then resulted.

Question 10: Evaluate the prognostic signs in relationship to neurological status, pulmonary status, renal function, and DIC.

Discussion: The continued worsening of seizure activity and the fact that Ellen never regained full consciousness after two weeks are poor signs. The hypoxia that had initially been present was corrected and a reasonable electrolyte balance restored by dialysis, making it more likely that Ellen had suffered a brain infarct secondary to DIC, and the extent to which this damage could be reversed was questionable.

Her pulmonary status, on the other hand, had improved. For the most part, all elements of respiratory insufficiency were secondary to non-pulmonary processes. Hypoventilation was a reflection of diminished consciousness, pulmonary edema a reflection of fluid and protein imbalance, and the original pleural effusions due to the abdominal infection. Once those problems were corrected by mechanical ventilation, dialysis, and chest tube drainage, adequate pO_2 and pCO_2 levels were readily achieved. It is therefore reasonable to conclude that no intrinsic pulmonary disease or irreversible damage had occurred.

Renal function remained essentially unchanged, as indicated by the volume of urine output and consistently elevated creatinine and BUN levels. However, ATN is a reversible process, and renal function could begin to improve. There is no reason, at this point, to believe that permanent damage has occurred.

Despite adequate heparin, the process of DIC continued. Data leading to this conclusion includes the persistent thrombocytopenia, bleeding from the ileostomy stoma, and conjunctival hemorrhages. Other laboratory studies, such as prothrombin time, are not valid because they are altered by the use of heparin. The appearance of fragmented red blood cells would be another indication of continued coagulopathy.

Question 11: Discuss ways in which the nurse could be supportive to Mrs. C. (Ellen's mother).

Discussion: In addition to the crisis of having a child seriously ill, Mrs. C. apparently was experiencing some feelings of guilt related to her perceived delay in treatment. Although this perception could also be related to a need to see this event as able to be controlled or affected by her actions, it would be important to assist Mrs. C. in limiting this self-reproach. This could be accomplished by providing her with a better understanding of the disease process, the gradual development of symptoms, and consistent reassurance that, at all stages, all reasonable measures had been undertaken.

Given Ellen's appearance, with numerous tubes and equipment attached, multiple bruises, and frequent seizures, it would be essential that the nurse stay with Ellen's parents during their initial visits; later, as they became more accustomed to her appearance, the nurse might wish to give the parents some time to be with their child alone. Throughout Ellen's illness, however, the nurse should plan to be with the parents at the start of each visiting hour, to answer questions and assess how *they* are doing. It would be even more helpful to meet them outside of Ellen's room to talk for a moment and prepare them for any changes in her condition.

Ellen's mother should be encouraged to talk to her daughter. Although it is unlikely that Ellen could hear, that cannot be definitely established. In addition, Ellen's mother needed the chance to express her feelings to her daughter, for her own sake.

In terms of preparing Mrs. C. for what was to come, it is difficult to outline any specific plan. Certainly both Mr. and Mrs. C. should be accurately appraised of significant changes in their daughter's condition; throughout her illness, the prognosis for Ellen's survival was quite poor. Providing them with the information necessary to anticipate the most likely outcome would allow them to prepare for this eventuality as they were able. However, in order to tolerate the situation, to continue each day, they also would need to maintain some hope; this could be supported in the same way, by providing honest information about improvements. For example, Mrs. C. would have no way of knowing Ellen's pulmonary status had improved if the nurse did not take the time to explain.

Depending upon Mrs. C.'s wishes, the nurse could also assist her in performing some care measures for Ellen, such as wiping her face with a cool cloth, re-positioning her arm, etc. This would provide her with some way to help her child.

In the next few days Ellen's condition suddenly grew much worse. The bleeding from her ileostomy increased and fresh blood began to drain from her nasogastric tube. The blood infusions were increased to two units every day. By May 29, she no longer tolerated dialysis for more than two hours at a time, despite saline infusions. Her potassium level began to rise and frequent ectopic beats occurred. Her WBC dropped precipitously, probably as a result of overwhelming endotoxemia. On the morning of May 30, her parents were called. The monitor alarms were turned off and the nurse who had worked most consistently with Ellen sat with them as she died.

REFERENCES

1. Biggs R: *Human Blood Coagulation, Haemostasis, and Thrombosis.* 2nd Ed. Blackwell Scientific Publications, London, 1976.
2. Bone RC, et al.: Intravascular coagulation associated with the adult respiratory distress syndrome. *American Journal of Medicine* **61**:585-589, 1976.
3. Brown BA: *Hematology: Principles and Procedures.* 2nd Ed. Lea and Febiger, Philadelphia, Pa., 1976.
4. Bull BS: Disseminated Intravascular Coagulation. In Weil MH and Shubin H (Eds.): *Critical Care Medicine Handbook,* John K. Nolen, Publishers, New York, 1974.
5. Coe NP, Salzman EW: Thrombosis and intravascular coagulation. *Surgical Clinics of North America* **56**:875-890, 1976.
6. Colman RW, et al.: Disseminated intravascular coagulation (DIC): an approach. *American Journal of Medicine* **52**:679-687, 1972.
7. Colman RW, et al.: DIC: a problem in critical care medicine. *Heart and Lung* 3:789-796, 1974.
8. Deykin D: The clinical challenge of disseminated intravascular coagulation. *New England Journal of Medicine* **283**:636-642, 1976.
9. Guyton AC: *Textbook of Medical Physiology.* 5th Ed. W.B. Saunders, Philadelphia, Pa., 1976.
10. Hasson HM: The role of enzymes in DIC—an overview. *Journal of Obstetric and Gynecological Nursing* May-June:27-29, 1974.
11. Lerner RG: The defibrination syndrome. *Medical Clinics of North America* **60**:871-880, 1976.

12. Mayer GG: Disseminated intravascular coagulation. *American Journal of Nursing* **52**:679-687, 1972.
13. Rappaport SI: Defibrination Syndromes. In Williams WJ (Ed.): *Hematology.* McGraw-Hill, New York, 1972.
14. Rocco F, et al.: DIC—disseminated intravascular coagulation. *Nursing '74* November:66-71, 1974.
15. Simpson JG, Stalker AL: The concept of disseminated intravascular coagulation. *Clinics in Hematology* **2**:189-198, 1973.

Index

Index

DATE DUE

JAN X 5 1980			
Jan 12			
APR 3			
APR 3 0 1981			
AUG 5 1981			
JAN 1 8 1982			
FEB 2 3 1983			
FEB 2 3 1983			
FEB 4 1985			
JUL 8 1985			
JAN 2 1 1987			
GAYLORD			PRINTED IN U.S.A.

THIS IS NOT A TALE OF OUR OWN WORLD.

It is a world like ours in many ways, but one where dragons live in their own lands, wary of humans. One with Sorcerers, light and dark. One where Pipers can control things around them merely by playing a Song.

Yet tales of other worlds can reach us, sometimes. All it takes is a little magic, and the Pipers have always known something that—for us—is easy to forget:

There is magic in music.
Listen . . .

TO MY SON ELIAS,
WHO HEARD IT ALL FIRST

Published by
PEACHTREE PUBLISHING COMPANY INC.
1700 Chattahoochee Avenue
Atlanta, Georgia 30318-2112
PeachtreeBooks.com

Text © 2018 by S. A. Patrick
Cover and inside illustrations by George Ermos
Title typography by Leo Nickolls

First published as *A Darkness of Dragons* in Great Britain in 2018 by
Usborne Ltd., Usborne House, 83–85 Saffron Hill, London EC1N 8RT,
England. *Usborne.com*

First United States version published in 2022 by Peachtree Publishing
Company Inc.

First trade paperback edition published in 2023

Composition by Lily Steele
Imported by Jonah Heller

Printed and bound in January 2023 at Thomson Reuters, Eagan, MN, USA.
10 9 8 7 6 5 4 3 2 1 (hardcover)
10 9 8 7 6 5 4 3 2 1 (trade paperback)
HC ISBN: 978-1-68263-376-2
PB ISBN: 978-1-68263-521-6

Cataloging-in-Publication Data is available from the Library of Congress.

A DARKENING OF DRAGONS

BOOK ONE OF SONGS OF MAGIC

S.A. PATRICK

PEACHTREE
ATLANTA

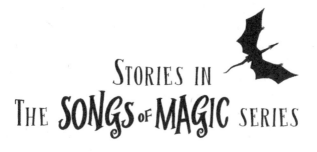

STORIES IN
THE SONGS OF MAGIC SERIES

A DARKENING OF DRAGONS

A VANISHING OF GRIFFINS

A THUNDERING OF MONSTERS

In a world of dragons, song-spells, and pipers, three accidental
heroes find themselves thrown into an epic quest.

★   ✶
★

Join 13-year-old Patch Brightwater as he and his friends Wren,
a girl cursed to live as a rat, and Barver, a fire-breathing dracogriff,
set off to vanquish the sinister Hamelyn of Piper.

Can this unlikely trio prevent a madman from
conquering humans and dragons alike?

1

THE ICE BEAST

The screams of the children brought the villagers running.

The little ones often played among the tall pines at the southern edge of Patterfall. This high in the mountains, winter was always hard; the pines offered shelter from the icy winds that blew through the valley.

As the villagers ran toward the sound, the panicked children emerged from the trees and came rushing through the snow. The first to reach them was Frer, the eight-year-old son of the baker.

"It's come! It's come!" said the boy.

"Steady, child," said Greta, the village Elder. "Tell me what it is. A bear?"

He shook his head. "No, Elder. It's the Ice Beast!"

With that, he ran past them to safety.

"The child is just scared," the Elder told the other villagers, because the Ice Beast was a legend, nothing more. A legend as old as the village itself, about an extraordinary creature formed of snow and ice—a creature that absolutely *did not exist*.

There *were* extraordinary creatures in the world, of course. Some, like dragons, were at least as intelligent as humans; others, like basilisks and manticores, were terrifying monstrosities.

But there was nothing like that anywhere *near* Patterfall. Dragons lived on a different continent, far to the east. As for the terrifying monstrosities, they were thankfully rare and limited to the remotest parts of the world.

Only those foolish enough to get lost on the valley roads in deep winter ever claimed to have seen the Ice Beast— people who were exhausted and frightened, seeing things that weren't really there.

Yet the villagers could see movement a short way inside the forest.

Something large. Something white. "*No*," the Elder said aloud. "It can't be!" But it was.

The Ice Beast was the height of a large man and seemed to be made entirely of snow. Its legs and arms were as thick as tree trunks. The head was a featureless white ball, but every villager could imagine where the terrifying mouth was, fangs dripping, ready to sink into the flesh of anyone who got too near.

Its slow steps drew a heavy *crunch* from the snow underneath. From its head came a steady moaning.

And the villagers kept moving toward it.

"Go!" they called to the children as they passed them. "Run to your homes!"

There was one child left, though. One small boy too frightened to move, standing directly in the creature's path—Hap Werner, only four years old.

"Little Hap," called the Elder. "You go home now! Go on with you!"

But Hap shook his head, rooted to the spot. The creature was getting closer to him.

With no time to waste, the Elder raised the shovel she was carrying. "I'll have you, Beast!" she cried, and ran toward the creature. The other villagers followed, wielding what weapons they had—hoes, pitchforks, brooms.

The Elder was first to reach it, and she swung her shovel hard, hitting the Ice Beast's head. The creature made a strange noise before falling to the snowy ground with a *thud*.

There it lay, motionless, as the villagers surrounded it, ready to hit it again if it moved even a fraction.

But where the shovel had hit its head, a few chunks of ice and snow were now gone, revealing something underneath. The villagers stared at what they saw: a very cold, very red nose, and below that, a very human mouth.

"*Ow* . . . ," the mouth groaned.

For a moment the villagers looked at each other in shock. Then they began to scrape away what they could of the ice and snow that clung to the stranger. With each chunk removed he was smaller, lighter, yet what they found underneath was a curious giant, the legs and arms unnaturally thick. Only when more ice was cleared did it make sense to them.

Clothes.

Layer upon layer of shirts and trousers: dozens, perhaps more. The stranger's neck was thick with a hundred scarves, the hands and head puffed out by gloves and hats. Torn strips of material were densely wrapped around the face, gaps left only for the mouth, nose, and eyes.

Too heavy to carry, they dragged the unconscious stranger to the village, his legs and feet still ice-bound. In the village hall a fire was roaring, and they propped him up in a chair in front of the blazing logs, then began cutting and unraveling the layers with care. In one corner of the hall, the pile of discarded garments grew, while the unconscious stranger shrank, until all that was left was a thin figure slouched in a chair, with a long coat over his simple clothing.

It was a *boy*, his hair dark and scruffy.

"Look how young he is, he can't be more than thirteen!" said a villager. "How did he survive his journey?"

"A good question!" said the Elder. "To emerge from the forest where he did, he must have come through Andig's Pass. An icy hell this time of year."

"It's certain death for anyone crazy enough to go that way!" said the villager.

"And yet this boy made it through," said the Elder, thoughtful. "There must be more to him than meets the eye!" She reached inside the boy's coat and searched the deep pockets within. After a moment, she slowly pulled out her hand. With it came a wooden flute, the length of her forearm. Those watching gasped as they saw.

It was *not* a flute, of course. The small finger holes were far more numerous, the layout much more complex, than on any flute they had ever seen.

This was not a flute. It was a *Pipe*.

The Elder lifted it up. "The Piper has come," she said in awe, and the people cheered. The doors of the village hall were flung open, and the news was passed on to those waiting outside. Everyone took up the call:

"The Piper has come! *The Piper has come!*"

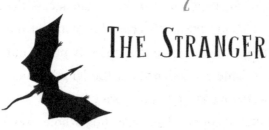

2
THE STRANGER

When the boy finally opened his eyes, he found himself on a small bed, in a room he didn't recognize, wearing a simple nightshirt that he was certain didn't belong to him. He sat up and tried to recall how he'd got there, but nothing came. Nothing but a sense that there was something very important that he needed to remember . . .

"You're awake at last," came a voice. Startled, the boy turned and saw an old woman sitting in a chair in the shadows of the corner. She stood and brought the chair over to the bedside. "My name is Greta," she said. "I'm the Elder of Patterfall."

"Of where?" said the boy.

"Patterfall," said Greta, looking worried. "This village."

"I'm sorry," he said. "I don't remember much. About anything."

Greta nodded. "Perhaps that's to be expected. The stress of your journey here has robbed you of your memory."

"Will it come back?"

"I've seen this kind of thing before," said Greta. "You're not the first to have stumbled out of the forest close to death, although you're certainly the youngest. Your memory will return soon enough. Something will spark it back to life. Do you remember anything about your journey?"

He thought for a moment, but all that came was that terrible dark walk through the forest, one step after another with no end. His eyes widened. "I don't even remember my own name!"

"I think I can answer that one," said Greta. She stood and fetched a coat that was hanging on a hook on the far wall. "When we found you, you were snowbound from head to toe, and wearing layer upon layer of clothes. Underneath them all was this coat. Is it yours?"

The boy smiled when he saw it, feeling relief at remembering even such a small thing. "Yes," he said. "It is."

"Then here," said Greta. She turned back the collar of the coat to reveal a name embroidered in neat stitches. "I suspect this is your name."

The boy read the name aloud: "Patch Brightwater."

It felt right, and with the name came another small piece of his memory. "My grandmother stitched it in my coat, so I'd not lose it."

Greta smiled. "It's very good to meet you, Patch Bright-water!" she said. "It's *more* than good. You see, I know why you came here." She reached into Patch's coat pocket and pulled out the Pipe. "You came to save us!"

Patch stared. "Me?" he said, and Greta nodded. "I'm a Piper?" He reached out slowly and took the Pipe in his hands. As he held it, more memories came back to him, precious fragments and images. Moments, he realized, from his training at Tiviscan. *Yes,* he thought, *Tiviscan Castle, the home of the Pipers' Council.* The place where those hoping to become Pipers go to learn the Piper's Art.

There was still so much missing, but as his fingers moved over the holes in the Pipe, he knew that the Songs were clear in his mind.

"I *am* a Piper," said Patch at last, and now the tears came, flowing down his cheeks and past his broad smile.

Greta gave him a kindly pat on his hand. "You're much younger than we expected, I admit . . ."

Patch was filled with a sudden worry—the same feeling he'd had when he'd woken, that there was something very important he still needed to remember.

"But no ordinary traveler could have made it through that snow!" said Greta. "We summoned a Piper, and here you are!"

Another memory came to him then. "Wait . . . There was an emergency. I was in a hurry." He looked to Greta, and she nodded to encourage him. "I think . . . there was a trader. He had the only cart heading this way, him and his family." His eyes narrowed as he concentrated. "The road was blocked, the snow too deep. As we turned, the cart's axle snapped. The trader unhitched his horse, mounted it with his wife and child, and rode off."

"They left you?"

Patch sighed. "Who can blame them? I looked in the cart for food, and all I found was clothing—the trader's wares. At first, I stayed in the shelter of the cart and played a heating Song on my Pipe to keep me warm. But the cold became too great; my fingers grew numb and I had to stop. So I put on layer after layer of clothes and waited for the weather to improve, but it just kept getting worse. Finally, I started to walk. There's a simpler heating Song that can be whistled—lip-playing, we call it. I used that for a time, until my dry lips cracked in the chill and I was forced into silence. I kept walking, all through the night . . ." He thought of how *long* that terrible icy walk had seemed. *Endless.*

"And you reached us!" said Greta. "You mentioned an emergency, Patch, and that's exactly what our village has! One that will leave us all in poverty and perhaps end our lives. As soon as we knew how dangerous things had become, we sent a messenger to Wassil, the nearest town. The messenger took the only horse strong enough to make it through the deep snow. His mission was to summon a Piper. You!"

9

"Tell me, Greta," said Patch. "Tell me what I've come here to do."

Greta paused, looking weighed down with worry. "In summer," she said, "the fertile valley gives us enough grain to last a year, for our cattle and our bellies and for seeding the next year's crops, with some left over that we can sell. Each winter, the roads become impassable. The village remains isolated until late spring. Our dogs and our cats deal with any vermin from the forest. But not this year. One by one, our dogs went lame, our cats grew fearful, and the food in our homes was plundered. At first, we couldn't understand what was doing it. They were not seen, and they left no signs."

Patch's face grew pale. "What . . . what was it?"

"Rats," said Greta. "More than we've ever known. Bigger than we've ever known. Smarter than we've ever known. Anything we did, it wasn't enough. They ate no poison. They triggered no traps." Greta shook her head, visibly distressed. "Nothing we've done has stopped them. They are frightening, Patch. And now they're all in the grain storehouse in the center of the village, but we dare not attack them. They like it there, protected from the cold, with enough food to last them a few weeks. But when that's done, they'll find all our hidden stores. They'll consume everything we have. And then—" She closed her eyes, unable to speak for a moment. "None of the villagers have been hurt by them, yet. Not one. But when the grain is gone that will surely change."

Patch stared at her in horror. "Change? What do you mean?"

"We are trapped in the village, but so are the rats. When they're hungry enough, they'll come for us! You can see why we're desperate."

"Rats . . . ," he said, thinking. What had he been taught? "Infestations are a common thing for Pipers to deal with, be it rats, mice, cockroaches." He let his fingers move over the Pipe and smiled as he realized they were already marking out the notes of the Song he needed. "It's strange," he said. "There's so much I don't remember, but my training comes back to me easily."

"We should have called for a Piper weeks ago," said Greta. "But some of the villagers were afraid to."

"Afraid?" said Patch. "They have nothing to fear from me!"

"They thought of what happened in Hamelyn."

Patch opened his mouth to answer, but then the memory of the Hamelyn Piper returned to him like a slap to the face.

It was the greatest shame of Pipers—ten years ago, the town of Hamelyn had been infested by rats. A Piper came, a Piper with nothing but evil in his heart; once he had got rid of the rodents he played another Song and led the children of Hamelyn off into the night. And what had become of them? To this day, nobody knew. Even after the Hamelyn Piper had been caught and thrown into the deepest dungeon, he had never revealed the truth.

For centuries, Pipers had been trusted completely, their honor beyond question as they wandered the lands, seeking work—helping crops to grow, say, or finding the right place to dig a well. A price would be agreed, and the work would be done.

The events in Hamelyn almost destroyed that trust. Never again would a Piper be able to simply turn up and offer their services. Now, Pipers had to be officially summoned, so that people could be sure that the Pipers who came were qualified and trustworthy.

"They have no need to worry," said Patch. He pulled back the blanket that covered his lower half and swung his legs out of the bed. "There's no time to waste. My clothes?"

"The clothing you wore under your coat has been cleaned in readiness," said Greta. "But I think you need to eat and rest first, to regain your strength."

"Nonsense," he said. "Waiting just means the rats eat more of your precious grain!" The rats, Patch thought, couldn't be as bad as Greta had made out. They were scared, these villagers, and their fear had made everything seem so much worse that it really was. He would cure them of their rats—and cure them of their fear!

He tried to stand, but his legs gave way at once and he fell back onto the bed, breathless.

"You see?" said Greta. "You've been unconscious for two days. You must eat and drink and rest some more. Only then will you have the strength to deal with those rats. Tomorrow!"

Patch knew she was right; he was only just getting his breath back, and the mention of food had made him realize how hungry he was. "Tomorrow it is," he said.

Patch ate his fill and slept well.

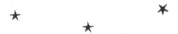

In the morning, after a bowl of stew for breakfast, he got dressed and spent some time exercising his fingers. Nothing more of his memory had come back yet, but he was confident about his Piping—and that was all that mattered.

Greta knocked on the door and entered. "Are you ready?" she asked.

"Almost," said Patch. "First, though, we need a plan—a way to kill the rats! Somewhere to drown them, say."

"Follow me," said Greta.

Beside the village was a river twenty feet across, a simple wooden bridge spanning its fast-flowing water. They followed it a short way downstream until they came to a cliff edge. There, the river became a roaring waterfall.

"This is where our village gets its name."

"Patterfall?" said Patch. "I would have expected something more gentle."

"The village has been here for three hundred years," said Greta. "Back then, the river was little more than a stream. Things have changed."

"No kidding." He crept forward to the precipice and looked over. The drop was at least a hundred feet, and the base of the waterfall was littered with jagged rocks. The falling water would dash the rats against the sharp stones, so a quick death was assured. "This will do it," he said.

When they got back, everyone had gathered around the oak tree that stood in the heart of the village. They cheered at the sight of the Piper.

Patch waved to them, and Greta led him to the front of the large grain storehouse where the rats had taken up residence.

The cheering fell away to silence as the people of the village waited for the Piper to begin.

Greta walked to the doors of the storehouse. She removed the chains that had been thrown across the doors, then placed a huge key into the lock and turned it. She looked to Patch, who nodded. Slowly, Greta pulled the doors open, returning quickly to Patch's side. All eyes watched as he studied his quarry.

Then Patch, his body completely rigid, fell backward in a dead faint.

3

THE PIPER OF PATTERFALL

Patch came to, the flagstones cold under his back. He opened his eyes and saw Greta's worried face.

"Take my hand!" she whispered, supporting him as he stood.

"Let's try that again," said Patch, but his breathing grew more and more rapid, and his grip on Greta became ever tighter.

He didn't want to look through the storehouse doors again, but he had no choice.

He looked. Rats!

Sleeping among mounds of grain and bags of seed and sacks of corn, sleeping in groups of three and groups of ten and—Patch shivered—groups of far *more* than ten. Brown rats, white rats, speckled rats, long rats, short rats. One had a tail with curious markings, ringed with red hoops all down its length.

All were asleep, but nowhere, not anywhere he looked, could Patch see a rat that could be called "small," or "thin." Some were too fat even to curl up for their sleep, looking like big, furry squash or hairy loaves of bread. The fattest of all was a great rat pumpkin that surely couldn't have moved even if it wanted to, its feet sticking straight out, high off the ground, its belly making a dent in the grain where it lay.

Not a sound came from them—except perhaps, if he'd been brave enough to step inside and listen with a careful ear, the noise of little ratty snores and burps.

Rats, content and asleep.

Huge rats.

A vast number of huge rats.

He turned to Greta and opened his mouth to speak.

No words came.

"You thought I was exaggerating," she said.

Patch nodded. He took a very long breath and let out a very long sigh.

"Is it too hard a task?" said Greta.

Patch saw hope drain from the Elder. *No,* he thought, *I won't give in.* These people needed him, and they had saved his life.

But he could hardly pretend this was a selfless act. *He* was trapped here, just as the villagers were. Yet the rats did seem oddly cozy; they were so peaceful that it was a bit of a stretch to imagine them bearing down on him with blood-drenched maws.

He shivered. His mind had already started to imagine it. He turned and addressed Greta. "The Art of Piping," he started, but it came out squeaky. He cleared his throat and tried again. "The Art of Piping," he repeated, in the confident voice that came from reciting such a well-learned passage, "has many magics. The Song most often used for clearing pests of whatever kind is called the Dream. This magic fills the target's mind full of the wonderful things that they most desire, and makes them think those things can be found by following the music of the Pipe." He looked at the rats, his mouth suddenly dry. "There are . . . *more* than I expected, I admit, but you avoid thinking about the number, you see. Then it's just as if there were ten, or twenty, rather than—" He gestured toward the rodents, then reached into his coat and took out his Pipe.

The Dream, he thought, grateful that he could remember his training. His fingers were already moving against the Pipe, rehearsing the intricate patterns that would draw the rats to their doom.

He put the Pipe to his lips and began.

It started with a simple melody, six notes repeated with a little variation. Patch played this half a dozen times, then took his mouth from the pipe.

Yet the music continued. Greta's eyes were wide with astonishment. "It . . . it keeps *playing*—"

"Of course," said Patch. "Otherwise you couldn't add layers, and it's the layers of a Song that make it so powerful." Now, Patch started another melody—overlapping the first, seeming to shift away from it, then toward it again.

Beside him, Greta was smiling, *grinning*, at the sound.

With the second melody holding, Patch added another sequence, then another and another. The real work was being done. There was a change in the overall sound, a change that spoke of things that *could be*.

The Dream. The Dream was forming.

Patch's fingers moved in what seemed like effortless complexity. Suddenly he frowned and stopped playing. His hands fell to his sides, the Song starting to fade. He looked at Greta, anxious.

"What's wrong?" she asked, but Patch's attention was stolen by the sound that started among the villagers. The sound of cheering and applause.

He looked from the villagers to Greta, confused. "Why are they clapping?"

"They've never heard anything like that," said Greta.

"It was . . . It was—" She shook her head, grasping for the word. "It was *beautiful*."

"Maybe so," said Patch. "But it didn't *work*." He nodded toward the storehouse. The rats hadn't even stirred. "I don't understand! They should be filled with the knowledge that their dreams, *all* their dreams, await them if they follow the sound!" He began to mutter to himself.

It was Greta who realized what was wrong. "Patch, look at those animals." They both looked. "Do you think they *could* find somewhere better? They are warm and sleeping in a building full of food! Don't you think they're already in their dream?"

"Of course!" said Patch, putting a hand to his forehead. "Think, think!" he said to himself. He began to stride up and down, his Pipe clenched behind his back. "Wait!" he said at last. "There's another way. But it's a little bit"—he paused for a moment, before finishing—"a little bit *unusual.*"

"Unusual" wasn't the first word that had come to Patch's mind.

When Greta had pointed out the reason for the Dream's failure, he'd hunted around in his memory for an alternative. *Maybe I can't remember enough of my training after all*, he'd thought, and that was a *terrible* thought, because part of his mind had got really very *good* at imagining how the rats would go about feasting on him if he botched this whole thing.

But eventually one idea *had* come, a Song that was so clear and so strong, something he *knew* would work, because he somehow knew that he was particularly good at it. Unfortunately, there was one other thing that he knew about the Song.

He knew that using it was absolutely against the laws of Piping, and had been ever since the Hamelyn Piper had played it to such devastating effect.

In short, it was *illegal*, and "illegal" was the word that he'd almost said to Greta. "Unusual" seemed a lot less alarming, so he'd gone with that instead.

He tried to recall what "illegal" meant for a Piper, and images came to him, images of very serious-looking Pipers in black-and-purple robes. *Oh, yes*, he thought. *Them.*

The Custodian Elite, they were called. If a Piper was to break the laws of Piping, the Custodian Elite would be the ones who brought them to justice.

Still, this was an emergency, and surely even the Custodian Elite would understand.

"This one is called the Dance," he said, then he raised his Pipe and started to play.

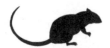

4
THE DANCE

Layer upon layer, the Dance took shape in his Pipe. At the sound of it he felt a familiar joy grow in his heart.

Soon the Song had formed. At first, the sleeping rats seemed oblivious to it. Then one of them stirred—the strange rat with the red-ringed tail. With a yawn it stood and sniffed the air and saw Patch. Its paws came up to its mouth in a way that was strangely human, as if it was shocked. It waved frantically, shaking its head and squeaking, almost as if it was trying to warn the others.

How peculiar, Patch thought.

The strange rat clamped its paws tightly over its ears, attempting to shut out the sound—as if that would make any difference! But after a few seconds the animal's rear paws were tapping to the rhythm, its agitation vanishing as it started to whirl and swish from side to side, caught in the Dance. All thought of escape had gone, Patch knew. The only thing it would know, from now until the moment it hit the rocks at the bottom of the waterfall, was the joy of the music.

In the center of the storehouse floor was a small clearing, and that was where the red-ringed rat made its way. One by one, the other rats woke and followed, hopping and marching in time to the Song that Patch played. A circle of rats formed in the clearing, all on their hind legs, their little paws grasping those of the rats either side of them. As the ring completed, another larger ring started to link up outside the first.

It's working, Patch thought, thrilled and relieved in equal measure. *It's working!*

It wasn't long before ten circles of rats danced around and around, more rodents joining them every second. The circles danced one way, then turned and danced the other. The faces of the rats were happy, and gleeful squeaks could be clearly heard over the music.

The center of the floor was almost full, so the rest of the rats formed groups in the hollows and spaces where they found themselves. The fattest rats, unable to dance, waggled their paws and heads and feet with smiling eyes and loud cheering squeaks.

All the rats were caught in the Dance now.

It's time, he thought. *Time to take the Dance outside to the river—and the waterfall!*

He backed away from the storehouse. In each of the dancing groups, the rats paired up and began skipping to the exit, with the fattest being rolled out by some of the others.

Patch glanced toward the villagers; anxiety was written on their faces. They wouldn't have to worry for much longer. He turned toward the bridge that crossed the river. From there, he would guide the rats into the water and keep them entranced until they went over the precipice. Greta was already heading to the bridge—the sight of the rats streaming out of the storehouse was enough to make anyone want to get away as quickly as they could.

Patch couldn't hurry, though. As he played, he took slow steps and kept glancing behind him, making sure his pace was right.

Hundreds of rats—*thousands*—were pouring out of the doors, following Patch in a line ten rats across, spinning and jigging their way along, twenty feet behind him.

Had he been walking at normal speed he would have reached the bridge within a minute. Matching the pace of the rats, it took five times longer to get there, his fingers racing over the Pipe.

He reached the middle of the bridge and sent the rats toward the water. Line by line, the rats waded in, and each line kept dancing as they swam, forming a little circle as the strong current carried them downstream. Entire circles of rats would turn one way then another, before diving under the water, their tails and feet sticking out and moving from side to side in perfect time, before they brought their heads back up and danced on.

When a third of them were in the river, Patch looked to the waterfall's edge; so did Greta, who was now standing beside him.

"It almost seems cruel," said Greta. "Look at them, with no idea what's coming!"

Patch shook his head and took his lips from the Pipe. "They'll dance all the way down to the sharp rocks below," he said. "The whole time, they'll be happy."

"And we'll be free," said Greta, suddenly overwhelmed. "The village is saved!" She stepped forward and embraced him, then quickly stepped back again with an apologetic nod.

Patch smiled. He was almost overwhelmed, both with emotion and fatigue. It was only excitement that was keeping him on his feet, he knew. It would be a while yet before he fully recovered from his icy journey to the village, and he was still close to exhaustion.

Greta waved to the cheering crowd. Patch waved at them too, but only briefly—the Song could start to unravel if he didn't maintain its melodies. He turned back to the rats, nearly half of them now in the water.

He'd glanced so briefly at the villagers, he couldn't be blamed for not noticing one *very* important detail . . .

The villagers' feet had started to tap.

Almost there, Patch thought.

The frontmost rats were floating downriver and close to the point of no return, where the water quickened before hurtling into the void. The rearmost were just entering the water now.

He looked at Greta, expecting to see triumph on her face, watching the rats get ever nearer to oblivion.

Instead, Greta was staring past him, back down toward the villagers. Patch turned to follow her gaze and gasped.

The people of the village were dancing!

Dancing in a column that was speeding toward the river, their grinning faces lit up with absolute glee.

"Oh no!" said Patch, horrified. "What's gone wrong?" said Greta.

"The Song spilled out beyond the rats," he said. "The villagers are caught in the Dance!"

He looked to the rats near the waterfall, then back to the people. He played his Pipe, trying to add in a separation, to keep the rodents on their way and send the people back.

He quickly realized that it wasn't working.

Next option, he thought: *wait until most of the rats have gone over the falls and bring the Dance to an end.*

But the people were so much *faster* than the rats, and many would be in the water by then. *Too risky,* he thought. There were children among the dancers. The water could sweep them to their deaths, however short a time they were in the river. Besides, could everyone even *swim?*

He added counter-rhythms that should slow the Dance down. That way, most of the rats would simply drift to their fate.

It had no effect. Closer the villagers came. Closer to the river's edge.

Greta grabbed his shoulder. "Patch! You have to do something!"

If he merely stopped playing, the Song would take too long to fade. As the first line of people stepped into the icy water, Patch knew there was only one option left.

He took the Pipe from his lips and snapped it in half.

At once, the Dance died.

The grins on the faces of the villagers dropped away. Those who found themselves standing in the ice-cold river looked at their sodden legs, baffled. Panicked squeals came from the rats, who were now scrabbling their way toward the riverbank, finding purchase at the river's edge. The villagers watched as the rats helped each other and emerged from the water, scurrying back toward the village.

Patch's heart sank. He had come so close to success, but would have to start again once he'd recovered enough strength to . . .

The villager nearest the bridge raised a trembling arm, pointing right at Patch.

"He tried to kill us!" the villager screamed.

"Uh, no, I—" said Patch.

"He almost drowned us all!" cried another.

Greta stepped forward. "Wait!" she shouted. "That's not what happened!"

But the accusations kept mounting. Soon it seemed as if the whole village wanted his blood.

"He's like the Hamelyn Piper!" they cried. "Twisted, evil! Lock him up and throw away the key!"

"Um, Greta?" whispered Patch. "Maybe I should, uh, run away . . ."

She shook her head. "If you run, they'll chase you down like a mad dog! Your only chance is to reason with them."

"He's got Greta under a spell!" a villager cried.

Greta's eyes narrowed with anger. "*I'm not under any spell!*" she shouted, and the villagers fell silent at once, looking at her like children caught misbehaving by a parent. "Now all of you just calm down and listen! Angry decisions are bad ones, don't I always say?"

Nods and grumbles came from the villagers. Some agreed with Greta, but it was clear that many didn't. For Patch it was torture. Wherever he looked he saw suspicion and hate-filled eyes. It proved too much for him. Thinking this was his only opportunity to get a head start, he made a terrible mistake.

He began to run.

Over the bridge he went. The villagers were taken by surprise, but soon most were giving chase.

"Don't hurt him!" yelled Greta.

Patch hadn't yet realized the madness of his action—indeed, as he ran and found the road leading out of the village, he was hopeful. It didn't look impassable by any means! Pure white snow, flanked by trees, running straight on into the distance. He could outrun the villagers! He could keep ahead of them, and . . .

Suddenly the snow was too deep to run through. Too deep to *walk* through. He lost his balance and stumbled, falling facedown into white. His limbs felt impossibly heavy as he looked back to the villagers.

"Send him over the waterfall," one of them yelled, fist in the air. "See how he likes it!" It got a hearty cheer from the others.

Perhaps Greta could talk them out of it. Perhaps not.

Patch was so tired he almost didn't care.

The villagers fell suddenly silent and halted, staring past him. Patch looked at the road ahead. In the distance, the tops of the trees were shaking. The movement came nearer; the air itself was twisting, spinning.

The deep snow in the road was being hurled out to either side, as a corkscrew of white approached.

"He's summoned the Devil!" screamed one villager, running away. Some followed, terrified, but most were transfixed by the sight.

He could hear it now—a harsh whirring, almost like the

buzz of wasps. And under that sound was another: rhythm and melody blending together in a Song for the wind.

When the twisting air broke through the last of the snow, Patch wasn't surprised by what he saw. Two horses, on a road that was clear of snow behind them. The riders wore the black and purple garb of the Custodian Elite.

Exhausted, he let his head fall. He half-laughed, and half-sobbed. He was safe. The villagers couldn't harm him now.

He heard the horses stop, then the crunch of boots in snow as one of the riders approached. Patch lifted his head and strained to look up. The face looming over him was young; with a shock, Patch realized it was familiar.

"Patch?" said the young man. "Patch Brightwater?"

Patch squinted at the young man's face. *I know you*, he thought. *How do I know you?*

Ever since he'd woken in Patterfall, he'd known there was something very important that he needed to remember. At long last, that very important thing came back to him, and with it came everything else, all his lost memories returning at once.

"Oh no," he said. His head dropped back down to the snow.

He wasn't a Piper, not really. He'd fled from Tiviscan in disgrace before completing his training.

And now he knew just how much trouble he was in.

5

A RAT
OF DISTINCTION

Patch woke from a dream.

He'd been walking hand in hand with his mother, feeling the kind of total happiness that he'd not felt in a long time. He'd only been three years old when both his parents had died, leaving him to be raised by his grandparents. He'd been left with no memories of his father at all, and only that single precious memory of his mother: holding her hand, looking up to see her smiling at him.

He was in a small room with a bare flagstone floor; there was a little window and a thin mat for a bed. It was cold. A fleece and a blanket covered him, and without it he suspected he would freeze.

He could feel a heavy weight around his ankle—it was a manacle. Wrapping his covers around his back, he followed the chain to an iron ring on the wall. Out of the window, he could see the grain storehouse, its doors locked tight once more. He was wearing the clothes he'd fallen unconscious in, but his coat had been removed. On the floor was a tin bowl with a few hunks of stale bread, and a cup of water.

Hearing a clatter of keys, Patch turned to the door, and when it swung open he saw the face of the Elite Piper who had brought his memory rushing back. Erner Whitlock was his name; two years his senior, at fifteen. One of the three best Pipers that Patch had trained with.

"Erner," said Patch, looking at the robes Erner wore— rich purple on thick black cotton. "The Custodian Elite! The clothes suit you. I knew you'd pass your final trials."

Erner nodded. "I wish you'd been there to see it," he said. "Three of us went through the trials, and all three succeeded!"

"Who were the other two?"

"Mort and Kara. Mort is apprenticed with the Marinus Pipers in the Eastern Seas, but Kara turned out like me— Custodian Elite. She's gone to Skamos."

Patch could picture them both. Mort was a tall, strong lad with a love of the sea; Marinus Pipers were keenly sought by merchant ships and needed a knack for whipping up winds and fending off pirates, which the Eastern Seas had plenty of. Kara, meanwhile, had been Erner's match in every task they'd ever done. Skamos was an important place, the only human city left on the continent known as the Dragon Territories. Peace between humans and dragons had always been fragile, but problems at Skamos had almost tipped things into war more than once. The Custodian Elite there had a crucial role in stopping that from happening.

"Pirates and dragons," said Patch. "Exactly what they wanted. It's good to hear."

Erner stepped forward and gave him a sudden, brief hug. "I've missed you, Patch. We all did."

For a moment, Patch couldn't speak. The thought of all he'd left behind in Tiviscan was too much. Six months ago, just like Mort and Kara, he had known exactly what lay in his future—for him, it would be a glorious career in the Custodian Elite, bringing justice and help to those most in need. Then he'd thrown it all away, leaving Tiviscan behind, struggling to make ends meet. And now . . . the future wasn't something he even wanted to think about. "So," he said at last, changing the subject, "*Apprentice* Whitlock then!"

"It still sounds strange to my ears," said Erner.

An apprenticeship lasted two years, after which the title changed from "Apprentice" to "Fortis," which was the first proper rank of the Elite. Patch thought of the other figure he'd seen in the snow: "Who are you apprenticed to? What rank are they?"

"A Virtus," said Erner.

"Impressive!" said Patch. "Virtus" was the highest rank of all, and it was rare for them to take on an apprentice. "Which Virtus is it?"

Erner smiled awkwardly, and Patch could tell he was almost embarrassed to say it. "Virtus Stone."

Patch stared. "Good God, Erner. *Rundel* Stone?"

"Himself," said Erner.

The name of Rundel Stone brought two strong emotions to Patch. First, a deep sense of pride that his friend had been taken on as apprentice by such a legendary man— Stone was one of the Eight, the group of heroes who had finally captured the Hamelyn Piper.

The second emotion was utter despair, that the very same man held Patch's fate in his hands. Pity, the story went, was not a word Rundel Stone knew.

"Virtus Stone is making preparations to deal with the village's rat problem," said Erner. "While he does that, I'm to question you about . . . recent events."

"Hang on," said Patch. "Elite Pipers, dealing with rats?"

"With this many rats, people think of Hamelyn," said Erner. "The pride of all Pipers is at stake! We came to Patterfall because we happened to be in Wassil when the call for help was received, and the Virtus immediately volunteered. We arrived just in time to stop you being lynched. According to the villagers, you burst out of the forest half-dead and with amnesia. They assumed you were the Piper they'd sent for, and you assumed the same. What were you doing in the forest?"

"I, um, just happened to be traveling nearby," said Patch. "The merchant's cart I was getting a ride on broke, and I was abandoned. The merchant hadn't known how dangerous the region was at this time of year."

"The villagers told us what happened to them, when you tried to deal with the rats."

Patch hung his head. "I broke the law," he said. "I played the Dance, yes. But I didn't mean for the people to get caught up in it!"

Erner nodded, sorrow in his eyes. "There's something else, Patch," he said. "It's the reason Rundel Stone and I were in Wassil. There was a great mystery we'd come to solve."

"Um . . . go on." Patch didn't like where this was going.

"A few months ago, the Pipers' Council became aware of tales of traveling musicians whose music was said to be the best anyone had ever heard. Witnesses all said the same thing: people danced like they'd never danced before. It seemed that the musicians had a mysterious Piper among them, and that the Piper had been play-ing the most illegal Song of them all. The Song that you played for the rats, Patch. The *Dance*. Forbidden, since Hamelyn!"

"Er . . . gosh," said Patch. He *really* didn't like where this was going.

"The Council grew even more concerned, because every description of this mystery Piper was different. In one place, people had seen a tall, thin woman. In another, a short, wide man. One week, old. Another week, young. The Council was scared, Patch. Scared! A Piper who played the Dance even though it was forbidden! A Piper powerful enough to change physical appearance from one day to the next! Unheard of! A dark and evil Piper, the Council assumed. *Toying* with us. So they sent Rundel Stone to hunt this villain down. And myself, of course."

Patch coughed. When he'd fled from Tiviscan, earning money for food and lodging hadn't been easy. Piping was all he knew, but as a failed student fleeing in disgrace, working as a Piper was impossible. After a week on the road, hungry and tired, he'd met a traveling band of musicians who were barely scraping a living themselves. He'd offered to play the flute for them, but they already had a flute player.

That was when he'd had the idea.

He told them of a wonderful tune he knew, a sea shanty they'd never heard before, and convinced them to try it out. While the band performed, Patch stayed hidden and played the Dance in secret, making sure the audience had the time of their lives. Tips flowed, of course, and the grateful band gave him some of the money. They asked him for another tune, and so it went on.

That was how he had spent the seven months since he'd left Tiviscan: staying with a band for a few weeks, then parting company and setting off to find another band before anyone got suspicious.

He thought of all the bands he'd been with, and of the flute players in them—a tall, thin woman; a short, wide man. Old, and young.

Meanwhile, the Council had heard rumors of an evil Piper, and the varying descriptions they got were simply those of the different flute players.

I scared the Council, he thought, amazed.

He opened his mouth to confess, and stopped. There was a pained look in Erner's eyes.

"You already know it was me," said Patch.

Erner nodded. "Changing the bands you played with was clever," he said. "It made it difficult for us to track you down, but we got word from Wassil and headed there at once. It seems you'd left the town just before we arrived."

Patch sighed. "Someone had been asking too many questions. I figured it was time to get out of town, and the merchant who gave me a ride was the only one leaving that day."

"Yet fate led all of us to Patterfall," said Erner. "Virtus Stone has examined your broken Pipe, and the history of its Songs was still there to hear. I can't tell you how shocked I was to discover that it was *you* we'd been chasing all along!" He shook his head, saddened. "Why, Patch? Why would you take such a risk? Playing the Dance to deal with the rats was one thing, but playing it to entertain *people*?"

"It was the only way I could earn money, Erner. Nobody was harmed, and I didn't think anyone would find out." The look of disapproval on Erner's face was almost unbearable. "So," said Patch, "you'll take me back to Tiviscan, then. To certain imprisonment."

Erner seemed utterly deflated. "The Dance is absolutely forbidden. Ten years is the penalty." He walked over to the small window and looked out, silent for a moment. "There's some room for hope, though. The Lords who preside on your case can reduce the sentence by half—the rash actions of a trainee Piper without a malicious bone in his body."

"Five years, then," said Patch. "If pity is taken." He wondered if it might have been better if he'd died in the snow.

After Erner left, Patch lay down on his thin mat and despaired. Exhausted, he fell into an uneasy sleep. A curious sound, somewhere between scratching and rubbing, dragged him slowly back from slumber. He became aware of a gentle weight on his chest.

He opened his eyes and saw a rat.

It was the rat with the red-ringed tail, and it was looking at him.

The part of his brain that had done such a good job of imagining the rats *attacking* him went into overdrive. With a sudden yelp he sat up and backed away as far as he could, flinging the rat off him. It landed and gave him a very obvious glare, then raised a paw out to its side.

"I'm sorry! I'm sorry!" said Patch, gathering his blanket around himself. "Don't kill me!"

The rat looked to the ceiling and let out a tiny sigh, then nodded in the same direction as its paw.

"You're . . . you're not here to kill me?" said Patch, looking around frantically to see if the other rats were about to pour out of every crevice and devour him.

The rat shook its head and impatiently jabbed its paw toward the wall, its glare intensifying.

Patch stared at the rodent. He followed the line of its paw. On the flat stone of the wall beside him, written in chalk, were the words *Help me.*

The rat picked up a small piece of chalk from the floor and scurried over to the wall, ignoring Patch's whimper.

Patch wondered if he was still asleep or if madness had taken him. All he could do was stare at the animal as it wrote more letters on the wall. At last it squeaked at him, and he read aloud what the rat had written.

Help me. I am the young daughter of a rich nobleman. I have been cursed by a Sorcerer into the shape of a rat. You will be well rewarded!

Patch looked at the rat, and the rat nodded. "Right," said Patch, and he hid under his blanket. He clearly wasn't asleep, so madness seemed the only possibility.

After a few seconds he could feel the rat on top of him. He peeked out. It had its paws clasped together, pleading. "No!" he said. "You're not real!" The animal kept looking at him, forlorn and pitiful. A tiny tear formed and fell down the side of its face.

Patch felt a horrible stab of guilt. "Okay, enough!" he said. "Stop crying! I'll help." The rat gave a little jump for joy. "But why me?"

As if in answer, there was a sudden cheer from outside. Both Patch and the rat looked to the small window. Patch stood, and as he did the rat scampered up onto his shoulder. Patch walked to the window and looked out; a crowd of villagers had assembled by the oak tree, watching Virtus Stone and Erner as they approached the storehouse.

Patch turned his head to the rat. "The other rats all just went back to the storehouse?" he said. The rat nodded and slapped a paw to its forehead. "Not the smartest, are they?" said Patch, and the rat shrugged. Then the penny dropped. "*Ah!* You need protection from the Pipers, and who better to provide it than another Piper?" The rat nodded. "You'll be safe here," he said, wondering what Rundel Stone would play to get rid of the rodents. Stone had studied Patch's broken Pipe, so he probably knew the Dream wouldn't work.

Which Song would he try?

Stone took out his Pipe, and Patch could see that it was very dark in color. There was an old rumor that Rundel Stone's Pipe was made of obsidiac, one of the rarest magical substances in the world. It was a form of obsidian—black volcanic glass—only ever found in the Dragon Territories. Stone's Pipe couldn't actually be *made* of obsidiac, of course—no piece big enough had ever been found, and even if one had been, the material was impossible to carve. But it could certainly have been coated in an obsidiac glaze, if the obsidiac was finely ground and mixed with resin. Such a glaze had once been highly prized in Pipe-making, as the resulting Pipes were immensely powerful. However, obsidiac was considered holy by dragons; as a result, the Pipers' Council had banned its use in new Pipes long ago, in an effort to keep peace.

The Virtus raised his Pipe and began.

Patch listened carefully to the first notes, trying to identify the Song. He frowned. "I'm not sure what that is," he said. "The safest thing would be to wrap you in my blanket, little rat. Then, however the Song tries to compel you, you'll be unable to move and—"

He stopped talking.

The Virtus had started a rhythmic section, complex and primal. It was ringing a bell in Patch's mind. A great big worrying bell, one with *panic* written all over it.

"Oh," said Patch. "Oh no."

He had placed the rhythm. He knew the Song.

It was called the Dispersal, and it was a Song of execution—a terrifying thing, one of the most difficult Songs to perform.

Yet here was the Virtus, using it against a vast pack of rats.

The effect of Dispersal was simple. Every part of the target, every tiny *fragment*, would be utterly destroyed, the target reduced to its components—a devastating, instant unraveling that left nothing behind. Those components were widely dispersed, spread so thinly that not even a speck of blood would remain. Only dust, scattered across a thousand miles.

Patch listened in horror. The Dispersal was a highly selective Song, and the Virtus was allowing it to spread out, knowing that only his target—the rats—would be affected, without risk to the villagers. *All* rats within the bounds of the village would be killed, and perhaps for some distance beyond.

Patch had no idea if any defense was possible. "Uhhh . . ." he said. "Um . . ." The rat put its paws over its ears so it couldn't hear, as it had done with the Dance, but Patch shook his head and it put its paws down again. "A Song isn't just heard with the ears," he said. "Every single *part* of you hears it." The rat stared at him, terrified.

Patch looked around the small room and his eyes settled on the tin bowl the bread was in. "Worth a try," he muttered. He grabbed it, tipping the bread out. "Quickly," he said to the rat. "Under the bowl!" The rat ran to him, and he turned the bowl upside down on top of it. "Keep entirely inside," he said. "And whatever you do, whatever you hear, don't come out!"

He placed his hands on the bowl and thought about what he could do. To keep the rat safe, he needed to play a counter-Song and create a bubble of protection that surrounded the animal. He had no Pipe and would have to play it by lip, which made it harder—especially since his lips were still cracked and sore—but the bubble wouldn't need to be big.

Time was running out. Virtus Stone's Song was building. Patch could hear the chatter of the nervous villagers, as they sensed the sheer force of the music.

Here goes, he thought. With one ear on the Song outside, he began. The counter-rhythm he whistled was almost identical to the core rhythm of the Dispersal, but with a few carefully chosen added beats. Next, he whistled a modified version of the Song's secondary melody. Without a Pipe, all he could do was switch from rhythm to melody and back again, faster and faster, his lips getting ever closer to the upturned bowl.

The protective bubble began to form just in time. He could sense it surrounding the metal of the bowl, a bubble that would guide the flow of the Song safely away, and not let it penetrate.

He tensed, knowing the moment was close. The bowl started to vibrate as the counter-Song struggled to hold together. On the floor nearby, the piece of chalk began to shake, then it rose up onto one tip, spinning. Patch felt his hair stand on end, and the chain around his ankle grew oddly warm.

The Dispersal reached a sudden crescendo and the force of it hit him, almost knocking him over. He managed to keep his hands firmly on the bowl, but he despaired as he felt his counter-Song shatter. From outside came the anguished cries of terrified villagers.

Then silence.

Shaking, Patch took his hands away from the bowl, wary of lifting it. Who knew *what* he might find there. "Hello? Little rat?" There was a pitiful squeak. "It's okay," he said. "You're safe. You can come out now." The rat peeked out, trembling, looking at him for more reassurance. "Really," said Patch.

Outside, the shocked silence of the villagers was broken by hesitant cheers. "They've gone!" cried a voice. "Look! The rats have all gone!" The cheers grew.

The rat emerged from under the bowl and looked at Patch, a question in its eyes. Its companions were all dead, Patch realized—turned to dust and scattered across vast distances. "Yes," said Patch. "The other rats . . . They've all gone."

The rat slumped.

Patch waited a moment before he spoke again. "I have two questions," he said. "First, were any of the other rats human too?" The rat shook its head, which was a huge relief. "And second," he said, lifting the piece of chalk from the floor and offering it to the rat. "What's your name?"

The rat took the chalk and wrote two words on the wall. Patch looked at them and smiled. He held out his hand, taking the rat's paw and gently shaking it. "Good to meet you, Wren Cobble," he said. "I'm Patch Brightwater."

Wren dashed up Patch's arm to his shoulder and gave his neck a grateful hug.

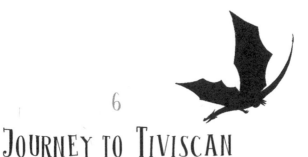

Journey to Tiviscan

"How old are you, Wren?" said Patch.

Wren ran down from his shoulder, and wrote *13* on the wall.

"Same as me!" he said. "And educated enough to read and write! A benefit of your wealthy family, I suppose. I was in training at Tiviscan Castle from the age of ten. It's a free education, for those with the gift of Piping. That education will come in handy now that I'll never be a real Piper—"

Wren frowned at him.

"Oh, I mean it," said Patch. "I've played an illegal Song. The Custodians will take me to Tiviscan, I'll be put on trial, and jailed for five years at the very least! As a criminal, I'll never be permitted to work as a Piper." He sighed; his gaze moved to Wren's chalk-written plea for help, and he read the last part aloud: *"You will be well rewarded!"* He turned to Wren. "I'm thankful that your parents are rich. Don't think me greedy, but when I'm released from the dungeons in five years, I'll need that reward." He gave her a weak smile, then bowed his head and closed his eyes. If he'd still been looking at her, he would have seen a curious expression cross Wren's face: a mixture of guilt and worry.

Patch opened his eyes again. "You'll have one heck of a story to tell your parents," he said. "When you get back home."

Wren shook her head and started to write again, Patch waiting patiently as she slowly drew out each letter: *Not until curse lifted.*

"I'm sure your parents—" started Patch, but Wren jabbed at the words she'd written and added an exclamation mark. *Not until curse lifted!*

"Fair enough," said Patch. He could sympathize, really— his grandparents thought he was still training to become a Piper, and the idea of them finding out the truth made him feel ill. He would leave them to their happy ignorance for as long as he could. "We'll have to get help from the Custodian Elite, then. They're in the best position to know what can be done for you."

She shook her head firmly.

"Saving you from that Song is one thing, Wren," he said. "But as a prisoner, I won't be able to do anything more to help you. You'll need the Custodians. Let me talk to them."

Wren shook her head again and mimed a lumbering monster. Patch laughed, because he understood who she meant.

"He's *Rundel Stone*," he said. "One of the Eight who hunted down the Hamelyn Piper. There isn't a more respected Custodian in the world! He's no monster."

Wren put her hand to her chest before taking it away sharply, as if it was painful. The Cold Heart of Justice, she was saying—Stone's famous nickname.

Patch sighed. He could understand why Wren would be wary of putting herself at the man's mercy. There were plenty of stories about how Stone sometimes applied the law far too strictly, and as a rat, Wren had certainly been guilty of stealing food and scaring the villagers. "Yes, but who can blame him for his cold heart?" said Patch. "He vowed to find the children of Hamelyn and bring them home, safe and sound. Rundel Stone and the rest of the Eight did all they could: they caught the Hamelyn Piper and brought him to Tiviscan to be imprisoned. But the children weren't found, and their fate is still unknown. Rundel Stone couldn't keep his vow. That's enough to leave anyone with a cold heart."

Wren was standing with her arms folded. She wasn't having it.

"Very well," said Patch. "We'll leave Stone out of it. I know his apprentice, Erner Whitlock. Honest and decent.

You'll like him. When I get a chance to talk to him alone, I'll *have* to tell him about you, okay? There's no other choice."

After a long pause, Wren gave him a reluctant nod. "Strange to think I'll actually *meet* Rundel Stone," said Patch. He recited the rhyme every child knew—the names of the Eight, the heroes assembled by the Pipers' Council to capture the Hamelyn Piper. "Palafox, Corrigan, Kellenfas, Stone," he said. "Casimir, Hinkelman, Drevis, and Throne. My grandmother has a way with stories, and she told me their adventures every night. A race against time, hunting across every nation of these lands and into the Islands of the Eastern Sea, until they finally caught the Hamelyn Piper and locked him away to rot in the dungeons of Tiviscan Castle." He paused, knowing that it was in those very dungeons that he would be spending the next five years—or maybe ten! "To be jailed by one of my heroes . . ."

Wren nodded, downhearted. She set down her chalk, climbed onto his shoulder again, and curled up.

Patch was glad of the company. "It's at least a week's journey to Tiviscan Castle from here by horse. Ever seen it?"

Wren shook her head.

"It's impressive," he said. "It sits on a cliff, and the dungeons extend deep into the rock. The deepest of the dungeons is called the Dark. No natural light reaches it." He sat on the floor, miserable. "The Hamelyn Piper is imprisoned in the Dark, of course. At the deepest point of the deepest dungeon. It's said

48

that each night the prisoners in the dungeons can hear him scream—scream until he's hoarse and can cry out no more."

He fell silent and closed his eyes.

After a while, Wren ran down to the ground and picked up her chalk. She wrote, but Patch was lost to his misery. She squeaked to get his attention.

You're too young for prison, she'd written.

"I'm not," he said. "Children younger than me have been jailed there." The Tiviscan dungeons were mainly used for those who broke the laws of Piping, so almost all the prisoners were Pipers themselves. Even the youngest child, discovering their own Piping ability for the first time, could accidentally break the law and end up in a cell. Although, Patch knew, it would often be just for a day, to scare them and make sure they didn't do it again. He honestly didn't know the longest time someone his age had been imprisoned for. Perhaps he would be setting a new record.

He could see that Wren was trying to think of something else to write.

"Look, I know you're trying to cheer me up," he said. "And thank you. But the only things that are important are that you're okay, and I'm not alone."

Wren nodded. She set down her chalk and clapped her paws together to get rid of the chalk dust, coughing as a little cloud of it engulfed her.

"It'd be easier with a quill and paper," said Patch. An

image of a tiny feather cut to a quill came into his mind, and he smiled. "Perhaps Erner will get you that. Although . . ." A thought had occurred to him. "Have you heard of Merisax hand speech?" Wren shook her head. "Merisax is a language used by mercenaries and pirates. My dream was to join the Custodian Elite, and they're required to be fluent, so I spent a lot of time learning it." Ah yes, his dream . . . Long since shattered. He sighed. "Anyway, with Merisax you only use your *hands* to talk. It allows for total silence in setting an ambush—you can hold a conversation without giving away your position. It's also useful in battle. Or in a loud tavern. Or any time you can't speak—" He gestured toward Wren and paused, waiting for the penny to drop. When it did, Wren's face lit up. "How about I run through some phrases, to give you a feel for it?"

She gave him a brisk nod and sat facing him, eager to begin.

"*Yes. No*," said Patch, thumbs up, then thumbs down. "*Hurry up. Slow down. Come over here. Go away.*" With each example, he gave Wren enough time to mimic the sign he was showing her. "*Keep going. You're an idiot. Pass the rum.*" Next he made a throat-slitting motion. "*Kill,*" he said.

"Lots of variants of kill, actually. Lots. That's pirates and mercenaries for you, I suppose. *Kill quickly. Kill slowly. Kill everyone. Don't kill anyone.*" He thought for a second. "That last one's probably not used much. Let's see . . . *Don't do that here. I'm bleeding. You're bleeding. Please stop the bleeding.*

50

You're on fire. The ship is on fire. The ship is sinking. Oh no it's a shark. Maybe we should murder the captain."

Wren studiously copied each action, deep in concentration. Patch continued. "*You smell terrible. Run away. If you do that again I'll kill you.* The eyes are important for that one," said Patch. "Otherwise it's a bit too much like *Pass the rum.* I expect that's caused a few fights in its time. Anyway, that should give you the flavor of it. What do you think?"

Yes, kill everyone, oh no it's a shark, signed Wren.

"Well," said Patch. "It's a start."

It was several hours before Erner Whitlock returned, and by then Wren had shown herself to be exceptionally quick at learning Merisax. Patch reckoned she would soon get to grips with it—something that had taken Patch months to achieve.

When the keys rattled in the door, Wren hid under Patch's blanket. Patch stood as Erner came inside.

"Your coat," said Erner, handing it to Patch. "We'll be setting off shortly."

Patch put the coat on, immediately glad of its familiar feel. He looked at Erner and noticed that the Apprentice Piper was uneasy. "Are you okay?" he asked.

Erner smiled nervously. "I should be asking *you* that. Patch, I want you to know that I—" He stopped and shook his head. "I'm sorry, about how things are."

Patch put his hand on Erner's shoulder. "I know," he said. "It's the way it must be, though. How's your boss?"

"Virtus Stone is unusually quiet," said Erner. "He's even moodier than normal."

"I could have guessed he was in a bad mood when he chose the Dispersal to deal with the rats," said Patch. "A bit over the top, don't you think?"

Erner shrugged. "The Virtus is the best Piper I've ever seen, by far. To him, the Dispersal is *easy,* and it was certain to do the job." He paused, before lowering his voice. "To be honest, it *was* overkill. I think he's cross from all this traipsing across frozen terrain, chasing you."

"I hope he cheers up on the journey back," said Patch. It seemed like a good opportunity to mention Wren. "Actually, there's something I need to talk to you about—"

"Silence!" came a voice. Rundel Stone swept through the doorway, and Patch took a step back from Erner. Even given the circumstances, Patch felt awed to be in the presence of a legend. "We leave in five minutes. The weather conditions are deteriorating. I've purchased another horse from the villagers for our *burden.*" He looked with disdain at Patch when he said it; instinctively Patch opened his mouth to object, but the glare from the Virtus stopped him. "No speaking!" said Stone. "Understand? Not now, not while we travel. *Never.* You are a criminal. A *disgrace* to Piping. Oh, I know all about you, Patch Brightwater. I make it my business to know. A promising young student, you wanted to join the Custodian Elite, but instead you embarrassed yourself and vanished with your tail between your legs. Then you chose to *misuse* the skills you'd managed to learn, to lead me on a merry chase while my time would have been far better spent elsewhere, dealing with problems that—unlike you—*actually matter*."

Patch opened and closed his mouth in silence, like a dying fish.

"Five minutes!" said Stone. He turned to Erner. "Come, Apprentice," he said, and left. Erner gave Patch a regretful look and went with his master, locking the door behind him.

Wren poked her head out from her hiding place.

"So much for meeting your heroes," said Patch. "We'll get to speak to Erner on his own, sooner or later." He held his coat open. "Handmade by my grandfather, this coat. Deerskin. His gift to me when I first went to Tiviscan. A little big back then, but now it's perfect. Cool in summer, warm in winter, with endless pockets. Come on then, hop inside."

Wren wasn't too sure.

"I will *not* squash you," said Patch. "I promise."

When Stone and Erner came back a few minutes later, Wren was snuggled up in his pocket. Patch was led outside. The Elite Pipers' horses stood waiting, a smaller horse beside them. Next to the horses stood Greta, the only person there to bid him farewell; the other villagers of Patterfall had stayed indoors.

"Good luck, Patch," said Greta. She looked at Stone. "Don't be harsh on the lad. He meant well."

Rundel Stone said nothing in reply.

As Stone had instructed, Patch stayed silent as they rode. It made him miserable. He had too much time to think—about his past, and about his future. Neither was a place he was keen to visit. With Stone's expert Piping to clear the snow, it only took a day of travel for them to get out of the valley and reach lower altitudes. Heading south, winter's icy grip weakened quickly. Wren was a little pocket of extra warmth near his heart.

Each night, they camped in the cover of woods and forests, using three of the traditional Piper's shelters that had been part of Patch's training—tiny oilskin tents that, when folded up took hardly any space in their horses' packs, but when assembled gave just enough room for a single, curled up sleeper. The tents kept out the cold, but even better was how the privacy let Patch help Wren learn her Merisax signs at night, until the light from the fire dwindled.

Each morning, Erner hunted for prey soon after dawn, when rabbit and fowl were more vulnerable to one of the various luring Songs. While he was gone, Stone got to work lighting a fire. Only on the third morning did they swap roles. When Stone went to hunt, Patch realized the chance had come to talk to Erner.

"Morning, Erner," said Patch, emerging from his little tent.

Erner had just struck his firesteel to light the fire. "Morning, Patch," he replied.

"Um, Erner?" said Patch.

Erner looked up, the fire doing well. "Yes?" he said, at which point Wren emerged from Patch's pocket, scurried to his shoulder, and waved.

"A rat!" said Erner, startled. Wren signed something, and Erner's surprise turned to astonishment. "That's Merisax hand speech!" he said. He watched the rat intently as she repeated what she'd signed. He stared in shock. "You want me to *what?*" he said, appalled.

"She didn't mean that," said Patch. "She's learning." He turned to Wren and signed: both hands opening and closing in fists. "*This* is 'Help me,' Wren," he said. "What you just signed . . . Well, it's very much *not*, and I don't want to *ever* see you do that again."

Wren grumbled.

"No, I *won't* tell you what it means." Patch turned back to Erner. "Erner, this is Wren. She's human, she was cursed by a Sorcerer, and she needs help. She lived among the rats in the village, and I suspect she was the reason those rats were so successful at avoiding traps and poison." He glanced at

Wren, who was trying to look as innocent as possible, but given how bright she'd shown herself to be, Patch had no doubt about it.

Erner's eyes widened in horror. "Wait . . . there were *people* among the rats?"

"None of the other rats were human," said Patch. "Luckily. Wren came to me when the Dispersal was about to happen, and I protected her from it, but with me in prison she'll need someone else to—"

"You *protected* her?" said Erner. "From *that* Dispersal? I felt how powerful it was."

Patch waved away the compliment. "Trust me, it wasn't easy. Look, we'd rather not involve the Virtus and he'll be back any minute."

"Why don't you want to involve the Virtus?" asked Erner. Wren signed something incredibly rude again, and Patch thought that this time she knew *exactly* what she was saying. He turned to Erner. "She thinks that Rundel Stone is so stubborn he'd probably arrest her for being, I don't know, a talking rat without a *license*. Or something."

Erner laughed wholeheartedly, then suddenly stopped. "Ah. I see your point."

Patch nodded. "Exactly," he said.

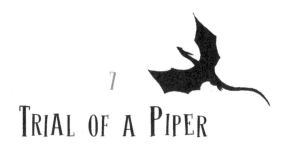

Trial of a Piper

Erner agreed to keep Wren's presence a secret and to begin investigating a cure for her curse the moment they reached Tiviscan.

As they continued their journey, Wren's grasp of Merisax grew in leaps and bounds, and teaching her provided Patch with a welcome distraction from what awaited him when they reached their destination.

At last, ten days after setting off from Patterfall, the three horses trudged through rain on the rising road; ahead, they could see the sheer cliff on which Tiviscan Castle sat, overlooking forest. To the rear of the castle was Tiviscan town, a ramshackle spread of buildings that flowed from the castle's gates toward grassy plains and hills.

The castle rose high and seemed larger than was possible, since at its base it continued *into* the rock of the cliff. It was hard to tell where the castle ended. Some parts of it were ancient beyond measure, older even than Piping. Originally, it was a village carved into the rock itself— networks of tunnels, tombs, and homes that lay within the cliff. As the castle grew, it grew down as well as up.

The oldest and deepest of those tunnels formed the dungeons where Patch would soon find himself. He thought of them and shivered.

They reached the castle gates, passing under the massive double archways and through the courtyard market, which was busy despite the rain. They dismounted at the vast central Keep, and Virtus Stone led them through the ironclad Keep gate, into a dim stone entrance hall.

There were two sets of steps ahead. One set was plain stone, leading downward. The other led up, and was far grander: the steps were marble, and the walls beside it were carved with images from the history of Piping.

The first carving showed the earliest days when Pipers knew only the simplest Songs. They were more like monks or knights back then, and traveled the world bringing help where they could, for no reward but food and shelter. A simple life, based on a proud code of honor—an ideal which was reborn much later, when the Custodian Elite were founded.

The next few carvings showed the discovery of new Songs and new skills, as the Piper's Art was refined over centuries.

A great and glorious history, Patch thought, *is carved into those walls.*

And then he saw a carving that depicted a battle: army facing army, but only one side had Pipers in their ranks. It took Patch a moment to realize which battle was being represented, and when he did he sighed with sorrow.

The Pipers in that battle had been paid to fight. The opposing army was being slaughtered.

The history of Piping was not always great or glorious, thought Patch.

Stone stopped walking and looked at him, raising an eyebrow. He followed Patch's eyeline to the carving. "Ah," he said. "The Battle of Dornley Flats. I see you disapprove."

"Of course I do," said Patch. "Before then, Pipers could only fight for causes that were *just,* not for money."

"Pipers didn't invent war, boy," said Stone. "The many nations of these lands have always quarreled with each other. Sometimes those quarrels grow. Sometimes they become wars. If Pipers have skills that are useful to an army, shouldn't they be able to profit from them?"

Patch didn't answer.

"Besides," said Stone, "no ruler—no king, queen, baron, or overlord—wants the Pipers' Council as an enemy, for without the Council's approval they could hire no decent

Pipers to help in their battles. They'd be forced to use *outcast* Pipers, poorly skilled, poorly trained! Their forces would be at a severe disadvantage. That fact keeps the Pipers' Council safe, and all Pipers too, something you'd be wise to remember."

"Maybe," said Patch. It might have been the truth, but it left a sour taste in his mouth.

"Up past those carvings lies the Chamber of the Council," said Stone. "That's where you would have graduated if you'd proved your worth. Think how different your life could have been! As it is, your trial tomorrow could be the last time you ascend those stairs." He shook his head with a sigh and raised his arm, pointing ominously to the other steps. "We go *that* way."

Stone led them down the spiraling steps, followed by Patch, with Erner at the rear. It got darker as they descended, and a horrible stench rose from below.

They came to a locked gate. Stone knocked, and a burly man opened it.

"Prisoner for trial," said Stone. "By the name of Patch Brightwater." He turned to Erner. "Accompany him to the holding cell. I'll inform the Council of our success."

"Come on through," said the burly man. He closed the gate once Patch and Erner were inside. "My name's Furnel, lad," he said to Patch. "This way."

Furnel led them to a dank corridor lit by oil lamps. Patch saw a row of small cells, with one door open. Furnel pointed to the door, and Patch went inside. There was just enough space to lie down, and a sickly light came through the bars in the door. On the cold floor was some straw, and a rough blanket that at first touch felt like it might give him splinters. The door was shut behind him and he could hear Furnel and Erner walking away.

Wren came out of his pocket and ran up to his shoulder. *Horrible place*, she signed, anxious.

Patch nodded. *Five years*, he thought. Five years in a cell that would probably be even worse than this. And that was if he was lucky enough to have his sentence reduced.

A few minutes later, Erner opened the door and handed him a bundle of clothes. "The jailor insisted you change into these," he said. "Prison clothing must be worn by the accused at a trial."

Patch took them. Rough cloth trousers, rough cloth shirt.

"You can keep your boots," said Erner.

"What about my coat?" said Patch.

Erner shook his head. "I'll look after it until your release."

Patch set Wren on the floor and changed, then handed Erner his clothes and coat. "There's one other thing I want you to look after," he said. He turned to Wren, whose eyes widened.

What are you talking about? she signed.

"I'll take good care of her," said Erner. "You have my word."

No chance! signed Wren. *I'm staying with Patch! Someone has to lift his spirits!*

"You can't stay with me, Wren," said Patch. "The dungeons are no place for you." She folded her arms and avoided eye contact. "Please, Wren. Erner will find the help you need. I'll make it through. In five years, I'll be out. And you can bring me that reward!" When he said it like that, it almost sounded *possible.*

Wren looked to Patch, then to Erner, and back again. Her shoulders sagged, and her head dropped. She nodded. *I'll miss you,* she signed.

Erner was carrying a satchel, and he kneeled down and opened the flap. "There's room in here," he said.

"Keep out of sight," said Patch. "People have a thing about rats. Safest to stay hidden!"

Wren hopped inside, with one last sad look at Patch. She waved, and Patch waved in return. "Look after yourself, Wren," he said. Erner closed the door, and Patch listened as his friend's footsteps faded.

He was alone.

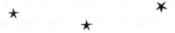

After a long restless night, Patch was awoken with a bowl of hot stew.

"Is it morning?" he asked the jailer—Furnel, the same

burly man who'd been on duty the night before. Given that no natural light seemed to reach his cell, he had no way to tell if it was daytime.

"It is," said Furnel. "Your trial begins in an hour."

Patch ate the food, his last meal before perhaps ten years of confinement, or five if he was lucky. When he finished, Furnel manacled himself and Patch together.

"I know you're not thinking of escape now, lad," said Furnel. "But things change when the sentence gets passed and the reality of it hits home. Trust me."

He led Patch up the central steps of the Keep until they reached the ornate door to the Council chamber. Furnel knocked, and the doors swung wide to a cacophony of voices.

The chamber was full.

Around the walls, rising rows of seats made it feel like a theater.

Rundel Stone sat in a chair at one side, and Patch was led to a stool in the middle of the chamber. He sat and looked around the room quickly, trying to find Erner—and there he was, three rows up on the left, satchel in hand. Patch thought he could see a tiny nose peeking out from the bag.

He would be judged by members of the Pipers' Council, usually two of them. A door in the far wall opened, and his judges started to come into the chamber. He watched, anxious to see who was going to rule over his fate.

He stared as all five members of the Council came in and sat at the judges' bench.

Lord Drevis entered first, followed by Lord Pewter, Lady Winkless, Lord Cobb, and Lady Rumsey.

All of them would preside over his case. They wore ceremonial robes, fold after fold of garments stitched with gold, silver and brilliant indigo.

Patch turned to Furnel. "Isn't it supposed to be just *two* judges?"

"For something this infamous?" said Furnel.

Patch gave him a wary look. "Infamous?"

"Aye, lad. You were big news for a time, when the rumors started about a rogue Piper. People were scared! They thought the Hamelyn Piper himself might have escaped! I'm not surprised the whole of the Council is here. And look at the size of the crowd!"

The clap of a gavel sounded from the judges' bench, and the chatter of the audience began to settle. The gavel was in the hand of Lord Drevis, the head of the Pipers' Council. Drevis, like Stone, was one of the legendary Eight. Indeed, he had *led* them in their successful capture of the Hamelyn Piper, and as a result was probably the most famous Piper in the world. Another two claps of the gavel, and silence was finally achieved.

"The Court of the Council is gathered," said Drevis. "Accuser, state your case."

Rundel Stone stood from his seat. "This prisoner before you is Patch Brightwater."

"Prisoner shall stand!" called Drevis, and Patch stood, chain rattling.

"Thirteen years of age, Brightwater trained in this castle," said Stone. "Last midsummer, his own failings led him to abscond after bringing shame on himself. He left the castle, abandoning his training." The audience murmured darkly. "As the Council is aware, rumors began of a rogue Piper, playing the Dance throughout the land. A Piper able to change *form*!" The murmurs grew. "It transpires that Brightwater was at the root of the affair. However, the rumors of shape-changing were misplaced. He merely played the Dance in secret at various inns and taverns, to extract *moneys* and *favors*!" Stone addressed his next words to the audience and spoke them with some relish. "His actions brought *disrepute* to the pure and glorious Art of Piping!"

The audience booed.

"The evidence?" said Lord Pewter.

Stone held up the two halves of Patch's broken Pipe. "The history of his crimes lies within the Pipe he used, one he had clearly crafted himself."

Lord Pewter gestured for Stone to bring the pieces to the bench. He took the broken Pipe and examined it carefully, then passed it to his colleagues. "A very traditional Pipe, but easy to get wrong," said Pewter. "I'm pleased to see how well you learned your carving, Patch Brightwater."

"Uh, thanks, Lord Pewter," said Patch. "It was cured over a hawthorn fire. Makes all the difference."

Stone glared at him. "The prisoner is to remain silent!"

"Come, come, Rundel," said Pewter. "I addressed him directly. His comment was allowed." He turned to Patch. "Think carefully, now, Patch Brightwater. Do you confess to your crime? Did you Pipe the Dance as the Virtus claims?"

There seemed little point denying anything. "I did," said Patch. A gasp came from the audience. "But it was not through greed, Lord. It wasn't riches I sought, only food and a bed to sleep in."

The Council turned to one another and entered muffled discussions. Finally, Drevis clapped the gavel and spoke. "Patch Brightwater, you have confessed your guilt. We must now consider the case for leniency. You have misused Piping, but I know your tutors thought well of you, and that previously you had shown yourself to be honest and of good nature—although not always of good judgement. Now, as you have done before, you have gone astray and chosen poorly." He looked to his colleagues. "We are all agreed?" They nodded. "This crime demands ten years in the dungeons of Tiviscan. The mercy of the Court allows us to reduce this to five years."

The audience murmured, nodding their heads. Erner gave him an encouraging glance. Patch looked to Erner's bag and could just about make out a thumbs up from a certain small paw.

Then a voice spoke: "Wait." It was Rundel Stone.

"Yes, Virtus?" said Lord Drevis.

Stone got up from his chair and strode to the center of the chamber. "I agree with your assessment of the prisoner. To my mind, he is indeed a *fool* more than a villain." Sniggers came from the audience. "However, there is one matter that I strongly disagree with."

"Go on," said Drevis, his eyes narrowing.

"This is a serious offense," said Stone. "When the Hamelyn Piper was imprisoned, the Dance was forbidden at once. In all these years, nobody has broken that law. Until now. Yet you wish to give the perpetrator a slap on the wrist?"

"Look at him, Rundel," said Lady Winkless. "There's no evil in the lad. Five years in the dungeons is already a severe punishment."

Stone shook his head, and when he spoke again there was a hint of anger in his voice. "You look at Brightwater and see a boy who came here to study, a boy who then strayed from the path. I see *danger*. Here was a boy willing to play the Dance and ignore the law. Time has passed since Hamelyn, and people are starting to forget the horror of it. That cannot be allowed!" He looked around the chamber, the audience utterly silent. Yet, Patch noticed, Stone didn't look at *him*. "There has been *fear* since these rumors of a Dark Piper emerged, but before that, something curious had happened to the story of the

Hamelyn Piper. On my search for Brightwater, for example, I saw an inn called The Piper and the Rats. The inn's sign showed a *jolly* scene, but it was the Hamelyn Piper that was depicted! Smiling! *Benevolent!*" His hand formed a fist as he spoke. "I spoke with some who even thought he might have been a hero. Who said the children had been taken to a wondrous place, to live happy lives. Who said that the people of Hamelyn must have done something to provoke him, or had treated their own children so *terribly* that the Hamelyn Piper needed to rescue them!" He paused, his anger seeming to overwhelm him for a moment. "How can that be? How can we have forgotten?" He looked around the chamber. Most would not meet his gaze. "The notion that the Hamelyn Piper was not evil cannot be allowed to stand," he said. "And so we cannot be lenient now. We cannot show pity. We must reassert the seriousness of what occurred in Hamelyn ten years ago. Brightwater's crimes must be treated with grim brutality. As such, I invoke the rule of multiple infractions!"

The Council all looked at Stone with stunned expressions, as the audience broke into uproar.

Patch bent down slightly to Furnel. "What does that mean?" he whispered.

"I think you'd best sit down, lad," said Furnel. "This ain't going to be pleasant."

Patch stayed standing.

"It's your right to insist, Virtus," said Lord Drevis, sounding almost dazed. He turned to the other Council members to discuss the matter, as the din from the audience continued.

At last, Lord Drevis clapped the gavel and the commotion in the chamber settled. "It is with sorrow that we must accept your request, Rundel," he said. "Patch Brightwater, your sentence will still be treated with leniency and reduced by half. However, the basic sentence is now ten years for *each time* you broke the law and performed the Dance." He looked to Rundel Stone. "In studying the broken Pipe, how many times did you assess?"

"One hundred and two," said Stone.

There was total silence in the chamber now. The faces of the Council paled, as the implications became clear to all.

"We will take it on ourselves to verify the figure, Rundel," said Drevis.

"Naturally," replied the Virtus.

"Patch Brightwater," said Drevis. "The sentence is ten years for each of the one hundred and two occurrences of your crime. You are hereby sentenced to one thousand and twenty years in the dungeons of Tiviscan, reduced to five hundred and ten by the clemency of the Council. Jailer, take him down." He clapped his gavel, looking somewhat ill.

The audience began its din once again. "God have mercy on you," shouted someone, "because Rundel Stone certainly won't!"

Patch fell back onto his stool, unable to take in what had just happened. He looked up to where Erner sat and could see him struggle with his bag as Wren tried to escape. "No!" Patch shouted at Wren. "Please! Don't!"

Someone from the audience laughed: "Beggin' won't help you!"

Patch kept his gaze on the bag. He saw Wren's paws, briefly. She signed something to him, then hid back inside.

Furnel dragged him out of the chamber and led him back down the steps, and through the dungeon gate once more, but instead of heading back to where he'd spent the night, Patch was taken to another spiraling staircase.

Down they went into the gloom below, passing level after level, and Patch thought, *How deep will I be put?*

Furnel took him down a long dank passage, one that reeked of decay and was lined with cell doors. As they passed each door, shouts started up from behind: "Who d'ya have? Eh? Who've ya brought us?"

Furnel stopped at the last door in the corridor. There was a folded blanket on the floor, and Furnel picked it up and gave it to Patch. The burly jailer was subdued and could hardly make eye contact. "It's not often I feel sorrow when I bring a prisoner down," he said, shaking his head. "This cell is the best I can do for ye, lad, given your sentence. Deep, sure enough, and at the very edge of the Dark. But it's by the outside wall of the castle—so you have a window, such as it is." He unlocked the door and swung it open.

Patch stared. The door was several feet thick, as were

the walls of his cell. He looked inside and saw that the cell was larger than he'd expected, perhaps five strides across. The "window" was an open hole barely the size of his hand, allowing a narrow band of light in from outside. The depth of the window showed that the outer wall was at least six feet thick, even thicker than the cell door. A bundle of rags was in one dark corner.

The stench in the cell was appalling.

"Your toilet is there," said Furnel, pointing to a hole in the floor. "You get food and water most days. There's your bowl and water jug." He pointed to a clay bowl and jug over by the rags. "Food and water tubes come in those holes by the door, see? Be sure you're ready to catch 'em." Patch noted small holes in the wall, and a mound of decayed food on the floor underneath. No wonder the smell was so bad. Furnel unlocked the manacles on his and Patch's wrists.

Patch rubbed at his chafed skin. "What happened to the last prisoner who was in here?" he asked.

"Oh, that reminds me," said Furnel. He walked across to the corner where the bundle of rags was and lifted it up in his arms.

It wasn't a bundle of rags. It was a *corpse*.

Furnel carried it to the corridor and set it on the ground. Patch saw the dead man clearly now—ancient, and thin to the point of being just a collection of bones. "Innocent Jack, they called him," said Furnel.

"Why did they call him that?"

"On account of him being *innocent*," said Furnel. "Found guilty of murderin' a man through Piping, then the man showed up alive only last year." He shook his head. "Shame Jack died. His review was only a couple of months away. They'd probably have let him out!"

"How long had he been here?" said Patch, looking at the old face, its skin like parchment. *Must have been a long, long time*, he thought. *Perhaps it's possible to live long enough for the Council to come to their senses and let me go . . .*

"Jack was convicted when he was twenty," said Furnel. "So, let's see now"—his eyes went to the ceiling as he worked it out—"he'd been here almost fifteen years."

Patch stared at Furnel in shock.

"Time in here takes its toll," said Furnel. "Well, good luck, lad." He swung the huge cell door closed, and Patch heard the man's heavy steps vanish back along the corridor. Then he could *feel* the walls, unbearably heavy, crushing him . . .

He ran to the tiny window, stretching up on tiptoes to put his mouth to the slight draft that came in. Breathing deeply, he waited for the panic to subside.

He thought back to the message Wren had signed to him in the Council chamber: *Don't give up.*

But how could he not? Right now, there seemed to be only one thing that Patch Brightwater was certain of.

Like Innocent Jack, he would be in this place until he died.

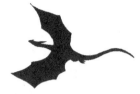

8

THE HAMELYN PIPER

Patch's panic was just starting to lessen when he heard something that didn't help at all.

"Hey!" said a man's voice.

Patch pulled back from the window. "Who's there?" he said, looking around.

"Down here!" came the voice again, but it seemed to be coming from *everywhere*.

Aren't things bad enough, thought Patch, *without having to share my cell with the ghost of Innocent Jack?* "Who are you?" he said. "Please, just leave me alone!"

"Look, mate," said the voice. "We're going to be spending a *lot* of time together, so let's try and get along, eh? My name's Vague Henry."

"Are you . . . are you *dead?*"

Vague Henry sighed. "I'm your *neighbor*. Just look at the bottom of the wall. See the hole?"

Patch looked at the wall to his right. There was a dark area, smaller even than the five-inch window. It was level with the floor, and as he moved toward it he realized it actually *was* a hole. "I see it," he said.

"Stick your eye up to it and say hello!"

Patch put his eye to the hole. It was a long, dim channel cut through the thick stone wall, but at the other end— perhaps five feet away—was another eye, looking back at him. "Hello," he said.

"You've only got me as a neighbor, since you're at the end of the row," said Henry. "The holes are part of the plumbing, but it's a handy way to chat without having to shout and annoy everyone. So you're Patch Brightwater, eh?"

"How do you know who I am?"

"Word travels fast down here! Pleasure to meet you, Patch. We've not come up with a nickname for you yet, though. Not like Jack, your cell's previous resident."

"Innocent Jack," said Patch.

"Indeed! Used to be *Murderous* Jack, of course, before the whole innocence thing happened. Your nickname usually has something to do with why you're in the dungeons, see."

"So why do they call you Vague Henry?"

Henry paused. It was a long pause, and a strangely awkward one. "Dunno," he said.

Patch waited, but nothing more was forthcoming. "Uh . . . okay," said Patch at last, wondering if his question had been answered.

"What'll we call you?" said Henry. "Doomed Boy Patch? Bleak Young Patch? We'll get it. We've got plenty of time."

"Right," said Patch, the words "plenty of time" filling him with horror. He pulled away from the hole and lay on his back, staring up at the rough stone ceiling.

"Some advice for you," said Henry. "First up, when feeding time comes, the guard calls out 'tubes.'"

"Furnel mentioned those," said Patch. "Why do they use tubes?"

"So they don't have to open the doors, lad," said Henry. "Be ready to catch it when it comes—especially the water! When it rains, you'll see the rainwater come in through holes like this one and run through grooves in the floor. See 'em? See where they lead?"

Patch looked to the floor and saw them. Grooves a couple of inches across ran toward the hole in the floor that Furnel had pointed out previously—the toilet. "I see them."

"Exactly. We get some of the, er, *waste water* from above us, and we're five levels down. So don't drink the rainwater, however thirsty you get, however clean it looks! And for your sake and ours, make sure your hole doesn't block up!"

"Will do," said Patch. "Henry, is it true that you can hear the Hamelyn Piper scream at night?"

"Oh, you'll hear him all right," said Henry.

"Doesn't it frighten you? Being so close to him?"

"The Hamelyn Piper? He's a wreck. His brain is nothing but mush by now. But no, I'm not frightened, not by him or any other Piper here. It doesn't matter how well a prisoner can lip-play to whistle up a Song. Hell, even if someone managed to get hold of a Pipe, it'd do 'em no good. They have precautions."

"Precautions?"

"Haven't you seen the depth of the doors and windows? If you look close, you'll see that every way out of your cell is lined with little furrows."

Patch looked into the hole that led to Henry's cell. Dark as it was, he could make out a slight twist here and there on the stone, a pattern carved into the rock. "Sound baffles?" said Patch. He'd heard of them in training—they confused any Songs you played, and took the edge off the magic enough to render them useless. They only worked for conduits that were long and thin, so they were no good as a general defense; they were more a curiosity of Piping theory. In here, though: perfect.

"Precisely," said Henry. "The workers down here are almost immune to Piping, lip-Piping at any rate, but the baffles make sure. It's why the walls and the doors are so thick, and why they feed us with the tubes. Inside your cell, you can't affect anyone else. So don't let the Hamelyn Piper frighten you. He's harmless now. Especially with what they did to him!"

"The Iron Mask," said Patch, nodding to himself.

When Patch was younger, his grandmother had often told him the story of the Hamelyn Piper, but only when he pestered her. She preferred to tell him about the adventures of the Eight as they hunted him down and caught him, rather than the horrors that had led to their quest in the first place.

She would say, "I don't want to frighten you, Patch." And he would insist, "It doesn't scare me, Nan."

Eventually she would give in, and Patch would thrill at the tale. But he had lied to her about it not scaring him. He knew that once she was done—the instant his candle was blown out and the door shut—his courage would fail and he would lie in his bed and tremble, wondering when the long bony fingers of the Hamelyn Piper would wrap around the door handle.

She always began with the same words, words which, even when he thought of them now, brought back a strange combination of adventure and terror: *Have you heard of the town of Hamelyn, Patch? It was once overrun with rats . . .*

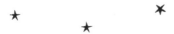

Of course, *every* town has its rats, but one summer there were so many that the Mayor of Hamelyn brought in rat-catchers from all around, and they did their work. In the past, this had always done the trick.

But not this year.

At first, the rat-catchers were happy. The more rats they caught, it seemed, the more rats they *saw*, and as they were paid for each rat they killed, there was real money to be made!

Then they began to grow nervous.

"It's not natural," they said to one another. "We catch a thousand a day, yet their numbers just keep rising!" They began to think the town was cursed, and one by one the rat-catchers left.

The townsfolk were angry with the Mayor for letting them leave, but what else could the Mayor do?

A Piper!

Much more expensive than rat-catchers, yes, but a Piper was the answer.

One thousand gold coins were raised and locked in the Town Treasury. By early evening the Mayor was sitting in the Town Hall surrounded by the most powerful people in Hamelyn, writing a letter to summon a Piper: *one thousand gold coins*, it said, *to the Piper who rids us of our rats*.

As he was placing his seal on the envelope, the door to the hall opened wide. There stood a Piper so tall and so thin that he seemed to be built entirely of edges.

"I heard you had a problem," said the Piper.

"You did?" said the Mayor, wary. He looked at the letter in his hand. "And *how* did you hear?"

"From the twenty rat-catchers I met along the road," said the Piper. "But now I've arrived, and the rats will soon be gone! For five hundred gold coins."

The Mayor nodded, and tried to stop himself from grinning. *Five hundred!* he thought. *Only five hundred!*

He carefully placed the letter in his pocket before standing and walked over to the Piper. "A hefty price," he said, looking up at the considerably taller man.

"Well, if you'd rather find another Piper—" began the stranger.

"We accept!" said the Mayor. He offered out his hand, and the Piper shook it.

The Piper smiled. Those in the hall smiled back, even though they all thought that the Piper's teeth seemed a little sharp . . . and the smile a little cruel.

The Piper cleared his throat. From his coat he produced a long thin Pipe, and began to play. As he played, he took slow strides out of the hall, then along the street outside.

The first rats appeared from the shadows, watching him, but soon they followed in the same slow rhythm: step—step—step!

More and more rats poured out from every house, every street, and by the time the Piper reached the edge of the town there was a vast shifting carpet of rats coming after him.

The Mayor and all the people watched this huge procession leave, cheering that the town would soon be free of its rat plague.

The River Weser lay ahead, beyond the walls of the town. At the river's edge, the Piper stopped walking. He raised his arms out to his sides, and the rats reached him.

The townsfolk shuddered, seeing from a distance how the wide column of rats engulfed the Piper, crawling up his coat then down the other side into the water to drown. It was almost an hour before they had all completed their final journey and the Piper was revealed again.

He lowered his arms and returned to the town. The townsfolk cheered and applauded. The Piper took an extravagant bow and smiled. The Mayor stood outside the Town Hall, waving to the crowd to make sure he would always be remembered for such a great success.

As the Piper reached him, the crowd fell silent.

"My job is done," said the Piper. "I will take my payment."

The Mayor summoned the Town Treasurer, who brought a bag that was so heavy it needed its own cart. "You have counted the coins?" asked the Mayor, and the Treasurer said he had. "Here is your payment," said the Mayor to the Piper. "Five hundred gold coins!"

The Piper opened the fastening at the neck of the bag and thrust in his hand. When he pulled it out, it was only *sand* that ran through his fingers.

A shocked gasp spread through the crowd. The Mayor stared at the Treasurer. The Treasurer stared at the bag; he darted forward and tipped the contents of the bag out. Nothing but sand!

"You try to trick me?" said the Piper.

"No!" said the Mayor, terrified by the malice he saw in the Piper's gaze. The Mayor looked to the Captain of the Town Guard and pointed to the Treasurer. "Arrest this man!" he cried. "And bring five hundred gold coins from the treasury vault!"

The Treasurer protested as he was taken away. Soon, the Captain returned and shook his head. "There is only sand in the vault, sir," he said.

The Mayor was speechless. He looked at the Piper, who scowled.

"I see you have a thief in your midst," said the Piper. "I will return tomorrow to collect my payment."

The Piper turned and walked out of the town.

The Mayor looked to the Captain. "Find the money!" he said. Then he turned to his most trusted advisor. "You are now the Treasurer! Raise more, in case we can't find the missing coins!"

The next morning, the River Weser burst its banks downstream as the rat corpses blocked the flow of water. Fields of wheat and barley were destroyed. The townsfolk set about clearing the corpses and built pyres to burn them on. By afternoon the air was thick with the smoke of the pyres and the stench of burning rat flesh.

The stolen money was not found; the previous Treasurer had refused to admit taking it, whatever unpleasantness was done to him. In the end, the Captain of the Town Guard stopped torturing him and concluded that he was innocent.

The new Treasurer, wary of the fate of his predecessor, managed to raise enough for the Piper's pay, but it was difficult. When the money was gathered, it was all witnessed by trusted men of the Town Guard, who then stood watch over the vault.

As dusk approached the Piper was seen coming along the road to town. This time the crowd was silent as he came. There was a fearfulness that was shared by all.

The Piper was brought to the treasury, where the vault stood closed. It had not been left unattended, not even for a moment.

"Greetings, Piper," said the Mayor.

"Greetings, Mayor," said the Piper. His smile seemed dangerous. "My payment?"

The Mayor nodded to the new Treasurer, who opened the door of the vault and handed the Piper the first of the bags that were inside. The Piper untied it and tipped it out.

Sand.

"No!" cried the Mayor.

"No!" cried the Treasurer.

The Piper shook his head, tut-tutting. "Such a *terrible* crime problem you have here," he said. "What *are* we to do?"

The Piper's eyes were aimed directly at the Mayor, that sinister gaze drilling deep. The Mayor could see a darkness there, unlimited and uncaring. He cleared his throat. "We have no more money," he said. Suspicion and fear almost overwhelmed him. He thought of how the rat-catchers had been so wary of the rats, some of them believing the infestation was unnatural; he thought of the money disappearing repeatedly, with no apparent culprit.

He could see suspicion in the eyes of others around him too, all looking at the Piper. But what could they do? People looked from the Piper to the Mayor, waiting for someone to speak.

"Don't worry," the Piper said at last, but in a voice that was far from soothing. "Tonight I will take my pay. I will take things that are often unwelcome. Things that *everyone*, at some point, wishes were gone. Could I be fairer than that?"

The Piper turned and left. Silence filled the entire town until he was far in the distance.

The Mayor looked to the Captain. "Ready your men," he said. "Guard the gates. Let *nobody* in tonight."

Night came.

In the distance, the pyres still burned.

The guards were ready. The townsfolk locked their doors. It was midnight when the sound of Piping began. The music grew louder. The people of Hamelyn could hear their own children stir from their beds, laughing. The children came out, unlocked the doors, and danced into the streets.

The adults all found that they could not move, could not even *speak*.

They could only watch.

And the Piper, his eyes burning like the distant pyres, danced by each house and smiled a wide, sharp smile, and the children of the town followed him toward the town gates, dancing with unbounded joy. The gates were flung open by an invisible force, and the Piper led the children out of Hamelyn.

It was not until morning that the townsfolk could move again. They fell to the ground, wailing in horror at what had happened. Then they ran, seeking their children, following the road, seeing where the grass at the edges had been trampled by the dancing.

On and on they went, until the trampled grass veered onto a smaller pathway that went up Koppen Hill. Near the top of the hill, the trail ended by a sheer face of rock.

The children were not there.

The townsfolk heard the sound of sobbing and found one small boy, who had been lame since birth.

"I couldn't keep up," he cried again and again, despairing.

"Where are the others?" asked the adults. "Where are all the other children?"

"He promised us a Land of Play, with all the toys and sweets we could want," said the boy. "When the Piper reached this point, a doorway opened in the rock and they all danced inside. But I couldn't keep up! I was too late!"

He burst into angry, desolate tears. "The door shut before I got to it!"

They found no sign of a doorway. In all, one hundred and thirty children had been taken by the Hamelyn Piper.

It took over a year to catch him.

The Pipers' Council assembled a group to track down this evil creature who had brought shame on their kind—a group who became known as the Eight, their exploits now legendary.

When the Piper was finally caught, he refused to reveal what had become of the children. Many wanted to see him die for what he had done, convinced he would never reveal the children's fate, but the Council kept him alive, and gave him the cruelest punishment they could devise. The Iron Mask: fastened around the head of the Hamelyn Piper, it prevented him ever using his abilities again, as no magic could escape it, Song or otherwise.

But it had one more function. Once put in place, whatever the Hamelyn Piper said next would be the only thing he could ever say again, unless he was to tell where the children had gone. When the Mask was fitted to the Piper's head, the Council addressed him.

"Piper of Hamelyn!" they said. "Do you still refuse to tell what you did with the children?"

"Aye!" the Hamelyn Piper cried, his eyes at first defiant; but then his eyes became defeated, and lost, as he finally knew that his reign of evil was ended, and the world would be forever safe from him.

They locked him in the deepest, darkest place within the dungeons of Tiviscan, and "Aye!" is still the only word he speaks.

For he has never revealed where the children went.

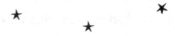

"Sleep well," said a voice, bringing Patch crashing back to the present. He realized the voice belonged to Vague Henry, but those were the words his grandmother had always said to him as she left him in his bed.

He was a long way from there now, in this cold cell in the dungeons of Tiviscan. The dungeons that would be his home for the rest of his days.

"Goodnight, Henry," said Patch. He stood and looked around to see where best to sleep. The corner where the corpse of Innocent Jack had lain was, for the moment, ruled out, so Patch chose the opposite corner.

He lay down and closed his eyes, trying his best to cover himself in the meager blanket he'd been given. Rather than consider what the future held, he thought back to the past again.

There was so much more to the Hamelyn Piper's story, of course; the quest of the Eight to catch him was, in itself, an epic tale of courage. But of all the things he'd learned during his training, the most shocking was the Hamelyn

Piper's *next* crime, and how close it had come to triggering another war between dragons and humans.

It was shocking, because Patch's grandmother had never told him about it.

One week to the day after the children of Hamelyn were taken, there had been another atrocity: in the Dragon Territories, young dragons had vanished from an isolated school. One hundred dragon children, gone. The ten adult dragons who were their teachers and guardians were poisoned, and only one of them survived, managing to reach another settlement and reveal what had happened.

"A human came," the dragon had said. "A *Piper*, riding a griffin! He played his Pipe and the children followed him, flying over the horizon, laughing as they went."

The Hamelyn Piper had struck again.

When the evil Piper was finally captured, the dragons wanted him executed for his crimes. The refusal of the Pipers' Council was absolute, however, and tensions between Pipers and dragons, high at the best of times, increased. The dragons threatened war against the Pipers. One by one the many nations of the world made their choice: they would stand with the Pipers, whatever happened.

The last war between humans and dragons had been hundreds of years ago, and the loss of life had been horrifying; but suddenly, a new war seemed inevitable.

Yet war was averted. Just.

Among humans, meanwhile, the notion that the Hamelyn Piper had taken the dragon children was treated with suspicion, as if it was only a rumor invented by the dragons to stir up resentment. It was rarely spoken of, and this was probably why Patch's grandmother hadn't included it in her tales.

Humans had always feared dragons, and *fear* could easily turn to *hate*.

For many people, the hatred they had for dragons was so great that they could never have sympathy with them, whatever the situation. Even if their children had vanished.

For some, having fewer dragons would always be a good thing.

It took a while before he stopped feeling so cold, but Patch finally started to doze on the floor of his cell. Then, as sleep was beckoning, he heard it: from elsewhere in the dungeons came a terrible sound.

"There he goes," sighed Henry. "He'll keep at it until he's hoarse."

"Aye!" screamed the Hamelyn Piper, again and again, deep in the Dark. "*Aye!*"

Patch trembled, hands over his ears, but nothing he did blocked out the noise. It was two hours before the screaming stopped.

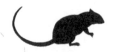

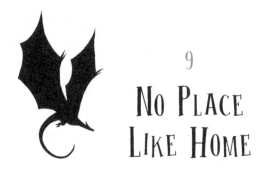

9

No Place
Like Home

"T*ubes!*"

Patch's eyes snapped open. All he could remember was the nightmare he'd been having, the Hamelyn Piper's long fingers creeping along the floor toward him.

"*Tubes*, Patch!" yelled Henry. "Come on, get up! Tubes!" Everything came back to him. He hurried to fetch his bowl and jug, turning to the door just as the metal tubes came in through the holes two-thirds of the way up the wall. Sludge oozed from the wider of the tubes, and water came from the other. He reached them in time to collect half of his meal, the rest having joined the rancid pile on the floor.

He looked cautiously at the contents of his bowl, pushing the food around with his fingers. It was a thick gloopy mush, with gristly bits dotted through it. Wary, he raised his fingers to his mouth and tasted it, ready for the most horrible flavors he'd ever encountered, but it was mercifully bland. Even after eating all of it, he was still hungry. He looked at the food that had fallen before he'd reached it, glistening on top of the rank heap that had been there yesterday—the remains of all the food Innocent Jack had presumably failed to collect before they'd noticed he was dead.

Surely he could salvage the rest of today's meal? Just scrape it off carefully, not taking any of the moldy food below, or the *maggots* that were squirming in amongst it?

"No," he said to himself. But how long might it be before he took that next step and ate the maggots and moldy remnants without a thought?

What would he become in a year? In ten years?

He set down his empty bowl and walked to the tiny window, his only view of the outside world. The sun was bright, and on his tiptoes he could see the forest on the distant hills. He would never walk in a forest again, he realized; never feel the sun on his face.

He fell to his knees, sobbing hard, and there he stayed, lost to his misery. When he heard footsteps approaching up the corridor he was unaware of how much time had passed.

The footsteps halted, and the lock in Patch's door clunked. He got up and went to the middle of his cell as the door swung open, and the first thing he saw was the purple and black of a Custodian Piper's robes.

It was Erner, carrying his satchel and a parcel. Behind him stood a guard even larger than Furnel.

Erner stepped into the cell and the door slammed closed, the noise reverberating for a few moments. He looked around and spotted the hole in the wall that led to Henry's cell. He walked over and fetched Patch's blanket, then went to the hole and blocked it up.

"Do you mind!" Vague Henry shouted, his voice muffled. "I'm trying to hear what's going on in there!"

Erner walked back to Patch. "Better if we can talk in private," he said. "I didn't come alone."

Wren's head peeked out of Erner's satchel. Patch held out his arm and she hopped onto it, then along to his neck, which she hugged.

Patch grinned, tears falling. "It's so good to see you," he said. "*Both* of you."

Erner nodded, smiling. "I've been enjoying Wren's company very much," he said. "Her Merisax is very good, considering how short a time she's been learning."

"She's a bright girl," said Patch. He glanced at Wren, who gave a proud nod.

"She is," said Erner. "Virtus Stone and I have been assigned duties elsewhere, and I fear Wren would be in too much danger if she came with me. I suggested leaving her with a trusted colleague, but she insists that I tell nobody else about her yet. Besides, she's desperate to keep you company.

She should be safe enough with you, now that you're in your cell. I'll be back in two or three weeks."

"What about curing her of her curse?" said Patch.

"By the time I'm back, I hope to have a reply to *this!*" he said, and with a flourish he produced an envelope, complete with an official Custodian Elite wax seal.

Patch read the address. "Brother Tobias, Marwheel Abbey," he said.

"Indeed," said Erner. "I asked Virtus Stone if he knew of anyone capable of curing a Sorcerer's curse, given how . . . well, you know how it is with Pipers and Sorcerers."

Patch knew very well how it was. While the obvious course of action might be to ask a *Sorcerer* for help, the notion of a Piper doing so was almost unthinkable.

Sorcerers were few and far between, secretive and wealthy. They used a different, older form of magic that they thought was far superior to Songs, and so they looked down their noses at Pipers. In return, Pipers didn't have much liking for Sorcerers; they also didn't *trust* them. Sorcerers often had questionable morals and little regard for laws, although if it ever came to a clash between them and the Custodian Elite, the Custodians had the advantage of greater numbers—Sorcerers always worked alone.

"Didn't Virtus Stone want to know why you were asking about curses?" said Patch.

"An apprentice is expected to extend their knowledge as much as possible," said Erner. "I ask him so many strange questions, he didn't bat an eyelid at that one. He just told me to contact Brother Tobias at Marwheel Abbey. I've kept my letter vague and explained that a victim of a shape-changing curse needs help."

"Well, let's hope that Brother Tobias has the answers," said Patch, looking at Wren.

He'd better, she signed. *I want to be human again soon!*

Patch smiled at her, overwhelmed with gratitude that she would choose to stay with him. "In the meantime, we can work on improving your Merisax," he said.

There was a heavy knock on the cell door. "Time!" came a shout.

Erner sighed. "Visiting prisoners is frowned on," he said. "And even when it can be arranged, they keep it brief. So, here"—he handed Patch the string-tied parcel he was carrying—"the wrapping is a new blanket, a warmer one, and there are a few other items inside. They're strict about what can be given to prisoners, so if I were you . . ." He leaned closer and whispered. "Unwrap it in secret!"

The door started to open again. Wren gave a tiny squeak of panic and ran down Patch's back, her claws digging through his thin clothing and into his skin. She clung there, out of sight, and Patch grimaced.

"Come on," said the guard to Erner.

Erner looked at Patch. "I'm sorry," he said. "I still can't believe what happened at the trial. I'll do what I can for you, but . . ." He shook his head.

"Thank you, Erner," said Patch.

Erner nodded, silent, then stepped out of the cell. The door closed with another thunderous slam.

Patch sighed with relief as Wren's claws stopped digging into his skin and she climbed back up to his shoulder. "Right then," he said quietly, raising the parcel. "Let's see what we've got here!"

Quietly in the corner of the cell, with Wren on the floor beside him, Patch untied the string. Inside was one of the tiny oilskin tents they'd used on the journey to the castle, which folded up smaller than a fist. Patch found himself staring at it. No more cold nights, he realized, as long he was careful not to let the guards see it. There was also an apple, a curious little wooden box, and a small bag of wheat grains that had Wren's name written on it, in a scratchy style that Patch guessed was Wren's own writing. "Yours?" he said.

She nodded, with narrowed eyes. *Touch it and you're dead!* she signed, then pointed at the apple. *That's for you.*

Patch smiled and set the bag down beside her. He looked at the strange wooden box. "What's this?" he asked.

Fox and Owls, signed Wren. *Ever play it?*

"My grandfather tried to teach me once," he said. "I

couldn't get the hang of it." He fiddled with the box until the top popped open. The inside of the box lid was a game board, and a dozen little pegs were the playing pieces.

Well, now I can teach you, signed Wren.

"We have plenty of time," said Patch, and the phrase didn't fill him with horror the way it had when Henry had said it. As he ate his apple and tried to remember how to set the board up for a game, Wren wandered off into the cell. After a while, Patch heard a crunching sound. Wren was on the top of the rancid food pile, merrily picking up the maggots and eating them.

Wide-eyed, he watched her as she polished off another of the wriggling grubs.

Wren noticed him watching. *You don't mind if I . . . ,* she started.

"No," said Patch. "You go ahead. Is it just the maggots, or are you going to eat the rest of the pile?"

Wren screwed up her little face in revulsion. *What, this moldy old stuff?* she signed. *Don't be disgusting!*

They settled down for some Merisax practice, and after taking Wren through the signing of numbers Patch could tell she was distracted by something. "Are you okay?" he asked. "Do you want a break?"

Wren shook her head. *I've just been dying to ask a question,* she signed. *But it might be upsetting for you.*

"Go on," said Patch. "Ask away."

Why did you leave Tiviscan and abandon your training? she signed. *At the trial, they mentioned bringing shame on yourself.*

Patch took a deep sigh. "Ah," he said. "That."

You don't have to tell me if you don't want to, signed Wren.

"You may as well know," he said. "It happened at the Trials Ceremony, just before summer."

The trials?

"Each year, all the trainee Pipers engage in trials to show how well their studies have gone, and to demonstrate their abilities. When a trainee reaches thirteen, though, it's a special time. That's when they can be chosen to begin training for the Elite."

Like with Erner? she asked.

"Yes. He was chosen and did two years of training before passing his final trials to become an apprentice. But it's not just the Custodian Elite. There are other specialties, you see. Those who excel in Arable Piping, for example, might be accepted into the Arable Elite. If a nation faces famine, say, or disease wipes out entire crops, the Arable Elite will help prevent disaster. I was like Erner. I wanted to join the Custodian Elite. They enforce the laws of Piping, but that's only part of what they do. They also act like the Pipers of ancient days. They help those most in need, and bring justice to places that justice has forgotten. For that, a trainee has to be among the very best."

And you are, aren't you?

He shrugged. "I hoped so. Even when I first found I had a talent for Piping, I knew what I wanted to do. Pipers are mainly used by the wealthy. The bigger towns and cities can maybe afford them regularly, and the richest farmers, but for most people they're too expensive. The Custodians were always different. They're not paid by anyone. I mean, every Piper is expected to do their duty, do what's right, but Custodians apply basic laws of justice, even in countries that don't *have* those laws. In every civilized nation, the Custodian Elite have the power to make a difference, and defend the defenseless! If only there were more Custodians, the world would be a much better place to live."

And that was your dream? signed Wren. *To become one? Make the world a better place?*

Patch nodded. "When I first came to Tiviscan, the Tutors were very excited. I showed great skill in the Piping of *people*. Unprecedented, I was told! It's why I'm so good at the Dance. I could even affect *myself* with what I played, which I'd thought was normal, but for most Pipers it's nearly impossible. It's like trying to tickle yourself—it just doesn't work. They told me I could be anything I wanted to be, so I studied as hard as I could, and I tried my very best, because I knew that the *only* thing I wanted was to join the Custodian Elite. And then last summer, the Trials Ceremony came. With all the trials over, the ceremony began, and I knew I'd done really well. Every trainee, every Tutor, and the Pipers' Council themselves, were all gathered together, and at the very end of the ceremony the list of trainees selected for Elite training was read out."

Oh no! signed Wren, looking anxious. *They didn't call out your name!*

Patch shook his head in sorrow. "They called my name, all right. Just not as a Custodian. I couldn't believe what I'd heard, and I stood up, and I shouted. 'The Custodian Elite! It has to be the *Custodian* Elite. No other will do!' But my trial results weren't quite good enough, and that was that. It felt like my world had ended." He paused, then looked at Wren. "Have you ever wanted something so badly that anything less just wouldn't do?"

Absolutely, she signed. *What happened next?*

"Being chosen for *any* Elite training is such an honor, you don't turn it down. Nobody had *ever* turned it down."

You turned it down? signed Wren, and Patch nodded. *That's all you did? It doesn't seem so bad.*

Patch winced. "I turned it down very, *very* rudely. To the faces of the Pipers' Council; in front of everyone. My disappointment had turned to anger, you see, anger that just bubbled out of me before I even knew what was happening. I called Lord Pewter a stupid old drunkard who stank of rotting cheese; I yelled at Lady Winkless that she couldn't Pipe her way out of a sack. And I didn't stop there."

Oh dear, signed Wren. *That doesn't sound good.*

"The Council watched me in disbelief, with their mouths hanging open, as I insulted them one by one. When I finished there wasn't a sound. Everyone—the Council, the Tutors, the students, *everyone*—was staring at me. I couldn't believe what had happened! I did the only thing I could think of. I turned and ran. Away from Tiviscan. Away from Piping."

Wren put a paw on his hand. *You must have wanted to be a Custodian very much.*

"It was everything to me. A few days later I thought of returning, but I couldn't face it."

Wren nodded. *What branch of the Elite had they offered you?* she signed. *Arable?*

Patch shook his head. "It doesn't matter now." He felt a little distant for a moment, before snapping out of it. "My turn to have a question answered," he said. "How did you manage to get a Sorcerer angry enough to curse you like this?"

I was kidnapped, she signed. *The Sorcerer wanted a maid-servant. This was last summer too. As your life was changing, so was mine. When I almost managed to escape, he caught me, and that was that.*

"He turned you into a rat."

Exactly. I fled into the forest, terrified of the dangers around me from hawks and the like. I was even fearful of other rats at first, but they proved to be generous creatures. Stupid, but generous. I found a little rat community near some local wheat fields and stayed with them for a few weeks. Ten rats, terrified of the farmer's dog, half starved. They knew there was something unusual about me and started to follow my lead. The dog was easy to outsmart, and soon everyone was well fed, but it came time for all of us to move on. As we traveled, we'd come across other rats, and they'd tag along. We snuck onto a barge transporting barley and spent a week on it. I'd hoped we would make it to a warmer place before winter, but we were discovered and had to flee the barge. Turned out we were in the middle of the Breydram Valley, and winter came faster than I'd expected.

"Patterfall was your only refuge," said Patch.

Yes. We tried to push further downstream, but gave up in the end and stayed put. At first, I thought we had plenty of food to last us through winter, but a population explosion put an end to that idea. Rats will be rats, and they just wouldn't be told.

"The villagers were terrified that you'd eat them. So was I, come to that."

They're much more mild-mannered than people believe. The villagers needn't have feared, but the rats didn't get the chance to prove it . . . She looked at Patch. *Would they have suffered?*

He shook his head. "I know the Dispersal is horrifying, but as far as I know the effect is instant. They wouldn't have suffered at all."

She nodded, tears in her eyes. *I didn't make a very good leader in the end,* she signed.

He picked her up and put her on his shoulder. She snuggled down, and they sat together in silence for a time, until they both felt ready to get back to the Merisax number system.

In the afternoon, shortly after the food and water arrived, Vague Henry shouted loud enough and long enough that he couldn't be ignored, and Patch removed the old blanket from the hole between their cells.

"Thank the stars!" said Henry. "Set something in front of it if you want to stop me peeking in, but please don't block it up like that. God help me if it rained!"

"Sorry," said Patch. "I forgot it was there." He gathered up the blanket and left it a little way in front of the hole, perched over the narrow channel in the floor so Henry couldn't see into Patch's cell. "That okay?" he said.

"That's fine," said Henry. "No harm done." He didn't waste time moving on to a subject he was clearly more interested in: "So, um, your visitor? A Custodian Piper, then? I saw that much."

"A friend," said Patch. "He came to commiserate with me on how things turned out."

"Oh," said Henry. "I just wondered if you were holding up okay? I mean, I thought he'd given you more bad news or something, since—"

"Since?"

"Since you've started to talk to yourself. And don't say you haven't!"

It occurred to Patch that if Henry thought he was crazy, he could chat with Wren as much as he liked without worrying about how loud he was talking. "Let me deal with things my own way, Henry," he said, smiling. "I'll be fine."

After a little more Merisax practice, Wren was eager to get started on Fox and Owls. She took the game board and rearranged Patch's failed attempt at placing the pieces.

Which do you want to be? she signed. *Fox or Owls?*

Patch shrugged. "Remind me of the difference."

Okay, signed Wren. *I'll start with the basics. There's only one fox piece and two owls. Say you be the fox, then you move, and I move one of the rabbits, then I move both owls, then you move a rabbit and it starts again. Easy!*

Patch smiled, bewildered by the game but curiously happy. The cell around him had suddenly stopped being so oppressive.

He looked at the pile of rotting food and vowed to get it cleaned up soon. He faintly wished for a chair, or a mirror.

It feels more like a home than a prison, he thought. *Just because I'm here with a friend.*

10

Unwelcome Arrivals

Overnight it started to rain heavily. When they woke, the importance of Henry's warning about not blocking the hole in the wall became clear—the channel in the floor had turned into a murky stream, flowing toward the toilet hole.

Patch saw the opportunity to clean things up. He gritted his teeth and scooped up handfuls of the rotting pile of food, carrying it to the toilet hole and letting the filthy rainwater wash it away. Once finished, Patch used a little of the water from mealtime to clean his hands.

Outside, the weather kept getting worse, and with it the murky stream threatened to overflow its channel, but as the hours passed the flowing water became a little less filthy, and the stench in his cell began to fade.

Henry, meanwhile, kept trying to get Patch to converse. He seemed sure that Patch was falling apart, talking to himself and—God help him!—actually *laughing* occasionally.

"I'll be okay," Patch told him.

"I'm just worried," said Henry. "I asked some of the others if they could help, and all I managed to do was land you with your nickname."

"Which is?"

"The Mad Piper, I'm afraid."

Patch laughed out loud, which presumably didn't settle Henry's nerves one bit.

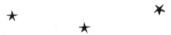

The heavy rain continued unbroken for the next two days. Patch, meanwhile, was improving at Fox and Owls. At the start, Wren had always won within a dozen moves, but now it was taking perhaps twice as long for her to be victorious. In one game, his owls had taken *four* rabbits, and he'd clapped with excitement.

Then, after a particularly vicious thunderstorm that continued until dawn, the rain faded at last. The dungeon seemed oddly quiet with the rain gone. The drainage channel in the cell had little more than a trickle running through it.

When chatter started to grow from the prisoners along

the corridor, it was hard to miss in the relative silence. With Wren on his shoulder, Patch went over to the hole in the wall. "Henry?" he said. "What's the fuss about?"

"All this rain has caused serious flooding lower in the dungeons," said Henry. "They're having to move some prisoners from the deepest levels until it's sorted out."

There were footsteps in the corridor. For a moment Patch wondered if it was Erner again, but this time the sounds stopped short of Patch's door. It was Henry's turn for a visitor.

"Henry Trew!" called a voice.

"Yes?" said Henry.

"Ready your things, you're to be moved up a level." Other prisoners called out to ask if they would be moved too. "Shut up!" yelled the guard. "None of you lot are going anywhere."

The whole corridor complained.

"We'll be bringing a prisoner up shortly from a flooded cell," said the guard. "Keep the noise down or you'll not get a meal today! Now, hurry up, Trew!"

"I'll just fetch my things," said Henry. He came back over to the hole. "Patch! Did you hear? I'm getting an upgrade! Moving up a floor, until it's sorted out. Maybe they'll let me stay up there!"

"I'll miss you, Henry," said Patch. "Good luck upstairs!"

"God bless you, Patch. And I'm sure whoever they put

here in my place will, um—" Henry paused, and Patch knew why—*any* prisoner from the deeper levels would likely be unpleasant company.

"It'll be fine, Henry," Patch said. He looked at Wren, who seemed fretful. "Don't worry," he told her. "I mean, how bad could it be?"

It wasn't long before they found out.

An hour later Patch heard the sound of rattling chains in the corridor, soon followed by the shouts of the other inmates: "Who's your prisoner, eh? We don't want no scum here!"

The clanking stopped at Vague Henry's cell. Patch and Wren heard the door open, and they both went to the hole and looked through. A narrow shaft of light from the window fell on the prisoner, who was shuffling into the center of the cell.

You want me to go in there and take a look? signed Wren.

"No!" whispered Patch. "Stay here, where it's safe."

The prisoner stood in the light, but all Patch had sight of was the legs, chained together, thick manacles at the feet. The prisoner was facing the window, and Patch presumed the light was so unfamiliar that they were mesmerized. They might not have seen any sunlight in years.

The cell door slammed shut, catching Patch by surprise. He'd expected the guard to remove the chains before leaving, but apparently not. The prisoner's arms came into view, wrists also manacled with a long chain between them. That was when the sobbing began, deep and agonizing, as the prisoner fell to their knees and out of the shaft of light. After a while, the prisoner's hands came back into the light, twisting around, almost playing with it. *Yes*, thought Patch, *this is someone who hasn't seen daylight in a while.*

Wren sneezed. Suddenly the shape in the gloom snapped up into a sitting position, chains clanking.

Patch and Wren pulled back from the hole.

Sorry! signed Wren.

Let's wait a bit before we have another look, Patch signed back.

The chains in the other cell rattled as the prisoner moved around within. Eventually the rattling stopped, and after a few minutes of silence Wren and Patch glanced at each other and nodded.

They looked through the hole.

An eye was looking back at them, full of desperation. And there was something around the eye, Patch saw.

Some kind of metal.

Iron.

Patch pulled back, and so did Wren. "Oh," said Patch. "Oh no."

"Aye?" came a quiet voice through the hole. It sounded like pleading. "Aye?" More sobs followed, and then the prisoner spoke again, louder and louder, becoming more and more angry, the same word every time. "Aye! *Aye!*"

The other inmates knew immediately what this meant. "Guard!" came the shouts. "Take him away! You can't do this! Anyone but him! *Anyone but him!*"

"*Aye!*"

"Guard! You can't leave him here!"

"*AYE!*"

"*Show us some mercy!*"

Patch grabbed the old blanket and stuffed it into the hole, pulling his hand out quickly—fighting the childish terror that the fingers of the Hamelyn Piper would close around his wrist. He lifted Wren from the floor and ran to the little tent at the far side of the cell. They stayed there all night, awake and shivering with fear as the Hamelyn Piper screamed.

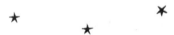

Soon after dawn, Patch took the sleeping Wren from his lap and set her on the soft blanket Erner had brought. He went to the hole and pulled out the old blanket, then looked inside the other cell.

The Hamelyn Piper was asleep near the hole, and Patch could see the Iron Mask clearly. It seemed to be made from many smaller sections, forming a mesh that wrapped around the back of his head and obscured most of his face, save for his eyes and mouth. It looked grubby and tarnished, unsurprising after almost a decade of imprisonment. The Hamelyn Piper's beard—if that was a word that could be used for such a jumble of hair—had grown through the mask, and seemed to have been haphazardly cut quite recently. The guards had probably taken advantage of the move to do this most basic of maintenance.

As the other prisoners awoke, the complaints about the new arrival started up again, growing in volume all morning. The response from the guards came later—when the tubes arrived, it was only water that came and no food. That night the Hamelyn Piper screamed again, and the prisoners complained again, and the only difference was the hunger that gnawed at Patch. Wren nibbled at her grain, offering Patch some, but he refused to take it from her.

"They'll feed us tomorrow," he said. "They'll have to."

But the next day, the food was still withheld. Complaints about hunger were now almost as loud as the complaints about the Hamelyn Piper.

The day after, the prisoners had learned their lesson. Any grumblings were quickly silenced by a scolding from the others, and the food came at last.

Once Patch's bowl and jug were full, Wren asked to sit in the tiny window as she sometimes did. Patch was quietly jealous, as Wren could scurry to the far end of the six-foot-long hole and see much more than Patch, who was limited to a tiny piece of sky and distant hill.

As he finished his food, he heard Wren squeak urgently. He came to the window.

You need to see this, she signed, looking worried. She hopped onto his shoulder and he went up on his toes, straining to look out of the window. It took a moment for his eyes to adjust to the bright sky, but eventually he saw dark spots against the blue: birds flying.

"Starlings?" he said. Wren shook her head, agitated. He looked out again at the dark spots in the sky. It had to be starlings, he thought, with so many of them—a vast flock, coming over the distant hill.

Wait. The *distant* hill?

The trees on that hill were so far away they seemed tiny, yet he could see the individual birds, see them *flap* . . . How was that possible? He froze, staring at the dark cloud. He looked at Wren, and she nodded.

You understand now? she signed.

"Yes," said Patch, watching the dark cloud come ever closer. It wasn't a flock of birds.

It was *dragons.* Thousands of them.

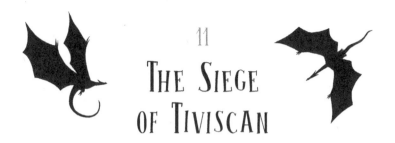

11

THE SIEGE
OF TIVISCAN

Warning bells rang out on the castle battlements, something Patch had heard in the occasional drills during his training.

"It's been centuries since anyone dared attack Tiviscan," he told Wren. "They'll be readying the castle defenses now, with the garrisoned Pipers preparing the Battle Horns." Those huge horns were mounted permanently on the roof of the Keep, able to create barriers of turbulent air strong enough to protect against flaming catapult attacks, say—or to knock dragons out of the sky. He shook his head, stunned. "*Why*, though? Nobody wants war. What could they hope to achieve? Sending such a huge army?"

The dragons were obscuring more and more of the sky as they came ever nearer, the flock filling their little window now.

No, thought Patch. It wasn't a *flock*. That wasn't the right word.

The right word depended on the creatures in question: a *flock* of birds, a *swarm* of bees, or a *pack* of dogs. There was a word especially for dragons too, and until now Patch hadn't understood why that word had been chosen, instead of something more appropriate for fire-breathers. Surely, he'd always thought, a *burning* of dragons would make more sense? Or a *firestorm*?

But seeing the dark cloud approach, blocking out more and more light, he understood at last why the right word was *darkness*.

A darkness of dragons was coming. And it wouldn't be long before they reached the castle.

Wren scurried up to the far end of the window for a better view. After a moment, she came back. *Some of the dragons are carrying something,* she signed.

Patch looked past her, trying to make it out. Yes, there it was—small groups at the front were linked in some way, a shape hanging down below them.

"Are those . . . ?" said Patch, squinting. "Are those *rocks*?"

Wren nodded. She hopped onto Patch's shoulder. Closer and closer the dragons came.

"What would they need huge rocks for?" He looked at Wren. "Not to—"

Wren nodded again.

Patch stepped back from the window and kept going until he reached the cell door.

The other prisoners were yelling to be released—"So we can help defend the castle!" cried one, although Patch very much doubted their sincerity—and the general air of panic and doom was overwhelming. He sat at the base of the door, Wren on his shoulder, and waited.

The sounds of shouted commands, fearful cries, and angry prisoners were soon joined by another sound.

The beating of giant wings.

"Here they come," said Patch. He cupped his hands around Wren as a roar of fire came. Flame lit the window and the cell, then a black shadow flew past, heading up. After a moment there were screams and explosions. The dragons they'd been watching couldn't have reached them so quickly. He realized that some must have come in low, unseen, then shot up at the last instant to surprise the garrison. Certainly, he couldn't hear any sign of a barrier Song being played on the Battle Horns.

"I wonder if—" he started, but then the wall exploded and everything went black.

Patch felt something hitting his nose repeatedly, but all he could hear was a high-pitched continuous tone. He opened his eyes. The air was thick with dust. Wren was on his chest, slapping his nose with her paw.

Sit up, she signed.

"What happened?" Patch said—or *tried* to say, as his voice didn't seem to work. He clapped his hands but couldn't hear it. He was temporarily deafened; time to switch to hand-speech. *What happened?*

The dragons used their rocks, Wren signed, pointing at the wall.

Patch coughed as he looked. At least now he couldn't complain about having a small window. A large chunk of the wall had gone, taking the window with it.

His hearing was starting to recover. Wind howled past the damage in the wall, and there were groans and shouts from the prisoners and beyond, but it seemed that there was a definite lull in the attack. He set Wren on the floor and went to the hole, climbing up into it. The view was dizzying. The forest and hills were now home to the many dragons, bursts of flame coming here and there as shows of bravado. He looked up at the outside wall above him. "My God," he said.

The damage was considerable. Huge slabs of stone had fallen away, but the attack had been tightly targeted. He climbed back down to the cell floor and realized he was shaking. "This is madness," he said. "What could they possibly want—?"

He stopped talking and slowly turned his eyes to the wall of the cell next to them.

"They've come for *him*," said Patch. "They've come for the Hamelyn Piper. All these years they've waited, and finally they've come. Somehow they heard he'd been moved, and they must have known exactly where he was moved to!"

What will they do next? signed Wren.

Patch laid out his blanket and started to put his belongings on top, preparing to turn it into a parcel again. "I'm not waiting to find out," he said. "We're lucky that attack didn't kill us. If they do it again we're dead!"

Wren jumped onto the Fox and Owls board as he reached for it, his hand trembling. *What are you doing?* she signed.

"We're leaving."

How?

Patch pointed at the newly created hole in the wall. "That way." He nudged her off the game board and packed it up.

Wren looked at the hole. She stared at Patch. *We're climbing down?* she signed. *You're not serious!*

Patch nodded, trying to sound confident rather than terrified. "They'll assume I died in the attack, Wren! This is my chance of freedom."

You're crazy, she signed, and he thought she was probably right.

"I can lip-play a bit of courage into both of us," he said.

"And there's a climbing Song I know that'll help." He wrapped the blanket-parcel to leave plenty of string spare, and tied it around his waist.

But at that moment, the warning bells rang out again.

Outside, a lone figure was flying toward the castle from the assembled dragons. Patch wondered how much damage the previous flaming assault had done to the huge Battle

Horns. Not enough to put them out of use, it seemed—as the solitary dragon approached, the low pulsing hum of the Horns began, building a defensive Song. They'd been caught by surprise once before, and this time they were taking no chances.

The dragon representative carried a white flag in one front claw and something else in the other.

A scroll! signed Wren.

"Their demands, I assume," said Patch. He climbed up into the hole again to keep sight of the dragon. This time, Wren scampered up with him. She seemed confident enough, he saw, climbing on the shattered wall, even in the blustering wind. A rat, he knew, could fall from such an enormous height and walk away after landing. For him, the result would be very different. *Messier*, for a start.

Patch watched the dragon as it came closer to the castle. It wore a battle harness—a hardened leather chest plate on the front, and packs and straps on the sides which held equipment and supplies. The animal certainly looked fearsome enough. Patch could see what he thought were battle scars, discolored areas on the creature's underbelly and flank. There had clearly been some trauma affecting its muzzle. And wings.

And tail, come to that.

It was male, Patch could tell, lacking as it did the giveaway spines on its back. It—or rather, *he*—came within a hundred feet of the battlements and stayed there, wings beating steadily as he tucked the white flag into the top of the battle harness.

The dragon unrolled the scroll he carried and began to read in an impressively booming voice. "By the authority of the Triumvirate of the Great Circle of the Red Sand, I demand that you hand over the prisoner known as the Hamelyn Piper. Failure to do so will be met with the displeasure of the dragons here gathered. You have thirty minutes to respond." He rolled up the scroll and turned to fly back to the other dragons.

"We have to go right now," said Patch. "If we're here when they attack again, we'll be killed."

Wren jumped onto his shoulder and gave him a thumbs up; Patch found the water jug on the floor, on its side but still with some water in it. He rinsed the dust from his mouth and licked his lips, ready to whistle up some courage.

But before he could begin, a deep rhythmic melody filled the cell. It was coming from the Battle Horns.

"That's an attacking Song they're building," said Patch, looking out to where the dragon with the scroll was still flying away from the castle, barely a fifth of the distance back to the rest of the dragons. "Don't tell me they're going to—" The melody suddenly picked up pace, the underlying low hum from the Battle Horns pulsing now, rapid and deep. "They *are*!" he said, shocked. "They're sending their answer already! They're going to bring that dragon down!" The dragon messenger looked over his shoulder and started to flap his wings harder. Too late, though—the sound from the Battle Horns grew so loud and so strong that it made the air shimmer and twist, and the space in front of the castle took on a multicolored sheen. The colors shot out toward the lone dragon like a rainbow turned into a torrent of flame, making a sound that was half-thunder, half-scream. The dragon was engulfed by the blast, and he tumbled hundreds of feet down through the air, vanishing into the dense pines in the forest far below.

The crunch of impact made Patch wince.

Cheering began from the castle walls, but in the dungeons a shocked silence fell. One prisoner shouted out: "We're dead! The fools have killed us all!"

The Battle Horns maintained their deep pulsing rhythm. Out of range in the distant trees, dragons were taking off and circling, gathering their numbers. "There are just too many of them," said Patch. "The Battle Horns won't be able to stop them all. They'll get through and the Horns will be abandoned. We'll be defenseless."

And then he heard a voice that had been silent all this time.

"Aye?" said the Hamelyn Piper, his voice almost mournful.

Patch looked out of the gaping hole and saw the rock-wielding dragons closing in. Behind them he saw *other* groups of rock-wielders, who were rising sharply at high speed, releasing their rocks well out of range of the Battle

118

Horns. The air shimmered as the Horns did their work, but the rocks were flying up, arcing, coming down again, this time within the castle walls.

There were crashes and screams, and the Song of the Battle Horns was silenced.

The dragons had already taken out the most important defense.

Cannons thundered from the battlements high above, but it was the rock-wielders heading right for the dungeon walls that Patch was watching now, almost hypnotized by the sight.

Wren's piercing squeal snapped him out of it. She scampered to the outer wall in the corner farthest from the Hamelyn Piper's cell, and Patch dived toward her as the rocks hit their target.

Impact after impact came. The cell shook violently. Stones shattered and flew. He tried to shield Wren with is body as he covered his ears with his hands. He yelled in terror, certain that he was moments away from a painful death.

The attack stopped.

Patch stood, shaking. On the floor under him Wren was holding her paws around her head. She peeked out and looked around.

There was no dust this time. It had cleared quickly in the strong breeze, because there was almost no wall now. The only remaining part was the small piece beside them that had miraculously remained intact. Patch looked up at the ceiling and saw a worryingly deep crack in it. He looked across to the Hamelyn Piper's cell. Much of the wall between the two cells had collapsed, and the external wall in that other cell was entirely gone. The Hamelyn Piper was on the floor, half-covered in rubble. A single word came from him, frail and almost lost to the wind. "Aye . . ."

Patch found himself staring at the most dreaded of Pipers, yet somehow he felt no fear of the masked man and started to walk toward him. He was aware of movement out in the distance. He turned and saw dragons holding their position in the air higher up, making sure of no further defensive assaults from the castle, while a line of dragons formed some kind of honor guard, maintaining their height. Past the end of that line a group was coming closer, at the center of which were three who wore incredibly ornate battle harnesses, flanked by black-armored dragons.

The Triumvirate and their guards, Patch guessed. The rulers of the Dragon Territories, here in person to claim their quarry. They would reach their target soon, but Patch still walked toward the edge of the Hamelyn Piper's cell, drawn there by an irresistible need to *see*.

The attack had wounded the man badly. A large slab of stone had crushed his legs. The Iron Mask was visibly damaged at the front. Patch watched with horror and fascination as the Hamelyn Piper's hands came up and tore at the Mask, until the front opened outwards and it clattered to the cell floor.

Patch stared at the thin face, the Hamelyn Piper's eyes now locked with his own.

"Aye . . . ," said the man, with a cough of pain that brought up blood. But the Mask's protective charms, the charms that had forced him to repeat the same word over and over, had no more hold over him now. "Aye . . . am . . . ," he said.

Patch marveled at how he felt no terror, even though he was in the company of the most evil Piper ever to have lived. And he realized what the man had actually said.

What he had *always* been trying to say.

It wasn't "Aye." It wasn't the single word of defiance that the story claimed. Instead, it was only the first word in a sentence that he had never been able to finish.

Until now.

"I . . . am . . . ," said the man, relief in his voice. He swallowed and took a breath, still looking directly at Patch. "I am not the Piper of Hamelyn."

The sound of wings announced the arrival of the black-armored dragons. Patch stepped away quickly, knowing he was at their mercy, but they ignored him. Instead, they lifted the slab the man was trapped under and yanked their quarry from the rubble.

There was no fear written on the man's face, Patch thought, only a sense of *release*.

A short way from the castle, the Triumvirate waited. They gave their guards a nod. The dragon carrying the prisoner let out a deafening screech and flew high into the air, higher than the castle battlements. The other dragon guards, together with the Triumvirate themselves, formed a circle. When ready, the prisoner was released, falling toward the circle in silence.

The circle of dragons aimed upward and breathed their fire, creating a blast of flame that caught the man right in the center and tracked the path of his fall.

All that emerged from underneath the circle were the blackened chains that had held him. Of the man, there was nothing left but ash, drifting in the wind.

Patch looked back to where the Iron Mask had fallen. He climbed over what was left of the dividing wall, then took the Mask and returned to his own cell.

Wren was angry with him, squeaking loudly to get him to come back. Fragments of stone fell on his head as he ran to Wren, and the moment he reached her a loud cracking came from the stone around them. Wren climbed up to his shoulder, scowling.

You scared me! she signed. *Promise me you won't do anything that stupid again!*

But before he could make any promise at all, the floor shuddered under them and shifted outwards in a sudden jerk. Patch found himself dropping down, a scream leaving his lips as he fell.

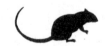

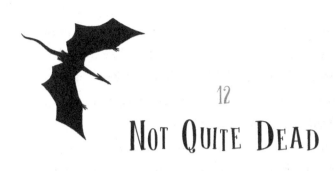

12

NOT QUITE DEAD

Patch came to an abrupt halt, sprawled on his knees on the small section of cell floor that had broken away. It had landed on a wide rocky ledge jutting out from the sheer cliff the dungeons had been built into; beside them, in the jagged rock of the cliff face, was a crevice about ten feet high and two across.

He shared a look of bewilderment with Wren. She suddenly squealed with terror and pointed up: above them another huge chunk of wall was falling. Patch grabbed Wren and scrambled off the ruined floor, into the crevice. He winced as the falling chunk crashed into the space he'd just stepped out of, then stood with his eyes shut, not daring to look as debris rained down behind him.

There were other screams. He opened his eyes and turned, staring as masonry and prisoners alike tumbled down past them. The piece of floor they had been on had already vanished, and the ledge that had stopped their fall had been sliced away from the cliff face.

They'd fallen fifty feet or so. Above them at least eight cells were open to the elements now—eight cells whose walls had gone, several having lost most of their floor. Shouts for help echoed around the devastation.

He put Wren on his shoulder and was suddenly aware of something in his other hand—he was still clutching the Iron Mask. He tied it to the parcel at his waist.

Very slowly, Patch bent his knees, keeping his back pressed hard against the rock. He worked his way as far into the crevice as he could, and found he could actually sit. Wren was staring ahead blankly, just as stunned as he was.

"I'll, um, wait until I stop shaking before I climb anywhere," he said.

It took a while.

As they waited, the shouts and calls echoing around the castle above them grew less and less urgent. Apart from the occasional piece of stonework tumbling past them, the structure of the dungeons held together.

Soon they could hear gruff voices hollering to each other, describing the damage and assessing what could be done to shore up the castle until repairs could be attempted. Patch wasn't shaking any more, but with all the activity that was going on he decided to wait until nightfall before risking the climb. As things stood, the Pipers would assume he'd died—certainly, he didn't imagine they'd be hurrying to hunt through the rubble for bodies. If people saw him climbing, that would all change.

In the distance, the dragon army was preparing to leave, apparently unhurried. There certainly didn't appear to be any sign of reprisal from the castle—the dragons had come here to kill the Hamelyn Piper, and now that it was done the fight seemed to be over.

Far below, the forest at the base of the cliff showed the scars where the largest chunks of masonry had crashed to the ground. There was another scar that Patch could see—a smaller area further out, where the broken tops of trees were visible. He pointed it out to Wren. "Is that where the dragons' messenger fell, do you think?"

Wren looked for a moment then signed her reply: *Could he have survived?*

Patch thought back to the dragon dropping out of the sky, and the crunch of the impact. "I doubt it." The dragons had presumably collected their colleague's body during the attack. Patch felt a wave of empathy for the messenger, accompanied by a strong feeling of shame at how the Pipers had attacked him from the rear while he carried a white flag.

The dragon army rose and began the long journey back to their homelands. The darkness of dragons receded, until at last it looked like a flock of birds in the distance, just as it had when Wren had first seen it approach.

Once the dragons had gone, the sound of hammer on stone and the bawdy conversation of workmen drifted down to them.

Patch set Wren down beside him in the crevice, and a moment later she lurched to one side and grabbed a juicy beetle that had blundered too close. She tucked in, ripping the insect's head off with her first bite. As she crunched into the abdomen, she noticed Patch's grim expression. She polished off the rest in two mouthfuls. *They're actually pretty good*, she signed. *A bit like caramel.*

"I'll take your word for it," said Patch.

As night fell, the work on the castle ceased. Patch and Wren risked a quick glance up and saw the roped-timber reinforcements that had been put in place, all rather impressive considering how speedily it had been assembled.

In the sky the moon shone through wispy clouds.

"I think it's safe to go," he said. He checked the parcel at his waist and took a moment to better secure the Hamelyn Piper's Mask. He lifted Wren back onto his shoulder. "If I fall, jump away from me. You'll survive the landing as long as I don't come down on top of you." Wren just gave him a hard stare. "Okay, okay. I won't fall. Right. Time to whistle up some courage. Quite a bit of it, I think."

Patch built the Song of Courage as best he could without a Pipe. As a very young boy, he'd stumbled onto some rhythms and melodies that made him feel a little braver; anyone who had ever felt emboldened by joining in a normal song of hope or patriotism could understand the kind of feelings he'd been able to create when he was young. The power of music was clear even to those who knew little of the Piping Arts. But as he'd learned the ways of the Pipe at Tiviscan, his eyes and ears had been opened to the *real* power that music could conjure.

He felt strength flowing through his blood. Confidence. Certainty. Courage.

I can do this, he thought.

He stepped to the edge of the crevice they had taken refuge in, and looked down.

I can't do this, he thought.

He stepped back from the edge. It was a *long* way down.

Long, and craggy, and *sharp.*

Are you okay? signed Wren.

Patch took a breath and nodded. "I've a little courage now," he said. "Next, I need help with the *climbing* part." He began the Song of the Climb, slowly building it up, the rhythm steady. In his mind, he could already feel the satisfaction of his hands moving over rock, finding purchase, knowing how much weight a handhold could support.

As he whistled, he put out of his mind the knowledge of

where many Songs came from, where many had originated and been refined.

War.

Pipers had accompanied armies for centuries, and had also ventured on smaller missions: infiltration, sabotage. The Song of the Climb, for example, would have helped a group of fighters tackle terrain that an enemy thought impossible.

And while not all Songs had such origins, most of those that affected *people* came from the battlefields of history.

He whistled, eyes closed, until he felt a kinship with the rock itself. It would show him where to place his feet. It would guide his fingertips to where they would cling. He was ready to start the descent. He kneeled and lowered his legs over the base of the crevice.

The moonlight was unnecessary; instinct alone was leading him down the face of the cliff. Only the rock seemed real. Everything else faded away, coming back into focus from time to time and prompting him to change what he whistled. Whenever terror crept into his bones, he whistled for courage; when his sure reach for handholds faltered, he went back to the Song of the Climb.

When at last they were safely down, he stopped whistling and stared back up, unable even to *see* the crevice where the climb had begun. How long had it taken? Somewhere between hours and centuries, it seemed.

He looked at Wren, her expression one of awe. She hugged his neck.

Patch took her from his shoulder and gently set her down. "We made it," he said, falling to his knees. Then he spent ten minutes retching, his last prison meal forced out of him in a thin stream of bile.

Where to now? signed Wren, when he'd stopped being sick. Patch wiped the spittle from the side of his mouth. "Erner's letter, remember?" he said. "We go to Marwheel Abbey, to find a way to cure you! Unless you've decided to remain a rodent?"

No chance of that, she signed.

Now that the climb was over, Patch noticed how cold he was feeling. Tiviscan always enjoyed a mild winter, but his meager prison clothing wouldn't do much to keep him warm. "I wish I had my coat," he said, rubbing his hands together. "Are you cold too?"

I'm all right, signed Wren. *Being furry comes in handy*. "Well as long as we keep moving, I should be okay on the journey to the Abbey." He pointed to the trees ahead.

"We go that way through the forest. We have to get far from Tiviscan without being discovered. I'm an escaped prisoner now, Wren. I have to be cunning and resourceful! A day's walk will take us to the Penance River, which we can follow north."

And after I'm cured, what about you? She pointed to his

waist, where the Mask was tied. *You're the last person to see the Hamelyn Piper alive. Perhaps you'll be famous!*

Patch shook his head, untying the Mask to take a proper look at it. "Obscurity is all that I want, Wren. If Rundel Stone found out I was alive, he'd make sure I went back to the dungeons." He held the Mask closer, peering at it. The parts that seemed damaged simply popped back into shape after some prodding, although the lock itself was beyond repair.

Every inch of the Mask's inner surface was covered in symbols that reminded him of the ancient magical textbooks in the Tiviscan library. He wiped it to see the runes more clearly, and was astonished at how much cleaner the metal was where he'd wiped. What he'd taken for tarnish seemed to be merely dirt. "The Mask came off the Hamelyn Piper's head just before the dragons took him," he said. "I don't even know why I picked it up. I should just drop this here and be done with it." Studying the metal, he could see that it wasn't welded together. It was made from overlapping pieces connected with *joints*, similar to the ones that allowed it to hinge shut over the wearer's face. He tried to move some of the pieces against one another, at first without success, but then parts of the Mask seemed to fold up. He tried again with another section, and this time the entire Mask flattened down into a rectangle the size of his hand.

He looked at Wren. "Interesting," he said. "Should I keep it, do you think?"

She nodded. *A souvenir,* she signed. *Of when you saw the most evil man in history finally get his reward!*

"I'm not sure that watching a man die is something I want a souvenir of, Wren," Patch said, but then it occurred to him—Wren hadn't heard what the man had said. *I'm the only one to know the Hamelyn Piper's last words,* he thought. *If I should even think of him by that name anymore!* Suddenly the knowledge was a terrible burden: the prisoner had suffered a great injustice, if those last words had really been true, and worse—it would mean that the *real* Hamelyn Piper must still be free.

And if that was the case, surely it was Patch's duty to tell the Council? *They'd lock me up again,* he thought. *Whether they believed me or not, I'd spend the rest of my days rotting in a cell.*

He tied the folded Mask to his waist. He would need money soon enough, he reckoned, and strange magical objects always had value.

He put Wren on his shoulder and made his way through the light vegetation at the forest's edge, then through thicker bushes until they were in amongst the vast pines. By the time the first hint of predawn twilight was visible in the sky, they were far enough from the base of the cliff—and from Tiviscan—for Patch to breathe easier.

A little further on, the undergrowth became more challenging. The sky was brightening rapidly, letting Patch look further ahead to spot the clearest path. He could see a much brighter area beyond a thicket. "Is that a clearing?" he said. Wren shrugged, but as they got closer they could see splintered treetops high up, and a dark shape on the ground ahead.

The messenger? signed Wren.

Patch paused. Surely the dragons wouldn't just have left their fallen comrade? Yet as they got closer, they saw that it *was* the messenger, broken and still. The dragons had abandoned their sole casualty of the battle. "I don't understand," said Patch. "Why didn't they retrieve the body?"

That's really sad, signed Wren.

"This poor soul was attacked from the rear," said Patch. "Seeing that happen made me ashamed to be a Piper. But now this lack of respect from his own kind!" He scowled, surprised by how angry he felt. "It's not like dragons at *all*. During training I learned quite a bit about their culture. When a dragon dies, the body is taken by members of the Order of the Skull—the most ancient and secretive part of their religion. The body is buried deep, in total secrecy, the location never revealed."

Wren frowned. *So a dragon's family don't even have a grave to visit?*

Patch nodded. "It's been that way for thousands of years. Mind you, humans have always thought various parts of a dragon have magical properties. There are plenty of idiots who'd buy any old potion if you pretended it had powdered dragon tooth in it. Can you imagine the trouble that'd be caused if there were dragon graves to rob?"

When Patch had first seen the messenger he'd noticed an odd discoloration on the scales, which suggested terrible old wounds; now, he could see the same thing around its closed eyes and mouth. The snout seemed misshapen, and was presumably broken. The wings were limply spread out, and one had a long bleeding tear near its base.

"A proud creature, reduced to this," he said. "Meeting its fate after showing true bravery, yet ending up mourned only by us, Wren. An escaped prisoner and a cursed rat."

He stepped closer. It wasn't very large for a dragon, he realized, its head perhaps four feet long and two across. Something nagged at him about the markings, especially those on the wings.

Couldn't we do something? signed Wren.

"Well, we couldn't exactly *bury* him," said Patch. "Unless we had a week or two to spare."

You could say a few words, she replied.

Patch nodded. He thought back to what he'd learned of their culture, then cleared his throat. "Today, we ask the Gods of Fire and Scale to look to the ground, and see this fallen warrior, that they may bring him to the Mighty Flame and—"

At that moment, Wren tapped his cheek. He glanced at her, irritated that she would interrupt such a solemn occasion, but she was pointing furiously toward the dragon. He turned his gaze to see what was bothering her. The dragon's eyes were open, and looking right at him.

"Could you *stop* all the mumbo jumbo, please?" the dragon said in a deep voice. "I've already had a terrible day, and the last thing I need is *religion*."

13

The Messenger

It took a few seconds for Patch to get his mouth to work. The sudden reality of standing next to a living dragon, especially an injured and obviously *irritable* one, had quickly pushed him close to panic. He racked his brains to remember the most respectful form of address, and came up with *seken*—roughly the equivalent of *sir*. "I'm glad to see you're alive, Seken!" he said.

The dragon eyed him carefully and grunted. "Don't call me that."

Patch's eyes widened. "I'm sorry, I thought it was the correct term—"

"Oh, yes, it's the correct *term*," said the dragon, sitting up. "For a dragon. But I'm *not* a dragon, and after today I suspect I'll have nothing more to do with the pigheaded *idiots*."

"*Not* a—" began Patch, then his voice trailed off. He looked again at the creature, and those nagging feelings he'd had before resurfaced. Aside from the obvious tear, the wings were discolored in places; the snout was misshapen, but he'd thought it had been badly injured in the fall and not looked at it too closely. Now that he *did* look closely, he saw a snout that ended in a hooked shape more reminiscent of a *beak*; he saw wings that were covered in the stubs of cut feathers, as well as areas of the thick leathery skin that dragons had. There were stubs of feathers around the snout too, but those were charred.

Now that the creature was sitting up, Patch could see that the legs each had densely packed brown feathers running down them. And while the front claws were very like those of a dragon, the rear were more like the feet of some enormous falcon, or . . .

Well, thought Patch. *Of course!* A smile crept onto his face as the truth dawned on him. The creature in front of him seemed to grow even more irritated because of the smile, but Patch couldn't help it.

Some features of a dragon, and some of a *griffin*. "You're a dracogriff!" he said. He glanced at Wren and saw the confusion on her face. "Half-dragon, half-griffin!" he told her. "I'm sorry, it's just I've never met a dracogriff before. Actually, I've never met a *dragon* before, not really, or a griffin come to that, but when it comes down to it they're two a penny! A *dracogriff*, though! Now that *is* an honor."

Why is it an honor? signed Wren.

The dracogriff sat up suddenly, looking at Wren with astonishment. "Your rat can talk!" he said, wide-eyed. "I know Merisax hand speech when I see it! I've spent the last seven years as a bodyguard-for-hire in the Islands of the Eastern Seas. Merisax came with the territory. Is *talking* the nature of its curse?"

"Curse?" said Patch.

"Yes. As you approached, you referred to yourself as an escaped prisoner and a cursed rat."

Patch blinked. He looked at Wren.

Oh great, she signed. *We've only been fugitives for a few hours, and we've already given ourselves away.*

"Please," said the dracogriff. "You have no need to fear that I'd hand you over. I'm certainly no friend to Pipers. Even if you *are* one." Patch stared at him, openmouthed. "I *also* heard you say that what they did to me made you ashamed to be a Piper."

"I did?" said Patch. "I did. Damn. I need to be more careful what I say in future. Being an escaped convict is harder than I thought."

"As I said, you've nothing to worry about from me," said the dracogriff. He held out his front claw. His *hand,* Patch corrected himself—that was what dragons and griffins called them, and it seemed impolite not to think of them as such. Patch offered his relatively tiny hand out in return, and they shook. "I'm Barver. Barver Knopferkerkle."

"Barver Nop-fur-ker-kill," said Patch, trying to get his mouth around it.

"That's it," said Barver. "Dragon surname, griffin forename. Your turn!"

"Patch Brightwater," said Patch. "Imprisoned a week ago, now free and hopefully presumed dead. This is my friend Wren Cobble, a girl cursed by a Sorcerer into the form of a rat. I taught her some hand speech when we met so that we could talk. She's a quick learner."

Barver looked closely at Wren. "Your markings *are* pretty," he said. "I especially like the red rings on your tail."

Thanks very much, signed Wren with a smile.

"A Sorcerer's curse, eh?" said Barver. "It always saddens me that Sorcerers are such *awful* people. Think of all the good they could do if they were nicer!"

Tell me about it, she signed.

Barver turned his attention to Patch. "Aren't you a little *young* to have been imprisoned?"

Patch felt himself bristle. "I'm thirteen," he said, as imposingly as he could manage. Wren suppressed a laugh, and he glared at her.

"I meant no offense," said Barver. "It just seems harsh, to experience such adversity so young." He looked up through the trees. Patch and Wren followed his gaze and could clearly see the damage to the castle through the branches. "I saw the flames burn brightly as the Hamelyn Piper was executed," said Barver. "I heard the screams as other prisoners fell to their deaths. Yet you lived. It seems fate has plans for you!"

"I hope not," said Patch. "I'd rather just find somewhere I can earn a living and get some peace and quiet. I reckon I've earned it."

"How did you survive the fall?" said Barver. "Humans must be hardier than I thought."

"I climbed down the cliff," said Patch. "How did *you* survive the fall? I heard the crunch when you hit the ground!"

"It was a bad one, I admit," said Barver. He slowly folded his wings up along his back and stretched his legs, wincing.

"Are you sure you should be moving anywhere for a while?" said Patch.

"I'll certainly not be flying for a few weeks," said Barver. "But apart from that it's just bruises."

"Incredible," said Patch. He and Wren shared an amazed look, and both raised their heads to the sky, through the broken treetops, thinking about how far Barver had plummeted.

"How much do you know about dracogriffs?" said Barver.

"That they're rare," said Patch. "Beyond that, not much."

Barver nodded. "There are two broad kinds. One is called a *higher*. The other is called a *lower*. Highers have a blend of the prettier aspects of dragons and griffins, but they're a bit delicate. Lowers have a blend of the more *durable* qualities.

We're ugly, but very hard to kill. Naturally, dragons and griffins prefer the pretty ones, but I know which I'd rather be!" He grinned, and as he did his strange blend of features suddenly seemed to make *sense*. Wren and Patch both found themselves grinning too.

I like him, signed Wren.

"Me too," said Patch.

"So, my new friends!" said Barver. "Where are you headed?"

"The Penance River flows through the forest," said Patch. "Following it will take us to the Collosson Highway, and then to Marwheel Abbey. We've heard that someone there can help lift Wren's curse."

Barver grinned. "Then we should set off at once!"

"We?" said Patch.

"You don't mind if I tag along? I seem to have been abandoned, and I'll not be able to fly for quite a while. The company would be appreciated."

Patch looked to Wren.

Why not? she signed.

"Why not indeed," said Patch. "Although I have to say, Barver, you don't seem all that cross about the dragon army leaving you behind. I think if I was you, I'd be *seething*!"

Barver waved his hand like he was swatting a fly.

"I won't waste my anger on that lot," he said. "They weren't very keen on me accompanying the army when we left the Dragon Territories, but it seems they were even *less* keen on me going back with them." He shrugged. "As I said, dragons prefer the pretty kind of dracogriff. They tend to look at me as some kind of unfortunate *mistake*."

Wren was outraged and signed some things that made quite clear what she thought of the dragons.

"You should mind your language," said Patch, wincing. He noticed that the scroll of demands Barver had read out was still tucked into his harness. "When I saw you approach the castle, I'd assumed sending you to deliver the demands must have been some kind of honor."

"I volunteered when nobody else came forward," said Barver. He frowned. "Makes me wonder if they all knew something I didn't." He shook his wings a little and stretched again. "Anyway, enough of all that! Which way is the river?"

Patch pointed toward an overgrown area of bushes that looked worryingly thorny. "That's the most direct way, so if we head over *there*"—he pointed toward a more accessible route—"it should be easier going."

Barver nodded and trotted off toward the wall of thorny bushes, flattening a path as if it were nothing more than tall grass.

Patch smiled at Wren, shrugged, and followed.

They could hear the soft murmur of flowing water as they approached the river. Barver paused and turned. "Can either of you smell something?" he said. "Bears, maybe? Or wolves?"

"Bears?" said Patch. He looked at Wren and she gave him a frightened glance, but following in Barver's trail made Patch feel about as safe as he'd ever felt in his life. "Oh, I don't think we've much to worry about on that score, Wren," he said.

"Actually, not a bear," said Barver. "Something *dead*." He lifted his snout high and sniffed deep and long, turning his head this way and that. "Over there," he said. "*Human*," he added, then led the way to a small rise covered in ivy-choked trees. He stopped and pulled at the ivy.

The corpse underneath was revealed. The skull grinned out at them, ragged remains of flesh clinging to it. It wore a long coat, which was torn in several places—gashes from sharp claws. Within the coat, little but bone remained.

Patch stared at the skull and couldn't help imagining his own skull there instead. "Have I mentioned how glad I am that you're here, Barver?" Wren, who was also staring, nodded in agreement.

"It's at least a few months old," said Barver. "Probably a bear attack. A gruesome enough death, but quick." He pulled at more of the ivy, and discovered a hardy shoulder-slung leather bag, similar to Erner's satchel. "What do we have here?"

Patch picked up the bag and untied the fastening strap. Inside was a simple cotton tunic, a sheathed knife, a fire-steel, a small waterskin, and the moldy remains of an old hunk of bread—which he took out and discarded. "He just carried the basics of survival," said Patch. "Perhaps the poor soul traveled along the river, in search of a new life." He shook out the tunic. It was a little musty, but basically clean, so he set Wren on the ground before taking off his coarse prison shirt and putting the tunic on. It was a vast improvement. He gave the torn coat a sorrowful look. "Shame about that," he said. "It seems well made."

Barver shrugged. "It's not beyond saving. And a good wash in the river will shift much of the smell." He gave Patch a look. "Speaking of which . . ."

"What?" said Patch.

"Go to the river, Patch Brightwater, and scrape the dungeon stench from your skin. It makes my eyes sting even more than the odor of this corpse." He turned to the gnawed jumble of bones on the ground and looked at it, thoughtful. "In the meantime, I'll see what can be done with that coat."

14

A CLEAN START

C old, was it? signed Wren.

Patch tried to nod in response, but it was hard because he was shivering so much. He'd stripped off and jumped into the river, but the water had turned out to be rather more chilly than he'd expected. Half-screaming, half-whimpering, he'd cleaned himself as quickly as he could before leaping out and returning to Wren.

He'd already untied his blanket parcel, leaving its contents on the fallen tree trunk next to Wren, so that he would have his blanket ready to wrap around himself. He dried off as best he could, then he dressed and put his meager belongings back into the damp blanket. Wren hopped onto his still-trembling shoulder, and they returned to where they'd left Barver.

To Patch's amazement, Barver was holding the dead man's torn coat, stitching up the rips. Patch had never imagined that the clawed hands of dragons and griffins were capable of much dexterity, but Barver wielded a needle and thread with the skill of an expert.

Barver reached into his harness and produced another reel of thread. He smiled when he saw them nearing. "A few large slashes and a couple of minor tears, that's about it," he said. "I'll be finished shortly." He looked closely at Patch, his expression suddenly concerned. "Should your lips be *quite* that shade of blue?"

"The w-water was a b-bit c-c-cold," Patch said. "I'm not k-k-k-keen on being c-c-cold."

"My apologies, I should have thought!" said Barver. He set down his sewing and took a few steps forward, then with a broad swipe of his tail cleared an area of the ground down to the soil. He made a small mound of earth at the center. "Stand back," he said, lowering his head to the mound. He opened his mouth wide and a gurgling noise came from his throat. He coughed and thumped his chest a few times. "Hang on, I'll get there," he said, and opened his mouth again.

This time, an intense flame poured from his throat, flowing over the mound of earth. It sounded, Patch thought, like a blacksmith's forge with the bellows being pumped. The heat reaching him was already significant, and very welcome.

Barver kept the fire coming until the earth started to glow, stones within it audibly cracking. "There you go," he said. "Get yourself warmed up!"

Around Barver's half-griffin muzzle there were blackened stubs, one of which was currently on fire. Patch licked his finger and thumb and reached out, pinching the stub to extinguish the flame.

"Thank you," said Barver. "My dragon and griffin features don't always work together. Griffin feathers on a fire-breathing face, for example. They don't last long, trust me."

Patch sat and let the heat fill him. On his shoulder, Wren stretched her paws out to the warmth. Barver held the coat up, examining his work. "I'll wash it when I'm done," he said. "Shouldn't take long to dry on a heated boulder." He returned to his stitching.

Patch and Wren watched him with an obvious bemusement. It wasn't long before the dracogriff caught their expressions. "Anything wrong?" he said.

"Sorry," said Patch. "But it's just . . . well, the sewing?"

"My mother taught me," said Barver. "For my wings."

He unfurled his left wing a little. Patch and Wren looked, and saw that the tear they'd seen when they'd first found Barver was now neatly stitched. Barver traced his fingers along the line of the injury. "I treat my wings *terribly*," he said with a gentle melancholy. "Always have. They're about as hardy as those of a typical dragon, but I'm used to the *rest* of me being so much more resilient." To underline his point, he picked up a thick fallen branch from the ground and smashed it over his own head. "See? I was a clumsy youth and my wings often got torn. They heal better when stitched, and my mother got tired of having to keep doing it, so she made sure I learned. And I've had plenty of practice, believe me."

For a few quiet minutes, Barver stitched the coat while Patch and Wren warmed up near the glowing mound of earth. Patch opened out the blanket he'd used to dry himself, setting his belongings to one side and holding the damp blanket up to the heat.

Oh, show him the Hamelyn Piper's Mask! signed Wren, pointing at it.

"I don't want any fuss," mumbled Patch.

Barver had seen what Wren had signed, though. "The Hamelyn Piper's Mask?" he said.

Patch shrugged. "I was in the cell next to him. Like you, I saw him die, although I was *much* closer. His Mask fell off him before he was pulled from his cell. I picked it up."

"The actual Iron Mask of the Hamelyn Piper?" said Barver, fascinated.

Patch picked up the Mask and demonstrated how it unfolded. He tossed it to Barver.

"Astonishing," said Barver, turning the Mask over in his hands. He reversed what Patch had done and the Mask folded up again. "We've seen history made today. A dark and evil thing, finally brought to an end." He shook his head slowly and gave the Mask back to Patch. "Well, the sooner I get this coat washed and dried, the sooner we can set off again." He picked up the coat and made his way to the river.

Patch put his belongings into the traveler's leather bag, and looked at the small pile of bones that was all that now remained of him. "This traveler was heading for a new life," he said. "Hopes and dreams, all brought to a terrible end." He shook his head. "Looking at those bones makes me think," he said, wistful. "However bad things have been, we're alive; we're luckier than that poor soul."

It makes me think too, signed Wren.

"What?" said Patch.

Wren grinned. *Stay away from bears*, she signed.

They made good pace alongside the river, and Patch was glad of his new coat. Barver had managed to clean it well, and although a slightly odd smell still clung to it, the warmth it provided was more than enough to compensate. Spring wasn't far away now, but the air still had a deep chill to it. As evening approached, Barver found a secluded clearing for their camp. Exhausted, Patch put up his little tent and lay down for what he thought would be a short rest before eating.

When Wren woke him with a loud squeak in his ear, night had fallen.

Patch came out of the tent. Barver was sitting by a small fire, holding a spit over the flames—rabbit, Patch saw. His mouth watered.

"Awake at last!" said Barver. "Wren was telling me all about your exploits, yours and hers both. She told me the story of Patterfall and of her own curse, and I gave her some tales of my adventures in the Eastern Seas." He took the spit away from the fire and sniffed the rabbit, then handed the spit to Patch, who tore off a piece of meat and ate it. It tasted sublime.

"That's *amazing*," Patch said around his mouthful.

"A few common herbs to bring out the flavor," said Barver. "Now, Wren . . . Shall we finish our game?"

Wren nodded and scampered over to where—Patch now saw—the Fox and Owls board was laid out. *I taught him,* signed Wren to Patch. *He picked it up pretty quickly.*

Patch ate his rabbit and watched the game, which was hard-fought by Barver. Wren's victory came in the end, but it was much closer than Patch had ever managed against her.

In the warmth from the fire, with his belly full, he realized with a degree of shock that he had a *future* to look forward to. Barver's mention of the Eastern Seas had made him think. The Islands of the Eastern Seas were mostly outside the influence of Tiviscan and, as such, uncertified Pipers could still work there if they were careful.

He could work there.

Of course, the Islands were also overrun with pirates and criminals, but it was something for him to consider: a future as a Piper, even if it wasn't the one he'd always dreamed of. But there was one thing he would need to do before even *that* future was possible.

He would need to make himself a new *Pipe*.

He'd already noticed plenty of mature boxwood bushes in the forest, so it wouldn't be hard to find some suitable branches that he could use.

A new Pipe, for a new life. That night, he slept well.

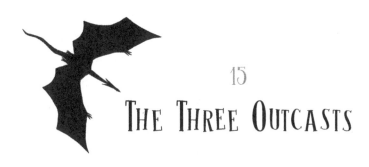

15

THE THREE OUTCASTS

The next evening, as dusk approached, they reached the Collosson Highway—a rather grand name for what amounted to a slightly-wider-than-normal muddy road. They were confronted with another smell in the air, but one that was rather more pleasant than a dead traveler: the smell of food cooking.

"Beef stew," said Barver, his eyes half-closed. His stomach gave a rumble so loud it echoed.

"Fresh bread," said Patch, his mouth starting to drool.

There must be an inn nearby, signed Wren.

"It's a shame the dead traveler wasn't carrying any money," said Patch, mournful. There was a curious tinkling sound to his left, and he turned to see a glorious sight. Barver was grinning, and in his hand was a small purse.

"Let this be my treat," said Barver. "Since I returned from the Eastern Seas I've not known many I'd care to spend time with, and now I meet a condemned criminal and a cursed rat and find them to be honest, decent, and agreeable company. What do you say? We'll have a feast, and I insist on getting you a proper bed for the night. Then we'll reach Marwheel Abbey fed and rested."

A bed, thought Patch.

A proper bed. He almost wept.

The inn lay around the next bend in the road, and it looked as perfect as it smelled.

The innkeeper was petrified the moment he saw Barver, but soon enough Barver's friendly manner—and his money—smoothed things over. "A feast, if you please," said Barver, offering up a shiny golden coin. "And beds for the night."

"Will the smaller of our stables do you for sleeping, my large friend?" asked the innkeeper. "It's clean and warm, and you'll have it to yourself."

"Sounds perfect," said Barver.

The innkeeper spotted the rat on Patch's shoulder and frowned. Wren gave him a wave and bowed.

"Trained rat, eh?" said the innkeeper. "Clever."

"You don't know the half of it," said Patch.

The innkeeper showed them to a table at the back of the inn. Patch had a tankard of small ale brought to him;

Barver had a bucket of the same, and insisted on a thimble for Wren, the innkeeper delighted by the level of training this "pet" rat displayed.

Patch looked at Barver's bucket. "I would've thought you'd drink something stronger," he said. Small ale was a very weak brew of barley and oats, tasty and thirst quenching with hardly any alcohol.

Barver shook his head. "Anything strong irritates my fire ducts," he said. "This is just about right for me."

Patch nodded. "A toast," he said, raising his tankard. "To you, Barver, and to you, Wren! Only days ago, I was alone and in despair. Today, I'm happy and with friends!"

"Thank you," said Barver. "But I'd rather we raise a toast to my mother. She was the reason I recently returned from the Islands of the Eastern Seas, and it is her gift to me that is paying for our meal. To my mother!" He raised his bucket. "May she rest in peace."

Wren's face fell, and so did Patch's.

Oh, Barver! signed Wren, distressed.

"It's good for me to talk about it," said Barver. "In the dragon tradition, she left me what's called a Vanishing Gift—the money now in my purse. In her honor, I must spend it all within one month." He shook his head, his eyes moistening. "But I'd not spoken to her in years. We'd fallen out, which was why I left for the Eastern Seas in the first place. If my father had still been alive things might have been different, but me and my mother never spoke again. By the time word reached me that she was dying, it was too late. Her funeral ceremony had happened, and the Order of the Skull had taken her body to its final secret home."

They fell into silence for a moment.

"Then we *must* raise a toast to your mother," said Patch. They raised their ales and took a drink. "I'm so sorry, Barver."

Barver nodded, grateful. "She left a letter for me. I'd hoped there might be some kind of apology for the way she'd acted, but instead it was instructions for a last wish. I feel overwhelmed by it all. Things have been so rushed, you see. The day after I got back to the Dragon Territories, they began raising the army to claim the Hamelyn Piper. My mother had always been fascinated with him—an *obsession*, really. It seemed fitting that I should volunteer and see with my own eyes what happened. I think she would have been appalled at how it turned out. Revenge is such an unpleasant thing."

Why was she obsessed with the Hamelyn Piper? asked Wren.

"She was an advisor to the Dragon Triumvirate. *Highly* respected. Even her relationship with my father hadn't tarnished her reputation, and dragons are very touchy about one of their kind falling in love with a griffin, believe me.

She'd first taken an interest in the Hamelyn Piper when the *human* children vanished, but when the dragon children were stolen her obsession was complete. And while the other dragons wanted war with the whole of humanity—as if it was their fault!—*she* was a voice of reason. Without her guidance, I think another war might have been unavoidable."

"Then we have much to thank her for," said Patch.

"True," said Barver. "But it was that same obsession which drove such a wedge between us. She became ever more distant and was often cold to me. One question burned within her, the most important question of them all! *Why* had the Hamelyn Piper taken the children?"

Because he was insane, signed Wren. *Me and Patch saw him, remember? We saw his eyes! Crazy!*

Patch felt his cheeks redden and wished above all else that he could just *forget* what the prisoner had said. He wanted to tell his friends the truth, but he also knew that doing so would lead to trouble. It was easier to pretend that the Hamelyn Piper *had* been mad, and so anything he'd said at the end was meaningless. "Did your mother ever suggest an answer to that question?" he said.

"Some claim the children were taken to a mysterious and beautiful place," said Barver. "To show that humans and dragons could live in harmony and prevent wars from ever happening again. Fairy-tale nonsense! It's a miracle it didn't *start* a war at once, instead of preventing them in future. No, my mother didn't think any of the popular theories made much sense. If she had her own ideas about it, she never shared them with me." He took a drink of ale and sighed. "Then again, she stopped sharing *anything* with me. That was why we grew apart."

The food was soon brought out, and it was impressive. A pair of roasted boars at its center, the table soon strained under the weight of cheese and bread and cake, nuts and fruit and bowls of spiced porridge, soups and stews and biscuits and salted fish.

Barver's table manners were almost a shock to Patch. He'd expected the dracogriff to consume the feast one vast mouthful after another, but instead he took his time and ate with delicate care. He didn't hold back on praise for the wide variety of dishes that had been cooked for them.

"Living out in the Islands of the Eastern Sea, you get used to decent food," said Barver to the delighted innkeeper. "This is all superb!"

They continued with the meal, Patch and Wren eating until they were almost in pain. Patch looked at his own plate, tempted by the various bits and pieces that were left on it. The idea of not eating everything he'd taken was unthinkable to him, but it would be a few minutes yet (and probably a belch or two) before he could fit anything else in.

He delved inside his bag and pulled out several pieces of boxwood that he'd cut from bushes as they'd walked. He studied the wood and chose the best pieces, straight and free of awkward knots. Before long, he'd planned out the new Pipe in his mind. The knife the dead traveler had carried in his bag was a good one, and Patch set about stripping the bark.

What are you working on? signed Wren.

Patch smiled. "A Pipe," he said. "I don't quite feel whole without one."

You've done this often? signed Wren.

"Twice before," he said. "Not everyone makes their own, but making it yourself lets you get to know it right from the start." He blew away some shavings. "I'll need some fine woodcarving knives, though, before I can really get to work."

I can't wait to hear you play it! she signed. She sat back and patted her stomach. *You know, after this meal I'll probably sleep for a month.*

Barver nodded. "It's a very welcome feast." He let rip with a thunderous burp that seemed to last forever. Done, he gave a satisfied smile, while Patch and Wren laughed.

Barver started loading his platter up with food again, two-thirds of the feast now gone.

Patch mopped up soup with some bread. "What will you do, Barver?" he asked. "When we go our separate ways?"

"I'll fulfil the last wish of my mother," said Barver. "Her letter gave me instructions—there is a place I must go and a second letter to open when I'm there. After it's done, I'll return to the Eastern Seas. There's nothing for me in the Dragon Territories. I've always been a bit of an outcast, but I think I prefer it that way." He smiled, and nodded to Wren. "And you, an outcast from your human form, but not for much longer! What will you do when the spell is reversed?"

I'll go home, she signed. *I miss my parents terribly, but I refuse to go back to them until I'm cured.*

"And you, Patch?" said Barver.

"Once Wren's free of the curse, I'll see her safely back to her home. Then—" He set down the stripped boxwood he was holding. "I'm making this Pipe because I feel incomplete without one, but I'll never be a true certified Piper. I'm an outcast too. I can make a living, but it must be far from Tiviscan. Far from its *dungeons*."

"Well," said Barver, "if you happen to find yourselves in the Eastern Seas, just ask for me at any inn on the Islands. They'll be able to point you in the right direction." He raised his bucket of ale. "To the three of us! Outcasts all!" They each took a drink. Barver wiped the froth from his mouth. "There's an old griffin tale called 'The Three Outcasts,'" he said. "Have you heard it?"

"No," said Patch, and Wren shook her head.

Barver looked wistful for a moment, then drew in a breath and frowned. "Probably better you haven't," he said. "It doesn't end well."

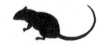

16

MARWHEEL ABBEY

The next morning, they saw the Abbey long before they reached it. The road took them up over a high ridge, and on the descent they could see a wide expanse of farmed land with cottages dotted throughout. At the center was a vast, ornate gray-stone building. A large, central, rectangular section was impressively high and topped with densely packed spires. Around it, smaller annexes had their own profusions of smaller towers and pinnacles. The overall impression was that the architect must have had a considerable fondness for hedgehogs.

"Marwheel Abbey," said Patch. "Down there, Wren, lies the answer to your predicament."

Wren peeked out from Patch's pocket, where she was sheltering from the morning chill. She looked and nodded, returning to the pocket without a word. Patch could understand—she was nervous. There was a lot riding on this visit.

They reached the Abbey entrance—huge wooden doors, the frame intricately carved with flowers and animals. The doors were closed, and a bell-chain hung down next to the frame. When Patch pulled it a delicate tinkling came from the other side, followed by the echoing approach of footsteps.

A small inset hatch opened in the door directly in front of Patch, revealing the face of a young monk. "Yes?" said the monk.

"Would it be possible to see Brother Tobias?" said Patch.

"If you give me a moment I'll find out," said the monk. He caught sight of Barver and let out a curious noise, as if someone had trodden on a vole. He looked petrified. "Oh. I . . . um. Back in a minute." The hatch shut. Hurried footsteps charted his rapid retreat.

After a while, the hatch opened again, revealing a different monk. He was much older, with blue, penetrating eyes on a lean and weathered face, the left side of which had a deep scar running from jawbone to forehead. With the man's gaze on him, Patch felt like a rabbit being sized up by a wolf. "I'm Brother Tobias," said the man. "Who exactly are *you*, lad?"

Patch opened his mouth and suddenly realized that giving his real name might not be the best idea. "Um . . . Henry," he said. "Henry . . . Smith." He felt a little wriggle in his pocket from Wren, and could almost *see* her exasperation; the way it had come out, calling himself "Archibald Fakename" would have sounded just as convincing. "And this is my friend Barver Knopferkerkle, a dracogriff."

Tobias nodded briefly to Barver, apparently unconcerned, then turned back to Patch. "I understand you wish to see me about something?"

"I'm a friend of Erner Whitlock, an Apprentice Custodian. He wrote to you about a problem regarding the victim of a curse?"

The man's eyes widened, and he looked at Barver again. "Lord, really? That's one *heck* of a curse."

Patch glanced at Barver, who seemed bemused rather than offended. "No," said Patch quickly, "Barver actually *is* a dracogriff." He held open his coat; Wren poked her head out of the pocket and waved. "This is Wren. She's the one who needs your help."

"A rat, then!" said Tobias. "That's more what I was expecting. You'd better come inside."

Tobias opened the large main doors and led them along a tall, arched corridor, which was spacious enough to give Barver no trouble moving around. Patch noticed a few fearful glances from the monks as they passed, but only a few ran off in terror.

"We've had some griffins here in our time," said Tobias. "But never a *dracogriff*. You're very welcome. Although, given recent events, you might find things a bit awkward for a while, being part dragon."

"Recent events?" said Patch.

"Yes," said Tobias. "Did you come to us from the south?" He nodded to Barver. "Did you fly?"

"A fall has left me too wounded to fly," said Barver. "For a week or two, at least."

"We came from the north," said Patch. "By road."

"Shame," said Tobias. "I'd hoped you could add to the news we've been getting from travelers on the West Road about an attack on Tiviscan Castle!"

Patch forced out a vaguely convincing gasp. "Goodness no," he said. "Was anybody hurt?"

"A dragon army assaulted the castle, it seems," said Tobias. "The only fatalities were a few of the prisoners in the dungeons, one of whom was particularly noteworthy. The Hamelyn Piper!"

Patch gasped again. "Gosh," he said.

"The dragons finally got their wish," said Tobias. "And the Hamelyn Piper's secrets have now died with him. There's understandable anger that the castle was attacked, but frankly the Hamelyn Piper's death is being widely celebrated. I suppose if he was ever going to reveal the truth about the children, he'd have done so by now . . ." They reached another set of double doors. "Ah! We're here. Come through."

The doors led outside to a walled garden. A solitary monk tended some of the plants, and looked anxiously at Barver.

"It's okay, Brother Jessop," said Tobias. "There's no reason to be scared."

"Morning," said Barver. The monk nodded without a word and turned back to the plants, trembling visibly.

"The infirmary garden," said Tobias, gesturing to their surroundings. "I'm a Healer, or at least I try to be. I've been running the Abbey infirmary for some years now, and we grow as many of the key herbs here as we can. Sit, sit."

There were stone benches in the middle of the garden. Patch and Tobias sat on them, while Barver hunkered down on the ground. Wren emerged from Patch's pocket and came out onto the bench. She stretched. *Come on then*, she signed. *Get down to business.*

Patch nodded. "So, Apprentice Whitlock wrote to you and explained?"

"That he had met someone who had been shape-shifted by a Sorcerer's curse," said Tobias. "That's the essence of it, yes?"

"It is," said Patch. "Rundel Stone himself suggested your name as Wren's best chance of finding a cure."

"Yes," said Brother Tobias, sounding annoyed. "Whitlock mentioned he was Rundel's apprentice. I'm afraid, Wren, that you have come here with false expectations. I sent a reply to Apprentice Whitlock telling him as much, but not soon enough to save you a journey."

Wren sagged, and Patch didn't know what to say.

"What?" said Barver. "You can't just snatch away the girl's hope like that!"

Brother Tobias shook his head in sorrow. "I'm sorry. Rundel had someone else in mind, I suspect. Someone we both used to know."

"It sounds like you and Rundel Stone are old friends," said Barver.

"Old friends?" said Tobias. "Rundel doesn't really *do* friends. We were colleagues. But it was this *other* person I spoke of that is the true expert in matters of sorcery. I think Rundel sent you to me in the belief that I could take you to them, but I cannot. I made a solemn vow, a long time ago." Wren was staring ahead of herself, tears falling. Brother Tobias looked at her, a pained expression on his face. "I really am sorry, Wren."

"Please," said Patch. "Tell us where this expert is, we'll go and ask directly."

Brother Tobias looked at Wren and seemed torn for a moment, but he shook his head. "That's not going to work," he said. "Even if I broke my vow and told you, it would do you no good. The danger is too great. It's complicated, but there you have it. For your own safety, I'm not going to say any more. There are others who I think can help, however.

Let me gather what information I can, and give you a list of names."

Patch put his hands out to Wren; she hopped onto them and went to his coat pocket to curl up.

Barver let out a deep sigh. "Well then, we must seek a cure elsewhere. Brother Tobias, we would appreciate those names as soon as possible."

"I think they are all a considerable distance away, I'm afraid," said Tobias.

"Not a problem," said Barver. "If I'm flight-ready soon, I'll take her wherever she needs to go."

Wren peeked out of the pocket and wiped away a tear. She shook her head. *You have your mother's last wish to deal with*, she signed. *I'm not going to make you delay that.*

"Nonsense," said Barver. He looked at Tobias. "Any hot springs around here? That tends to sort me out quick-smart."

"No hot springs," said Tobias. "But I'm sure we can do better than that." He called to the monk who was still tending the plants. "Brother Jessop? Could you find Brother Duffle and ask him to come out here?" Brother Jessop seemed only too happy to go. "Brother Duffle has experience with non-human healing. I insist you stay and let him help you, Barver. The Abbey can extend all of you hospitality for a few days."

Barver nodded. "I'd be very grateful," he said. He reached for his money purse and pulled out a coin. "I'll make a donation, naturally. Also, if there's any stitching or darning to be done I'll be only too happy to help."

Tobias gave him an odd look. "Uh . . . okay. The money is very much appreciated. The infirmary has been dealing with an outbreak of firefoot recently; various supplies are depleted. This will help considerably."

At that, a plump monk bearing an overwhelmingly excited expression entered the garden, heading straight for Barver.

"It's true!" cried the monk. He took Barver's hand and shook it repeatedly. "A dracogriff! Welcome! Welcome!"

"Brother Duffle," said Tobias. "This is Barver, our visiting dracogriff, and his friends, Henry and Wren—she is human, the victim of a Sorcerer's curse. A recent fall has left Barver unable to fly, and I thought you might take a look?"

"Absolutely!" said the monk. "Tell me, Barver, can you spread your wings a moment?" Barver did as asked, and Brother Duffle spent a few minutes looking over his new patient. As he did, he mumbled to himself. "I see, I see," he said at last.

"And your prognosis?" said Barver.

Duffle shook his head and tutted. "You've not been taking very good care of yourself! Your shoulder is in terrible shape, your wing skin is peppered with wounds that have never healed fully, and I suspect you've torn every muscle in your body at least once in your life."

Barver nodded, impressed. "You seem to know your stuff, Brother," he said. "But can you get me flying again soon?"

"Indeed!" said Duffle. "A poultice of my own creation will make short work of the old wounds, and a combination of hot rocks and massage will do *wonders* for your shoulder." He cleared his throat. "Um, could you just lie down for a moment, first?" Barver did, bemused. Brother Duffle stood beside Barver's head and took hold of his wing above the shoulder. "Just hold still," said Duffle. "This might . . . tickle." With unexpected force, he wrenched the wing back then pushed it forward.

There was a deeply unpleasant crunching sound, and Barver howled. He stood at once and backed away, glaring angrily at the monk. Brother Duffle toppled over, but the smile on his face was as broad as ever, and it soon widened even further—Barver started to move his shoulder, and suddenly grinned. "Good gods," said Barver. "What on earth did you just do?"

Duffle looked immensely chuffed. "Your *secundum humeri* had a dislocated *alae vallo*," he said. "Could have been like that for ages. I'm surprised you hadn't noticed."

"I have no idea what you just said," said Barver, stretching out his wings. "But you, Brother Duffle, are a genius!"

At the request of Brother Tobias, Brother Duffle led them out of the gardens and around to the side of the Abbey, which was dotted with a ramshackle collection of smaller stone buildings. He walked up to one and opened the door, revealing a large interior with a crudely built fireplace in one wall. Half the room was taken up by assorted piles of wooden boxes.

"The pigsties!" said Brother Duffle, smiling. "Oh, don't worry, we've not kept pigs at the Abbey for at least forty years. A fireplace was added so it could be habitable when necessary, although now it's mainly used for storage. Hence the boxes."

Barver peered into the nearest box and pulled out a piece of cloth, on which was embroidered "Grettings frum Marwel Abey." He looked in another box and pulled out a small misshapen lump of wood that, eventually, he identified as a model of the Abbey itself. A very *bad* model. "What is all this?" he asked.

"Souvenirs," said Duffle. "Handkerchiefs, little Abbey models, and other stuff. Some of our Brothers spend their days making them, and we sell them to visitors as a way to increase the Abbey's funds. Anything that's not quite up to scratch, we put in here. We might try and fix them, or, well ... find another use." He gestured to the fireplace. "The Abbot often says that a wasteful heart is the first step to evil! Although please don't burn anything salable."

"Understood," said Patch.

"I'll arrange a sleeping mat and bedding for later, and some candles," said Duffle. "For now, settle in and rest your weary feet. Barver, I'll return with my poultice shortly, and we can begin the rest of your treatment. The muscles in your shoulder will need a few days to settle before you can risk flight, but you'll soon be on the road to recovery." He bade farewell and left.

Barver chuckled to himself, moving his shoulder in circles and muttering, "Amazing!" every now and again.

Patch tapped gently on his coat, just where his chest pocket was. "Come on out of there," he said, gently. "Have an explore. I'm sure there'll be a nice beetle or two you can find."

Wren stuck out her head. Her eyes were still wet with tears, and her little nose was running. Patch went to the boxes and found one of the souvenir handkerchiefs. He tore a small square from one corner and gave it to her. "Here," he said. "More your size."

Wren took it and blew her nose. *I think I just want to sleep,* she signed.

"Don't be like that," said Patch. "It's not so bad. Once Barver can fly and Tobias gives us his list, it won't take long to get you cured."

She shook her head, despairing. *But what if none of those people can help me either?*

"Nonsense," said Patch. He was trying to sound as positive as possible, even though he was thinking the same thing. What if she *was* beyond help?

A distraction was needed, so he took off his bag and rummaged for the Fox and Owls board. "You and Barver should play." Beside the board were the boxwood pieces he'd stripped ready for his new Pipe. A thought struck him, and he looked over to the models of the Abbey. Bad as they were, surely it meant the Abbey had some woodcarving knives? "Actually, I think I might pop out for a bit and see if I can borrow some tools. I can spend the time getting my Pipe made."

Will your Pipe take long? signed Wren. *I imagine it needs weeks of work.*

"Goodness no!" said Patch. "Carving it only takes a few hours. Then I can cure it and decide on a glaze." The thought of his new Pipe was giving him some much-needed optimism. Wren blew her nose again, and set the mini-handkerchief down beside her. Suddenly, her stomach gave a little rumble.

She looked up at Patch with a fragile smile on her face.

You're probably right about those beetles, she signed, and she scampered off to hunt.

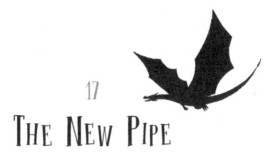

17

THE NEW PIPE

Patch returned to the pigsties a few hours later. He'd managed to borrow tools from the small group of woodcarvers in the Abbey, on condition that he stayed in the workshop as he used them. His Pipe was a joy to carve, the boxwood having a particularly good texture that made it almost soap-like to work with. The central airways didn't take long to finish with the tools at hand, and the headpiece likewise was completed very quickly. This gave him plenty of time to cut the finger holes—first the primary set, then the more intricate ones. Without feeling rushed, he took great care in their placement, although he was careful to keep his work out of sight to avoid awkward questions. As soon as he saw any of the other woodcarvers coming near, he swapped his Pipe for another piece of boxwood, which he whittled into a crude bird.

Before returning to Barver and Wren, he gathered a few more things he needed, including some hawthorn sticks and flat stones from the Abbey grounds. When he entered the old pigsties, an overwhelming smell assaulted his nose—a mixture of flowers, garlic, vinegar, and sulfur. Barver was sprawled on the floor with his eyes closed, as Brother Duffle worked the muscles of his weakened shoulder. Some of the boxes of junk had been moved to give Barver space to spread out his wings, which were smeared in places with a greenish gloop that, presumably, was the source of the stench.

Wren, meanwhile, was dozing in front of a fire built up mainly from rejected souvenir Abbeys. They burned rather well.

Duffle nodded a greeting and stopped his massage. "That'll do for today," he said. "I'm going to make a start on an ointment for tomorrow, Barver. I have a few ideas I want to try." Barver opened his eyes, rose onto all fours and folded up his wings. He stretched, and an alarming crack came from his spine. "No, no!" said Duffle. "You should stay flat for a while longer. Your back is much more delicate than you think!" He lifted his near-empty poultice jar and went to the door. "See you tomorrow," he said, and he left.

"See you, Brother Duffle," Barver called as the door closed. "Successful day, Patch? Or should I say, *Henry Smith?*" He winked.

"It went extremely well," said Patch. He set down his bag and produced his newly-carved Pipe, then played a simple scale and nodded, very happy with the sound. "I'm going to start the curing process now. How's your treatment coming along?"

Barver brought one wing up to his face and licked at the green gloop. "It's certainly *delicious*," he said, then grinned. "Brother Duffle gets *so* cross when I eat his poultice. It's doing my wings the world of good, I must say. Duffle told me it's laundry day tomorrow, so I'm going to sit in the laundry house and soak up some steam. It's the nearest thing to hot springs he can manage. A few more days, and he says I can try a small flight." He stretched his wings out as wide as the room allowed. "My shoulders and wings feel better than they have in years." He took another lick of the green poultice. "I know I shouldn't, but I just can't resist. It's too tasty."

Wren sat up and gave a big yawn. *I'll take your word for it,* she signed with a grimace.

"This from the one who loves maggots and beetles," said Patch, moving to the fireplace, where the model Abbeys burned brightly. He took the poker and tongs from beside the hearth and spread the Abbeys out. Once the fire was less fierce, he added his hawthorn and made a little chamber using the flat stones.

Is this for curing your Pipe? signed Wren.

"It is," said Patch. He produced a pot of sandy earth and poured half into the chamber, then laid his Pipe inside and covered it with the other half. He added a few more Abbeys around the sides and sat back, pleased with his work. "An hour in there, and the Pipe will almost be done." From outside came the tolling of the Abbey's bells. "That's dinner time!" he said. "I'm off to the refectory. You want me to bring a bucket of anything back, Barver?"

"Yesterday's feast will last me a week," said Barver, licking more poultice. "I really shouldn't snack."

Bring some for me, signed Wren. *I've already eaten all the beetles I could find.*

When Patch returned from the meal an hour later, Barver was sleeping in front of the fire, with Wren curled up beside him. She greeted Patch with a wave and ran over to see what he'd brought her—a little wooden bowl of stew, with a small hunk of bread. She tucked in as Patch checked on his curing Pipe. He prodded the stones and the sandy earth spilled out. With his hand wrapped in the bottom edge of his tunic, he removed the Pipe and let it cool for a few minutes before examining it carefully.

"A good result," he said, testing various combinations of

fingering. The notes from the Pipe were steady. "I've borrowed a pot of varnish, so I can get the glaze done once I've sorted out the other ingredients." He reached for his bag and took out the varnish. As he did, the folded Mask of the Hamelyn Piper clattered to the floor.

Barver opened his eyes and sat up. "Can I take another look at that?" he asked. Patch handed it to him. Barver twisted the rectangle, opening it out into the Mask and studying it. "To think, this was created by Casimir himself! My mother read me the stories of the Eight, and I think he was my favorite!"

"I didn't think dragons were interested in the Eight," said Patch.

"Not usually," said Barver. "But my mother certainly was." He had a dreamy look in his eye as he spoke. "At first, news of the Eight was only rumor—a special team assembled to find the Hamelyn Piper and bring him to justice! It was an exciting idea for a young dracogriff, all that adventure and intrigue . . . But it was only once they'd succeeded that the tales of their adventures started to come out. Every week, it seemed, a new part of their exploits would be told! With her position as an advisor to the Triumvirate, my mother got copies of the pamphlets as they appeared, and I still remember them all. First was *The Call*, when the Pipers' Council brought in a dozen of the greatest heroes they could find and tested them. Lord Drevis—a Virtus in the

Custodian Elite at the time, not a member of the Council—was chosen to lead them, and one by one the heroes proved their worth or were shown lacking, leaving the Eight we all know. Next was *The Terror of Imminus Rock*, where the Eight hoped to find a great Sorcerer to help them, but discovered instead an island full of monsters! And then came *The Caves of Casimir*, where—"

"Okay, okay," said Patch, laughing. "I was only three when it was happening and too young to understand, but by the time I was seven I knew every chapter back to front. My nan must have been tired of reading them to me."

I loved those stories, signed Wren. *Our village had a copy of the collected pamphlets.*

"*Palafox, Corrigan, Kellenfas, Stone,*" said Barver, reciting the names of the Eight. "*Casimir, Hinkelman, Drevis, and Throne.* Casimir was so mysterious! A Piper who spent decades trying to understand sorcery and called himself the Sorcerer Engineer."

Wren nodded with enthusiasm, but Patch decided not to comment. While Casimir had created the Mask and various other useful magical devices, Patch reckoned that the sheer courage and Piping skills of Stone, Palafox, and Corrigan had been more important.

Barver went to the boxes at the back of the room and took a handkerchief, using it to rub at the Mask. "There are fine symbols engraved on the inner side," he said. "I don't recognize them. Do you?" He passed it back to Patch, who looked closely at the parts Barver had cleaned up.

"They're an old runic language," said Patch. "No idea what it says, but . . . Oh, that's interesting." In the places Barver had cleaned, the darkness in the engraved lines was glinting. "I'd thought it was just dirt in the engraving," he said. "It's not." He passed the Mask back to Barver.

"What, then?" said Barver, examining it.

"I think the letters are inlaid with obsidiac," said Patch.

At once Barver let go of the Mask, dropping it as if it was red hot. "*Black diamond*," he said, sounding angry.

Wren looked confused. *Black diamond?* she signed.

"It's the dragon name for obsidiac," said Barver. "The first humans to chance upon it in the Dragon Territories thought it was ordinary obsidian, just simple volcanic glass. But soon they realized it had magical properties, and because it was only ever found in the lands of dragons they called it 'drac-obsidian,' a name which eventually became 'obsidiac.'" He shook his head slowly. "Dragons, though, have long known that it is a dark, evil substance. Corrupting. Black diamond is a much more suitable name. Just as diamond is a rare form of beauty, black diamond is a rare form of darkness."

Patch picked the Mask up again and fetched the knife from his bag. He used the tip of the blade to scratch at the dark glints in the runes. "Not leaving a mark," he said. "Pretty sure it's obsidiac."

Barver scowled.

Why do you hate it so much? signed Wren.

Barver sat down in front of the fire again and added some more model Abbeys. For a moment he watched the flames in silence, then he looked at Patch and Wren with sorrow-filled eyes. "For dragons, black diamond is so dangerous it's something only the *gods* can use. Digging it up is a kind of blasphemy."

"I thought you weren't religious," said Patch.

"I'm not," said Barver. "But most dragons *are*. There is an uneasy peace between humans and dragons, but there are those who dream of more, of cooperation and coexistence, working together. Truly sharing this world. Black diamond makes this impossible."

What do you mean? signed Wren.

"Humans come to the Dragon Territories to steal black diamond, and dragons hate them for the blasphemous theft. Dragons *burn* the humans caught stealing it, and humans hate them for the killing. Black diamond creates a circle of hatred. The world would be a better place without it."

He fell silent again, watching the fire.

Wren turned to Patch. *When I was the Sorcerer's captive,* she signed, *I read some of the books in his castle. One mentioned an old legend that obsidiac could give unnaturally long life. Is it truly that powerful?*

Patch shook his head. "Don't believe everything you

read. Sorcerers are *famous* for wasting their lives looking for immortality. It is very powerful, though. An obsidiac-glazed Pipe is supposed to be as good as they come. The obsidiac is powdered and flaked, then bound in a resin varnish and used as a Pipe glaze." Absently, Patch started looking closely at the Mask again.

"Don't even think about it," growled Barver.

"Oh, I doubt I could remove it from the grooves," said Patch, still looking at the Mask. "It's known for being extremely tough, so unless I—" He trailed off, the tone of Barver's warning finally sinking in. "No," he said. "Of course not."

There was a cold silence.

After a few moments, Wren broke the tension. *What else can you use as a glaze?* she asked.

"Some flowers are good," said Patch, flustered. "But they have to be fresh. This time of year, the ash of feathers might be the best bet."

Feathers? asked Wren.

"Yes," said Patch. "Eagles are particularly effective." He frowned, wondering where he would get any.

"Eagle, hmm?" said Barver, his voice softer now. "How about *griffin* feathers?"

"That's good too," said Patch. "Falcons as well, and buzzards. Has to be carnivores, you see, and—" He stopped, the penny dropping. "Ah," he said.

Barver was holding up three of his own feathers. "How many do you need?" he asked.

The following morning, Barver was awake the moment the dawn bells sounded.

"What's got into you?" said Patch, yawning. "Don't fancy a lie-in?"

"I'm off to the laundry," said Barver. "They get the fires lit early, so the water's hot by now. The laundry room fills with steam, Brother Duffle told me. I'll get half an hour before they need me out to get the laundry started. It'll do me the world of good."

"Well, I'll see you later," said Patch. With Barver gone, Patch went to where he'd hung his Pipe after glazing it the night before. The glaze, with its dracogriff-feather ash, had given the Pipe a rich, dark color, a deep reddish brown that Patch hadn't seen on a Pipe before. He touched it to test the varnish. "Dry!" he said, excited. He gave it a look over, then put it to his lips and played a few scales. "Good tone," he said. "Let's see if dracogriff feathers are up to the job!" He thought for a moment about which Song he should try. "A Lift, perhaps?" he said. "Yes. A Lift!"

And what's that? asked Wren, emerging from the folds of the blanket she'd spent the night in.

"Battle Pipers do it a lot," said Patch. "Lifts the mood. Raises morale." He paused, thinking back. "When I told you about the ceremony at Tiviscan, and the moment I learned I wasn't to join the Custodian Elite, you asked me what branch of the Elite they'd offered me. I didn't give you an answer."

I noticed, signed Wren. *I figured you'd tell me when you were ready.*

Patch nodded, feeling somber. "It was the Battle Elite. That was the branch that wanted me."

Not something you would consider? asked Wren.

"With Battle Piping, there are Songs with the power of cannon fire; Songs to set distant tents ablaze. But it's the Songs that increase hatred and bloodlust that are most valued. And I was so good at playing Songs that affect people, you see. That's why they wanted me. I'd dreamed of making a difference in the world, Wren. Making people better at *killing* each other wasn't what I'd had in mind."

Wren thought for a moment, then smiled. *I'm proud of you,* she signed.

"Thank you," said Patch. "Although I wish I'd just told them as much, rather than insulting them all and running away." He shook his head, then looked pointedly at Wren. "So . . . do I have a volunteer for the Lift?"

What, me? signed Wren. *No chance. That's an untested Pipe!*

"Oh, come on, you're perfectly safe. The chances of a new Pipe actually going *wrong* are tiny."

Find another idiot to try it on, she replied. She scurried over to the door, pointing through a knothole. *One of them,* she signed. *They always look like they could do with a bit of cheering up.*

Patch joined her and crouched low to peer out. There was the usual, solemn flow of monks, mostly individuals, sometimes pairs, quietly making their steady way around the Abbey in the time left to them before morning service. "I don't know," said Patch, although it appealed to a mischievous part of his mind. "A new Pipe is usually pretty weak. It might be hard to tell if it worked." He felt something tickle his hand and looked down to see an ant crawling over it. "Aha!" he said. "Perfect."

Wren was skeptical. *How do you tell if an ant's morale improves?* she signed.

"Trust me," said Patch. "Ants are always good for practice. Plus, I can keep my playing nice and quiet."

Fine, signed Wren. *Just make sure I'm not part of your experiment.*

"Don't worry," said Patch. "Stay beside me, we won't be affected. With things like the Lift, it's a simple matter of moderating the direction, range, and nature of your subject to guarantee that the Song doesn't spill out beyond the desired target. Easy peasy."

Easy? signed Wren. *Isn't that what happened to make the villagers dance in Patterfall?*

Patch winced at the thought. "That was a lapse of concentration," he said. "Could happen to anyone." After carefully placing the ant in the middle of the room, he put his Pipe to his lips, furrowed his brow, then started to play. The Lift was a very simple Song at its core, and Patch had always been good at it. No wonder, really—it shared many of its patterns with the Dance, although it didn't *direct* the subject in any way and was much less potent. All it did was perk them up, and the resulting effect varied considerably from subject to subject.

Patch built up the heart of the Song. It took him back to the days when he'd sat in the woods by his grandparents' home, whistling and seeing the effect it had on the wildlife as they drew near, intrigued and playful.

The little ant, which had started to march back toward the doorway, stopped. Its tiny head tilted up slowly, then moved down again; then up, then down. It started walking once more, but there was a definite *swing* to the motion, left and right, and it sped up and slowed down to the Song's rhythm. It began to take an extra little step to each side as it went, and from time to time it turned in a circle on the spot. It continued in the same way until it reached the door. Wren looked at it, delighted. *That's one happy ant*, she signed. The ant tapped out the music for a moment, then made its way under the door and outside. Wren watched its progress through the knothole. Suddenly she turned back to Patch.

Hold on, she signed. *I think your Song has spilled out a little!*

Patch stopped playing, and the Song faded gently. "Oooh, listen to that," he said, distracted by the Pipe. "The sustain is impressive! It usually takes a few more—"

Wren interrupted him with a cough and pointed at the knothole. Patch crouched down to look out again.

The monks were still making their way around the Abbey, but now their pace had picked up, oh-so-slightly; from time to time, some had a bit of a skip in their step. The clearest change, though, was that most were smiling. There were even, shockingly, a few laughs to be heard.

Did you have another lapse in concentration? signed Wren.

"Not this time," said Patch. The Pipe was silent at last, and he looked at it with genuine satisfaction. "This packs a punch, let me tell you. Dracogriff feathers are now *officially* my favorite."

How long will the Lift affect them? asked Wren.

"That depends on the monk," said Patch. "Some, I imagine, will decide that they're *far* too serious for all that smiling. Others, well . . . it might stay with them for a few hours." In the distance, through the meandering monks, he caught sight of someone who definitely did *not* have a smile on his face. "Look who it is," said Patch. "Brother Duffle."

Duffle had a stern expression, but there was a hint of puzzlement there too. He paused, looking at the smiling faces of the strolling monks. He shook his head and continued, making a beeline for the pigsties.

Wren frowned. *What's troubling him?* she signed. *I hope Barver's okay!*

"What is it, Brother?" asked Patch when Duffle reached them.

"There's a dire situation," said Duffle. "Brother Tobias needs you in the infirmary, right away!"

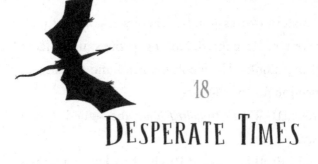

18

DESPERATE TIMES

With Wren in his pocket, Patch followed Brother Duffle to a small room within the infirmary. On one wall were shelves of old books, bottles, and containers. Brother Tobias was standing by a table on which sat various sizes of pestle and mortar and bunches of herbs and plants in the process of preparation.

"You can leave us, Brother Duffle," said Tobias. "Thank you."

"I'll return to Barver," said Duffle. "Some light massage as he takes in the steam, I think."

Once Duffle had gone, Tobias gave Patch a cold look. "*Henry Smith*," he said. "An interesting choice of name. As an escaped convict, you could have spelled trouble for the Abbey, Patch Brightwater!"

Patch felt his ears redden, but before he could ask how Brother Tobias had learned the truth, the monk turned and left the room through a second doorway. As he went, Patch could see he was holding something in his hand. He almost gasped to see it—a Pipe. What was a monk doing with a Pipe?

A moment later he *did* gasp, because through the doorway Tobias had left by, someone else entered.

Erner Whitlock.

"Patch!" cried Erner, hurrying over to him. Wren emerged from Patch's pocket and climbed up to his shoulder. "It's really you! And Wren! I thought you were both *dead*!" Erner flung his arms around Patch and gave him a hug, a look of immense relief on the Apprentice Custodian's face. When Erner let go and stood back, Patch stared at him.

"Oh no," said Patch. "Oh no, oh no, oh no . . ."

Erner looked at him, confused. "Why do you look at me with such horror? I can't tell you how thankful I am to see you alive! Virtus Stone and I were traveling to Yarmingly when news came through of the attack on Tiviscan. We heard that the Hamelyn Piper was dead and that some prisoners had died too. Including the young lad who'd only just been locked away, they said! The Piper of Patterfall!" He shook his head, clearly distressed. "An awful thing to hear, Patch. *Awful*. When we arrived at the Abbey just an hour ago, Brother Tobias told me that Wren was here, accompanied by a dracogriff and a young lad calling himself Henry Smith." Erner shook his head, smiling now. "I didn't dare hope, but here you are. Both of you!" When Patch and Wren still said nothing, Erner's confusion returned. "But still you look at me so strangely—"

Patch's mouth felt horribly dry. He kept glancing at the door, expecting Rundel Stone to enter at any moment. "Don't you understand? You've found me alive, and it's your duty to see me delivered back to the dungeons! Where is your master, anyway? I would have thought Rundel Stone would be *incredibly* pleased to be able to slap some manacles on me!"

Erner's smile dropped away. "My duty . . . yes. Perhaps it is. In all the relief of seeing you, it hadn't occurred to me. But Patch, please . . . I'll not tell a soul, not even the Virtus. Stay as Henry Smith, and you'll be safe. Nobody will know!"

Wren tutted. *Brother Tobias already knows*, she signed.

"Oh, ah, yes," said Erner, wincing. "Brother Tobias. I'm sorry. I blurted it all out when he told me you were here, Wren. I'll tell nobody else!"

"I know you mean well," said Patch, still glancing nervously at the doorway. "But Virtus Stone would never allow such a thing. Where is he, anyway?"

And what was the dire situation we were told about? signed Wren. *Was that just a trick, to get Patch to come here?*

Erner shook his head, looking grim. "No trick," he said. "You see, things have become rather complicated." He walked to the doorway. "Follow me, and I'll explain."

Erner led them through to the main part of the infirmary. Twenty simple beds were in a long hall, and each bed was full—there were men and women, old and young, being tended by three monks.

At the far end of the hall was a curtained area, and from there Patch could hear the sound of a Pipe. Once they reached the curtain, Erner pulled it aside. By the wall was a bed, and sitting on its edge was Brother Tobias, playing the Pipe he'd carried out with him.

Patch listened, impressed by the complexity of the Song Tobias played—a healing Song, and far more intricate than any he'd ever managed to learn. "Wow," he said.

Erner nodded. "Impressive, isn't it?" he said, his voice barely above a whisper. "Brother Tobias was a Piper before he took holy orders. He could make a fine living, yet he's chosen a life in the Abbey and to give his skills for free."

For the first time, Patch turned his eyes to the patient lying in the bed, and he almost jumped. There lay Rundel Stone, his eyes closed and his skin horribly pale. "What happened to him?" said Patch.

"We were called to the village of Yarmingly," said Erner. "There had been a death, and the dead man was a close friend of the Virtus. The cause of death was obvious, and gruesome—several blows to the back of the head. We'd been there only a few minutes when Virtus Stone cried out and collapsed to the ground. Half-conscious, he ordered me to bring him here. I had to stop often and play a healing Song, just to keep him alive. Brother Tobias and his monks have treated him since, but he has not woken, and the cause of his condition is a mystery."

Brother Tobias stopped playing and beckoned them. "Quickly, Erner! He's coming around!"

Erner rushed to the bedside; Patch moved to follow, but Wren squeaked at him from his shoulder.

You should keep your distance, she signed. *Better Stone doesn't see you!*

Stone gave a spluttering cough and opened his eyes. "Virtus!" said Erner. "It's me! Apprentice Whitlock! Can you tell me what caused your collapse?"

Stone gripped Erner's arm. "An *enigma enicatus!*" he said, struggling for breath. "A death puzzle. A *box*, Erner. A small metal box. I found it under a book on the floor, near to where Ural lay dead. I felt its sting as I grasped it and realized my mistake too late!"

Ural . . . thought Patch. The name of Stone's dead friend was somehow familiar, but he couldn't quite place it.

Brother Tobias checked Stone's hand. "There! A small mark, some kind of needle." He looked at Erner. "Did you see the box he speaks of?"

"Well, I did find this on the floor near the Virtus," said Erner. He reached into his pocket and pulled out a small metal cube, about an inch across.

"Don't touch it!" cried Stone. He knocked the box from Erner's hand. The effort was too much for him—he slumped back, and his eyes closed.

Erner looked at Tobias, shaking his head. "I already *did* touch it, Tobias, yet it did nothing to me."

"Death puzzles have specific targets," said Tobias. "You touched it without incident, but Rundel was stung. That means *he* was a target." He rushed to his room and returned with wooden tongs and a jar. He picked the metal cube from the floor and dropped it inside the jar, then held it up for a clear view.

Stone opened his eyes again, straining to speak. "Identify its targets, and you find the killer!"

"Forget finding the killer," said Brother Tobias. "Your *life* is the priority now, Rundel. Healing Songs can keep you alive for a time, but I fear I can't treat this, not fully. There's sorcery at work here." He paused. "You suspected as much, Rundel. You didn't come here to get help from me—you came to get help from *her*. Didn't you!"

Wren frowned at Patch. *Her,* she signed. *Who does he mean?*

"Yes," said Stone. "I sensed it was no simple poison. A Sorcerer's poison, needing a Sorcerer for the cure. You know where you must take me!"

Tobias looked away. "You're asking too much!"

"Please, Tobias!" cried Stone. "*Please!*" He tensed and cried out in agony, then went limp.

Tobias examined him. "Unconscious," he said. "And refusing to die. Stubborn as ever." He shook his head and hit the nearby wall in frustration. "That settles it, we have no choice." He looked directly at Patch. "I only pray that the expert we both seek has the answers we require."

"The expert we *both* seek?" said Patch. "Both?"

Tobias nodded. "You'll be coming as well. Wren's best hope is also Rundel's. I told you there was too much danger, and I meant it, but now Rundel's life is on the brink. Where we're headed, your dracogriff friend will keep us safe, to a point. We must leave at once. It's a full day's journey by horse, Erner, and while we're gone you must stay here and play that healing Song, to the best of your ability, for one hour out of every four. It'll be grueling work, but it's the only thing that will keep Rundel alive. Can you manage it?"

"I can," said Erner.

"And, um, where exactly are *we* going?" said Patch.

"You've heard of the Gemspar Range?" said Tobias.

Patch frowned. His training had involved studying notoriously treacherous locations throughout the world, and the Gemspar Range was high on that list. "Home of vicious criminals and unbounded danger," he said. "It has quite a reputation. There's also the mythical Witch who, legend says, makes the central peak of the range her home— Gemspar Mountain itself! A foreboding craggy deathtrap, by all accounts."

"Afraid of old myths, are you?" said Tobias.

"Oh please," said Patch. "I know there's no actual *Witch*, but the Gemspar Range is a hostile place, home to the worst smugglers and wrongdoers in the land. The Witch was just a story to frighten people away from the area. But those are all pretty *scary* old myths, Brother Tobias. Even *you* have to admit it."

"I'll grant they're unpleasant tales," said Tobias.

"Unpleasant?" scoffed Patch. "Horrible murders, horrible monsters, a horrible warty old hag of a Witch! Kept me up at night, some of those tales. She was said to have extra joints in her arms that she could make grow a hundred feet long. Her enemies would be strangled in their beds with their doors locked, the only clue being a sprinkling of soot from the fireplace. Her eyes were supposed to shine bright in the dark, so you could see her blink in the depths of the forest." He shivered. "Besides brigands, I'm surprised *anyone* wants to make their home somewhere so creepy! Your *expert* must really like privacy."

"That is certainly true," said Tobias. "She *absolutely* does."

"So, um, who exactly are we going to see?" said Patch, an awful feeling stirring in his guts.

Brother Tobias widened his eyes. "We're off to see the Witch of Gemspar Mountain!" he said.

Patch whimpered.

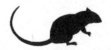

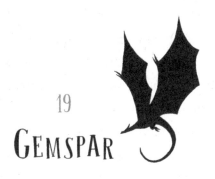

19
GEMSPAR

The Abbey possessed only five horses, and the group took three of them. Patch was given the smallest, a friendly black-and-white mare. He tied his bag to his saddle, and Wren opted to sit on his shoulder rather than be cooped up for the journey in his pocket. As well as Tobias, they were joined by a burly monk called Brother Madder, who was armed with a decidedly un-monkly broadsword.

Barver was reluctantly dragged from the warmth of his steam treatment and looked rather grumpy when Brother Duffle led him to the front of the Abbey to join the others. "Be careful!" Duffle told him. "Absolutely no flying, and if you *must* kill any brigands, don't strain your shoulder in the process."

"Okay, okay, I promise," said Barver, and Duffle waved him farewell. Barver looked at Patch and Wren. "Bit of a rude awakening to have to leave that lovely heat and come out here," he said. "Duffle was vague about where we're going. Can you fill me in on the details?"

Wren told him everything. When she got to the part about the Witch, Barver went strangely quiet.

The presence of Barver unsettled the horses a little, so he kept himself to the back of their column, with Patch next, then Tobias, and Madder leading. They kept up a rapid pace, riding mostly in silence.

They stopped to rest only once, letting the horses drink from a stream and graze its banks. Patch took his Pipe from his pocket to take a look at some of the lowest finger holes— while playing the Lift earlier, he'd felt some rough edges on the mouthpiece that he needed to fix, but he'd not had a chance to deal with it until now. He used the tip of his knife to gently smooth the wood.

Brother Tobias approached him. "Ah!" he said. "Erner Whitlock told me you were a trainee Piper before you were put in the dungeons. I suggest you put your Pipe away, though. I have my Pipe with me too, but I'll only use it if the worst comes to the worst. Be in no doubt: *Barver* is our protection in Gemspar. The brigands there have evaded capture from the Custodian Elite for a very long time. Anyone they see with a Pipe is likely to have a dozen arrows in them before a single note can be played. A dracogriff will give them reason to stay well clear of us."

Patch nodded. Before they set off, he made sure to put his Pipe in his bag.

By afternoon they could see the peaks of the Gemspar Range, and by evening they had reached the forest on the slopes of the first of the mountains. The path was rough, growing narrower with each passing mile, as the forest grew thicker.

Brother Madder held up his hand for the party to stop. "From here on," he told them, "there must be absolute silence. If anyone sees anything suspicious, they should draw my attention by clapping their hands together twice."

"And, um, what are we looking for?" asked Patch.

"Brigands. Bandits. Thieves," said Madder. "Given Barver's presence, anyone who attacks us will have to be especially crazed. That would make them especially *dangerous*."

Barver raised a hand. "I want to clarify the rules of engagement," he said. "Is fire breathing okay?"

"Feel free," said Madder.

"And am I allowed to *eat* anyone who attacks us?"

"Absolutely," said Madder, with a sly grin.

Patch and Wren stared at Barver. The dracogriff shrugged. "I'm kidding!" he said, although they weren't sure if he was.

From then on, Patch scanned the gloomy forest constantly. He saw nothing with his eyes, but his mind spotted dozens of nonexistent, cutthroat villains hiding behind every trunk, every bush, every pine cone, every leaf. He broke out in a sweat as his anxiety grew.

The peaks of the Gemspar Range towered above, but it was another hour before the razor-jag tip of Gemspar Mountain itself became visible: bare, black rock that seemed to cut and slice at the sky.

Behind him Patch could hear Barver's stomach gurgle continuously, the only sound coming from his otherwise stealthy friend. Patch slowed, dropping back a little from the others, and turned to Barver. Heeding Brother Madder's earlier warning of silence, he used hand speech.

Are you okay? he asked.

I think it's Brother Duffle's poultice, answered Barver. He rubbed his belly, looking queasy. *I don't think it agreed with me.*

Do you need to rest?

Barver shook his head. *It'll pass*, he signed, and sure enough it did seem to settle down.

The forest path began to weave as they ventured through a valley deep in the Range. Steep climbs became precarious drops, and the path led them through twisting high-walled gullies that Barver was only just able to fit through.

The narrow path, with high trees all around and little sky to see, gave Patch an increasing sense of claustrophobia. Then, as they rounded a series of tight bends, a clearing lay ahead. Patch smiled with relief and turned around to look at Barver.

Barver wasn't there.

Terrified, Patch clapped his hands twice. At the head

of the group, Brother Madder turned and stared, seeing at once that their main protection had vanished. He guided his horse to Patch.

"Where is he?" whispered Madder.

"I don't know," said Patch. "He was behind me a minute ago."

Madder eyed the trees warily and went back around the bends they'd just passed. After a few moments he returned. "No sign of him," said Madder, his intense gaze darting around the trees. "We may be in trouble."

"You think somebody—" said Patch, disbelieving.

Wren was horrified. *Somebody nobbled Barver?* she signed. *How?*

"To the clearing, quickly!" said Madder, taking his horse to the front and picking up speed.

It was too late.

The vegetation around them erupted into life. Fifty well-armed bandits burst from behind every tree and bush, with a huge cry of "*Yaaaaarrgh!*"

They were caked in grime, and a smell like month-old pigswill filled the air. The bandits shook their various weapons at the travelers, growling menacingly as the leader stepped forward and addressed their victims. He was especially grubby, his hair long and matted, his blackening teeth on display as he grinned. Patch very slowly started to reach back to his bag; despite the warning Tobias had given, if they'd hurt Barver he was going to try and take out some of them before he was disarmed.

"Welcome to our forest, wanderers!" said the leader. His fellow robbers jeered and waggled their blades some more. "A dangerous forest too! It's lucky that we chanced on you this day!" Another jeer came, with some coughing from the less-healthy members of the group. "Me and my friends wish to offer you protection against the evils here. A basilisk walks the woods!" A mock-scared "Wooooo!" came from the bandits. "An evil Witch haunts the mountain!" An "Ahhhhhh!" from the thieves. "Worst of all, the most feared band of murderous villains also prowls these parts!"

He paused for dramatic effect.

"And that's *us!*" he said, flourishing his sword as the brigands cheered long and loud. "Who better to offer you protection from our blood-keen knives, friends, than we ourselves? So if you would, a simple fee!" He paused again, and the grinning outlaws looked at him with anticipation, waiting for the punchline. "*All you have!*" cried the gloating leader, as every blade—long sword, short sword, knife and dagger—moved in to point steadily at the travelers, each blade-tip no more than a foot from flesh.

Patch's hand froze halfway to his bag. He looked at the brigand whose sword-tip was nearest his throat and slowly brought his hand back to his horse's reins. Playing a Pipe would be *much* harder without fingers.

Madder, his broadsword half-drawn, gave an angry growl and shook his head. "Without Barver we have no chance," he muttered. He put the sword back in its scabbard and reached into his cassock, producing a small pouch. He threw it to the bandit leader. "Take it, and let us be on our way!"

The leader caught the pouch and looked at the contents. He raised an eyebrow. "This is all you have?" he said. "I think not!" He stroked his chin for a moment then suddenly looked at Madder's horse, pretending to be surprised. "Goodness!" he said. "A horse! And another! And a third! These should cover your fee, I think." The malice in his voice was matched by that in his eyes.

Madder gritted his teeth. "So if we give you our horses too, we can go on our way?"

"*If* you give us your horses? When we *take* your horses, then we'll see! Right, lads?" A sinister cheer came from his fellows.

"Might I ask what you did with our companion?" said Madder. "Is he alive?"

"Companion?" said the leader. "What companion?" He dismissed Madder's question with a shake of his head, and at that moment spotted Wren on Patch's shoulder. She was standing defiantly with her arms folded, glaring. The leader was fascinated. "What on *earth* is that?" he asked, then smiled. "What curious markings!"

From behind him another bandit—face wide with fear—cried out: "Dragon!"

The leader turned to him with a look of complete scorn. "Don't be stupid, man!" he said. "It's obviously a rat!"

But by then all of his men were staring past him with widening eyes, their bravado gone. Patch and Wren turned to see, and grinned: Barver was striding around the bend in the path. His expression was one of outrage—although, Patch saw, there was also a hint of glee at the reaction he was getting.

The dracogriff stopped, eyeing up the terrified brigands who, for now, seemed rooted to the spot. "If you've hurt any of my friends," cried Barver, "I will have to eat you. *Alive*." There was a moment of silence, broken only by one or two sobs of dread. Barver let rip with a huge burst of flame and a thunderous roar, then charged forward. The thieves scattered at once, squealing like piglets as they fled. Barver had set his sights on the leader. He seized the man by his feet and dangled him upside down. "I wonder how *you'll* taste," he said, leering.

"They're all fine!" cried the leader. "Your pals! All fine! Just our little . . . joke! Yes! A joke!"

But they weren't *quite* all fine. The horses had been seriously scared by Barver's fiery entrance, and were in a panic—particularly Patch's, which was hurtling around the perimeter of the clearing, whinnying in terror.

Patch was barely able to hang on to the reins; Wren was off his shoulder and clinging on for dear life to the saddle. The horse wasn't slowing—indeed, each time it caught a glance of Barver, the animal managed to go even faster. Patch reached back to his bag, trying to grip the horse with his legs so he wouldn't fall. At last, his fingers wrapped around his Pipe.

"Yes!" he cried, almost losing his balance. "Don't worry, Wren! I've got this!"

There was a Battle Song he knew, one that could be used against cavalry. It slowed a horse down, whatever the plans of the rider or the horse. Patch quickly looped the reins around his left arm and gripped even harder with his legs, leaving his hands free to Pipe. "Hold on tight!" he said to Wren. Her little face grimaced with effort as she clung to the saddle.

This was no time to be subtle, he knew; he went for it, and built the Song up as fast as possible. Finally, he played the key melody that would slow the horse down.

It stopped dead. Patch kept going.

Over the horse's head he went, and the ground came up fast to greet him with a hard, stony welcome. When his head stopped spinning, he sat up and looked behind him. There was his horse, slightly confused, and on the saddle sat Wren, giving him a thumbs up.

Patch stood, trying to ignore the pain in his shoulder and

the smarting of his scraped knees. He went to the horse and took the reins, leading it back to Barver and the others.

All the brigands had abandoned their leader, who was now lying on the ground with his wrists and ankles tied, a gag in his mouth, and Madder's sword against his throat.

"So what happened to you?" Patch called to Barver.

"I had to go," said Barver, sheepish.

"What?"

"I had to *go*. Brother Duffle's poultice—" He rubbed his belly. "Sorry about that."

Wren jumped from the horse to Patch's shoulder and scowled at Barver. *We thought something had happened to you!* she signed.

"We're all okay," said Patch. "That's what matters." He looked at the brigand leader. "What do we do with him?"

Madder grinned, leering close to their captive's face. "What indeed!" he said. "All your friends have gone. And they won't be back."

The leader tried to speak through his gag. "Mmmpph!" he said. "Mmmph mmmpph!"

"A few years back I would've cut your throat on principle," said Brother Madder. "But I'm a man of God these days."

Tobias kneeled down beside him. "Maybe he can be useful," he said, pulling the gag down. "We're here to seek help from the Witch."

The leader laughed. "The Witch doesn't help people," he said. "Unless they want help to *die horribly*."

"You've met her?" said Tobias.

"None meet her and live!" said the leader. "We stay clear; she leaves us alone. You'd be wise to do the same. I've heard things screaming in the trees when I've got too close to her territory. You're idiots if you seek her out!"

Brother Madder pressed the blade of his sword a little harder against the man's throat. "Less of the backchat, scum. Is she easy to reach from here?"

"Follow the path until it splits, and you'll know which way to take. Trust me, you'll know . . ."

Madder took his sword away from the leader's neck and forced him to his feet. "You'd best run along now," said Madder. "Before I decide to kill you anyway. I'm sure God would grant me forgiveness if I asked nicely."

"Untie me, eh?" said the leader, his bound ankles making him wobble as he stood. "Please? Dangerous place this forest. Lots of undesirables, you know?"

Barver strode up to him and brought his head down until he was face to face with the trembling prisoner. For long seconds he studied the man. "You know what they say about the *eyes*," said Barver with a grin.

"They're the windows to the soul?" said the leader.

Barver shook his head and put the gag back over the man's mouth. "Tastiest part of the face," he said. The leader let out a muffled squeal and started hopping toward the trees, falling over every few hops. Barver watched him go, with a look of pure satisfaction.

Brother Madder swapped horses with Patch. "She knows me," said Madder, letting the animal nuzzle him. "And if I take her up to the front of the line, she'll not panic again."

Patch took Madder's horse, and went to put his Pipe in his pocket.

Tobias nodded to him. "Let me see it then, lad," he said. Patch handed the Pipe over, and Tobias examined it. "Your Song was a little stronger than needed, but given the situation it was impressive. Whitlock told me you were talented, and he was right."

"I have my moments," said Patch.

Barver tutted. "Listen to him! He's being modest. They offered him a role in the Battle Elite, but he turned it down, not wanting death and destruction to be his life."

Patch raised an eyebrow and gave Wren a pointed glance. "Do you share everything I tell you with Barver?" he said.

Friends don't have secrets, signed Wren.

"I too was in the Battle Elite," said Tobias, and Patch noticed the man's expression change suddenly, looking almost haunted. "You made the right decision, lad. The scars cut deep, and they stay with you for the rest of your days. And I don't just mean *this*." He gestured to the terrible scar that ran down the side of his face.

After another hour of travel, they came to the split in the path that the leader of the brigands had told them about. On the path to the right, the forest continued without change, and songbirds perched among the leaves and tweeted happily. To the left, the trees were stunted, diseased things, the bushes spiky, and blackened by fungus. The only wildlife Patch could see were crows, sulking in large groups on leafless branches.

"Well," said Madder, with a wary smile. "He said we'd know the way to the Witch when we saw it."

They took the leftward path.

The peak of Gemspar Mountain loomed high above them. Patch felt uneasy when he looked at it, as if the sharpness of the rocks was pricking at his eyes.

As dusk approached, Brother Tobias held up his hand and called for a halt. "We're almost there I think," he said, sounding anxious.

"How should we approach her domain?" asked Brother Madder.

"The two of us will leave our horses and proceed on foot," said Tobias. He turned to the others. "The rest of you wait here. We're taking a great risk, and I can't say for certain how the Witch will react. We'll be back by dark."

With the horses tethered, Patch and his friends were happy enough to watch Tobias and Madder walk off to meet the Witch, but their nerves grew frayed as the light started to fail with no sign of the monks returning. Moonlight was all they had, lending yet another sinister edge to the forest.

What if they've been killed already? signed Wren, on Patch's shoulder. *Or eaten? Or turned inside out and rubbed with salt and then eaten? While still alive!*

"They'll be back soon," said Patch. "There's no need to worry. Barver will protect us."

From behind that tree? signed Wren.

Patch turned to look. Sure enough, Barver was hiding behind a large oak, peering around it fearfully. "Oh, come out here, you big wuss," said Patch.

"I don't like it," said Barver, edging out from hiding. "All this creepy stuff. I just don't."

A low moan came from the forest ahead of them. Nobody said anything, but Patch stood up slowly and started to walk in the direction of the sound.

Wren squeaked at him. *You're going* toward *the sound?* she signed. *Count me out.* She scurried down his leg and ran to Barver.

"It might be Tobias and Madder," whispered Patch. "Maybe they need our help." He felt for his Pipe, whatever use it might be, then remembered it was in his bag. "Barver?" he said. "Come on!"

Barver shook his head. "Uh-uh," he said. "Absolutely no way."

There was another low moan, longer this time, followed by what could only be described as a *cackle*.

"Okay," said Patch. "So it's not Tobias and Madder."

Two bright circles appeared in the gloom, fifty feet from where they stood. Patch's legs wobbled. The light from the circles (Patch didn't want to think of them as *eyes*, not yet) made it easier to see the shape *around* the circles, and the two long dark lines on either side of it.

The shape was that of a bent figure. The two *very* long lines were about the width of arms, held out as if to embrace. Or to *grab*.

Patch backed away. The circles of light went off and came on again.

"It blinked!" said Barver.

The next moan was louder, longer, and far more ghastly. The cackle that followed was unmistakable. The dark figure shifted slightly, moving toward them one slow step at a time.

Patch kept backing off until he bumped into Barver, who was rigid with fear and staring at the wailing *thing* that was approaching.

Wren climbed over to Patch's shoulder again. They huddled together, the three of them, trembling and whimpering.

And the Witch of Gemspar Mountain drew ever closer.

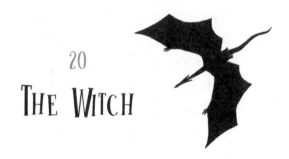

20

THE WITCH

The Witch was wearing a black cowl. Its arms, ten feet long, ended in deathly white claws that twitched with each step it took. The disc-like eyes glowed in the midst of a face as craggy as the mountain itself, and under the eyes an oversized mouth gaped open, revealing discolored teeth like ancient tombstones.

Patch could feel his sanity draining away, such was the terror he felt, and from the sound of her whimpers Wren was the same. The scariest noise of all, thought Patch, had to be Barver's hitched breaths: the dracogriff was paralyzed with dread.

Then the Witch let out a hideous screech and Patch decided that no, actually, *that* was the scariest noise of all. As one, the group answered with their own long, drawn-out scream, which only faded when another voice cut through the air.

"Alia, stop it! They're with me!"

The Witch instantly halted. Without moving her mouth she answered in a voice that didn't sound anything like the cackling wails she'd been making so far: "Who said that?"

From the trees to the far left of the cowering group, Brother Tobias emerged, Brother Madder beside him.

"It's me! It's Tobias!" he said. "We need—" He paused and shook his head. "*I* need your help, Alia. Please. For old times' sake."

The Witch's long arms slowly lowered until the claws were on the ground. The light in the eyes faded. From behind the Witch, a second figure emerged in a gray hooded robe. It walked in front of the Witch's still form, then over to Tobias and Madder. Its hands—on the end of ordinary-sized arms—reached up and pulled back its hood.

Patch gaped. The figure was a woman, and a beautiful one at that. She was looking at Tobias with a defiantly raised eyebrow.

"Brother Tobias," she said. "I always knew some day you'd come walking back through my door." She frowned and glanced around at the trees. "Metaphorically speaking."

As Tobias and the woman spoke, Patch looked again toward the Witch, squinting to try and see better in the moonlight. He had a moment of realization, and all his fear vanished suddenly. With one eye on the newcomer in the gray robe, he walked toward the Witch.

Wren was on his shoulder, and she wasn't happy. *What are you doing?* she signed. *Stop!*

"It's okay," said Patch. "Take another look, Wren."

As they got closer, it became obvious. The frightening face was just paper, glue, and paint; the terrible claws were jointed wood.

It's a puppet! signed Wren. *A big, horrible puppet!* She hopped off Patch's shoulder onto the "Witch" and vanished under the black cloth that covered it.

Barver arrived by Patch's side. "Never tell anyone about this," he said. "Not in the Islands of the Eastern Seas, anyway. I wouldn't live it down."

Wren reappeared on top of the Witch's head. *The eyes are lamps,* she signed, clearly impressed. *There are all sorts of levers back here!*

Barver reached out to one of the long arms and waggled it up and down. It broke off in his hand.

"Hey, leave that alone!" called the woman. She walked over, Tobias and Madder behind her.

"Um, sorry," said Barver. He half-heartedly tried to poke the arm back into position, and when he let it go it fell to the ground. "I didn't mean to break it."

The woman lifted the end of the arm and slotted it back

into place. "It's far more delicate than it looks," she said, tetchy. She stared at Barver. "And *what* are you?"

"The name's Barver," he said. "I'm a dracogriff."

She turned to Patch. "And you?"

"Patch Brightwater," he said. "Uh, human."

The woman shook her head, unimpressed, but then she saw Wren sitting on top of the Witch-puppet. "Ah! Now you . . . you're a different prospect entirely. Cursed, eh?"

Wren nodded. *I'm here so you can cure me,* she signed, but the woman waved a dismissive hand at her.

"No, no, stop all that," she said. "I don't understand a word."

Tobias stepped in. "Alia, this is Wren. She's part of the reason we're here. Everyone, this is Alia, the Witch of Gemspar Mountain."

"Obviously not the *original* Witch," said Alia. "So, the rat curse is *part* of why you came. What's the rest of it?"

"I need help with a patient who is close to death," said Tobias. "A poison runs through his veins, one that is dripping with sorcery."

Alia shrugged. "And why should I care?"

"The patient is Rundel Stone," said Tobias.

She scowled at him. "I say again, why should I care?" Tobias said nothing and just looked at her. After a few moments Alia sighed and shook her head, clearly irritated. "Oh all *right*. Give me a minute to pack up." She reached under the black cloth that covered the main bulk of the Witch-puppet, and pulled. The arms grew shorter and folded themselves under the cloth. She nodded at Wren. "Do you mind?" she said politely, and Wren hopped from the puppet to Patch's shoulder. Alia pushed down on the head, which retracted, and then shoved hard against what remained of the puppet. It pivoted down, and Alia gathered up the cloth and shut a lid. The entire puppet was now contained in a wheeled box, like a small handcart.

Wren couldn't resist giving a little round of applause.

"Everyone get your things and follow me," said Alia.

She nodded to Barver and pointed to the cart. "Make yourself useful and push that. Just try not to damage it!"

She led them through the trees to a forbidding path between high volcanic cliffs. They emerged into a large open area, most of which was desolate. The peak of Gemspar Mountain loomed over them like a constant threat, yet among this desolation, next to the entrance to a cave in the side of the mountain, was an expanse of grass, perhaps eighty feet across, with various fruiting bushes and a vegetable patch, all surrounded by a fence. It looked like the whole thing had been cut out of a different landscape and dropped here.

Alia saw their bemused looks and smiled.

"Welcome to my home," she said. "The cave is ancient, but the garden is my own construction."

Tobias was obviously impressed. "Does it not drain you, to sustain this kind of green magic?"

She shook her head. "The only magic needed for the garden was for the transportation of soil, Tobias. It gets plenty of sun and water, all free."

With the horses tied up, she led them into the cave. It seemed extensive, going back into the rock of the mountain for at least a few hundred feet, before bending away out of sight, the true extent impossible to tell. Lamps were burning everywhere, keeping it bright. Simple shelves were filled with glass jars of various contents, some of which were rather grim. Patch made an effort not to look at them too closely.

Barver still pushed the Witch-puppet, and Alia pointed to a spot by one shelf. "Over there, if you don't mind," she said, and Barver did as instructed. "The birds and insects around here are my eyes and ears. It's easy to tell when there are intruders in my part of the forest. Not very common, these days. My reputation seems to be enough discouragement."

"Why do you have the puppet?" asked Barver. "Surely you can just . . ." He made a spell-casting motion with one hand.

Alia gave him a warm smile. "Magic is an effort. I save my powers for the work that interests me. Lately I've not had need for elaborate magical defenses. *Witchy* there is rather effective at chasing off strays. Also, she's considerable *fun*." She walked across to a large trunk and opened

215

it up. It contained a vast number of little glass vials and bottles. "This is research," she said. "Out here, I refine my skills in peace." She gave Tobias a long, pointed glare. "In *peace*, Tobias. I wanted to be left alone, and never see any of you again. Why have you broken your word?"

Patch looked from Alia to Tobias and back again, feeling a very definite chill in the air.

"I kept my word," said Tobias. "Until I had no choice."

"And now you're here," she said. "Seeking help from the all-terrible Witch, even though I swore I would *kill* you if you came. *Any* of you."

Patch frowned, wondering who exactly Alia meant by "any of you." He shared a worried look with Wren and Barver.

Alia caught the look on Patch's face. She narrowed her eyes at him, making Patch's knees suddenly feel very wobbly. "Do I disappoint?" she said to him. "Did you want to see the old Witch, the *mad* Witch? I can pretend to be like that, if you want. I can be what the Council thought I was. A seeker of unnatural power, dabbling in things no Piper should touch! Things that even Casimir feared!" She clenched her fists and turned toward the cave entrance. As she went, the lamps within the cave dimmed as one.

Patch felt Wren's claws grip tightly to his coat, and he found himself putting his own hand on Barver for support.

Outside the cave, the moonlit sky was clear. Alia raised

her arms, and clouds seemed to congeal out of the heavens. "Power without limit!" cried Alia, and the clouds began to move in a slow spiral. Lightning flashed within them. "Unconstrained! Terrifying!" she cried, before shouting out a long series of incomprehensible words, each spoken with unmistakable rage. Lightning flared like none of them had ever seen before—tinged purple and red, it spread out in shapes like claws, bathing the whole forest in irate light. She lowered her arms. Gradually, the lightning faded, and the clouds vanished. The lamps within the cave grew bright once more. She turned to Tobias and heaved a deep sigh. "Is that *fear* I see in your eyes?" she said to him. "I don't know what hurts me more. That you broke your word or that you kept it for so long. That you really believed I could hurt *you*, of all people. You really did fear me."

Tobias suddenly looked rather fragile. "I kept my vow," he said. "I left you alone. But not because I feared you. I did it because you *asked* me to." She said nothing in reply, only looked at him with sadness. Tobias put his hand on her shoulder. "It's . . . it's good to see you again."

Alia seemed dazed for a moment. Then she stepped away, letting his hand fall from her. "I half expected a visit from someone," she said. "Given what happened at Tiviscan."

"You heard about the attack?" said Tobias.

She nodded. "A little bird told me. I'm not surprised Drevis didn't come. I *might* have killed him."

"It was the Council who expelled you, Alia, and that was before Drevis was one of them. He was always on your side. And while Casimir was your greatest champion, don't forget that Rundel was also outspoken in your defense."

"Ah," she said. "Rundel." She let out a long sigh. "I *suppose* I can't let the old goat die, if I can help it. Back to the business in hand, then. Tell me what happened."

Tobias nodded. "His apprentice brought him to me, close to death. My strongest healing Songs have kept him alive but are unable to deal with the poison." He went to the cave entrance, where his horse was tied, and fetched the jar containing the metal box. "Here," he said, handing her the jar. "*This* is how it was inflicted."

Alia held the jar up. "*Enigma enicatus*," she said.

Tobias nodded. "A death puzzle. Rundel said if we identify its targets, we might identify the attacker."

"An *enigma enicatus* is a booby-trapped magical device," said Alia. "Difficult to make." She opened the jar and passed her hand over the top, back and forth. "Mmm. The *style* of the spells within it is unusual. You should take this to Ural. It's a very *engineered* form of sorcery. It'd be right up his alley. He might recognize the style and point you to its creator. He knows much more about the Sorcerers of the world than I do." Tobias looked immediately wary. "Good Lord, Tobias, what is it?"

"Ural is dead," said Tobias. "Bludgeoned, without witnesses to what happened. Rundel was called to investigate and was poisoned by the box when he picked it up."

Alia was stunned. "Ural Casimir, dead?" She closed her eyes, visibly distressed by the news. After a moment she opened her eyes again, and Patch could see they were wet. "Come," she said, venturing to a table beside her trunk of potions. "We must investigate the box."

The others followed, but Patch found himself frozen for a moment, distracted by a sudden realization. He'd thought the name Ural was familiar, and now he knew why. It was Ural *Casimir*, the Sorcerer Engineer. One of the Eight!

And there was something else he'd thought of, something that was surely impossible, but which made him look at Tobias and Alia with fresh eyes.

Wren jabbed his cheek. *Snap out of it*, she signed. *They're waiting for us.*

He nodded without a word and went to join them.

Alia handed out pieces of rag to Tobias, Madder, and Patch, and took one herself. "Each of you must spit in your rag," she said, and as they did she went to a corner where a hunk of cured meat sat. She cut some pieces from the meat and returned. "You first," she said to Patch. She took his rag, and wiped his spit over the surface of one piece of meat. Then, using a pair of tongs, she thrust the meat into the jar and pressed it against the box. Nothing happened. "Now you," she said to Madder. She repeated the process, and again there was no reaction.

"Can you be sure this works, Alia?" said Tobias.

"Hush!" she said. She took the rag from Tobias and wiped it over the third piece of meat. This time, when she pressed it to the box there was an audible *click*. She pulled the tongs away just in time to see a small needle disappear back into the metal surface. Black liquid dripped from the meat. She gave Tobias a dark look, and then tried her own spit with the last piece. Again, the click, and the meat was injected with poison. "As I feared," she said. "The targets include Rundel and the two of us. I give you one guess who else might be a target."

"Let's not get ahead of ourselves," said Tobias, giving Patch and the others a wary look. Alia saw the expression on his face and nodded. To Patch, the meaning was obvious: let's not talk in front of *them*. His suspicions grew almost to the point of bursting out of him, but he held his tongue.

"Now to identify what the substance is," said Alia. "Give me a moment." She took samples of the black poison from the pieces of meat, then added various liquids from vials she took down from the nearest shelf. A few minutes later, she nodded with satisfaction. "Moon-rot," she said. "A nasty fungus, but the effect has been enhanced with sorcery as you suspected. No wonder your Song couldn't quite deal with it." She hunted through the vials in her trunk and selected one containing a bright purple liquid. "Aha!" she announced, standing up. "This should do it." She took a long metal rod and touched it to the black poison, then swirled the rod in the purple liquid. The color immediately changed to green. "This must remain absolutely still for at least eight hours," she said, placing the vial in a tiny stand on the table. "By then it will have transmuted fully, and Rundel's cure will be complete. I'll come with you to Marwheel long enough to administer it, Tobias, not a moment longer. He'll remain unconscious for a week, perhaps two, but he should live."

"Thank you, Alia," said Tobias. Brother Madder offered out the pouch of money he'd reclaimed from the brigand leader.

"No, no," said Alia. "Keep it. You have need of it, I know, running your infirmary. You've been treating a firefoot outbreak recently, haven't you? And doing a fine job too."

"You know about that?" said Tobias.

Alia grinned. "Oh yes, I've kept my eye on you, Palafox."

That was it—Patch couldn't hold it in any more.

"Palafox!" he barked. "I knew it! I *knew* it!"

"Oh," said Alia, wide-eyed. "Damn."

Barver and Wren were staring at Patch. *You knew what?* signed Wren.

"*Palafox, Corrigan, Kellenfas, Stone . . .*" recited Patch.

"*Casimir, Hinkelman, Drevis, and Throne.*" Barver and Wren gave him bemused looks, but Tobias and Alia were watching him warily. "The names of the Eight," said Patch. "Kellenfas, Hinkelman, and Throne died in the quest. Of the survivors, we have Drevis, now a Lord of the Pipers' Council. We have Stone, now a Virtus in the Custodian Elite. The other three sought new lives, away from the fame that their quest had brought. First, Casimir, the Sorcerer Engineer. Who does that leave?"

"Palafox and Corrigan," said Barver. "What are you saying?" He looked to Wren, and Wren shook her head and shrugged.

Patch heaved a sigh. "You two should have paid more attention to the tales of the Eight! Don't you know their first names?"

"Mmm," said Barver. "The stories only mention them once, but I *think* I do. Let's see . . . Palafox's name was T—" His mouth dropped open and he stared at Tobias. Then he stared at Alia. Then he fainted, crushing a chair.

Wren was staring too. *No way*, she signed.

Patch gestured to Tobias. "Tobias Palafox, Hero of the Battle Elite." He gestured to Alia. "Alia Corrigan, the Great Piper of Shielding Songs!"

And Rundel Stone's dead friend—signed Wren.

Patch nodded. "—was Ural Casimir, the Sorcerer Engineer."

Barver was back on his feet, looking groggy.

Patch looked at Tobias and Alia. *"That's* why you're all old friends," he said. "You were all members of the Eight. And someone's trying to kill you!"

Barver fainted again, narrowly missing a table.

"We don't know that for certain," said Tobias.

"I think it's clear!" scoffed Alia. "Someone finally decided to get rid of us, the last of the Eight. We ruffled too many feathers in our quest and stepped on too many toes!"

"We did make enemies," said Tobias, sounding oddly proud.

Alia nodded. "We did," she said. She looked at Patch and frowned. "And now you know our secret. You must choose: swear to tell no one, or die in *terrible pain.*"

"The first one," said Patch quickly; Wren gave an emphatic nod.

"A good choice," said Alia. She nudged Barver with her foot, but he didn't stir. "That goes for you too," she said. "Unconsciousness is no excuse." Finally, she turned to Brother Madder. "And what about you?"

Madder smiled. "I'm an old friend of Tobias, ma'am," he said. "I knew him before the Eight set off on their quest. I've never betrayed his secret. And if I can be open, while Tobias has never told me the Witch's true identity, I'd come to that conclusion some years ago."

"Really?" said Alia, her eyes narrowing.

"Indeed," said Madder. "Whenever Tobias had a little

too much brandy and someone mentioned the Witch of Gemspar Mountain or the name of Alia Corrigan, it was never long until Tobias spoke of a mysterious lost love, his voice filled with longing and sorrow. But you can trust me to keep it to myself, ma'am."

Tobias's cheeks were reddening.

Alia blinked for a moment, then coughed. "Well then," she said, and took a deep breath. Once she'd composed herself, she rubbed her hands together with purpose. "Glad that's all settled. We'll start out for Marwheel when Rundel's potion is ready, but in the meantime we have a certain curse to deal with! I must prepare!" She looked at Wren. "It's your turn, little one. Don't think I forgot you!"

Wren started to tremble. Patch rubbed the top of her head to reassure her.

"Have faith!" said Alia. "Ural Casimir saw that I had even more potential as a Sorcerer than as a Piper. Oh, *Ural* ... how can you be gone?" She looked up to the moon, tears in her eyes. She wiped them away. "He believed in me. It was my destiny. Even though the Council declared me a witch and cast me out, I don't regret it one bit."

"Can we do anything to help you get ready?" said Patch.

Alia nodded. "We need a large fire, as big as you can make it. Take lamps into the forest, all of you, and fetch as much wood as you can. I'll start my preparations." She went further back inside the cave, where the shelves were laden with books, and began to consult her texts.

Patch and Wren looked at Barver, who was still out cold. *Leave me on the table next to him*, signed Wren, and Patch did, taking a lamp and following Tobias and Madder outside.

After a minute or so, Barver's eyes opened. He sat up suddenly in near-panic. "Someone's killing the Eight!" he said. "One by one!" He blinked and looked around. "Where did everyone go?"

Wren gave him an affectionate smile. *Welcome back, big fella*, she signed. *Now go and get me some firewood!*

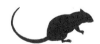

21

AWKWARD TRUTHS

There was plenty of dry wood among the creepy gnarled trees in Alia's part of the forest. Barver's contribution to the wood gathering dwarfed that of anyone else, which was no surprise given that he could carry half a dozen actual *tree trunks* on each trip. It wasn't long before they'd assembled the bonfire a safe distance from the cave entrance and Alia's garden. The wood took flame readily, and soon the bonfire was well ablaze.

Alia came out of the cave carrying a small leather pouch, paper, and some thin pieces of charcoal. She got everyone to sit facing the fire, then stepped closer to it and spoke a few garbled words. Taking a handful of some kind of powder from her pouch, she cried out in a high-pitched warbling voice and threw the powder at the flames.

There was a vast plume of yellow smoke, alive with sparks.

Alia walked to where Patch sat, with Wren on his shoulder as usual. The others were a few feet behind them, watching with interest. "Right!" said Alia, looking at Patch. She set down the paper and gripped a piece of charcoal. "I need background on Wren, please. You're her friend. You can speak this—" She waved her hands around madly.

"Merisax hand speech," said Patch.

"Oh yes!" said Alia. "That's it! I never quite got around to learning it. Go ahead, then. Ask her how this curse came about. I'll take notes." She was poised with her charcoal on the page.

"Oh, she's told me the story a few times now," said Patch. "She's the daughter of a wealthy nobleman, and last summer she was kidnapped by a Sorcerer and forced to work as a maid in his castle. She tried to escape and *blam!*"

"Rat curse!" said Alia.

Patch and Wren both nodded.

"Where was this castle?" said Alia. "What was the Sorcerer's name?"

Patch looked to Wren, who'd never told him those details. She signed, and he translated. "The village of Axlebury," he said. "The Sorcerer's name is Underath."

"Okay," said Alia, writing it down. "What we must do is look for a chink in the construction of the curse. If we find something to pick at, we can try and build a *counter*-curse. We may be able to shatter the curse outright, but I make no guarantees. Building a spell, a hex, a curse—these are similar to layering the parts of a Piper's Song. Building a counter-spell requires those layers to be understood, to allow them to be canceled out. First I need something of yours, little rat. Hair and nail." She produced a pair of sharp scissors, and Wren flinched. "Don't worry, I won't take much." Patch held Wren gently as Alia snipped a tiny bit of fur from her back. "Now, your paw." Wren held her paw out, trembling, and Alia cut the very tip from one claw. She put the clippings into a small square of paper, then folded it into a little parcel. "That'll do," said Alia. She handed the parcel to Wren. "You must throw it into the flames!"

Patch stood and carried Wren as close to the fire as the fierce heat would allow. She threw the parcel, but it fell short. "I've got it," said Patch. He set Wren down and stepped forward; braving the severe heat he grabbed the little parcel and went to throw it into the fire himself.

"Wait, she's the one who has to—" started Alia, but Patch had already let go and the paper was in flames. Alia shook her head as Patch came back with Wren and sat down. "Oh, fine. Ignore me, I'm just the expert." The fire erupted into more smoke, white this time, the sparks filling the cloud with an astonishing range of colors. Alia smiled.

"Oooh, hang on! We've got lucky!" She gripped her piece of charcoal, ready to take notes, then turned to the others behind them, who were whispering. "Shush!" she said. "It's starting!"

Everyone looked on in awe as the colored sparks in the fire began to gather into something recognizable.

A tiny run-down cottage in the midst of rolling fields. "Wren!" came a voice, and Patch almost *jumped*. But the voice was from the fire, booming loud; suddenly a woman's face appeared, kind and concerned. "Where are you going, young lady?"

And there she was, a girl of thirteen—Wren, as she used to be. Earnest and smiling, she wore a long skirt, which was a little threadbare, striped with rings of red and white. Patch looked at the red-ringed tail of his rat friend and knew it was no coincidence.

"Mum," said Wren. "The time's come for me to get work. I know how hard things are for you and Dad, and I'm an extra mouth to feed. I have a plan, and I won't be talked out of it!"

Wren's mother hugged her. "How I wish it wasn't so," she said. "Don't be gone too long."

"Six months at most," said Wren. "I'll save as much of my pay as I can!"

The smoke from the fire darkened.

Patch gave Wren—the *rat* Wren, on his shoulder—a pointed look. "Daughter of a wealthy nobleman?" he whispered. She was staring at the fire, looking mortified.

"Shhhh!" hissed Alia. "We'll miss something!"

The smoke lit up again, to show human-Wren walking through the countryside, a determined expression on her face. In the distance was a castle—far smaller than Tiviscan Castle, but impressive all the same. The viewpoint changed, and now Wren was at the castle door, knocking.

A weary-looking middle-aged man, dressed in an elaborate robe, opened the door and peeked out. "Yes?" he said.

"You are Underath, the Sorcerer?" said Wren.

"I am."

"Sir, I was hoping to offer my services as a maid."

Underath looked astonished. "I've been seeking staff here for twenty years. Nobody's ever come before."

"I'm here," said Wren. "Do you wish to hire me? Yes or no?"

"Yes," said Underath. "But be prepared! Of the hundred rooms in the castle I use only four. Those four are filthy with use, and the rest are filthy with neglect! Pick any bedroom you choose; keep yourself to yourself. The kitchen is always well stocked. Can you cook?"

"I can."

Underath seemed elated at the idea. "Good, for I cannot! I've been living on salted meats and cheese and bread and wine. Cook whatever you will, and I'll be grateful to end the monotony. Come!"

The view changed again. They now stood on a high wall that ran around a courtyard, in the middle of which was a large dark-gray griffin. It looked up at the two humans with a wary eye.

"That is Alkeran," said Underath. "The courtyard is his, and his alone. Do not speak to him. He is quick to anger." They reentered the castle, coming to a room where shelves of books filled the walls, potions and their ingredients cluttered tables, and sheets of paper littered the floor. "Here is my study. Keep the dust to a minimum, and tidy my papers. Beyond that, touch nothing."

Wren bent down and picked up some pages, looking at them with fascination. "Should I keep your writings ordered somehow, sire?" she said. "These notes are on necromancy, while these are on the history of prophecy."

"You can read?" said Underath.

"My parents taught me."

"How quaint to teach a girl something so useless to her! Just tidy the papers into one neat pile."

Wren betrayed no emotion, save for a brief narrowing of her eyes. She nodded and looked with interest at the bookshelves, reaching out to them.

"Do not touch the books!" warned Underath.

"As you wish, sire," said Wren.

(The smoke of the fire weakened, to disappointed sounds from those watching. Alia reached for her pouch and threw another handful of powder into the flames. The smoke billowed up again, and the images began to re-form.)

The days passed. Wren, wearing the simple clothes of a maid, entered rooms filled with dust and spiderwebs, and she cleaned them; she cooked, she ate, she slept.

One day she went to Underath's study to retrieve his dinner plates. She heard snoring. Underath was asleep in his bedroom.

Cautiously, she went to his desk. A great leather-bound volume of magic was lying open. She began to read it, concentrating hard. Then a light of understanding filled her eyes.

Again and again, as she collected the dishes from Underath's evening meal, she listened for the snoring and read what she could. At one point, deep in thought, she reached out to a spoon without touching it. She read aloud from the book and the spoon wobbled. A smile of utter delight crossed her face.

Day after day, she read; day after day, she could do more. She lit a candle without using a flame; she repaired a broken plate with words alone.

"Sire?" she said, as she brought Underath lunch one day. "I have heard it said that Sorcerers often take on an apprentice, yet I know that you never have. Will you ever do so?"

"Perhaps," said Underath. "Young men of talent are rare, though. Ah, lunch! Good." He started to eat. "Actually, I have something to tell you. I'll be gone for a week. I shall ride Alkeran to a distant land, so you shall be alone. You have nothing to fear in this place, and I shall see you soon."

When she returned to her room, Wren cheered. A week to study freely!

Once Underath had left on his journey, she began to scrutinize his most precious books late into the night. In her room, she stood before an old ragged mirror: "Sire? And what if *I* was to ask . . . to be your apprentice?" She closed her eyes. "You can do this, Wren, you can ask him when he's back."

Finally, a shadow in the sky announced the return of the griffin, and of Underath. She went to greet him. The door to the courtyard opened, and standing beside Underath was a woman of cold beauty. When the woman laid eyes on Wren, her smile contained nothing but malice.

"I have news, maid!" said Underath. "I am newly married! This is my wife. I have sought a companion even longer than I had sought a servant—a wife wise enough to keep within touching distance of my *superior* intelligence. I shall have no more need of a maid after today, but I will pay you well for the work you have done these last few weeks." He tossed a pouch of coins to her.

Crestfallen, Wren still had the courage to speak. "I was . . . I was going to ask to be your apprentice."

Underath laughed. His wife raised a sinister eyebrow. "You?" said Underath. "A girl?" He patted his wife's head, as if she was a pet. "It's not even right for a *woman* to be a Sorcerer, let alone a simple *girl*! Now run along and prepare a celebration meal for us!"

She did as she was asked. When she brought the first tray of food to the study, Underath guided her through to another room, one that used to be empty but which had been transformed into a dining room. An impressive table was laid out with plates and cutlery.

"See how I've been making changes to the castle already?" said Underath. "Nothing is too good for my beautiful wife!" He saw the food Wren carried—a wonderful-looking pie, bread, and soup. He smiled. "Thank you, maid. I know you're disappointed, but I wish you well, in all you do."

"I'll bring your best wines for the meal," said Wren. "And I've made some desserts too."

She brought the rest of the food and drink to the dining room. Underath's wife was there, smiling her malicious smile.

"There's no need for you to tidy after, maid," said Underath. "I grant you the night off, to let you gather your things ready to leave at dawn."

But that was not Wren's plan.

She returned later and, as she'd hoped, there was snoring from Underath's bedroom. This was, of course, why she'd made her meal with such care. They had eaten well, and now they would sleep well too.

Silently she went into the study and chose four of Underath's books on sorcery, smaller ones that she could carry more easily. She crept out of the castle into the gloom of dusk, dressed in the red-ringed skirt she'd worn when she first arrived.

She froze when a voice spoke up behind her.

"If I'd not seen it with my own eyes, I wouldn't have believed it," said Underath. "You were right, wife!"

Wren spun around. Underath was standing there, his wife by his side.

"I told you she couldn't be trusted!" said the woman. "Look! Look what she takes from you!"

Wren hung her head, angry and ashamed. She dropped the books and the pouch of coins at her feet. "Keep your books. Keep your money. I can become a Sorcerer! I've always known it! I only ever came here because I wanted to learn!"

Underath shook his head. "I thought you were loyal," he said, obviously hurt. "Go. *Go*."

"This is betrayal, my love!" said his wife. "She's the lowest kind of vermin! A *rat*! Why not make sure she never forgets it, dearest?" Grinning with malice, she placed her hand on her husband's arm.

Underath's expression was one of sorrow and regret, but it changed: oh so slowly, it changed. His eyes hardened, and he took on a look of spite and rage.

He muttered some words and began to wave his hands. A purple glow appeared around the tips of his fingers. He cried out, his arms pointing straight at Wren. The purple glow became impossibly bright and hurtled toward the girl, exploding around her.

The light faded, and when it was gone there was only a rat with a red-ringed tail. It squeaked in terror as it ran off into the trees, chased by the cruel laughter of the Sorcerer and his bride.

The sparks subsided. The smoke from the bonfire was now just ordinary smoke.

Wren hung her head. The silence was uncomfortable. Eventually Alia cleared her throat. "Ahem," she said.

"Yes. Um. There are details that don't *quite* match the account you gave, Patch."

"Don't I know it," said Patch, glum. He turned to Wren. "Kidnapped, were you? Wealthy parents, eh?"

Wren looked tearful. *I was desperate for your help in Patterfall,* she signed. *It seemed like such a little lie.*

Patch shook his head. "And you tried to steal his magical texts?" said Patch. "I can't believe this."

Wren gave him a defiant stare. *What?* she signed. *Are you upset that I can't reward you for your help? Is that why you became my friend? For the money?*

Patch was dumbstruck by the accusation. "Well!" he said. "Well, then . . . then I . . ." He felt very angry indeed, but he had a sudden fear that, perhaps somewhere deep down, he was guilty as charged. He hoped not.

"Enough!" said Barver. "You would risk your lives to save each other! Here we are, on the cusp of a cure for Wren, and you squabble over things that *don't really matter!*"

Long seconds passed before Wren and Patch found they could bear to look at each other.

"Sorry," muttered Patch. "I just thought you'd be more honest with me than that. *Friends don't have secrets,* isn't that what you said?"

There was a sudden *crump* from the fire. Everyone backed away as flames grew again, and colorful sparks exploded outwards with a loud bang.

"Something more for us to see!" said Alia. "Shush! *Shush!*"

The images in the fire resolved themselves, along with the sound of rock grinding against rock, and the cracking of masonry.

Patch's face filled the image in the smoke, coughing as the dust of the attack on Tiviscan Castle filled his cell.

"Uh-oh," said the real Patch, looking at the features of his past-self looming above him.

Alia seemed confused for a moment, but then she looked

at Patch and mimed throwing the parcel into the flame. "A little of *you* has crept into the spell, it seems," she said. "Looks like you were a prisoner somewhere. Wait a moment . . . is that Tiviscan dungeon? It is! You're a *criminal?*"

"It's fine, Alia," said Tobias. "He—"

"You knew?" she said.

"I did. There's nothing to worry about, we just—" Suddenly Tobias stopped talking. He stared at the fire, as did Alia.

As did all of them.

"Aye!" came a voice.

There in the smoke's magical images, the prisoner in the Iron Mask lay, his injuries obvious. His hands came up and tore at the mask, which swung open and fell to the floor.

"Aye . . . ," said the thin-faced man, coughing up blood as past-Patch drew closer. "Aye . . . am . . . I . . . am . . ." The man swallowed and took a breath. "I am not the Piper of Hamelyn." Then the dragons came. The man was taken, the expression on his face one of simple relief. He was thrown into the circle of fire the dragons made for him, and he perished.

With perfect timing, the images died and the smoke retreated. The bonfire's center collapsed in on itself.

Everyone was staring at Patch, even Wren. *Especially* Wren.

Patch coughed. "Um," he said. "Ah. Yes. Didn't I mention that bit?"

238

22

THE CHILDREN

You accused me *of dishonesty, eh?* signed Wren. *Take a look at yourself, you big dolt!* She hopped off his shoulder and went over to Barver, who was glaring at Patch.

Tobias seemed stunned. "You told nobody about this?" he said. "Even when you found out that Alia and I were part of the Eight, you still said nothing?"

Patch looked around at all the accusing eyes. "What *should* I have done? I'm supposed to be in the dungeons until I die. You want me to start blabbing about the Hamelyn Piper's last words and get thrown back into a cell? I'm happier not doing that, thank you!" He folded his arms and scowled.

Alia, who'd been pacing furiously up and down, stopped and looked at Tobias. "The Mask was *off* him," she said. "He could say anything he wanted and lie without restriction."

"You saw the same thing I saw," said Tobias. "You saw his eyes. Did it look like a lie?"

"Insane, then," snapped Alia. "He forgot what he was, perhaps. I don't *know*."

Tobias looked at her, a terrible doubt in his eyes. "Could we have imprisoned the wrong man?"

"Impossible!" said Alia. "We caught him with his Pipe, we knew the Songs he'd played! And the witnesses! The townsfolk of Hamelyn identified him, as did the child who was left behind—"

"The boy with the limp?" said Barver.

Alia gave a deep sigh. "That poor young soul." She clenched her fists. "You'd only need to see the look on that child's face to know we'd caught the right man."

"But his last words!" said Tobias, agitated. "He'd been trying to say that sentence, to deny he was the Piper of Hamelyn, for almost a decade!"

Alia put a hand on his shoulder. "You torture yourself for no reason, Tobias. Think back to the end of our quest. Think back!"

Tobias took a long slow breath, trying to settle himself. "We'd tracked the Hamelyn Piper down, in the Ice Fields near Port Hagen," he said. "He defended himself with a display of Dark Piping that was beyond anything I'd seen before."

Alia looked at him with an affection she'd not shown until now. "That was the day you got your scars. I thought

240

I'd lost you—" She drifted to silence for a moment. "The Hamelyn Piper was caught in the same blast, yet he escaped uninjured."

"But we *had* hurt him," said Tobias. "When we found him again, he was dazed, bewildered. Barely able to speak. But the evidence was clear: he was the Hamelyn Piper." He nodded, the uncertainty gone from his face. "Whatever he said just before his death, it means nothing. We must listen only to the evidence, and the evidence speaks with one voice. It was him!"

Patch was trying hard to believe that the prisoner's last words had meant nothing, but he was finding it difficult. There was something else worrying him, though—something Alia had mentioned. "Wait," he said. "You said you got his Pipe when you caught him, and you knew what Songs he'd played. In all the stories I heard of the Eight, the Pipe had been destroyed, so the history of its Songs was lost. Which is the truth?"

Alia and Tobias shared a long look. "She was, um, *mistaken*," said Tobias.

Alia frowned at him. "The Hamelyn Piper is dead," she said. "Perhaps the time for secrecy has passed."

"Alia," said Tobias, in a cautioning tone. "We *both* took a vow."

Alia looked to the ground, thinking. At last she shook her head. "We found the Pipe," she said to Patch. "And it told us what had happened to the children."

Barver, Patch, and Wren looked at Alia, openmouthed with shock.

Patch eventually managed to speak. "You know what happened to them?"

"The Hamelyn Piper had *tried* to destroy his Pipe before he was caught," said Alia. "There were only fragments left. Rundel Stone attempted to extract the history of the Pipe's Songs from those fragments, even though we all thought it was impossible. But he found two Songs of immense power. One had been played on the night the human children disappeared. The other was played after the dragon children were taken. I saw Rundel's face crumple as he found out the truth. I watched as his heart grew cold and bitter. Hope had left him."

Barver was staring at her. "What happened to the children?" he said. "What happened?"

"Don't, Alia," said Tobias. "Please."

Alia ignored him. "Both were Songs of execution, old Songs that were once used to carry out death sentences. For the dragon children, it was the Song of Endless Sleep. This slows the breathing of the target until they fall unconscious and die. For the human children, it was the Song of Dispersal. The children of Hamelyn were obliterated, their flesh and bones scattered like dust across the skies."

Barver gasped. "And the Pipers' Council have known this all along?"

Alia nodded. "Yes. And the dragon authorities too."

Patch shook his head. "But the Mask was going to force the Hamelyn Piper to answer that question! If they already knew the answer, what was the point?"

"The Mask's question wasn't about the fate of the children," said Alia. "We already knew their fate. It was about why he had done it, these senseless acts, these atrocities . . . *Why?* To get that answer, the Hamelyn Piper had to live—yet if the world knew the children were dead, his execution would have been impossible to stop! Then, the question of *why* could never be answered. So the Council ordered the fate of the children to be kept secret. The Dragon Triumvirate were reluctant to agree and brought us to the brink of war, but they did agree in the end."

"And now it is over, at last," said Tobias. "The Triumvirate must have decided that no answer would ever come, and when the opportunity arose they made their move and killed the Hamelyn Piper. Whatever the Council does in retaliation for the attack on Tiviscan, they'll be secretly relieved that their most hated prisoner is dead."

"Even so," said Patch. "With his final words the Hamelyn Piper denied his guilt. Surely you must tell the Pipers' Council about this?"

"I will tell Rundel and let him decide what to do," said Tobias.

"But you can't tell him about me!" said Patch. "Right now I'm listed among the dead. If he found out I'm alive, it would condemn me to a life of being hunted!"

"I'll not mention you," said Tobias. "It seems fair that we keep your secret, if you keep ours. I'll just say Alia conjured a way to see the Hamelyn Piper's final moments, and she told me what she'd heard."

"You think you could fool Rundel so easily?" said Alia. "Such magic needs a willing witness, and he'll want to know who that witness was."

"I'll tell him you have invented a new magic that needs no witness," said Tobias.

"He'll not believe you," said Alia.

Tobias thought for a moment. "He'll believe it if *you* tell him," he said.

Alia looked at him with a raised eyebrow. "You want me to wait around until Rundel wakens and speak to him? Just to keep this lad from the dungeons? Not likely! I have better things to do!" But the faces around her—Barver, Wren, and Patch himself—were looking at her with the pleading expressions normally found on cold kittens or hungry puppies. She glared back at them, defiant at first, but her defiance gradually ebbed away. "*Oh very well!*" she snapped.

Tobias nodded. "It's decided, then. We'll let Rundel choose what to do, when he awakens."

The word "awakens" made Patch think of sleep; he couldn't hold back a yawn, and the yawn spread to Wren, and then Barver.

"The night is deep," said Alia, looking up to the moon. "Sleep, everyone. Especially you, Wren." She bent down and gathered the pieces of paper she'd brought with her, which were covered now in circles and arrows and hastily scribbled words. "I have my notes to study, to seek a flaw in Underath's curse. I will see you at dawn!"

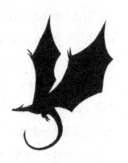

23

THE CURE

They slept near the embers of the bonfire. When dawn came, Alia woke them with a shout before walking off, a large earthenware jar in her arms.

Wren stretched and rubbed her eyes, but Patch knew she hadn't slept much. Neither had he.

Beside them, Barver was still snoring. Patch nudged him until he sat up with a start, one eye still shut. "How *dare* it be morning," muttered Barver.

Tell me about it, signed Wren. She looked over to where Alia stood, some distance from them, pouring salt from the large jar to create various shapes on the ground.

"She must have found a way to help you, Wren," said Patch.

I'm scared to ask, signed Wren.

They all watched Alia prepare, and at last she came over to them. "I'm ready," she said. "Wren, I'd hoped to be able to shatter the curse once and for all, but I fear it was too well constructed. Instead, I offer you this." She held up her hand, and in her fingers was a bracelet with intensely blue beads. "I did find a slight flaw in the curse, one that will let you be shielded from its power temporarily. This bracelet will give a few days at a time of human form. It's the best I can do." She put the bracelet around Wren's midriff. "Sadly it's not just a case of putting the bracelet on. It must be bonded to what is called your 'morphic countenance.' The process is painful." She looked at Barver and Patch with narrowed eyes. "And the two of *you* must not interfere, under any circumstances! It would put your friend in great danger. Do I make myself clear?"

They both nodded; Alia's stern gaze was enough to make anyone terrified of disobeying her.

"Make sure they do as they're told, Tobias," said Alia.

Patch felt almost sick with fear for Wren, yet he could do nothing but watch as Alia took his friend over to the salt symbols and set her down in the center. She poured more salt from the jar, forming an outer circle thirty feet across. The circle complete, Alia stepped inside and began to speak. Patch couldn't place the language, a harsh and guttural tongue, all phlegm and spit. Her words turned into a chant. *"Ree tee ko pak!"* she cried. *"Thagh pak skarra tak!"*

She raised her arms straight up as the chant grew in volume. A continuous low rumble began, and Patch could see the air within the circle shimmer.

Wren squeaked and scratched at the bead bracelet with her hind legs, clearly in discomfort.

"*Ree tee ko pak!*" cried Alia. "*Thagh pak skarra tak!*" Her arms swept down suddenly, open palms held out to Wren. The air above the salt circle seemed to have texture now, moving like oil spilled in water. Patch looked to Barver, both of them deeply uneasy. The low rumble grew ever louder.

Wren shrieked, twisting in agony on the ground. Smoke started to rise where the beads touched her fur.

Patch stepped forward.

"We can't interfere!" said Barver, but Patch ignored him and went even closer. He moved around the outside of the circle. There was heat coming from it now, and the light within seemed to redden suddenly. Alia's chant continued louder and louder, and Patch saw her face . . .

He ran and fetched his Pipe from his bag. As he rushed back, Tobias stood in his way.

"You heard her," said Tobias. "Interfering could harm Wren!"

Patch pointed into the circle. "*Something's wrong!* Look at Alia, Tobias! Look at her *eyes!*"

Tobias looked. "Dear God," he said, backing off.

Alia's face was a grinning mask and her eyes were glowing red. Her chant took on an edge of madness—laughter burst from her mouth after every few words, a terrible insane *cackle*.

Wren was screaming now, writhing in pain, smoke pouring from her fur. Everyone was frozen, staring as the light within the circle darkened, until only the red glow from Alia's eyes remained.

"She'll be killed!" said Patch. He got as close as he could to the circle and stretched his foot out to the textured air. As he'd expected, the air formed a barrier. He looked at the swirling patterns directly above the salt and remembered how Alia had described the intricate layers of a Sorcerer's work, and how it was not so different from the layers of a Song.

He started to play the same counter-Song he'd played to save Wren back in Patterfall. To his amazement, he could see patterns forming on the barrier, patterns that changed as he played. He tried to create something that matched the shapes already there, hoping it would somehow negate them. Again and again, he tweaked what he was playing and observed how the patterns altered, and suddenly he struck lucky—a tiny gap seemed to open up and widen. He intensified his playing, then reached out his hand. It *was* a gap, a break in the barrier wide enough for him to fit through, if he dived! He steeled himself and made the attempt, passing through the gap and landing hard inside the circle. He looked back at the barrier and saw the gap closing over. The noise was overwhelming, as if he was in the center of a howling storm, Alia's yelling and Wren's screams only just audible. Wind whipped the black earth into his face, and he could barely see.

He tried to move toward Wren, but it felt like moving through deep mud. Then Alia's face leered at him, inches away. From this close, her eyes were even more terrifying—Patch could see a fire within, churning and flaring up.

"The deed is done, Brightwater!" she cried, cackling. "Look! The bracelet is bonded to her! She changes!"

"Wren!" he yelled. His friend's body was surrounded in smoke. "*Wren!*" He made to go to her, but Alia's hand gripped his shoulder.

"Leave her be, boy. Let me take a look at *you!*" Patch trembled with fear as Alia examined him from head to toe, those fiery eyes emitting a fierce heat. Loud as the winds around them were, Patch could hear her perfectly, as if she was speaking directly into his mind.

"I see you!" she said. "Your past! Your future! I see Tiviscan Castle!"

"That's in my past," cried Patch. "*Absolutely* my past."

"Perhaps!" she said. "Know this: should you ever return to Tiviscan, there will be a heavy price to pay! And what else do I see"—she studied him again, her grip on his shoulder painful now—"I see betrayal!"

"Betrayal . . . ?"

"Yes, betrayal! The words come to me now, the *betraying* words. Listen and remember! The words I say next, Brightwater, burn them into your memory. There will come a time when you hear these words! A mouth that speaks them is a traitorous mouth and will betray you to that which you fear most! When you hear them spoken, get away as quickly as you can! *Run!*"

Her frightening grin faded and she closed her glowing eyes. The wind dropped as she spoke in a gentle singsong voice: "They thought they had us. But we're almost clear. Just the ridge to go. What's wrong with you? What's wrong?" Her eyes opened again and she stared at him. "An odd set of words, don't you think?" she said. Her voice shifted in tone, as if she was having a conversation with herself. "I agree, very odd! What say you, Patch? The lad's gone so very pale. The day's been quite a strain, I imagine." She let him go and began to cackle once more as the howling wind returned. Patch fell to his knees, bewildered by what she'd said. Suddenly a hot blast of air hit him hard, flinging him backward out of the circle.

There was silence.

He sat upright as a shadow fell across him. It was Alia, offering him a hand up. Her smile was utterly normal now, as were her eyes.

"That's got a bit of a kick, hasn't it?" said Alia as she helped Patch to his feet. She dusted herself off, seeming rather high-spirited.

Patch looked to the salt circle. All signs of the barrier had vanished, and a dense mist was starting to dissipate. In the middle lay Wren: human, wearing the clothes they'd seen her wear as she'd tried to flee from Underath.

"It worked . . . ," Patch said.

"It did," said Alia. "She'll be fine in a minute or two. I said you could trust me."

"Ye-ess," said Patch, not *quite* over how things had gone. "It was the glowing eyes and the insane laughter that were worrying me."

"Glowing eyes again, eh?" said Alia. She gave him an apologetic smile. "I lose track of things when it gets intense, so I can't remember what happens. Sorry if I scared you. I'll admit it gives me the heebie-jeebies, but that's just how it works." She frowned, as if remembering something. Then she whispered: "You tried to break into the circle, didn't you?" She leaned closer, squinting a bit as she looked at him. Her eyes widened suddenly. "You *did* break in! Fascinating! And very, *very* stupid of you."

"I was worried something had gone wrong," he said. "Sorry."

"Incredible that you managed it at all! But the *problems* it could have caused . . . For you, mainly. I didn't hurt you, did I? Or predict the day of your death, anything like that?"

"Um, what do you mean?" said Patch.

"You know. A prophecy. A warning. That kind of thing. I was really on form in there, I can tell you."

Patch thought of her prediction of betrayal, unsure what to tell her. "You really don't know what you did?"

"Not a clue. It often gets a bit intense, but that was a doozy."

"So . . . would giving me a prophecy be bad?"

"They're dangerous things, prophecies," she said. "Never straightforward. Tend to cause endless trouble." He was about to tell her the truth, when she added: "And I'd be absolutely *riddled* with guilt if I had, that's all."

"Ah," said Patch. It struck him that she didn't really need to know. Given that she'd been helping Wren, surely he could save her from her own guilt? "In that case, no. You didn't."

Alia smiled with relief. "Thank goodness for that."

In the center of the circle, Wren was starting to sit up.

Everyone turned to her.

"Hold on," said Alia. "Let her get her bearings."

Barver came to stand beside Patch, and they watched as Wren looked around her, nervous and confused. She scratched her nose, and then she stared at her hand for a good minute or so, bewildered.

Gradually, her wary expression was broken by a smile that grew and grew until, grinning broadly, she leaped to her feet. "Ha!" she cried. She jumped on the spot, then jumped again, laughing. She started to run and hop and leap, speeding around the salt circle and the ashes of the previous night's bonfire.

Suddenly her smile fell away. She looked down at herself, and the smile returned. "Phew!" she said. "Fully clothed!" She punched the air. "I was worried about that." She saw Patch and Barver, and her mouth opened in a look of utter delight. She ran to Patch and gave him a hug, then switched to hugging Barver. Then she hugged Alia and Tobias, before hurtling over to Madder and giving him a hug too, whooping and laughing as she went.

At last, thoroughly exhausted, she returned to where Alia was watching her with amusement.

"Happy?" said Alia.

Wren nodded rapidly. "What a result!" For the first time, she noticed that the beaded bracelet was now on her left wrist. "How does it work, then?"

"When the beads are all blue, concentrate, wish it, and you'll become human for a while. Once invoked, you will remain human until the power in the bracelet runs its course. When that happens, make sure you're somewhere safe, as you'll become a rat again! Then you must wait until the power of the beads has returned before you can be human once more. The time will vary—days, at least. You'll know when it's ready."

Wren nodded and took a closer look at the bracelet.

"A warning," said Alia. "Do not remove it or allow it to be removed. The spell would break, and the only flaw in the curse would be closed. You'd be a rat, immediately, and no amount of magic would shield you in the future."

"Understood," said Wren.

"See the color fading on one bead?" said Alia. "Each bead changes to white in turn. When all have changed, you become a rat again. As I said, make sure you're somewhere safe when that happens."

"And will it always hurt so much?" asked Wren.

"Yes," said Alia. "Becoming human and becoming rat, both will hurt."

"Every time?"

"Every time."

Wren let out a deep sigh and nodded. "Alia, is there any chance I might find a proper cure?"

"This is the best I can do." Alia looked to the ground for a moment, visibly upset that she had failed to do more. "At this point, only one other option remains."

Wren's eyes lit up. "Really? What?"

"Seek Underath," said Alia. "As the one who cursed you, he'll know exactly how the curse was constructed. He might agree to undo it himself."

Wren looked incredulous. "Isn't it just a *teensy* bit unlikely he'd help?"

Alia nodded. "He did seem the unforgiving type, I agree.

But I'd suggest flattery. Tell him how *amazingly well-made* the curse was, and how only a *wonderfully clever* Sorcerer could unpick it. You never know, he might say yes. Assuming he doesn't just kill you."

Wren despaired for a moment, but suddenly she smiled again. "Oh, I think he'll be only too willing to help! He'll know he has no choice when he sees what powerful allies I've brought with me! The greatest Piper in the world and the most fearsome beast you'll ever meet!"

She threw her arms out dramatically and gestured toward Patch and Barver, who instinctively looked behind them to see what Wren was talking about. It took a few seconds before they realized she'd meant *them*.

"Ah," said Patch.

"Um," said Barver.

Wren clapped, grinning. "Glad you're aboard!" she said. "Underath won't know what's hit him!"

24

AXLEBURY

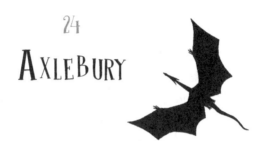

lia spent the next hour checking Wren for possible problems with the spell that had been cast, using an elaborate range of tests that included burning hairs plucked from Wren's head and making her balance pine cones on her elbow.

In the meantime, Patch found a blank sheet of paper and a piece of charcoal on one of the tables in Alia's cave, and wrote down the words she had spoken in the circle of salt.

The prophecy.

They thought they had us. But we're almost clear. Just the ridge to go. What's wrong with you? What's wrong?

He stared at the words he'd written. Someone would speak those words, someone who would betray Patch to whatever he feared most, and Patch would have to flee at once. Alia had mentioned how prophecies could cause trouble, and he had to agree—he was already worrying about it.

He began to fold the paper up nervously, as if it was dangerous.

"What do you have there?" came a voice.

Startled, Patch turned to see Barver. "Nothing," he said, putting the paper into his pocket.

Barver nodded to the cave entrance, where Alia was now getting Wren to hop for as long as possible. "Wren's serious, you know," he said, keeping his voice low. "About confronting Underath."

"I don't think that would end well," said Patch. "From what we saw in the fire, didn't you get the feeling his *wife* was the scary one?"

"Perhaps, but if I can speak with Alkeran, his griffin, I may be able to learn our best course of action. There might be something we could offer, in exchange for help. You know, something valuable. And magical . . ."

Patch stared at him. "You mean the *Mask*?"

"I notice you still haven't mentioned it to Tobias or Alia."

"Of course not!" said Patch. "It's valuable! And essential to my future, since Wren's parents aren't *quite* as rich as she'd suggested, and are actually very, very *poor*. The Mask is the only thing of value I possess."

"So you won't part with it, even to help Wren?"

Patch grumbled to himself for a moment, his teeth firmly clamped together. "Okay, okay. If the Mask will buy Underath's help, then . . . fine."

Barver patted him on the back. "You have very high principles," he said. "You should be proud."

"Proud and poor," muttered Patch.

As they left Gemspar, Wren rode with Patch, and Alia with Tobias. Patch found himself half wishing for bandits to attack again, just to see how the Witch of Gemspar Mountain dealt with them. *Spectacularly*, he reckoned, but in the end the journey was uneventful.

When they reached the Abbey, Patch dismounted and led the horse to the gate, with Wren still in the saddle.

Erner Whitlock hurried out to greet them, in his black-and-purple Custodian robes.

Patch was pleased to see his friend, and they gave each other a hearty hug. "Shouldn't you be arresting me?" Patch said quietly. "Before I run away again?"

"Why would I arrest you, Henry Smith?" said Erner with a wink. "How did it go?" Patch smiled and nodded to the rider on the horse, and Erner grinned. "Wren? Is that you?"

Wren jumped down from the horse and hugged Erner. "It's me! The less ratty version."

"You're cured then?" said Erner.

"Sort of," she said. "It's temporary, but I hope to remedy that soon enough."

Tobias and Alia joined them. "We have the medicine to heal Rundel," said Tobias. "How is he faring?"

"No deterioration," said Erner. "Your healing Song has been doing its job."

"Good, good," said Tobias.

"What are your plans?" Erner said to Patch. "Will you stay a while at the Abbey?"

"When Rundel Stone wakes, I want to be as far away as possible," said Patch. "The sooner we leave, the better."

"Do you know what you're going to do?" said Erner.

"I'm not decided yet," said Patch. "But a new life in the Eastern Seas is an option."

Erner looked anxious. "A dangerous place, my friend."

"He'll be fine," said Barver. "I'll look after him."

"I'm sure you can do that very well," said Erner.

"We have some errands to run first," said Barver. "The letter," he added, looking at Patch—his mother's last wishes.

"And I need to see Underath," said Wren. "The Sorcerer who cursed me. It seems he's now the only one who can fully undo his work, so I have no choice but to face him! I've vowed not to return home until I'm cured, and I intend to keep that vow."

Erner was horrified. "That sounds far too risky, Wren!" he said. "Please reconsider! If only I could go with you, but it's not Custodian business. Even the most *stupid* Sorcerer would think twice before incurring the wrath of the Custodians by attacking someone under their protection."

"If I might suggest something?" said Alia. She gave Erner a quick handshake. "Pleased to meet you. I'm Alia. Magic expert, friend of Tobias, long story." She held up the little jar with the death puzzle inside. "The box which poisoned Rundel has an unusual magical style. I studied Underath's curse and noticed similarities. Not quite the same, so I doubt Underath created the box, but he might have suggestions as to who *did*. It's a starting point if you wish to find the culprit. So, as a Custodian Piper, if you—"

"*Apprentice* Custodian," corrected Erner.

"Indeed, but it means that going with them to Underath *would* be on official Custodian business. Just an idea." She smiled, looking rather pleased with herself.

Erner grinned. "And a very *sensible* idea," he said. "It would mean a great deal to me, to be able to help my friends. I'll gather my things and return shortly."

As Erner headed back through the gate, Tobias stepped forward and shook the hands of Patch, Barver, and Wren in turn. "Now we must get inside and minister to Rundel," he said. "Good luck with the journeys ahead, all of you!"

Madder bade farewell too, then he and Tobias led the horses into the Abbey grounds.

"I'll follow in a moment," said Alia. She turned to Wren. "You went to Underath to become a Sorcerer. How long have you known that was what you wanted?"

"I think I've always known it," said Wren.

Alia nodded. "Watching you in Underath's castle as you learned the basics of sorcery from his books, I saw your potential clear as day. I could understand if your brush with magic has put you off, but in a year or so it's quite possible that I would consider taking on an apprentice . . ."

"Really?" said Wren, excited.

"Someone like me," said Alia, wistful. "Eager to study hard. Dedicated and obedient."

Wren's excitement seemed to drain away entirely. "Oh," she said. "I thought you meant me."

Patch put an encouraging hand on her shoulder. "She *does* actually mean you, Wren."

Alia smiled. "Perhaps I should reconsider?"

"No!" said Wren. "I can be all those things. Absolutely!"

Alia nodded. "Well, if you do decide that sorcery is still your future . . . come and find me."

Once Alia had left, they sat on the grass by the road as they waited for Erner to return. Wren's attention was suddenly diverted as a large beetle struggled through the grass near her feet. "Ooh!" she said, picking it up and biting into the juicy abdomen. "Blaaargh!" she cried, spitting it out. "That's disgusting!"

Patch shrugged. "It's always been disgusting, Wren."

"As a rat those things are delicious," she said. "But as a human . . ." She spat again and scrunched up her face. "Yuck! That's going to linger." She gathered herself for yet another spit.

Erner reappeared at the gate. He was leading three horses, and Brother Duffle walked beside him.

"I've commandeered Rundel Stone's horse for the trip," said Erner. "And I borrowed a third from the Abbey. It will speed up our journey." He handed one set of reins to Wren.

"Brother Duffle!" said Barver. "I'm glad you came to bid farewell!"

"You left this item in the pigsties," said Duffle, handing something to Patch.

Barver and Wren saw it and grinned. "Fox and Owls!" they both declared. Patch put it into his bag.

Brother Duffle gave Barver a serious look. "Now," he said, holding up a small glass jar. "An ointment for your shoulders and wing joints. Apply generously as required." He handed the jar to Barver, who placed it in one of his harness packs. "How about trying a few flaps to see how you look?"

"Okay," said Barver. "I'll try." He stepped away to give himself space, and then started to flap his wings—very gently at first, but giving a couple of really strong beats at the end. "Feels good."

"Everything looks fine," said Duffle. "You're almost there. Be careful though! Promise me not to overdo things! And can I say, it's been an absolute honor healing you."

"The honor was mine," said Barver, shaking Brother Duffle's hand. "And I promise to take things slowly."

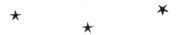

They arrived in Axlebury three days after setting off from the Abbey. Wren was keen to reach Underath before changing back into a rat, so she could let the Sorcerer know exactly what she thought of him. As such, she'd been eager to push on at every opportunity. It had meant taking only a few hours of sleep each night, and Patch was exhausted by the time they rode into the village.

Axlebury was busy, an early market drawing traders and shoppers in the central square. Barver attracted plenty of interest on their arrival, but his cheery greetings were enough to settle the nerves of the wary villagers.

"That's Fendscouth Tor," said Wren, pointing to a large craggy hill some distance away. "Underath's castle is on the far side." All but one of the beads on her bracelet was entirely white now, and even that last bead had only the barest amount of color left. "Oh hell's *bells*," she said. "I'm almost out of time."

Barver took a gentle hold of her hand, and looked closely at the bracelet. "You could change at any moment," he said.

"I'm afraid we must wait here until it's happened. Underath will have to make do with *our* sharp tongues, instead."

Wren muttered to herself, but Patch caught Barver's eye—they both knew it was better this way, as Wren would accept Barver and Erner taking the lead when they reached Underath's castle.

Barver reached for his money-purse. "That inn over there," he said, squinting to read its sign. "The Old Raven. I'll get rooms for each of you and a stable stall for me. We should rest for the night and see the Sorcerer tomorrow. And, right now, it'll be somewhere private for Wren to, um, change." As he spoke, he did some shoulder exercises that Brother Duffle had suggested. His flight muscles were almost back to normal, and once or twice on the journey he'd attempted flying for a few seconds at a time.

Wren nodded. "That'd be welcome, but I think two rooms are enough. I'll have changed back soon, and I won't need a bed. I'd also rather not be alone once it gets dark. I'll probably have nightmares about owls."

With the rooms arranged, Erner took the horses to the stables to tend to them. Wren went up to one of the rooms for privacy and refused Patch's offer to stay with her, so Patch and Barver ordered some small ale and sat in anxious silence at the front of the inn, sipping their drinks as they worried about her and waited for Erner to come back.

After a while, Barver took something from his harness and looked at it warily.

"Is that your mum's letter?" asked Patch.

Barver gave a big sigh. "Yes. The one I'm to open when I reach my destination."

"You haven't been tempted to open it in advance, then?"

"Of *course* I've been tempted," said Barver. "But I won't. Her instructions were specific. I must go to the place she's described, any time after the Scale Moon, and only read the letter when I get there."

"The Scale Moon?"

"The next full moon marks a special day in the Dragon Calendar, a few days from now. My wings are ready, I think. As long as I can remember the higher air currents at this time of year, I can ride the winds. If I set off soon I'll arrive just as the Scale Moon rises."

"And would you have the strength for a passenger?"

Barver frowned. "I appreciate the offer," he said. "The thought of going alone is—" Patch thought he could see his friend's eyes tearing up a little. "But my mother's instructions are to open the letter in a dangerous place called the Sun Canyon, in the middle of a desolate, harsh desert known as the Dragon Wastes. Nobody lives there. Nobody even *goes* there."

"I still want to come," said Patch. "If you can carry me for the flight?"

Barver shifted his wings a little. "That won't be a problem," he said. "But it's not *you* I'm worried about."

Patch nodded. "Wren," he said. "The last thing she needs is danger. If Underath cures her then she'll be happy for us to take her to her parents, but if not . . ."

"Then she'll insist on going with us," said Barver. "In which case, I think you must stay here with her. There's enough of my mother's Vanishing Gift left for you to stay at the inn until I return."

"You'd have to sneak off without telling her," said Patch. "And I don't relish the look she'll give me when she realizes what's happened."

Barver laughed. "Wren is courageous, loyal, and very stubborn. I can only *begin* to imagine her anger at us for being so protective."

"It's good that she means so much to you," said Patch.

"She does," said Barver. "She reminds me of someone, you see." He shook his head slowly, looking sorrowful. "I was a lonely soul as a child. As the only dracogriff, the other children both feared and mocked me. I had one great friend. My young cousin, Genasha. I'd known her from the day she hatched. Independent, short tempered, and rude!" He grinned.

"That *does* sound like Wren," said Patch.

"And honest, and loyal, and funny. Yes, Wren reminds me very much of Genasha." He fell silent for a moment.

"The year before I left for adventure in the Islands of the Eastern Seas, Genasha died. Her blood thinned. It's a common enough disease in dragon children, but most recover. She did not." He closed his eyes. "My mother behaved very oddly after Genasha's death. She never once mentioned her name, and if I spoke of my cousin she would become cold. It seemed as if her heart had turned to *ice*. It was the breaking point for our relationship. Genasha's death hit me very hard, but my mother didn't seem to care at all. That's why I left home and why I didn't speak to my mother again."

They finished their ales in silence, and the innkeeper came to fetch their empty tankards. "Another drink, lads?" she asked.

From above them came an awful scream, which was suddenly cut short and replaced by a few seconds of squeaking. Then there was silence.

The innkeeper looked up to the window of one of the rooms they'd rented. "That's your friend?" she said, eyes wide with panic. "We must help!"

Patch's throat was dry, hearing such a horrible noise coming from Wren. "I can assure you everything is fine," he said. "Our friend has . . . a severe terror of spiders." It was the best he could come up with on the spot. "She must have seen one."

"Oh!" said the innkeeper. "Fair enough. They do get very big in this old place."

"I hope Wren's okay," said Barver, once the innkeeper had left.

Patch nodded. "I'm thinking two things," he said. "The first is that we shouldn't wait until tomorrow. We need to get to Underath right away and free Wren from this curse, whatever it takes."

"Agreed!" said Barver. "What's the second thing?"

Patch shivered. "That I'll have to get rid of every spider in my room to have any chance of sleep tonight."

Patch left Barver and went up to check on Wren. He knocked gently and entered. Wren was on the bed, curled up. Patch sat next to her and she climbed onto his shoulder, still trembling. He could see markings in the fur running around her midriff and pointed them out to her: a series of gray circles, one of which was slightly blue. The bracelet was *part* of her in rat form, he realized—when the circles all turned blue, she would be ready to change again. "Is there anything I can do to make you feel better?" he said.

Absolutely, signed Wren. *Let's go and see Underath, right now.*

Patch nodded. "I was thinking exactly the same thing," he said. "First though, I have a little job I need to do here." He took his Pipe out from his pocket. "Let's see how my new Pipe handles these critters!"

Critters? signed Wren.

"You'll see," said Patch. He stood and opened the door, and also the door to the second room they'd rented, across

269

the corridor. He started to play. He built a gentle Dream, but it sounded very different to the one he'd made for the rats in Patterfall. The note lengths, for instance, were far shorter. His target, after all, was much smaller than a rat.

It was the money spiders who appeared first, dozens of the tiny dots coming out of the beams above them and drifting to the floor, where they formed a line. Then the larger ones peeked out, intrigued, perhaps ten or fifteen of them emerging from between floorboards. At last, the real *biggies* came out of hiding from under the bed and behind the few bits of rough furniture in the room. Patch's eyes went wide; Wren stared at them. There were only four, but four was more than enough when they were that size.

Patch changed the Song slightly, and the eager spiders traipsed across the corridor to the other room, where the Song made them think the juiciest of all the world's flies awaited them. Journey completed, Patch closed the other room's door and returned. "When we get back, we'll all spend the night in here, I think," he said.

I'm not good with spiders, signed Wren.

"Me neither," said Patch. "I pity whoever rents that room next."

270

25

UNDERATH THE SORCERER

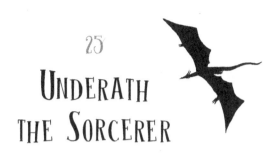

With Wren on Patch's shoulder, they set off to Fendscouth Tor. They'd left the third horse—the one borrowed from the Abbey—back at the inn stables, getting a well-earned rest that Patch was quietly envious of. The way was steep, through windswept scrubland. As they rounded the Tor, Underath's castle came into view, sitting on the edge of a forest that swept down toward a large lake.

"You two stay here," Erner told Wren and Patch. "This should be safe enough for you, while Barver and I speak to Underath and see how things are."

Wren grumbled, but conceded that it was for the best. Barver flexed his wings. "I think I'll try a bit of air time!" he said.

"Be careful, big fella," said Patch. "Are you sure you're ready?"

With a great leap and a huge grin, Barver took off. Patch watched with mixed feelings. It was a delight to see him enjoy himself so much, but being out of practice didn't lend itself to graceful flying. Soon, with a heavy landing, he was back on the ground.

"Feels good!" he said. He reached up and rubbed his shoulder.

Patch got off his horse and sat on a nearby granite outcrop. He was wearing his bag across one shoulder, eager to keep the Hamelyn's Mask close by rather than leave the bag tied to his saddle. Its value was too great—either Barver would manage to strike a bargain with Underath, with Wren's cure in exchange for the Mask, or the Mask would fetch a good price later and give Patch his chance at a new life.

Erner galloped toward the castle. Barver ran beside him, occasionally going airborne for a few seconds. At one point he veered off route and plunged down unnervingly before recovering.

Hmm, signed Wren. *I think I'll let Barver get the hang of flying again before I ask for a ride.*

With a while to wait, Patch reached into his pocket and unfolded the paper he'd written Alia's prophecy on. Wren stared at it.

I remember hearing those words! she signed. *I thought I dreamed it!*

"Alia spoke them in the circle of salt. She couldn't remember much and was worried she'd given me some kind of prophecy. She seemed so anxious about it, I didn't have the heart to tell her that she'd done exactly that. A prophecy that someone would betray us, but that we could recognize them by the words they would speak." He read the words aloud: "*They thought they had us. But we're almost clear. Just the ridge to go. What's wrong with you? What's wrong?*" He shook his head. "'Get away when you hear the words,' Alia said, 'as quickly as you can. *Run!*'"

Wren nodded. *I heard her*, she signed. *Then she spoke in a curious way, right?*

"Indeed," said Patch, thinking back. "Although pretty much *everything* was curious at the time. Her glowing eyes, for a start."

An odd set of words, don't you think? Alia had said, almost conversing with herself. *I agree, very odd! What say you, Patch? The lad's gone so very pale. The day's been quite a strain, I imagine.*

He shivered at the thought of the fiery red eyes.

The words on the paper seemed to taunt him. He groaned. "I wish she'd not said anything. I'll be listening out for it every day and it could be years before it happens. Decades, even."

So ignore it! signed Wren. *From what little I know, prophecy is usually more trouble than it's worth.*

"Ignore it?" said Patch. "Easier said than done." He folded the paper up and returned it to his pocket.

After a while, they saw Barver flying back toward them. Below, Erner was galloping on his horse.

Wren frowned. *Are they running away from something?* she signed.

Patch made sure Wren was secure on his shoulder before he mounted his horse, ready to speed off if necessary.

"Wait there!" cried Erner. He pulled up in front of them as Barver landed heavily, out of breath. Erner's concerned expression wasn't encouraging. "You need to see this," he said.

They left the horses grazing outside the main gate of Underath's castle and approached the entrance.

"The doors lay slightly open when we arrived," said Erner. "I called out and got no response, so entered carefully." He pushed the doors wide to reveal an entry hall. It was chaos inside. Every piece of furniture was upended. Glass littered the ground, and the smell of stale wine and ale filled the air. "This is what I found. Everywhere I looked is the same."

Wren stared at the mess in horror. *We have to find Underath,* she signed.

"His griffin is not in the courtyard," said Barver. "Whatever happened here, it was weeks ago," said Erner.

"There's rotting food on a table upstairs. I found his study. All his books were gone. I suspect the Sorcerer has fled."

Barver squeezed through the entrance and looked around. "We should search the whole castle. If Underath has gone, there must be clues as to his whereabouts." He sniffed the air, and moved toward another set of doors, flinging them open. The courtyard lay beyond. He pointed to a stone building within it. "The griffin's stable," he said. "There may be things we can learn about Underath there."

Erner nodded. "Patch, stay with Barver. You two take this half of the courtyard, check the various doors and cellars. I'll take Wren and search the other half."

"Agreed," said Patch.

Barver hurried across the courtyard toward the stable.

Patch let Wren climb onto Erner's shoulder, then went after Barver, finding him inside the stable hunting through shelves of the griffin's belongings.

"You see anything interesting here?"

"Plenty of books," said Barver. "Alkeran was an avid reader. Mostly tales of adventure, but some philosophy too. Wait, look!" He moved to one wall and lifted some kind of large ring from the floor.

Patch realized what it was: a locking collar, to which was attached a formidable iron chain. "Did Underath use that for his griffin?"

Barver shook his head. He raised the chain to show that it was short and not fixed to anything. "Presumably all that remains of a much longer chain," he said. "No, Alkeran was not a prisoner here. Griffins and Sorcerers are a good fit for each other, Patch. Both prefer isolation, and they can provide one another with a degree of safety. Alkeran and Underath are colleagues—perhaps even friends. The rust on this collar suggests it has not been in use for many years, yet Alkeran keeps it in his home. Interesting."

Patch nodded. "I'll start searching in the courtyard. I'll call if I find something." He left the stable and went to a nearby hatchway in the side of the castle. He opened it up, and there was coal inside. He looked to the stable again and saw a chimney, so the coal was presumably for the griffin's fireplace. Across the way, he could see Erner and Wren getting on with their search.

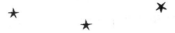

The courtyard had been out of bounds for Wren while she'd been living in the castle, so there was little advice she could offer Erner. They came to a row of doors, and Erner tried the first. It was locked; Erner took out his Pipe and played a rapid high-pitched Song. The lock thudded open.

Wren applauded, impressed. *I've not seen Patch do that kind of thing,* she signed.

"Thanks," said Erner, bowing his head. He opened the door and a terrible stench of rot came from within. Inside were barrels, from which liquid was seeping. He closed the door in a hurry.

These must be the food stores, said Wren. *Underath magically restocked the kitchen from them, and the stores were charmed to be cold. Not anymore.*

Erner frowned and went to the next door. Again, it was locked. Again, Erner played to unlock it. He opened the door and entered.

A yelp came from one corner, and Erner stepped to the side instinctively as something shot from the shadows and thudded into the door frame, a puff of some kind of powder coming from it when it hit. Wren looked to where the object had fallen—it was a small leather pouch. She looked over to the corner, and there, wearing his favored elaborate robe, stood Underath, terrified. He carried a bag filled with bread. Wren clenched her paws into little angry fists at the sight of him. She noticed how scruffy he seemed, his face and robes grubby, the hair on his head uncombed. He had always prided himself on his clean-shaven face, but now a ragged beard had grown.

Underath was distraught. "A Custodian Piper! Forgive me, I thought you were a brigand come to murder me! You caught me by surprise!" At that moment, he noticed Wren on Erner's shoulder. His face fell. "Oh dear," he said. "It's you, um, maid-person."

Wren scowled the deepest scowl she'd ever managed. "Her name is *Wren*," said Erner. "I assume you are Underath?"

The Sorcerer nodded.

Erner glanced down to the pouch that Underath had thrown. He gave the Sorcerer an angry glare. "A Kaposher Pouch, eh?" said Erner. "If you're going to use that, you can't afford to miss!"

Wren had read about Kaposher Dust in one of the many books she'd pored over in Underath's study. It was a sleeping powder, difficult to make and highly prized by thieves—throw a Kaposher Pouch at an unwary victim, and they would be rendered unconscious in moments by the dust that puffed out.

"I am Erner Whitlock," said Erner. "I represent the Pipers' Council in an important matter." He rummaged in his shoulder bag, then held up the jar containing the little box that had poisoned Rundel Stone. "We shall discuss Wren's situation in a moment. First, tell me everything you can about this."

Underath took it, wary. As he examined it through the glass, Erner reached into his bag and produced a cloth; keeping one eye on Underath, he gathered up the Kaposher Pouch in the cloth and placed it carefully in his bag. "In case you get any *ideas*," he said.

Underath waved dismissively. "I have others." He removed the lid of the jar and sniffed. After a moment, his eyes widened. "Oh no, this is a very nasty little thing. A death puzzle. Quite a complicated one."

"And did *you* make it?" said Erner.

"Absolutely not!" said Underath, sounding offended. He replaced the jar's lid and passed it back. "I don't make such weaponry. It's clumsy and brutal."

"I'm assured your style of magic is very similar," said Erner. "And remember, Sorcerer. I am here on Council business. I could make life difficult for you if you don't help."

"Make life difficult for me?" said Underath, with a sneer. "As if it's not hard enough already!" He glared at Erner, but soon bowed his head. "Very well. Look to the far north. Near Ygginbrucket, where a Master once lived. I was his pupil, and this *death puzzle* has his hallmarks. Hence the similarity to my magical style."

"The Master's name?"

"Sagharros. Died fifteen years ago. This box is of recent construction, so it definitely wasn't him. It may have been made by another of his students."

"And you're sure the box has nothing to do with you?"

"I swear it!"

"Mmm . . . ," said Erner, stroking his chin. "Perhaps I will trust you more, once you undo the cruel curse you set on my friend here."

Underath looked back at them, pale. "I can't, I'm afraid," he said. "I'm somewhat indisposed. I have no magic to spare."

"We saw the state of your castle," said Erner. "What happened here?"

Underath scowled. "My *wife* happened," he said, venom in his voice. "She's long gone now. She took my griffin and left!" He looked at Wren. "Did you notice anything odd about her? For example, did I mention her name at any point?"

Wren thought for a moment. She shook her head.

"There's a reason for that," said Underath. "I don't *know* her name. Isn't that strange? I know *nothing* about her. I don't think I ever did. There I was, off on a trip somewhere, and the next thing I know I'm married and *happy* and not thinking straight, with no memory of how it happened."

Erner raised an eyebrow. "Did you drink much wine on this trip of yours, by any chance?"

Underath looked at him with scorn. "If only it was so simple! That woman hexed me! I still don't know how she did it, but she got the better of Underath. *She stole my heart.*" He sagged, shaking his head in misery.

"Pull yourself together!" said Erner. "So you lost out in love! You must still make amends to Wren!"

"That's *not* what I mean," said Underath. He reached to his robe and unbuttoned it at the front. "She *stole* my *heart*," he said. He pulled his robe apart and exposed his chest. "Literally."

Erner and Wren gasped. In the middle of Underath's chest was a big hole, charred around the edges. "Nasty!" said Erner. The hole wasn't empty, though. "Is that . . . is that a *shoe*?"

"Yes," said Underath, seething. "She took my heart and thought me dead, but I had a little life left in me, and magic enough to keep death at bay. The shoe was a hasty replacement. All I had handy, really." He looked down bitterly at the hole in his chest, with its oddly pulsating shoe. "It takes every scrap of magic I have merely to keep going day by day. Slowly, the wound will close and the shoe will transform into a new heart, but it will take a year, perhaps longer."

"So you're refusing to undo Wren's curse?" said Erner.

"Look at me," said Underath. "I'm a wretch. I haven't the power to craft the undoing of a curse. Especially such a *fine* curse." He moved toward them and reached out to Wren. She squeaked and gnashed her teeth at him. "The circle around your waist... I see someone's had a go at fixing you already. Some kind of morphic deflector, I'm guessing. Interesting work, but not really a long-term solution." He looked up, a sly smile on his face. "There is one way I could help, however. For a price."

"What price did you have in mind?" said Erner, wary.

"My griffin," said Underath. "Get me my griffin back."

"If your griffin was happy to leave with your wife, then it's not for me to interfere."

"Happy?" said Underath. "*Happy?* Alkeran was her target all along. She told me as I lay there with my life's blood draining away. 'It was your griffin I wanted, Underath, not you!' For what purpose she wanted him I do not know, but that's why she took my heart—there is an old, dark spell to give control over a griffin. A spell that requires the heart of a friend, kept in a box, and tied around Alkeran's neck . . ."

There was a look of genuine loss in Underath's expression, a look that Wren had never seen nor expected to see on the Sorcerer's face. In all her time in this castle, she'd never known that Alkeran was anything more to the man than just a handy means of transport.

"He's a troubled soul," said Underath. "Nightmares plague him, of a time long ago when he was held captive. He's never told me more than that, but it's easy to see his pain and his fear. I promised to keep him safe, and I've failed him. So remove my heart from around his neck and free him. Bring my heart to me, and I can quickly regain my powers, but you must bring my *griffin* back too if you want me to create a cure."

Erner looked to Wren. "Can we trust him?" he said.

Does it matter? she signed, disheartened. *He obviously hasn't the strength to cure me, and we're not going to be able to bring back his griffin. I'm doomed!*

"Nonsense," Erner told her. He turned to Underath. "Do you have any idea where your wife may have gone?"

Underath frowned. "None, I'm afraid," he said. "Now if you don't mind, I'd like to gather some food and get back into hiding."

"Hiding?" said Erner. "Hiding from what?"

"From the mercenaries, of course!"

Erner's face fell. "What mercenaries?"

282

"Nastiest bunch of hired soldiers I've ever laid eyes on," said Underath. "My wife had some kind of deal with them. Gave them the castle when she left. They've made a terrible mess of the place. Didn't you notice them?"

Erner and Wren stared at him.

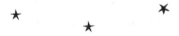

Patch searched a room that stored equipment for horses: saddles, martingales, bridles. It looked as though no one had been in there for decades. He came out and walked over to the largest of the doors on this side of the courtyard, and as he reached out to open it something ripped through the air. It pierced the sleeve of his shirt and the strap of his shouldered bag, pinning him to the door.

A crossbow bolt. He stared at it, gobsmacked.

"Aw, look at that," came a voice from behind him. "See, your aim's way off!"

Patch turned his head as he desperately pulled his arm, and saw a mean-looking pair of men clad in well-worn leather armor. One of them smiled, showing off a mouthful of broken teeth. "We'll be with you in a jiffy, mate," he said to Patch, leering. He turned to his colleague. "Come on, get that reloaded."

"I'm harmless!" said Patch. "Just looking for Underath, that's all!"

"The old Sorcerer? He's dead, mate. Like you'll be in a second. This is our castle now. You're trespassing!"

Patch yelped and pulled as hard as he could, but he couldn't free himself.

"I can't get the bolt in," complained the man with the crossbow. "Why do they make these things so hard to reload?"

His colleague scowled. "You need to pull that lever back more." There was an audible clunk as the mechanism fell into place. "There you go!"

"Ta!" said the mercenary. He turned to Patch, who was still frantically trying to get free. "Right then, just you hold still while I murder you."

Patch whimpered and closed his eyes. A moment later the unmistakable sound of roaring flame filled the air, accompanied by hearty screams. When Patch looked again he saw two smoldering corpses on the ground. Behind them, Barver was grinning.

"That was a bit brutal, wasn't it?" said Patch.

Barver shrugged. "They caught me in a bad mood," he said.

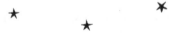

"Don't worry, Wren," said Erner. "Patch will be safe. He's with Barver." He turned back to Underath. "We didn't come across anyone in the castle. How many mercenaries are there?"

"A hundred, maybe. They have dogs with them."

"Dogs?"

"You know," said Underath. "The big ones mercenaries love so much. War dogs."

"War dogs," said Erner, looking anxious.

Is that a problem? signed Wren.

Erner looked to the door. "We have to warn them."

At that moment, they heard a roar of fire and screams. Erner ran out into the courtyard, Wren clinging tightly to his shoulder. Behind him, Underath hurried to the door and locked it, his muffled voice coming through the thick wood. "Good luck with that!" he said.

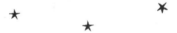

Barver came over to Patch and pulled the crossbow bolt out, freeing him.

"Thanks," said Patch. "That was a close one!"

The door the bolt had lodged in now started to swing open very slowly. The smile on Patch's face crumpled as he saw what lay in the large room beyond.

A long table, filled with bottles of ale and rounds of cheese, surrounded by benches on which dozens and dozens of unconscious mercenaries were slumped.

One of them snorted and opened his eyes. "Wha—?" he said. He looked at Patch. He looked at Barver. Then he looked at the smoldering corpses of his colleagues. "Awaken, lads!" he yelled. "There's trouble!"

Patch backed away as the mercenaries began to stir. He reached for his Pipe. He could try some battle Songs and take out a few of them, he knew.

"Oh don't worry," said Barver. "I can handle this lot!"

Then the growling started.

From the shadows within the room, two vast dogs emerged, almost as tall as the men around them. Their gray skin looked as tough as leather and much of it was without fur, giving them the appearance of being riddled with mange. Saliva was starting to drip from the mouths of both dogs. Their teeth were horribly long.

Barver was staring fearfully at them. As Patch watched the massive dogs approach he knew the odds were firmly in the mercenaries' favor.

War dogs hadn't actually been bred for war, originally. They had been for *hunting*, and the prey they'd been bred to hunt gave them their other name.

"*Dragonhounds*," said Patch. He heard a shout and turned to see Erner running across the courtyard.

"Time to fly," said Barver. "Quit fiddling with that Pipe and get on my back! I'll grab Erner and Wren on the wing."

"Are you sure you can carry us all?"

Barver frowned. "We're just about to find out," he said.

Patch jumped on and held tight to the straps of Barver's

battle harness. Barver launched himself into the air, straining hard to get speed. Ahead of them, Erner braced himself, arms raised. Barver grabbed him around the midriff and gained height immediately, setting Erner on his back.

"Where's Wren?" cried Patch, and then he saw her head poking out from Erner's robe. He took her and set her by Barver's neck, where a notch in the harness would give her some protection. She put her arms around a strap and held tight.

The dragonhounds prowled in the courtyard, and the mercenaries readied their bows. A bolt shot past them, and Barver attempted to get higher. Up they went, until they could get over the castle wall to the forest beyond, but below them the mercenaries opened another gate and allowed the hounds out.

"Tenacious, aren't they?" said Erner.

"We, um, killed two of their colleagues," said Patch. "I guess it annoyed them."

"Ah," said Erner. "I suppose it would."

"Where should I head for?" panted Barver.

Wren started to sign frantically, and Patch relayed the message. "See the lake in the forest?" he said, pointing. "If we fly over it, a large gorge lies on the other side of a ridge. They won't be able to cross it."

Soon they were flying just over the treetops, but the hounds were closing fast. If the dogs got ahead, it would only take them two leaps up a tree and Barver would be within reach.

"Go higher, Barver!" yelled Patch.

"I'm trying!" yelled Barver.

Erner took out his Pipe and tied his bag to Barver's harness. "Patch, we should ready some defenses! If the hounds jump for us, a Push Song should be enough to deflect them! Hook your feet under the harness like this."

Patch nodded and watched Erner slide each foot under parts of Barver's harness straps. He tied his own bag to Barver and did the same as Erner with his feet. It was uncomfortable, but it gave him both hands free to Pipe. He set about building a Push Song, a simple defensive force that was the first battle Song any Piper learned.

Barver roared and picked up the pace, his great wings straining. On his back, everyone was watching as the hounds narrowed the gap, those frothing jaws even more horrible from such a short distance, the snarls terrifyingly near.

Then they were over water. Barver roared again, this time in triumph. Wren cheered and Patch laughed with relief. The hounds barked with rage for a moment before pounding along the side of the lake, but by now they were so far back Barver could just keep his current speed.

At the far end of the lake, the forest rose sharply. "That must be the ridge," cried Erner. "Safety lies on the other side!"

"You hear that, Barver?" said Patch. "Head over that ridge, and you've saved us all!" He looked back and grinned at Erner. They both put their Pipes back in their pockets and unhooked their feet, holding on with their hands again.

"They thought they had us," said Erner. "But we're almost clear! Just the ridge to go!"

Patch froze, his blood turning to ice as Erner's words sank in. The words of the prophecy.

They thought they had us. But we're almost clear. Just the ridge to go. What's wrong with you? What's wrong?

He looked to Wren. She had one paw over her mouth, horrified. She shook her head slowly, back and forth.

Patch could hear Alia's warning: *There will come a time when you hear these words! A mouth that speaks them is a traitorous mouth, and will betray you to that which you fear most! When you hear them spoken, get away as quickly as you can! Run!*

It can't be, thought Patch. *It can't be.*

A moment of hope came to him: Erner hadn't said *all* of it, not yet.

"What's wrong with you?" said Erner, baffled.

Patch shook his head, not wanting his friend to say anything else; not wanting him to complete the prediction.

"What's *wrong*?" said Erner.

It was done. The traitor Alia had warned them of was Erner, however much Patch wanted to deny it. A terrible emptiness filled his heart as he realized what he had to do. Erner was watching him with utter confusion.

"I can't do it," said Patch, his vision blurred with sudden tears. "I *can't*." But he had no choice. "I'm sorry," he said, desolate.

He gave Erner a sudden shove, sending his friend flying off Barver's back and into the lake below.

290

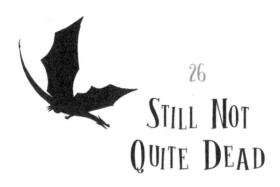

26
STILL NOT
QUITE DEAD

Barver started to circle back. "What happened?" he yelled.

"Keep going!" shouted Patch.

"We can't go without him!" said Barver.

"*Leave him!*"

Barver turned his head to look directly at Patch, and he saw that Patch meant it, even if he didn't understand. He faced front and, jaws clenched, turned toward the far shore of the lake and the ridge beyond it, flying harder than he'd ever done before.

Patch looked at Wren, clinging to Barver's harness. She was glaring at him, eyes wet, shaking her head and trembling, but there was nothing he could say to her. He glanced back and saw Erner swimming toward the lake shore.

There was movement just inside the trees. The dragon-hounds had made up most of the ground they'd lost.

"They're closing on us," said Patch.

"I know!" cried Barver.

"You need to go higher!"

"I *know!*"

It would be tight. If they were going to beat the hounds to the ridge, it wasn't going to be by much.

"I can't get the height," wailed Barver.

"You can do it!" said Patch.

Wren squeaked at him. *Your Pipe!* she signed. *Get ready to hit those dogs with something!*

Patch took out his Pipe and hooked his feet under Barver's straps again. He started to build another Push.

They reached the shore. The hounds were heading for the peak of the ridge. Barver was almost screaming now, putting all his might into squeezing out that last drop of height and speed. Wren and Patch watched the hounds.

The ridge: closer, closer.

The hounds: gaining, gaining.

The Push was ready. Patch held it, seeing the hounds get slightly ahead, watching them bound up the elm trees in front of them, and then . . .

Barver saw them leap, and swung right. One dragon-hound had managed to jump higher than the other, and it was almost on top of Patch when he loosed the Push.

The Song hit the beast hard enough to stall its trajectory, and it fell just under Barver, howling as it flailed with its claws and plummeted out of harm's way.

Breathless, Patch turned to see what had happened to the second hound. His heart sank—it had found purchase. Its jaws were clamped around Barver's neck, and it was shaking its head violently to work its teeth under the scales. Its back legs were fending off Barver's arms, stopping him from wrenching the hound away. Blood was already flowing. Barver roared with pain, but he was managing to stay in the air.

The trees vanished under them. Suddenly they were past the ridge and over a deep gorge. Patch raised his Pipe again, but he wasn't sure what he could use without risking Barver too. He decided to try something more direct: beside him, tied safely to Barver's harness, was his bag. He undid the fastening strap and took out his knife, putting his Pipe inside before fastening it again.

"Hold on tight," he told Wren. He unhooked his feet from Barver's straps and lunged past her, gripping Barver's harness as he swung the knife at full stretch, thrusting it deep into the dragonhound's paw. The blade went through until it scraped Barver's scales.

The dragonhound yelped. Livid, it pulled its jaws from Barver's throat and snapped toward Patch, snarling with rage, gobbets of bloody froth flying from its slavering mouth.

It was the respite Barver needed. He pulled higher just in time and they reached the other side of the gorge, skimming the treetops. As Barver gained a little more height, the hound clamped its jaws around his throat again and they veered suddenly to one side.

Patch's grip wasn't quite enough. He slipped forward, and the hound swiped at him with its injured paw. The claws caught on Patch's shoulder and yanked hard.

Patch fell. Above, he saw that the dragonhound still had its grip on Barver's throat. Wren, barely managing to cling on, stared forlornly after him, just as they had watched Erner plunge barely a minute before.

He braced himself, but the first branch he hit took all the wind from him and knocked the knife from his hand. He knew there would be plenty of other painful branches before he reached the ground.

Patch stood as quickly as his shaky legs and rattled head would allow. He was in agony from head to toe, but nothing seemed broken; without the branches to slow his fall, he would certainly have fared much worse.

Although he'd been preoccupied with plummeting, he was certain he'd heard a crash nearby. He reckoned the battle in the air had lasted only a few more seconds after he'd left it.

Ahead, the tops of the trees had been broken here and there. He feared terribly for Wren and Barver. There was no noise, not even birdsong. Aware of every breath, every step, every crunch of leaf and snap of stick underfoot, he started to walk.

The treetops showed more and more signs of damage as he went. Then, there it was: a massive oak, once tall and proud, had been ripped apart by a great impact. The top third of the trunk had fallen to the ground, and the next third had been shattered. At the base, covered in broken branches and blood, was the still figure of Barver.

Patch remembered the first time he and Wren had met their friend, and how they'd assumed the dracogriff was dead, but this was different. The wounds on his neck glistened with fresh blood, and his head was twisted at an angle that filled Patch with dismay.

Yet the greatest fear of all struck him when he noticed one other detail.

The dragonhound was nowhere to be seen.

Suddenly Patch realized that his own breathing sounded horribly *loud*. He held his breath and listened; the only thing he could make out was his heartbeat. Something small hit him on the head. He looked up and saw nothing, but another object came out of nowhere and got him square on the nose. This time he saw it hit the ground: an acorn.

"Wren?" he whispered, squinting to see if there was any sign of movement above him. He raised his voice a little. "*Wren?*"

He heard a distinct squeaking from above and peered harder, shading his eyes from the sun that was coming through the leaves. Nothing there . . . nothing *there* . . .

There! He could just about see Wren on a high branch, waving frantically.

"It's all right, I see you!" he said. His reassurance did nothing to calm her down. "I'm okay! A little bruised and battered, but—" He stopped, sensing something. Wren's squeaking grew even more urgent, and he realized that what he'd taken as *waving* was actually *pointing.*

A little whimper came from his throat when he heard the sound of the dragonhound's harsh panting behind him. He turned his head to see.

It was ten feet away, its muzzle soaked in Barver's blood. There was red on its flanks from open cuts. He turned fully to face the massive beast, its head higher than Patch's own. A vicious growl started up in the creature's throat as it edged closer to him.

He felt oddly *calm* as he watched slobber drip from the jowls of the massive dog. Its eyes narrowed, and the growl became even more sinister. The animal was preparing to devour him. The calmness he felt was the expectation of death.

He hardly noticed the high-pitched squeal from above, even as the squeal grew louder and louder, nearer and nearer . . .

As one, Patch and the hound looked up to see a small shadow falling from the sky. Wren flopped onto the confused dragonhound's head and clamped her teeth deep into the fleshiest part of its ear.

The hound let loose a terrible yowl and shook its head this way and that with greater and greater violence, trying to dislodge the insolent rat. Wren's grip was firm, however, all four little claws clinging to the beast's sparse fur, her mouth dripping with the hound's blood just as the hound's had dripped with Barver's.

Back and forth the hound swung its head, yelping and angry, gnashing at the air. Patch backed away and watched in awe. The hound moved closer to the nearest tree and swung its head hard at the trunk, trying to catch Wren in the middle, but Wren was too quick, jumping to the other side of the head just in time. Without her toothhold on the ear, though, she was struggling to keep hold of the animal's fur.

The hound sensed she was in trouble and quickly spun for another attempt at crushing her against the tree. With a howl it smashed its head at the trunk once more.

Patch closed his eyes, unable to look, but when he opened them again he couldn't understand what he was seeing. The hound was motionless, its head pressed against the tree trunk, while Wren was on the back of its neck jumping up and down with her arms in the air.

Celebrating.

Then he saw: jutting from the beast's neck was the sharp end of a broken branch, still attached to the trunk. Blood started to gush from the wound. The hound gasped, and its legs buckled, but it remained skewered to the tree. A final sigh came from the dragonhound as it died. Wren took a well-deserved bow, and Patch applauded the monster-killer rat. *Nobody messes with Wren!* she signed, before her triumphant expression turned to concern. *Patch, you're bleeding!*

"I'm fine," he said, but the encounter with the hound had made him forget the all-over pain he'd been feeling after the fall. His shoulder was the worst. Wren was right, he saw—there was blood seeping through his shirt. He put his hand to his shoulder blade and felt where the dragonhound's claw had caught him. He pulled his hand back and saw the bright scarlet that covered it.

He wasn't good with blood at the best of times, but when it was his *own*, he was absolutely useless. "Oh," he said, and he fell away in a dead faint.

Patch came around with Wren on his chest, squeaking at him.

Get up, she signed. *We need to check on the big guy.*

As he sat upright, she climbed up to his uninjured shoulder. He stood and started walking toward Barver's motionless form, and each step felt like the ringing of a death knell. He could see the fear on Wren's face too.

Please let him be okay, she signed. Patch didn't even attempt to reassure her. Things were bleak, and he didn't think there was any chance at all that . . .

Barver sat up with a start and raised his arms defensively. "Yaar!" he yelled, his eyes still half-closed. "Where are you, foul creature?"

Wren squeaked with relief.

"Hello there!" shouted Patch. "We thought you were a certain goner this time!"

Barver blinked. "Where is it?" he said. His eyes settled on the dragonhound's corpse. He flinched, then realized that the beast was dead. "Wow. How did that happen?"

"Wren killed it," said Patch.

A slow grin spread across Barver's face. He looked at Wren, and she told him the story of the dragonhound's death.

All hounds shall tremble when they hear me squeak! she signed.

Barver let out a delighted laugh. "I'll make a legend out of you, Wren!" he said. He stretched, turning his head from side to side; a great crack came from his neck joints, making both Patch and Wren wince. The blood on Barver's neck looked appalling.

"Hold on, Barver," cried Patch. "You should lie still for a while yet. You're badly injured!"

"What, this?" said Barver, gesturing to the wounds. "This is nothing. Looks much worse than it is, believe me." He turned to the massive tree he'd collided with, and whistled. "Now *that's* impressive! Luckily my head took the full force of the impact."

There was no answer to that.

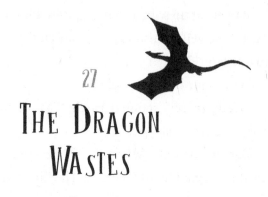

27
THE DRAGON WASTES

It seemed somehow wrong to Patch. There he sat, while Barver—covered in a ridiculous amount of his own blood—treated the gouge on Patch's shoulder, using the ointment Brother Duffle had given him.

"I can't believe that jar survived," said Patch, as Barver packed the ointment away again.

Barver smiled. "I'm very careful." Patch couldn't help but look at the smashed oak beside them. Barver ran his hands over his own bloodsoaked neck and winced.

"How is it?" said Patch.

"It smarts a little," said Barver. "But I heal quickly. My wings and shoulders have always been the exception. If the hound had gone for those instead of my throat, it would have been a very different result." He stretched out his wings and gave them an experimental flap. "They seem fine," he said. His expression grew serious. Patch could see something in his eyes—a question that he'd known was coming. "I think it's time you told me," said Barver, grim. "What happened with Erner?"

With a heavy heart, Patch explained about Alia's prophecy. Wren sat next to him, gloomy and silent.

"A tragic thing," said Barver when Patch finished. "I always thought I had a good sense of people. On our journey from the Abbey, I had no such inklings about Erner. Still, you two knew him far better than I did. Could the prophecy have been wrong?"

It was very specific, signed Wren. *Every word he spoke was as Alia predicted.*

"And his betrayal, Patch?" said Barver. "What could that have been? Would he have sent you back to the dungeons, did you think?"

"I didn't have *time* to think," said Patch. "In my mind I could just hear Alia's instruction to get away as fast as possible. Now that it's done, I don't know if it was the right thing." He hung his head. "It certainly doesn't *feel* like it." In his mind, he could see Erner swimming to the shore, and wondered if his Pipe had been lost as he fell. If so, he'd surely been captured by the mercenaries; what fate lay ahead for him?

"We must move on," said Barver. "We can fret about such things later, but first we must decide on our plans. What are we going to do now?"

Wren explained everything that had happened when she and Erner had seen Underath.

"Then our course is clear," said Barver. "I pledge myself to bring Underath's griffin home. And you, Patch? Will you join me?"

"Of course," said Patch.

I'm grateful, signed Wren. *But not until you've completed your mother's last request, Barver. I know how heavily that weighs on you. And then we must rest, for several days at least, before we set off to find the griffin.*

"It might be longer than a few days," said Patch. "We'll need time to prepare. And more money." He reached into his bag—still tied to Barver's harness—and took out the Mask. "Should we head to the Islands, Barver? We'll arrange to sell this as soon as possible."

"And so a plan emerges," said Barver. "To the Dragon Wastes for my mother's last wish, and then on to the Islands of the Eastern Seas. Sell the Mask, cure Wren, and have adventures along the way!"

"Some *safer* adventures would be appreciated," said Patch.

Barver grinned. "Understood! I'm sure we can manage that."

Wren suddenly scampered up to Barver's neck and gave him a hug.

Thank you! she signed. *I thought you two were going to take me to my parents and make me stay behind!*

"Leave you behind?" said Barver. "Unthinkable!"

Patch nodded, putting the Mask back in his bag, and as he did he noted Erner's bag was still tied beside it. He could hardly even *look* at it. They had left Erner behind, and the thought made him feel sick. Never again.

"We stay together," he said, "whatever happens."

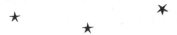

The flight to the Dragon Wastes was a revelation. Without the need to race ahead of certain death, Barver could take his time, making use of rising heat and wind coming off hills to maintain his height. The speeds they reached seemed impossible to Patch, traveling in a single day what might have taken months on foot. By nightfall they had landed at the coast, overlooking the sea from a high cliff.

The sea crossing would be the most dangerous part of the journey, a hundred miles without a place to land. With the sun setting behind them, the darkening waters ahead looked ominous.

They camped and foraged some berries before the last of the light had gone.

Patch and Wren were anxious as they set off over the sea the next morning, but the weather stayed calm and the air was warm. For hours they soared, and at last the land came into sight. Vast cliffs rose out of the water, the rock a mixture of oranges and reds.

"The Dragon Wastes!" announced Barver. "Rock and desert, a bleak wilderness. We fly on until we see the Hands of the Gods. There, we'll stop and locate the Sun Canyon." He was in his element, relishing the updrafts as he glided effortlessly above the dramatic and barren terrain. Soon, shapes rose on the horizon: features that dwarfed everything else in the landscape.

The Hands of the Gods.

Patch was awestruck. It was a formation of rock stacks, but even at this distance it was clear that they were immense. There were six wide stacks; on each, a further five stacks climbed high and ended in what seemed to be impossible curls and points.

Six hands, each with five fingers that ended in a *claw*. "Impressive, aren't they?" cried Barver over the noise of the wind. "Tradition holds that the gods were once defeated by the great Lords of the Night Kingdoms, who turned them to stone. They reached to the sky as they died. They came back from the dead, of course, and had their vengeance. My mother taught me that the stones are a natural formation, worn down by ancient seas, but looking at them in person I can understand believing the old tale. We land on the highest claw!"

"Uh . . . on *top* of it?" said Patch, terrified; it seemed such a delicately balanced thing, but as they flew nearer he could see that there was no need for fear. The tip of the claw was at least a hundred feet across and had stood solid for untold centuries.

Barver roared in glee as he touched down on the rock. "Feel free to dismount," he said, but he said it playfully.

No chance, signed Wren.

Patch was in complete agreement. Solid as the rock was, the sheer height was terrifying and the wind gusted hard. In the circumstances, the edge of the claw could never really be far enough away for his liking. "I think we'll stay on your back," he said. "If you don't mind."

Barver smiled. "Not at all." He broke out some of his rations and offered them around, little flecks of dried meat that had a strong fishy odor. Patch and Wren were reluctant at first, but it tasted rather like mackerel. They drank from their waterskins, and it was several minutes before Barver spoke again. "The Sun Canyon should be visible from here. It's almost as impressive in size as the Hands, but it's still very far away."

Wren was already squinting into the distance. *What does it look like?* she signed.

"It's a huge circle," said Barver. "With additional smaller canyons feeding into it like the rays of the sun." He strained to see, and at last pointed. "I have it! Are you both secure?"

Wren and Patch made sure of their grips. "We're good," said Patch. Barver ran to the edge of the great claw and leaped.

They landed where the instructions from Barver's mother indicated: at the northernmost point within the Sun Canyon.

Patch climbed down onto the brutal heat of the sandy ground, and Wren got onto his shoulder. "So, what next?"

"My mother's instructions say that there is a triangular rock. We dig under the rock until we find something, and then I am to read the sealed letter." They glanced around, and Barver's eyes settled on a chunk of stone five feet high, a rough triangle. "You two had better get back," he said, as he leaned down and took the strain. With a roar of effort he flipped the stone over. He reached to his side pack and untied a short-handled shovel, offering it to Patch.

"Me?" said Patch.

"I . . . I don't know what's there," said Barver. "I could damage it."

Patch and Wren shared a look, but they said nothing. They were both thinking the same thing, though—Barver was wary of what he might find. Patch took the shovel and made a start, Wren standing nearby in the shade of a rock.

It wasn't easy work, as the sides of the hole kept collapsing. Once he was down three feet or so, the hole kept its shape. Patch stepped down into it and got on with the digging, as the pile of excavated sandy earth grew behind him.

Four feet down. Five. Then he saw something.

He lifted out a tiny black pebble and held it up to the light, his eyes wide. "Volcanic glass," he said, looking at it in awe. "It could even be *obsidiac*. Black diamond." He set it on the side of the hole and continued to dig. "We could sell that too."

"We'll do no such thing," said Barver. "Be very careful with it! We must return it to the soil when we've finished."

Wren scoffed. *You shouldn't be so superstitious,* she signed.

"I can't help it, Wren," he replied. "From an early age, they drill into dragon children that taking black diamond is a terrible crime."

Patch dug a little more. "Oh, hang on, I've got something else." It took him a few moments to free his new find from the dirt, then he lifted it up. It was a large shiny black chunk as big as his hand, very like the pebble he'd found before. "There's our answer," he said. "It can't be obsidiac. As far as I know, the biggest piece ever found was about the size of a chicken egg. This *must* be plain old volcanic glass, nothing more."

Barver stared anxiously at the black lump. "Is there a way to be certain?"

"Perhaps," said Patch. "They say it can make a Pipe sing by itself, but that could just be a myth. Give me my Pipe from my bag, would you?" Barver reached into Patch's bag and pulled out the Pipe, tossing it over. Patch brought the lump closer and closer to his Pipe until they were less than an inch apart. He shook his head. "See?" he said. "Nothing." But then he caught a slight whisper. He let them *touch.*

A sudden explosion of noise came from the instrument, deafening him—he dropped his Pipe and tossed the lump to the side, but the Pipe played on, intricate layers that he recognized from the Songs he'd already played on it.

The sounds faded. He looked up at Barver and Wren. "I, um, think that was a definite reaction," he said.

Barver was horrified. "My mother has led us to a stash of black diamond?" he said. "What was she thinking?"

"Well," said Patch, continuing to dig. "There's one way to find out. Read the—"

Suddenly he yelped and scrambled out of the hole. Wren held her hands to her mouth in shock.

"What is it?" said Barver.

"Nothing," said Patch. "A . . . an insect startled me. Read the letter."

"An insect?" said Barver. He started to walk toward the pit.

"No!" yelled Patch, moving toward him to intercept. "*Read the letter.*"

Barver frowned. He was reluctant but stayed where he was. He opened the letter from his mother and read aloud.

My Dearest Barver,

This is the hardest letter I have ever had to write. I love you, my son, and yet I drove you away. I drove you away to save you. I owe you an explanation. Where else to begin, but with the

Hamelyn Piper? That evil man rots in the dungeons of Tiviscan Castle, yet for me that wasn't enough. My need to understand his crimes became an obsession.

The question gnawed at my soul: why would anyone kidnap children, human and dragon, never to be seen again? There was never an answer that made sense to me.

And then, the year before you left, I discovered something. I may yet be proved wrong, but if I am right then there is one simple fact that outweighs all else:

I finally have the answer I sought. I know why the Hamelyn Piper did what he did.

Barver stopped and looked up from the letter, his eyes wet. "What have you seen?" he asked. "What's in the pit?"

Patch said nothing.

Go on, signed Wren. *Read it all.*

Barver looked back to the letter and continued:

One year after the Hamelyn Piper was captured, a novice scholar arrived at our home and asked that I follow him. I left you sleeping, my son, and did as the novice asked, for there was something in his eyes that told me that it was important, and that questions would have to wait.

He brought me to a cave outside the city, and within the cave was an old dragon, eyes clouded by sheer age. The old dragon sent his novice outside to wait.

"You are Lykeffa Knopferkerkle," the old dragon said to me. "An advisor to the Dragon Triumvirate."

"I am."

"You saved us from launching a war against the humans, after the Hamelyn Piper. You worked with Lord Drevis of the Eight, and secured peace."

"I did. Who are you?"

"My name doesn't matter. I am a scholar, and I had to meet you in secret to tell you something. It is a burden I would pass to you, for I can do nothing more about it. You are familiar with the Order of the Skull?"

"A little," I answered.

Barver stopped again. "The Order of the Skull," he said. "The religious sect of dragons who deal with the burial of the dead."

"Yes," said Patch. "There are no graves in dragon culture, are there? The bodies are taken away and buried in secret."

Barver nodded and continued to read.

"The Order is based around a holy work, called the Book of Lost Names," said the old scholar. He produced a copy from beside him. "The rules for where burials may take place are specified in a single passage here: Chapter 4, verse 18." He opened the book and recited the passage. "The dry lands are not to be used for the rituals of burial. Only where plants may grow and the earth is

rich. In the dry lands, where heat is master, it is not just the dust of the ages that is left. There is also the shadow of memory; and for a child, this will be all there is." The scholar closed the book. "You see, burials must happen in fertile places, never in desert. Do you understand why?"

I shook my head. "I don't understand that part. What does 'shadow of memory' mean?"

The old scholar smiled sadly. "It means grief. The Order of the Skull believes that if they follow the rules in this ancient book, then the grief suffered by the relatives of the dead dragon will be lessened. If they break those rules, then the grief will be even worse, especially if it is a child who has died." He held up the holy book.

"But this is a translation," he said. "The ancient language the book was first written in is my area of expertise. Years ago, I realized that the translation 'shadow of memory' could be wrong. I kept my silence, however. I always thought it best that nobody knew."

I stared at the scholar. "Explain yourself," I urged. "What does nobody know?"

"The ancient word here translated as 'shadow' was more commonly used to mean 'dark,' or 'black.' The ancient word here translated as 'memory' was more commonly used for 'unbreakable,' or 'diamond.' Black diamond, Lykeffa."

"I do not understand," I told him.

"In the dry lands, where heat is master, it is not just the dust of the ages that is left. There is also black diamond; and for a child, this will be all there is." The scholar shook his head. "Don't you see? This text was never about grief. It was a warning. And it explains why the Hamelyn Piper took the dragon children!"

"Scholar," I told him. "I'm sorry, I don't understand what you're saying!"

The scholar had spoken with a quiet voice up to then. Suddenly, he shouted: "Black diamond is the bones of the dead!"

It seemed to Patch that the air had been sucked from around them; breathing seemed more difficult, as the weight of the words settled. All this, and Barver had yet to see what Patch had uncovered at the bottom of the pit he'd dug.

I fell silent, shocked.

"This passage tells us what happens if a dragon is buried in desert," said the scholar. "Some small part of its bones will darken and form black diamond. I believe this is why the Order of the Skull was created thousands of years ago, even before we first encountered humans—to ensure dragons are buried in ways that will not create black diamond, and so not create such terrible power to be misused. Yet the truth has been forgotten! 'And for a child, this will be all there is!' You see? The bones of a child, buried in desert! Pure black diamond! The dragon children were what he was after all along!"

"This is impossible," I told him. "What proof do you have?"

"Proof?" he said. "None! And now I am too old to do anything except pass the burden to you. Before the End of the Skies comes!"

The End of the Skies, my son. The old legend in which the earth gives up a vast store of black diamond, and all life is destroyed in the chaos that follows.

I left the old scholar in that cave and hurried home.

I was eager to forget what I'd learned, but again and again I would ask myself: why would anyone kidnap a hundred dragon children, never to be seen again?

And now the answer came: the bones of those children, buried in desert, will turn into the most dangerous magical substance that exists, in a quantity nobody ever imagined possible.

Yet why did the Hamelyn Piper take the human children? That I don't know, but I can guess. A war with the humans would have been unavoidable if only dragon children had gone.

I thought about what I should do. Without proof, this was just the ravings of a mad old scholar. Yet to prove it would require a terrible risk. If I was discovered, it would mean shame, imprisonment, even death—and perhaps not just my own. You too would be at risk, simply for being my son.

I drove you away to save you from that. To save you from having to see your mother brought down; to save you from suffering the same fate.

And so, I sought the proof.

Seven years ago, when your cousin Genasha died and the Order of the Skull took her, I followed them and watched as they buried her. When they left I committed an unforgiveable crime.

I stole the body from its resting place.

But I had to know.

Each year I have visited the site where you now stand, and so far no changes have occurred, but now illness has taken me. Soon it will be time to check again, and thereafter to return each year; this is what I ask of you.

I hope for all our sakes that the old scholar's fears were misplaced. I hope no change ever happens to those bones.

But if the worst comes to pass, you must find the bones of the stolen children and destroy them! You will need help, but the truth of black diamond must remain secret except to those who can be trusted completely.

I do not know how my dragon colleagues would react, so you must seek out Lord Drevis, the human I trust above any other. By capturing the Hamelyn Piper, the Eight saved us from far more than they ever knew. Imagine such evil power in the hands of so evil a man!

I love you. I wished to spare you this, but in the end it is a burden I must pass on. I know you have the strength to see it through.

You are all that stands against the End of the Skies. Forgive me.

Your mother,
Lykeffa Knopferkerkle

Barver let the letter fall to the ground. He looked up at Patch and Wren, tears flowing down his pain-stricken face.

"What's in the pit?" he said. Patch could only shake his head, lost for what to say. *"What's in the pit?"* cried Barver.

At last the dracogriff moved slowly around Patch and stood over the hole in the sand.

He kneeled and looked inside. There was the pebble of black diamond Patch had first found, and the larger chunk that had brought the reaction in the Pipe.

And beside them, beginning to blacken, was the skull of a dragon child.

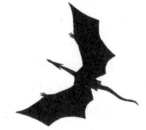

28

RETURN TO TIVISCAN

Barver let out a terrible roar of despair.

"*Genasha!*" he yelled. "How could my mother do this to you? *How could she do this?*" He plunged his hands into the pile of sandy earth beside the pit and started to push it all back into the hole, covering the horrors within.

Patch grabbed Wren and quickly moved away to give Barver room to vent his anger.

The letter from Barver's mother was on the ground nearby; Barver glared at it, then let loose with a burst of flame, incinerating it. He flung his head back, the flames still coming.

Patch and Wren looked on, almost *fearful*, unsure if Barver was even aware of their presence.

When the flames stopped, Barver sobbed. He replaced the triangular rock over Genasha's grave, then looked at his friends, heartbroken. "Genasha died holding my hand," he said. "When the Order of the Skull came to take her, it almost destroyed me. My mother made her excuses and left, telling Genasha's parents there was work to attend to . . ." He paused, then screwed up his face in disgust. "I tried to hate her, you know, for being so cold about Genasha's death. Eventually I left and didn't contact her again. I tried to hate her. And now . . ." He closed his eyes. "You should have told me, mother. You should have let me help you."

"She was protecting you," said Patch. "She hoped she was wrong about all this."

"But she wasn't wrong," said Barver. "My mother did what she knew was right, even though it caused such pain. She sacrificed everything in her quest for the truth—a truth that we are the first to really *know*. Somewhere in the world, in a dry and remote place, one hundred dragon children lie buried. And for what? For obsidiac. For black diamond. For power." He clenched his fists, visibly fighting his anger. At last he sagged, looking to his friends as he wiped away his tears.

We must do as your mother said, signed Wren. *Tell Lord Drevis.*

"Yes," said Barver. "My mother vouched for him, and that's good enough for me. But nobody else. The secret of black diamond cannot get beyond those we can trust."

Patch nodded. "Maybe Tobias and Alia would also be—"

"Nobody else!" said Barver. "Think, Patch! Can't you already *hear* the words, even from those we respect, those who mean well? 'We should take the black diamond and use it for good,' they would say. Tobias, perhaps, or Alia. Or Rundel Stone. That's a road to infighting, and the certain abuse of the black diamond's power. Not to mention war with the dragons—"

Patch thought about it, unsure—*couldn't* the obsidiac be harnessed for good? The dragons wouldn't have to know about it, and . . .

He shook his head, horrified by how easily his thoughts had taken that path. "You're right, Barver," he said. "The temptation would be there. It would always be a problem."

Barver nodded. "Some of Genasha's bones have already completed the change, and the rest is turning dark. It could be years before the bones of the stolen children have all transformed, or it might already have happened. Finding them will be a challenge! Still, the better it was hidden, the safer it remains, as it's unlikely to be *stumbled* upon. With the Hamelyn Piper dead, nobody knows where it is."

"If he truly *is* dead," said Patch.

"Enough of that!" said Barver. He sounded tired. "Tobias and Alia were certain of it. You're just tormenting yourself! The bones of the dragon children must be found and destroyed. We go to Lord Drevis at once. Agreed?" He looked to Wren.

Agreed, she signed. *Tiviscan it is, but I'll have to be the one who goes to meet Drevis.*

Patch heaved a sigh, and nodded. "True," he said. "I'd probably be recognized and arrested before I could even *see* Drevis, and Barver would cause utter panic. How long do you think it'll be before you can change into human form?"

Wren looked down at the circles in her fur, over half of them blue now. *A couple more days, maybe.*

"There is one more thing," said Patch. "Alia warned me there would be a heavy price to pay for returning to Tiviscan. That might not just mean *me*. We could all be in danger. Are you both absolutely sure you want to do this?"

Wren stood proudly on her back legs and solemnly quoted Barver's mother. *You are all that stands against the End of the Skies!* she signed. *I think that has to be more important than our safety.*

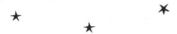

They landed well before dawn in forested hills over a mile away from Tiviscan, after two days of almost nonstop flight. Barver's shoulders had started to cause him discomfort, but with the help of Duffle's ointment he'd kept going.

During their journey, almost all of the beadlike markings on Wren's fur had become blue again. It wouldn't be long before she could change into human form; then she would set off to Tiviscan Castle and contact Lord Drevis.

In the meantime, they rested. Barver was exhausted and fell asleep within minutes of landing. He was restless as he slept, muttering Genasha's name often, and calling for his mother. Patch took his little tent from his bag and set it up for himself and Wren, and soon they were asleep too.

When Wren awoke, she roused Patch and showed him that her band of markings was completely blue. Patch sat up and stretched. He looked outside the tent and reckoned it was mid-morning. They'd had three or four hours of sleep at the most and could have done with far more, but they had a job to do.

Soon they were all up and ready. They looked at each other, wary of how important their task was.

"We should get on with it," said Barver.

Wren nodded. *Time to change!* she signed. *Back in a minute.* She scampered off into the privacy of the trees. There was a blood-curdling shriek, and a few moments later Wren reappeared in human form, brushing down her clothes and looking somewhat flustered.

"Right," she said. "So *that* still hurts."

"How bad was it?" asked Patch.

"Like being turned inside out while somebody hits you with a mountain," she said. "Here I go, then. Wait here for my return, hopefully with Lord Drevis by my side. Wish me luck!"

They muttered a reluctant farewell, and as she went they found it very hard not to follow.

Wren walked through the forest and joined the road to Tiviscan. She could see the castle ahead; wooden scaffolds encased the lower walls and the cliff face, as the work to repair the damage from the dragon attack continued.

For mid-morning, the town seemed empty and subdued. When she reached the main castle gate, there was almost nobody around, and it set her nerves on edge. The gate itself was shut, so she knocked at the guard door.

The wooden flap in the door opened, and a Piper in Custodian uniform looked out at her.

"Yes?" he said, sounding fed up. He looked Wren up and down. "What is it, young peasant?"

Wren glanced down at herself, and had to admit she was a bit grubby. "I'll give you that one," she muttered under her breath. "But don't push your luck."

"I didn't quite catch that," said the Custodian.

"I have an important message to deliver to Lord Drevis," said Wren.

The Custodian frowned. He turned his head behind him. "Hey!" he called. "Dana! Get over here and listen to this!" He turned back to Wren, and she really didn't appreciate the dismissive look on his face. Another Custodian joined him—a woman, looking just as dismissive as he did.

"What's up, Klaus?" asked Dana.

Klaus smirked. "This . . . *person* wants to give Lord Drevis an important message." The two Pipers looked at each other for a moment, then turned to Wren and burst into laughter.

Wren felt a nugget of anger building inside her. She glared at them. "I mean it," she said. "It's important."

When the laughter faded, the woman sighed. "Lord Drevis is attending the Convocation, girl. He should be back here this evening. Who shall I say is asking after him?"

"My name is Wren Cobble," she said. "What did you say he's attending? A Convoc-what?"

The Pipers smirked, and Wren's nugget of anger grew.

"A Convocation, girl," said Dana. "A gathering of the greatest Pipers in the lands!"

"Okay," said Wren. "Can you just point out where the Convocation is happening, so I can go and find Lord Drevis?"

Klaus shook his head. "Honestly, child. Just get yourself off home. We don't have time for games."

"I warn you!" said Wren. "This is of the *utmost* importance!"

The smiles vanished. The Pipers both narrowed their eyes. "*Listen*, you insolent little pig," said Dana. "Run along, if you know what's good for you. Understand?" She shut the flap.

Wren seethed for a moment, then stepped forward and knocked repeatedly. This time, it wasn't just the flap that opened—it was the whole guard door. Wren took a few wary steps back as both Pipers came out. They didn't seem at all friendly.

"That's *it*," said Dana. "You're coming with us. A night in the cells will teach you to show respect to your betters."

Wren let out a huge sigh. "You really did ask for this," she said. In her right hand were half a dozen daisy chains.

She calmly threw one at each Piper as they watched her with bemused scorn.

She'd made several stops as she'd come through the forest, so that she could gather and prepare a selection of useful flowers and plants. Underath's books had many complicated spells, far beyond her understanding, but she'd memorized a few humble little enchantments.

With the daisy chains, she'd tried a simple cooperation spell. She wasn't entirely sure it would work, but she kept her fingers crossed. As long as the targets didn't regard her as much of a threat, and so had their guard down, she reckoned she had a good chance.

Klaus bent down and picked up a daisy chain; so did Dana.

"What's this?" said Klaus, wide-eyed. His voice was oddly singsong, like a dreamy child.

Dana grinned at her daisies. "Pretty!" she said.

Wren smiled. Her spell had certainly done *something*. "So, where is the Convocation taking place?"

The two Pipers nodded, their grins not slipping for a moment.

"In the Monash Hollow," said Dana. "The Council members are all there, as are most of the Elite Pipers from the

323

castle and many more who have traveled far." She waggled her finger at Wren. "Not us though. *We're* not there. We're *here.*"

"It's not fair!" said Klaus. "A big party to celebrate the Death of the Hamelyn Piper, and we're missing it all! I mean, we've been helping out with preparations all week, but do we get to enjoy it?"

Dana shook her head. "Nuh-uh!"

"Feasts and dancing!" said Klaus. "Games and challenges! And we have to stay here and watch the castle." He frowned in a way that a grumpy five-year-old would have been proud of. "We're missing all the fun!"

Dana stuck out her lower lip and nodded. "Yuh-huh!"

"Fair enough," said Wren. She was done here. She turned around and started to walk off.

"Hold up!" said Dana. She looked at Klaus. "Weren't we going to chuck her in a cell?"

The two Pipers blinked and shook their heads as if they had water in their ears. The spell was slipping and *rapidly.* Wren delved into a pocket where she'd put some little bunches of clover stalks that she'd bewitched for an emergency. Quick as a flash, she snapped a bunch in two. "I can go about my business!" she said. "You should go and have some tea now!"

Dana nodded. "You can go about your business. We should go and have some tea now."

Wren felt a surge of pride at how well that one had gone, but Klaus was scowling at her.

"Hang about!" he said. "Is she . . . is she using *witch-craft*?"

Dana scoffed. "What, a good-for-nothing ruffian like that? Get a grip, Klaus!" They both shared a laugh, and then looked around with surprise. Wren, it seemed, had vanished.

"Where'd she go?" said Klaus.

"Fast runner," shrugged Dana. "Good riddance to her." She walked back through the guard door.

"I don't remember there being a tree out here . . . ," said Klaus. He moved toward the tree for a closer look.

Wren felt like a bit of a fool, standing there with her arms stretched out to her sides as the Custodian Piper peered at her. The tree-glamor was the only magical disguise she'd managed to learn in all her time poring over Underath's books, and while the birds had always been fooled by it, she felt a huge relief that it had worked on the Piper too.

She felt something land on her arm. "Ooh!" said Klaus. "A woodpecker!"

Wren gulped.

"Come on, Klaus," called Dana. "Your turn to make the tea."

"Yeah, okay," said Klaus, and off he went into the castle, closing the guard door behind him.

Very carefully, Wren turned her head and stared at the bird. "Really?" she said.

The woodpecker blinked. For a moment it looked confused, and then, decidedly embarrassed, it flew away in shame.

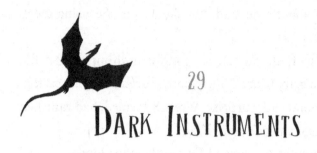

29

DARK INSTRUMENTS

Wren returned quickly to Barver and Patch and told them about the Convocation. She was still rather cross about the way she'd been treated by the two Custodians, but she didn't mention it; nor did she say anything about the spells she'd cast. Tempting as it was to boast, she wanted to keep that kind of thing quiet for now.

Barver wasn't exactly impressed by the news. "Pah!" he said. "A celebration of the Hamelyn Piper's death is hardly a strong message of anger to send to the dragons, is it? They badly damage the castle, and what's the response? 'You did a terrible thing, dragons, but also we're really happy about it thanks.'"

Patch nodded. "They clearly *are* happy about it," he said. "A Convocation is rare. There's an annual Spring Festival held in Monash Hollow, but turning it into a Convocation makes it a much larger affair—with the greatest Pipers from near and far, not just ordinary Pipers and trainees."

"Well, that's where Lord Drevis is," said Wren. She looked at Patch. "Lead the way!"

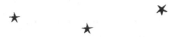

Monash Hollow was a wide circular area of grassland to the east of Tiviscan, surrounded by woods. Barver, Patch, and Wren took position on a neighboring hill, giving them a good view of the Hollow that let them appreciate how big it was—at least half a mile across.

Even so, every part of it was covered in tents and people. There were plenty of non-Pipers at the Convocation, including people running food and clothing stalls. It was no wonder Tiviscan had seemed so quiet; most of the population was here, either making a little money out of the huge event or simply enjoying the spectacle.

The sounds that reached them contained celebration and excitement and—naturally enough—music. Patch could hear the playing of the Garland Reel, a traditional spring melody that accompanied the Garland Dance. He spotted those who were dancing and smiled as he watched. The Garland Dance was essentially a game—pairs faced each other holding hands, dancing quickly sideway in a long line, and at different cues in the music the pairs had to change what steps they were doing. Those who got it wrong had to leave the dance, and as the music sped up the changes grew more frequent until only two dancers remained.

In the middle of the Hollow was a series of temporary structures, including a vast and impressive stage, which had been decorated as a towering mock-up of Tiviscan Castle made of painted cloth and scaffolding. It must have been at least a hundred feet high.

"Wow," said Wren. "Whoever did that has put in a *lot* of effort."

Patch looked at the throng, astonished by the sheer number of people. With a slight tremble he imagined how bad the toilet pits would be by the end of the day. "I loved the Spring Festival each year," he said. "But they were nothing compared to this! Look at how many Elite Pipers are attending! Such an opportunity for them to pass on their knowledge and experience. See that side?" He pointed to a fenced-off area where sheep grazed. "The Drover and Arable Elite are demonstrating their farming skills there. And if you look to the left"—there was a wide expanse of ground that had been churned up into crater-pocked mud—"the Battle Elite are showing off what they can do." He thought back to his own battle training. He'd learned that what generals most valued was anything that boosted morale or—when a fight was at risk of being lost—gave the fighters a frenzied bloodlust.

Patch had hated those lessons. The role of the Battle Elite in war typically meant treating soldiers as nothing more than weapons: using Songs to stop them caring about their own lives. Yet he'd been fascinated by Songs like the Push, and its close relatives—blasts of destructive force could be launched with incredible precision by the best of the Battle Elite. Patch had never quite mastered the *precision* side of it, but the destruction part was fun, when lives weren't being threatened. "Whatever Song you can think of, somewhere out there will be a place for interested Pipers to learn more."

"What's the massive pretend castle for?" asked Barver.

"Spring Festival always has a central stage for a tournament," said Patch. "I imagine the Convocation Tournament will be even *more* thrilling, given how many Elite are present. I mean, they've really pulled out all the stops with that stage, haven't they? Look at the size of it!"

"A thrilling tournament?" said Wren. "What kind of things do they do?"

"Lots of contests to pit the best against the best," said Patch. "For Custodians it might be chasing someone over obstacles, say. It can get very exciting."

There were Pipers on the stage as they spoke, but little movement. "They're not *doing* very much," said Barver, frowning.

Patch squinted until he recognized the uniform. "They're Arable Elite," he said. "It could be a race to see who gets some seeds to germinate and sprout first, or who can get water to flow uphill the fastest."

The three of them watched intently. After a few minutes without any activity to speak of, a whistle blew and one Piper celebrated by leaping up and down.

"Germination race, probably," said Patch.

Wren shook her head in disbelief. "Gripping entertainment," she said. "*Gripping.*" Then she set off to find Lord Drevis.

When she emerged from the trees at the edge of the Hollow, Wren was half expecting to be stopped and questioned by some more surly Custodians. Instead, the people were friendly and smiling, enjoying their day.

She headed for the mock castle stage first, thinking that perhaps the Council would be near the center of the action. The stage itself was empty at that moment, so she went around toward the rear to see if she could spot anyone important-looking. She was sure she could hear activity going on further within the structure and took a closer look at one of the large sheets hanging down around the exterior— canvas, it seemed, painted to resemble castle stonework. She was about to have a peek behind it when a hand grabbed her shoulder and firmly turned her around.

A large man was giving her a very disapproving glare. "No access," said the man, his voice oddly emotionless. "Go."

"Oh, I was just—" started Wren, but the man clearly wasn't going to take any nonsense.

"Go," he said again, in that same impassive way. Wren noticed that his eyes didn't seem to carry any emotion either—not anger or annoyance. Not even boredom.

"Go," said the man once more, giving her a shove.

"Okay, okay," said Wren. "No need for that. I'm going." She thought about trying another part of the stage area, but there were other men around, dressed almost identically to the one who'd shoved her. Instead, she headed out into the crowd, passing a woman selling iced buns.

"Pay him no mind, my sweet," said the woman, smiling.

"You saw?" said Wren.

The woman nodded. "They've been helping set all this up, but they're not the friendliest souls. I suppose they just don't want anyone messing about near their centerpiece! Think of the work it took!" The woman looked up at the mock castle looming high over them.

Wren's gaze followed. "I suppose you're right," she said.

"Here," said the woman, handing her one of her iced buns. "No charge! You deserve some kindness after that."

Wren grinned and thanked her. She ate her bun, glancing around the Hollow, looking for any sign of the Council.

At last she saw a group of Custodian Pipers emerge from a particularly impressive tent. They were followed by five overly serious-looking men and women in robes that must have weighed a ton. As they neared the stage, she could see their faces clearly and recognized them from Patch's trial. The Pipers' Council! Her opportunity to speak to Lord Drevis would come soon enough.

Once they reached the stage, the Custodian Pipers and the Council members walked up some steps at the side. Wren watched from a little way back as the Custodians held up their hands, signaling for quiet. When the general hubbub had settled down, a Custodian spoke up with a loud, clear voice. "Ladies and Gentlemen, and Pipers in Attendance!" he called. "The Lords and Ladies of the Council will hereby make an announcement regarding the events to be held this evening! I give you Lord Drevis!"

There was a round of respectful applause. Lord Drevis stepped forward and addressed the crowd. "Welcome to you all! Today is the day that we shall celebrate an end to the saga of the Hamelyn Piper. It is with delight that I announce that tonight's feast shall be followed by a spectacle of fireworks and wonders arranged by the Battle Pipers of Kintner!" There was a great cheer from the crowd. Drevis settled them down with several waves of his hand. "Those yet to lodge their horses in the stables at Tiviscan please be sure to do so in advance of the display. Also"—Drevis pulled out a sheet of paper and looked through it—"I've been asked to . . . to . . ."

He drifted off into silence. Wren frowned, puzzled.

There was a very low droning sound in the air, which varied rapidly as if an insect was attempting to fly into her ear. Wren looked around, expecting to see a swarm of bees or something similar nearby, but there was nothing.

Instead, she noticed curious behavior in those standing near her. Slowly, everyone bowed their heads in silence, including Drevis and the others on the stage. The low droning grew louder and more rhythmic, and a melody began to take shape. Wren could see that it wasn't just those nearby who were affected. Within the vast Hollow, every single person was now standing utterly still, head bowed.

She looked to the person next to her, a Piper with a blue and gray uniform; she took the woman by the shoulder and shook her vigorously. "Wake up!" hissed Wren. The Piper didn't open her eyes. Worse, she felt stiff as a corpse, muscles locked in place.

This wasn't good.

Suddenly, the people gathered around the stage began to stride backward in unison. Wren did the same, not wanting to be left standing alone. When they all stopped, the ground around the base of the stage was empty.

A group of men, dressed just like the one who had shoved her earlier, spread out along the back of the stage, then reached up into the cloth drapes beside them and seemed to *pull* on something. The meticulously crafted mock castle began to come apart. Painted canvas fell away from the wooden scaffolds, and then those scaffolds fell away too, landing on the newly vacated ground.

What Wren saw being revealed underneath—something that had been hidden there all this time—made her tremble with a fear that was almost overwhelming.

Where the mock castle had stood was a curious collection of huge cylindrical shapes. The tallest and widest of them, in the middle of the structure, was a hundred feet high and four feet wide; the cylinders became ever smaller out to each side.

It was a *Pipe Organ*, and each of the Pipes was deep black in color.

Wren stared at it, openmouthed. The sound was coming from those Pipes.

On the stage, one final canvas sheet was pulled away to reveal a figure wearing a long hooded robe, sitting at a multitiered panel of keyboards and pedals that would have been more at home in one of the great cathedrals. Hands and feet started to fly up and down the keys and levers, and the low droning sound grew more and more complex, with higher notes added now, to create intricate melodies.

The hooded figure stood and walked to the center of the stage to take a bow, and even though the keys of the organ weren't being played, the music kept going—just as it did whenever Patch paused while playing his Pipe.

Wren looked around at the silent people and felt a deep chill as she realized what was going on. She tried hard not to react—drawing attention to herself could be disastrous. "Time to go," she muttered. She backed away one slow step at a time. When she felt that she was at a safe enough distance from the stage, she made for the trees as fast as she could.

Once in the woods she ran, plunging blindly through bushes. When something loomed up just ahead of her, she screamed.

It was Barver. "Are you okay?" he said, looking just as panicked as she felt.

Barver was alone. "Where's Patch?" she asked.

"He fell into some kind of trance," he said. "I could hear those odd sounds, so I moved him down the other side of the hill until they faded. He went limp and collapsed. Then I came to find you." There was dread all over Barver's face. "What's happening, Wren?"

"Didn't you see it?" she said. "It was hidden underneath the fake castle."

"I left our vantage point to get Patch to safety," he said. "*What* was hidden?"

She told him.

They found Patch where Barver had left him, sitting behind an outcrop of rock. He was rubbing his head and moaning. Wren knelt beside him. "Patch!" she said. "Snap out of it! We need you!"

Patch looked at her, finding it hard to focus. "Did I fall?" he said. "I don't—" He flung a hand to his mouth in shock: while they were far enough away for the organ music to have lost its power over him, it was still audible and he was able to pick out some of the familiar rhythms and melodies that lay within the intricate sounds. "Oh. Oh no."

"It's a Pipe Organ!" cried Wren. "The Pipes are vast, and they're dark black, Patch! The black diamond, the bones of the dragon children! It's already been harvested, and turned into a huge Pipe Organ! Everyone in the Hollow is under its spell!"

Patch stared at her, despairing. "An obsidiac Pipe Organ?" he said.

"Exactly!" said Wren. "There was someone at the keys, and surely there's only one person it could be!"

Patch shook his head, dreading what she would say.

"It's the *true* Hamelyn Piper!" cried Wren. "It must be!"

Patch wanted to run away, to just leave and not return, but he forced himself to take a deep breath. He slapped the side of his head quite hard. "Think!" he said to himself. "Think!" He looked at Barver. "You're immune to the Song being played?"

"I seem to be," said Barver.

"It may be human-targeted, then," said Patch. "But why is Wren unaffected?"

She shrugged and held up her wrist, waggling her

336

bracelet. "I guess I'm technically still a rat," she said. "With modifications."

Patch thought for a moment. "In that case, this is going to be up to you two," he said. "I can't get closer to the music or I'll be just as useless as everyone else in the Hollow."

"So what do we do?" said Wren.

"I'll fly down and incinerate him," said Barver. Wren smiled. "I like that idea."

"No," said Patch. "He'll be ready to defend himself. The moment he saw you, he'd knock you out of the sky. Probably kill you in the process."

Barver tutted. "This is *me* we're talking about."

"Please, Barver," said Patch. "That Pipe Organ could have incredible power. It'd be like the Battle Pipes at Tiviscan, but ten thousand times stronger."

Another sound joined that of the organ music. *Voices.* "Go and take a look, Wren," said Patch. "Tell us what's happening."

She hurried up the hill and returned a minute later. "Some of the crowd are standing in rows and columns, like soldiers," she said. "They're moving suddenly every few seconds—both arms up, then to the sides, then down. They keep shouting every time they move, something I couldn't make out. The rest of the people are at the edges of the Hollow, standing motionless with their heads bowed."

Patch listened carefully to the music. He could feel it

pull on his mind, but he knew he was just beyond its range. "Like soldiers . . . ," he said, an idea forming. "Does the Pipe Organ look like it could be moved around easily?"

"Not a chance," said Wren. "It's just as big as the castle mock-up."

Patch frowned. "Then he needs an army. Unthinking, and controlled utterly by him. But the control would have to continue even after the Piping stopped or they could never *go* anywhere."

"Is that possible?" said Barver.

"The permanent domination of the mind of another person," mused Patch. "A Song of absolute control, of *puppetry*. Making someone a mindless slave! That kind of thing isn't *supposed* to be possible."

"Wait!" said Wren. "A man stopped me going too close to the back of the stage, and I swear he was in some kind of trance. There was something *wrong* about him. Apparently he and others like him helped build the stage in the first place."

"Puppets!" said Barver. "It would make sense for the Hamelyn Piper to recruit some before he came here, to help him prepare."

"Then such a Song must be possible after all," said Patch. "And he's attempting to enslave everyone in the Hollow, all at once!"

"Not everyone," said Wren. "Half of the people had taken themselves to the Hollow's edge."

"Did you notice a difference between them?" said Barver. "Those at the edges, and those being controlled?"

Wren thought for a moment. "Pipers!" she said. "It was the ordinary people at the edges, Pipers in the center!"

"An army of Pipers," said Patch, dread filling him. "And among them the best of the Elite . . ."

Wren's eyes widened. "And surely he would arm them all with obsidiac Pipes!" she said.

"They'd be invincible," said Barver.

Patch listened to the Song again. Parts of it seemed familiar enough—he thought he could unpick those aspects if he had a chance. "He's gradually taking them over," he said. "How long it requires I don't know, but if he succeeds then silencing the organ won't be enough. They'll already be his soldiers."

"So we strike now, before it's too late!" said Barver. "Let me toast his noggin!"

Patch shook his head. "No incinerating unless absolutely necessary," he said, to Barver's disappointment. "The very *minds* of his victims could be at terrible risk if the Song simply collapses! We need a way to disable the Hamelyn Piper safely. Knock him unconscious, maybe, so I can get down there and try to reverse the Song."

The three of them thought in silence.

"I've got it!" cried Wren. She went to Barver's side and delved into Erner's bag, pulling out a cloth and carefully unwrapping something.

A leather pouch.

"This might be just what we need," she said. "Kaposher Dust. Underath had it."

"Ah!" said Barver, nodding. He took the pouch from Wren, feeling its weight. "I can throw the pouch at the Hamelyn Piper if I get close enough, but it's a risk. As long as it still has potency there's plenty here, but Kaposher goes stale easily."

"We should test it," said Patch, taking it from Barver. He reached to the ground beside him and picked up an acorn. With extreme care he untied the mouth of the pouch, then dipped the acorn inside and tied the pouch shut again. He tossed the acorn high into the branches of a nearby tree.

They waited.

They heard a squeak and a squirrel dropped out of the leaves, falling like a stone. It was out cold.

Satisfied, Patch gave the pouch to Wren. "You'll both have to do this," he said. "Barver, you must focus on flying. Wren, you open the pouch up fully and throw it. Don't breathe the dust, whatever you do."

"And how do we get close, if he'll swat me like a fly?" asked Barver.

"I'll try to draw his attention," said Patch. "But I can't promise much, from so far way." He reached into his bag for his Pipe, but his fingers touched something else. He pulled out the Hamelyn Piper's Mask and unfolded it.

340

"If only we could slap *that* thing on him!" said Barver.

"Would it work?" said Patch. "Casimir built the Mask to block Songs passing through it, purely to stop the Hamelyn Piper from lip-playing his way to freedom. It wouldn't prevent him playing that organ."

There was a thought buzzing in his head, however. He thought back to the stories of the Eight, as his own words echoed around his mind: *this was designed to block Songs passing through it.*

But that wasn't quite true—it wouldn't let Songs *leave.* The Songs of another could still affect the prisoner while he wore the Mask, so that the Pipers guarding him could use whatever was needed to restrain him.

It was a one-way barrier to the magic of music.

Patch folded the Mask, then unfolded it again. The action was smooth and took very little pressure. Fold, unfold. He did it once more, but this time he twisted it in a slightly different way, and the Mask was inverted when it opened. The curious markings in the metal—those runes that Casimir himself had engraved and inlaid with obsidiac—were on the *outside* of the Mask now, not the inside.

Barver and Wren were staring at him. "You don't think—?" said Wren.

"It's worth a try," said Patch. He raised the Mask to his own head and put it on. He had an immediate sense of claustrophobia. With the Mask's latch broken he had to keep it closed with one hand. He strode toward the hilltop, Barver and Wren following. As he walked the music grew louder, but he could already feel the difference.

The Obsidiac Organ was having no effect; the Mask was protecting him.

"Do you have twine, Barver?" said Patch.

Barver nodded and produced some from his side pack. "Hold still," he said, and gently secured the front of the Mask.

Patch was the Piper in the Iron Mask now.

He took his Pipe from his bag. "But can I Pipe while wearing it?" he said. "I'm going to play you some courage. Tell me if it works."

He began to create the Song of Courage; as he played, Barver and Wren straightened up and thrust out their chins, looking to the sky, determined and fearless. Yet for once, Patch himself didn't get any benefit from his Song.

"It's *definitely* working," said Wren.

"Good," said Patch. "I'll be your distraction. I'll hit him with everything I've got. It should give you a window of opportunity. But whatever happens, once the Kaposher is thrown, get out of there as fast as you can and leave this place! Don't wait to check he's unconscious, just go! Get back to Marwheel Abbey: to Tobias and Alia and Rundel Stone. Make sure the world knows what's happening here!"

Barver and Wren both shifted uneasily, saying nothing;

Patch hoped their courage wasn't about to override common sense. "Do you understand? Whatever happens, get away from here as fast as you can!"

Wren frowned. "But what if you—?"

"Swear it!" cried Patch. "Even if I get into trouble, there's to be no *rescuing* of any kind!" He fixed his gaze on them both. Eventually they nodded.

"I swear," mumbled Barver.

"Me too," said Wren, reluctantly.

"When the Hamelyn Piper is unconscious I'll tie him up and put the Mask on him," said Patch, taking the rest of Barver's twine. "Then I'll see if I can use the Organ and reverse the Song's effects. Now go! Hide at the rear of the Hollow, then wait for my signal. The Pipe Organ itself should give you some cover as you fly at him."

"What's your signal going to be?" asked Wren.

Patch grinned through the Iron Mask. "Chaos!"

30

The Song of the Hamelyn Piper

Patch watched from the edge of the Hollow.

The civilians were standing around the perimeter with their heads bowed, all but forgotten by the Hamelyn Piper, whose focus was entirely on his new army. Now that he was so close, Patch could make out what it was these "soldiers" were shouting each time they changed position: "We obey you, Lord!"

The Hamelyn Piper was sitting at the organ, his arms moving in a frenzy over the keys. Standing along the back of the stage were a dozen large men, identically dressed; Patch assumed they were the ones Wren had mentioned, the Puppets. The organ's Song kept growing in complexity, the movements of the sleeping army becoming more refined as the Song grew ever richer. The Hamelyn Piper's control of his victims was increasing.

Patch gripped his Pipe. The Iron Mask felt more uncomfortable every second, making it hard for him to concentrate. He thought of that poor innocent prisoner, who had worn it for almost a decade, and scolded himself. He needed to ignore the Mask and focus!

His plan was simple enough. He'd promised chaos, and if there was one Song that had caused chaos in his own life, surely it had to be the Dance. And while the Hamelyn Piper had an army, Patch realized he could have one too— the unconscious civilians were no longer the target of the organ Piping. If Patch could reach them with the Dance, then delivering the chaos he'd promised would be within his grasp!

The Dance was a flexible Song; that was how Patch had been able to match it to the reels and jigs he'd taught the various bands he'd played with, after fleeing Tiviscan. Whatever the tune, he knew how to play the Dance underneath it. If it was a familiar tune for a well-known dance, those caught in the spell would perform the moves that the tune required.

He watched carefully as the Pipers in the Hollow repeated their movements again and again. A plan had taken shape in his mind.

He put his Pipe to his lips and started to play, hoping he was too far from the stage for the Hamelyn Piper to notice anything amiss. The feet of the civilians nearest to him began to tap out the rhythm he played. As expected, none of the Pipers were responding—they were lost to the Song of the Pipe Organ.

He risked playing a little louder to draw in more civilians, and then he moved along the perimeter of the Hollow. The civilians followed behind him in a line, like sleepwalkers, taking rhythmic steps with their heads still bowed. Each had a dreamy smile on their lips as, deep in their slumber, they enjoyed their dancing.

With perhaps two hundred recruits gathered, Patch turned and walked into the Hollow. He led his followers along the space between two columns of Pipers, who continued to follow their commands, oblivious to Patch and the civilians. When he was halfway to the Pipe Organ, he changed his Song to include the melody of something everyone would know.

The Garland Reel.

At once, the civilians did as the reel required. They paired up and faced one another, two lines of dancers just fitting into the gap between the columns of Pipers.

Patch paid close attention to the sequence of movements the Pipers were following. It included a section where they raised one leg, balanced on it for a few seconds, then lowered it, before doing the same with the other leg.

Timing would be everything. He waited for that first leg-raise to happen again, and when it did he played the musical cue for the dancers to separate and take three quick steps backward. The civilians did just that, but now they bumped hard into Pipers who were all standing precariously on one leg.

Here it was: Patch's attempt at chaos. He could hardly bear to watch in case his idea simply fizzled out, but the line of Pipers teetered back and toppled—right into the next line, who also fell.

And the next. And the *next*.

Patch couldn't contain his glee as the wave of toppling Pipers spread out and kept on going. The Pipers let out grunts and yelps as they fell, still trying to perform the movements that the Organ was commanding them to do. Unable to stand up again, they twitched their limbs and shouted, "We obey you, Lord!"

By the time the toppling petered out, a third of those in the Hollow lay on the ground flapping like landed fish. At the center of the confusion, Patch let out a triumphant shout, laughing as hard as he could. He saw the Hamelyn Piper suddenly freeze, hands stopping above the Organ keys.

He had finally noticed.

The Hamelyn Piper jumped up from his seat and strode to the edge of the stage, his mouth gaping open. The toppling had failed before reaching those closest to him, and as the music continued to play within the Pipe Organ they kept on with their bizarre drill. "Who dares to defy me?" he shouted. "*Who dares to defy me?*"

"I do!" yelled Patch. He raised his Pipe and started to build another Song—a Push, just to rile the man even more. He launched it and for once his aim was good enough to knock the Hamelyn Piper off his feet, even from such a distance.

The man was stunned for a moment, but snapped out of it and pulled a dark Pipe from his belt, quickly weaving notes together, taking Patch by surprise with the speed and strength of the result. A pocket of air shot from the Pipe straight at Patch, sending him flying before he could move out of the way. Winded, he quickly picked himself up off the ground.

The Hamelyn Piper roared in anger and started to build another attack; Patch was building one too. They launched simultaneously and the two Songs hurtled toward each other. At the midpoint the Songs collided, and a deafening thunderclap echoed around the Hollow. The two Pipers set about forming yet another attack.

Suddenly Patch saw Barver closing in fast from behind the Organ. If the Hamelyn Piper hadn't been focusing on Patch, Barver would have been the target of those powerful Songs, but instead he and Wren had a clear run. It was only as Barver flew over the tops of the organ Pipes that the Hamelyn Piper saw him, and by then it was too late.

The open pouch of Kaposher hurtled down toward him and exploded. A cloud of dust obscured the man, and some of the Pipers closest to the stage collapsed as the Kaposher reached them.

Barver and Wren saw Patch and started to head toward him.

"Go!" shouted Patch, waving at them to leave the Hollow. "*Go, now!*" He looked at the huge cloud of Kaposher obscuring the stage. The way that the pouch had *exploded* left Patch feeling very uneasy indeed. "*Get out of here!*"

They seemed to get the message, and began to turn.

Then Patch felt the cold edge of a knife at his throat, and a strong grip on his arm; his Pipe was wrenched from his hand. He didn't dare move, but he could see the sleeve of the arm holding him, with the colors of a Custodian's uniform.

The Hamelyn Piper's voice boomed through the air. "You fly *anywhere*, dragon, and he dies!"

A swirl of air began to spin on the stage, taking the dust cloud higher and higher until it dispersed. The Hamelyn Piper was standing there, the hood of his robe still hiding most of his face, but not his malicious grin. He was surrounded by a shimmer of air, the telltale sign of the protective shield he'd managed to create. The shimmer faded as the short-lived barrier vanished.

All around the Hollow, fallen Pipers were recovering and rising to their feet.

"Let him go or I will *burn* you," shouted Barver, maintaining his height.

"My *soldier* will slit his throat if you make any such attempt," cried the Hamelyn Piper. He waved a hand in a carefree gesture. "By all means try!"

Barver scowled but did nothing. On his back, Wren glared at the man.

The Hamelyn Piper gestured to his "soldier." Patch was pushed toward the stage and forced up onto it. He saw the members of the Council standing on the grass nearby, their faces blank.

"Now isn't *this* interesting," said the Hamelyn Piper. He pulled back his hood, and ran his fingers over the Mask covering Patch's face.

With the man's hood down, for the first time Patch got a good look at him, and all he could do was stare. Terrible scars covered his face, long healed-over but deep. The man's right ear was ragged, half-gone. But that wasn't why Patch stared.

He'd seen that face before, without the scars, but filthy and bearded. "My God," he said. "You . . . you look exactly like him."

"What are you babbling about?" said the man, raising an eyebrow.

"The prisoner in the Iron Mask."

The man's eyes narrowed for a moment, and then he smiled. "Oh, very good! *Very* good. You do seem to know a lot, don't you? And you have his Mask. However did you come by it? I thought it hadn't been found. I must try not to kill you, so you can tell me all about it later!" He looked more closely at the Mask, and his smile became a sneer. "Ah, I see what you did! Inside out, I'm impressed! Very clever. I wonder if Casimir originally made it that way, as a device for his own protection?" He looked around at his soldiers, only half of whom had managed to stand again. The rest were lying still. "You're little more than a *boy*, and look at all the trouble you've caused me. That will take time to fix." He shot Patch a look of sheer malice. "His Pipe if you please!" he ordered, and the Custodian—the *soldier*—holding Patch handed it over. "Beautifully made," he said, studying it. "The glaze is unusual." He raised it to his nose and sniffed. "Not sure what it's made of, but look at mine!" He held his own Pipe up for Patch to see. "Obsidiac glaze, of exceptional thickness and quality. Better than yours, lad." He put his own Pipe away and gripped Patch's with both hands. "Shame," he said, snapping it in two and tossing the pieces to one side.

Patch felt as if he'd been punched in the stomach.

He'd been getting to *like* that Pipe.

"I suppose you must be a trainee, studying at Tiviscan," said the Hamelyn Piper. "Imagine! Tiviscan's last hope, a child!" He leaned close to Patch, leering at him. "I know a way to deal with children, lad." Patch squirmed in the grip of the soldier holding him, and the Hamelyn Piper backed away. "But yes, of *course* the prisoner looked like me," he said, smiling. "Our mother would have been *so* disappointed by what I did to him."

"Your own brother?" said Patch.

"My twin, no less! It was always my plan to have him punished in my place. I played a Song of Forgetting and Piped away his memories, then kept him safe in a secret location. All I had to do was lead the authorities to him when the time was right! But the Eight made everything *so* much more difficult. They kept closing in on me, hundreds of miles away from where I was keeping my brother. It was tiresome! They almost got me too. Left me with *this*." He ran his fingers over the scars on his face. "A present from the Eight. I've wanted to repay the favor all these years, but I had to be patient and not draw their attention. And what patience I have shown! Then some idiot started messing around, playing illegal Songs and making everyone worry about Dark Pipers. I'd intended to put my plans into action *next* year, but I decided to bring everything forward. Rundel Stone had started to ask awkward questions! I couldn't take the risk that he'd stumble onto something, or get the other remaining members of the Eight involved."

Patch gulped. The idiot messing around and playing illegal Songs had been *him*.

"Why are you doing this?" said Patch.

"To rule! This world needs a ruler who's truly worthy of the responsibility."

"And that's you?"

"Of course! There are so very *few* people deserving of power. The rest"—he looked out across the Hollow, at all the people under his control—"cattle. *Sheep*." He leaned close again and smiled. "Now, I *could* tear that mask from you and make you just another of my soldiers, but I wouldn't want you to miss the rest of the performance. I think you'll appreciate it. Right now, they obey my will for as long as the Song plays, but when I am done they will be mine *forever*."

Patch saw the fearful look on Barver's face and on Wren's. They had to escape, he knew, escape and warn the world—and Patch had an idea, a way he could help them do it. "I have one question," said Patch. He made sure he sounded absolutely defeated. "Did you ever think of your brother, condemned in the dungeon?" His voice grew quieter with every word, and the Hamelyn Piper drew closer to hear better. "Did you ever think about what he suffered?" whispered Patch. "Have you no *compassion*?"

The Hamelyn Piper put his lips right up to Patch's ear. "No!" he snarled with glee.

His glee was short-lived. Patch turned quickly and flung his head forward with as much strength as he could muster, catching the Hamelyn Piper on the nose with the full force of the blow. There was a satisfying crunch as the metal Mask hit home. The Hamelyn Piper fell to his knees with a howl, his hands covering his face, blood pouring out between his fingers.

At once, Patch flung his head backward, connecting hard with the soldier holding him; the soldier's grip weakened and Patch tore free. He ran toward the rear of the stage where the Organ Pipes loomed high above him.

"Get him!" screamed the Hamelyn Piper, and more of his soldiers—the Puppets—strode with terrible purpose toward Patch. The Hamelyn Piper brought his obsidiac Pipe to his lips and began to play a Song that Patch recognized at once. A battle Song, and a powerful one—it wouldn't take long to complete, but Patch realized it wasn't going to be aimed at *him*: the Hamelyn Piper had turned to face Barver and Wren.

"Barver!" Patch yelled. "Do as you swore! Get out of here!"

He could see the hestitation on Barver's face, but there was no other choice. The dracogriff flew hard; seconds later the Song was launched, catching Barver with a glancing blow. He tumbled; Wren only just managed to stay on, but Barver kept them airborne.

The soldiers were closing in on Patch, and only one route was left: onto the very Pipes of the Organ itself. He leaped high and got his fingers on the edge of the smallest Pipe, pulling himself out of reach just in time. His pursuers hoisted one of their number up after him. He backed away, climbing the taller Pipes as he went; ahead, he could see more soldiers climbing the smallest Pipes on the other side of the Organ.

On the stage below, the Hamelyn Piper was working on another battle Song to throw at Barver, but after a few seconds he stopped. "No, no," he said. "That's boring. I've got a much better idea, and I do love a challenge!" He put his Pipe away and hurried to his keyboards. He sat and rubbed his hands to warm them. "Let me see . . . ," he said, and he feverishly worked the keys and pedals, adding more layers to the Song.

Barver and Wren were halfway to the edge of the Hollow. The Hamelyn Piper turned to look at them and frowned. "Nothing?" he said, disappointed. "Mmm. That really should have worked on a dragon. Hang on! Were those feathers I saw? Was that some kind of beak? A griffin?" He played a slight variation on what he'd added before, then stopped and frowned again. Barver was at the edge of the Hollow now. They were almost free!

The Hamelyn Piper grinned. "Of course!" he said. "How stupid of me!" He looked up to where Patch was scrambling to ever-higher Pipes, always just out of reach of his pursuers. "Taking control of a mind is so much easier one-to-one," he called. "Even if the target is a dracogriff!" He began to play again, laughing as he did.

Dismayed, Patch watched as Barver turned and started to fly back, helpless against the power of the obsidiac Pipe Organ. Patch felt a hand grab at his ankle, and he kicked it away, almost losing his balance. There was only one Pipe left to climb now—the largest of them all. He had little strength remaining in his arms, but he hauled himself up. This last organ Pipe was four feet across. He could feel the deep notes reverberate in his *bones*. Its edge was only a few inches thick and he struggled to stand, almost toppling into the gaping hole at its center.

Barver reached the stage, level in height with Patch. The dracogriff's eyes were blank; on his back, Wren pleaded with him. "*Barver!*" she cried. "It's *me! Please!*" She met Patch's eyes and shook her head in despair. The Hamelyn Piper smiled at Patch, then looked to Barver. "Let's deal with your rider first!" he said. "Fly until you are above the rocks over there. Drop your rider onto them from a *great* height. Then come back here and eat your friend."

"NO!" shouted Wren. She tried to jump from Barver, but he grabbed her by the arm and held her dangling under him as he flew off.

The Hamelyn Piper looked to Patch's pursuers. "Leave him where he is," he instructed. "Let him watch his friend die."

Patch looked on in horror. Barver flew away from the Hollow until he was directly above a wide rocky outcrop.

Up, up he went, a hundred feet higher, two hundred, three, all the while ignoring Wren's screams.

At last he stopped climbing. He held Wren up in front of himself and looked at her.

Wren was distraught, tears flooding down her cheeks. She could see no emotion in his eyes, only cold obedience.

"Please," she said. "Barver—"

He dropped her to a certain death below, then turned back to kill Patch.

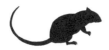

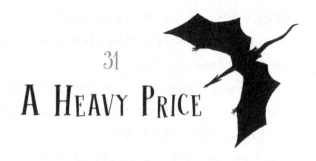

31
A HEAVY PRICE

Wren screamed as she fell. Above her she saw Barver flying off, and she knew his target was Patch. She wondered if her dracogriff friend was still conscious of what was happening. If so, he would be suffering horribly. She tumbled down through the air. She could see the rocks below her as she hurtled toward them, and she knew what she had to do.

Wren reached to her wrist and took hold of the bracelet that let her take human form. Alia's words of warning echoed in her head: *Do not remove it . . . You'd be a rat, immediately, and no amount of magic would shield you in the future.*

She pulled hard, and the bracelet came apart. The beads scattered in the air, becoming ash. Pain coursed through her body as she changed—immediately, and forevermore—into a rat.

At this size, she was safe. She could fall from any height, and the air would slow her down, cushion her.

Wren Cobble, *rat*, flopped onto the rocks and looked across to the Hollow. Barver had almost reached Patch. She closed her eyes, unable to watch.

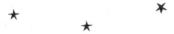

Patch saw her change and understood at once what she'd done. Tears poured down his cheeks, knowing what it had cost her.

Get away from here, Wren, he thought. She was the only one who could warn the rest of the world now.

Barver would be on him in moments. Below, the Hamelyn Piper's laugh became ever more insane as Barver approached his target. There was nothing he could do, except stand and wait for the end to come, keeping his footing on the vast organ Pipe and its gaping core.

The *Pipe*.

Patch gasped as the thought came to him. He shook his head, angry with himself for not thinking of it sooner.

Taking a deep breath, he lifted up his right foot and gathered all the courage he had. He stepped forward into empty space and fell, plunging into the darkness of the Pipe's interior. It grew narrower lower down, jamming him inside; the sense of claustrophobia was unbearable.

He could hear the Hamelyn Piper's laugh falter, hear him scream at Barver to stop. But it was far too late.

Barver would seek his prey, whatever it took.

Patch closed his eyes. A moment later, everything exploded around him.

32

AFTERMATH

Patch opened his eyes and found himself looking straight at the face of a rat: Wren was sitting on the Mask peering into an eyehole.

Get up! she signed and moved off him.

He sat up slowly. Pieces of debris fell from him—smashed organ Pipes and chunks of wood. He groaned, every part of him in pain. His lip felt swollen, and he had cuts and bruises aplenty. He started to work at the twine securing the Mask, eager to get out of it, but Barver had tied it too well.

Any bones broken? signed Wren. She was perched on a large section of smashed Pipe, a few feet away.

"I don't think so," said Patch. He looked right at her, and felt tearful. "I saw you fall," he said. "I know what you had to do. I'm so sorry . . ."

Yeah, signed Wren. She pointed to the markings around her midriff. The pattern of beads was still there, but they were all solid black now. *Being a live rat is better than being a dead girl.*

Patch reached out his hand to her, and she ran to his shoulder.

He stood, and they looked around. Everywhere in Monash Hollow, people were on the ground, out cold. In places, some were stirring, or sitting up and holding their heads. The Council members were on the grass near the stage, starting to rouse themselves.

"How long have I been unconscious?" said Patch.

I got back here a few minutes ago, signed Wren. *It was a long way to run on little feet. Half an hour maybe? I thought you were never going to wake up.*

Just in front of them a large pile of debris suddenly rose up, startling them both. A very familiar head emerged from underneath.

"What happened?" said Barver, blinking. "Why is everything blurry?"

"You plowed headfirst into the organ Pipes," said Patch. "Don't you remember anything?"

Barver frowned. He stood up, the debris falling away from him. "The last I remember I was escaping with Wren on my back!" he said. "And then I—" His mouth opened wide with horror. Huge tears welled up in his eyes.

362

"Wren!" he wailed. *"No! I killed her!"*

"It's okay!" said Patch. "She's here!"

"I can't see properly," said Barver, sniffling. "Talk to me, Wren! Let me hear your voice!"

Wren squeaked.

"She's a rat again," said Patch. "She had to break her bracelet and change back to survive the fall."

"But that means she'll never be able to change again!" said Barver, blinking away his tears. "We'll find a way, Wren. We'll find that griffin, and—" He was cut off by a shout from nearby.

"We have been attacked!" came the shout. "Get the rest of the Council back to the tent!"

Patch looked across and saw a group of Custodians; standing among them was Lord Drevis, who suddenly pointed right at Patch. "He wears the Mask of the Hamelyn Piper! Seize him!"

The Custodians ran directly at Patch. He held his arms in the air. "Hold on!" he said. "I'm not—" One of the Custodians tackled him; they hit the ground together, and the Mask popped open and came off. The Custodian pinned him down, but the relief of being out of the Mask was immense. Then Patch realized Lord Drevis was looming over him, staring.

"Good God," said Drevis. "Patch Brightwater. What have you done? Explain what happened here!"

"You were under a controlling Song, Lord," said Patch. "Everyone was! Try hard, and you'll be able to remember!"

Lord Drevis glared at him, but then his glare faded.

"There was another man . . . ," he said. He looked around at the debris. "He played a vast Pipe Organ. He tried to seize everyone's minds! You fought him!"

"That's it!" said Patch. "It's coming back to you!"

"He was—" started Drevis, but then his eyes went wide. "No. *No*." Drevis looked horrified. "Let him up," he ordered, and the Custodian released Patch and pulled him back to his feet. "I remember it now," said Drevis. "The Hamelyn Piper. How is that possible?"

"The prisoner in Tiviscan was his brother, Lord," said Patch. "He'd tricked you into imprisoning his twin, all those years ago."

"An innocent man," said Drevis, stunned. "I condemned an innocent man. Is the true villain dead?"

"He was at the keys when the organ was destroyed," said Patch. "He must have been crushed."

"Clear this area!" yelled Drevis. "Find the corpse! *Now!*" They watched as the Custodian Pipers worked to clear the debris. Patch felt a dread building deep within him. As each piece of shattered Pipe and broken timber was thrown to the side, his dread grew.

When the stage was cleared, no sign of the Hamelyn Piper—and no sign of his Puppets—had been found.

They had vanished.

Lord Drevis ordered that the search be widened. He looked at the Mask he now held, then turned to Patch. "You were thought to have died when the dragons attacked," he said. "Instead, the chaos gave you the chance to escape. But why take the Mask?"

Patch shrugged. "I honestly don't know. But I'm glad I did."

Drevis folded it, inverting it again. "It protected you," he said. "Smart lad. And it's lucky for us that you came back to Tiviscan. Now, there's much you have to explain to the Council. Come with me."

Patch looked across to Barver and Wren, who were clearly anxious. He signed to them: *Wait here.* Then he followed Drevis, who led him across the Hollow to a sumptuous tent where two Custodians stood guard outside. Drevis held the tent flap open for Patch. Inside, the other four members of the Council sat on wooden stools around a central table. Each of them bore scratches that showed how near the stage they had been when Barver had destroyed the Pipe Organ. Some held small glasses filled with a brown liquid that Patch suspected was brandy; he could see more than one hand trembling a little.

Patch stayed by the tent entrance, but Drevis strode over to the others.

"Your memories have returned?" Drevis asked them.

"More or less," said Lord Cobb. "Imagine, all this time. An innocent man in the dungeons!"

Drevis said nothing, but Patch knew the comment must have pained him.

"Those Pipes were obsidiac glazed," said Lady Winkless.

"Impossible!" cried Lord Pewter.

"No, no, he's correct," said Lady Rumsey. She held a fragment up. "I've yet to do the sums, but the glaze is thick. There must have been a vast store! Goodness knows how he got all that obsidiac."

Patch kept silent—he would tell Lord Drevis what he knew about the source of the black diamond, nobody else.

"Wherever it came from, it's ours now," said Lord Cobb. "It's a source of unspeakable power, and it will be researched. I'll put our top people on to it!"

"The dragons may have something to say about that," said Lord Drevis.

"Let them," said Cobb. "One thing's for certain, that amount of obsidiac will be very handy in rebuilding the castle defenses."

Patch had listened to this madness long enough. "You must destroy every fragment!" he cried.

Lord Cobb frowned. "Who's this? We're discussing sensitive Council business! This is no place for a boy!"

Drevis gestured for Patch to come closer, and Patch saw Lord Pewter sit up sharply, eyes wide.

"This is Patch Brightwater," said Drevis. "*This* is who was wearing the Mask and fought the Hamelyn Piper."

"Brightwater?" said Lady Rumsey, peering at Patch. "Didn't we lock him up?"

"We did," said Drevis. "He was in the cell next to the Hamelyn Piper—well, the Piper's *brother*, as we now know. Brightwater was presumed dead after the dragon attack."

"Well then, there's only one course of action!" said Lady Rumsey. "Guard!" One of the Custodians entered the tent. "Throw this criminal in a cell at once."

"What are you doing?" said Lord Pewter.

"The law demands it!" Lady Rumsey replied.

"Enough!" said Drevis. "He saved us all. I believe a suitable reward is appropriate for his courage." On the table in front of him was a small chest, which he opened. He took out paper and a quill and wrote for a few moments. When he was done, he stood and showed what he'd written to each member of the Council. "Any objections?" he said. There were none, although Lady Rumsey looked slightly peeved. "Good."

Drevis passed the paper to Patch, and Patch read it.

It was a pardon. It absolved him of all guilt and meant he was free. Tears rolled down his cheeks, and he didn't care. He folded the pardon up and placed it in his pocket, his fingers brushing against another piece of paper—Alia's prophecy, and an unwelcome reminder of Erner. Even so, the joy and relief he felt at being pardoned was so strong he thought his legs might buckle.

"Wait!" cried Lord Pewter, rummaging in the chest where Drevis had found the paper. He took out a small block of wood and what looked like an ink pad. "It still needs stamping with the Council Seal to make it official."

Drevis smiled and held his hand out. "My mistake. Can I have it back for a moment, Patch?"

Patch reluctantly took the pardon out of his pocket and returned it, feeling like it would burst into flames or simply vanish, but it was stamped and back in his grasp within seconds.

Drevis smiled at him. "When this immediate chaos abates, we must talk more. I'd like to know just how a disgraced trainee saved Tiviscan, and the world."

"The Hamelyn Piper is still out there, Lord," said Patch. "The world isn't saved yet."

"You saved it for today, at least," said Drevis. "That's all a hero can ever do."

At that, the tent flap opened and an out-of-breath Custodian entered. "Lord Drevis, your presence is needed."

"Good," said Drevis. He looked to the Council. "The hunt for the Hamelyn Piper is being organized in the castle as we speak, and I must oversee it."

"But there are things I must tell you—" said Patch.

"It will keep until later," said Drevis, and he left.

"I suppose we too should make our way to the castle,"

said Lord Cobb. He stood slowly from his stool and began heading out.

"Oh, please wait," said Lady Winkless. "I need to sit a moment longer. I'm too old to be in such a hurry."

"Indeed," said Lord Pewter. "Allow us to finish our brandies, at least."

"Oh, very well," said Lord Cobb. He turned back to the table, then stopped, gesturing to something on the ground near Patch's feet. He looked at Patch. "Did you drop your pardon, lad?"

But Patch still had the pardon in his hand. He looked down and saw what Cobb meant, and realized at once what it was. He checked his pocket to be sure, and yes—the pocket was empty. When he'd removed the pardon to be stamped, the paper with Alia's prophecy had come out too and fallen to the ground.

Lord Cobb picked it up and unfolded it. Patch had a curious sense of unease.

"'They thought they had us,'" Cobb read aloud, in a monotone voice. "'But we're almost clear. Just the ridge to go. What's wrong with you? What's wrong?'" Lord Cobb looked up from the paper. "An *odd* set of words, don't you think?" he said.

Patch felt every drop of blood drain from his face. He could hear Alia's voice in his mind, saying exactly the same thing: *An odd set of words, don't you think?*

"I agree," said Lady Winkless. "Very odd."

"What say you, Patch?" said Lord Pewter.

Patch stayed silent too stunned to answer.

"The lad's gone so very pale," said Lady Rumsey. "The day's been *quite* a strain, I imagine!"

An odd set of words, don't you think? I agree, very odd. What say you, Patch? The lad's gone so very pale. The day's been quite a strain, I imagine.

The precise words Alia had spoken. Patch had thought that those words were mere ramblings, but instead they had simply been a continuation of the prophecy.

There will come a time when you hear these words, Alia had told him. *A mouth that speaks them is a traitorous mouth. This* was the first time the words had been spoken in their entirety. *This* was the moment the prophecy had warned him of.

This moment and no other.

He felt sick with guilt. Erner had never been a traitor. The *Council* were the ones who had spoken the words. *They* were the ones who would betray him to whatever he feared the most.

When Erner had said it, Patch had most feared returning to the dungeons, being put back into the Dark by Rundel Stone.

But now . . .

His mouth went dry as he thought about what he feared most now. It was the leering face of the Hamelyn Piper that came to mind.

He looked at the Council, trying hard to keep his emotions from showing.

Get away as quickly as you can, Alia had said. *Run!*

The Council were still awaiting an explanation of what was written on the piece of paper. "Just the words of a song I heard," said Patch. "I wrote them down. Odd words indeed. Now, if the Council will permit, I think I need to go and get some rest."

"Indeed!" said Lord Cobb. "We'll speak again later, as Lord Drevis said."

Patch managed to smile. He prayed that it seemed genuine, because at that moment he wanted to scream and run from the tent.

"Absolutely," he said, and left.

Somehow he kept that smile going all the way out of the Council tent and across the Hollow.

He reached his friends. Barver was lying face down on the grass, his wings outstretched and badly cut. Wren was perched on his snout. "Ah, there you are!" said Barver. "How did it go?"

"Um," said Patch. "Yes. It went . . . fine. I was pardoned. Which was good." He coughed. "How's your eyesight? Still blurry? Can you fly, do you think?"

"Oh, my eyesight's recovered," said Barver. "But flying? I doubt it." He sat up and used his hand to lift one wing, then let it drop. It was completely limp. "Something's broken in there." He picked the tip up and bent it right back, making Patch and Wren wince. "It shouldn't be able to do that, either," he said, with a shrug.

"Perhaps we should, um, journey to Marwheel and call in on Brother Duffle to treat you?" said Patch. "Right now?"

"Oh, I'd rather rest for a few days," said Barver. "We all should! You seem agitated, Patch. Do you need to empty your bladder or something?"

Wren frowned with concern. *You do seem agitated,* she signed. *What's wrong?*

And even though there was nobody close enough to eavesdrop, Patch leaned over and whispered to them both, explaining what had just happened.

Barver stared at him. Wren stared too.

"Alia warned me that prophecies were dangerous things," said Patch, frowning. "Never straightforward, she said. Tend to cause endless trouble."

"She was certainly right about *that,*" said Barver. "So," said Patch. "Marwheel Abbey, anyone?"

Wren hopped from Barver's snout to Patch's shoulder.

We should leave at once, but how can we get away unseen?

Patch nodded to the edge of the Hollow farthest from Tiviscan. "We can reach the Penance River from that side," he said. "If we can sneak into the trees, it's forest all the way."

"Avoid the roads," said Barver. "Good."

We've done it before, signed Wren.

"Are we sure about this, Patch?" said Barver. "The prophecy already led us astray once. You say the Council will betray us to the Hamelyn Piper, but how? And what about Lord Drevis? My mother trusted him."

Patch shook his head, uncertain. "Drevis left the tent before it happened. Perhaps he's trustworthy, perhaps not. That must be for Tobias, Alia, and Rundel Stone to decide, when we tell them what's happened here. Let *them* deal with the Hamelyn Piper. We have our own business to attend to."

"Yes!" said Barver. "Our own business—to find Underath's griffin!"

Wren looked dejected. *Alia said breaking my bracelet would leave me permanently changed. Nothing can be done for me now.*

"What kind of talk is that?" scoffed Barver. "We'll find that griffin, Wren, and all will be well."

"There's something we have to do first," said Patch. He pictured Erner's shocked face as he'd fallen from Barver and into the lake below, swimming for shore to an uncertain future at the hands of those mercenaries. "We have a friend to rescue," he said. "Agreed?"

Agreed, signed Wren.

"Agreed," said Barver.

The Hollow itself was emptying, people going back to the town and castle. Patch led the way to the far edge of the

Hollow, and they waited. When they thought it would be safe, they walked into the cover of the trees.

Their departure went entirely unnoticed.

So it was that the three friends—Piper, dracogriff, and rat—began the journey that would take them, eventually, back to Marwheel Abbey. Even after they reached the Penance River, each step they took was leaden, as they fretted about Erner, and the Council, and the Hamelyn Piper.

"Look at us," said Barver. "Together we saved the world, but we're weighed down by worries!"

You should play a Lift and lighten our mood, Patch, signed Wren. *Like you did to the little ant and the monks in Marwheel.*

"My new Pipe was destroyed," said Patch, thinking of the terrible feeling of loss he'd suffered when it happened. "I hope you can spare a few more feathers, Barver, when I make a new one?"

Barver nodded. "As many as you require."

Can't you play the Lift without a Pipe? signed Wren.

"I can try," said Patch. But his lip, injured when the Pipe Organ was destroyed, was too swollen. When he tried to whistle, all that came out were flubs and raspberries. "Sorry," he said.

"Never mind," said Barver. "Do you know the shanty 'Farewell the Winter's Frowning'? It's popular in the Islands."

"It's popular everywhere," said Patch. He cleared his

throat and started to sing, his voice unsteady. *"Farewell the winter's frowning,"* he began. *"The sun's smile comes again."* As Patch sang the rest of the verse, Barver sang too.

Wren joined in with tuneful squeaks.

They gave voice to the lyrics of hope and renewal, and as they did their singing grew ever more heartfelt. Soon enough, hope had truly bloomed within them; they smiled and laughed once more. And all from a simple shanty.

For there is a truth, one that is all too easy to forget: There is magic in music.

Listen . . .

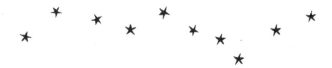

Patch, Wren, and Barver return for a second
spell-slinging, shape-shifting, flame-throwing

✦SONGS OF MAGIC✦

adventure in . . .

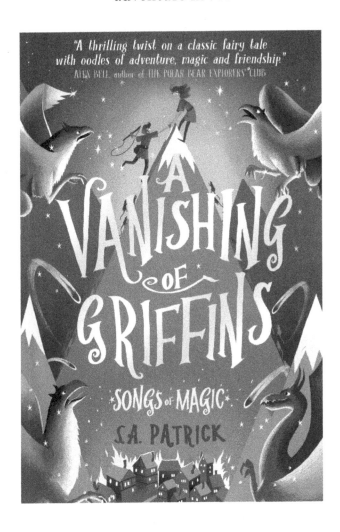

"A thrilling twist on a classic fairy tale
with oodles of adventure, magic and friendship"
ALEX BELL, author of THE POLAR BEAR EXPLORERS' CLUB

A VANISHING OF GRIFFINS

✦SONGS OF MAGIC✦

S.A. PATRICK

1

Whatever Happened to Erner Whitlock?

Erner woke, as he did every morning, from a nightmare: being pushed off the back of a dracogriff, into a cold lake far below. In his nightmare, the face of the person who had pushed him was smiling a terrible smile, cruel and cold, *laughing* as Erner tumbled through the air and into the icy water, his Pipe slipping from his fingers and lost to the depths.

When it had actually happened, though, there had been no smile on Patch Brightwater's face: he had looked utterly terrified.

A question had burned inside Erner ever since that fateful day, and he knew that there was only one way he would ever get an answer.

He would have to find Patch Brightwater, someone he'd always thought was a friend, and ask him *why*.

Why did you push me into the lake?

Erner's journey since then had been eventful. It had brought him, eventually, to the Islands of the Eastern Sea, and to the court of one of the many Pirate Kings and Queens. Here on the island of Pengersick was an old fortress, where the King of Pengersick had his palace. It was in the heart of that fortress that Erner was imprisoned now: hanging in a tiny cage next to the throne of a Pirate King.

The King snored on his throne. He always slept there when he threw a party, and he'd thrown a party almost every night since taking the crown. The floor of the throne room was covered in sleeping pirates and empty rum bottles.

Erner's legs were going numb. He shifted his weight, working his feet out from under him, trying not to make his cage swing—if the cage swung, the rope it hung from would creak, and the creak might wake the King.

That was never a good idea. Two nights before, one of the pirates had let out a belch that was long and thunderous as everyone slept. He'd woken the King. Worse, he'd *laughed* about it.

In front of the throne were a dozen wooden spikes, and on the top of each spike was the severed head of someone who had displeased the King. The head of the belching pirate was there, the freshest of the bunch.

Yes, waking the Pirate King was never a good idea. He was *not* a morning person.

Arpie Noss was his name—King Arpie to his subjects. He hadn't been King long. Two months, that was all, but it had been a *busy* two months. Pirate rulers didn't tend to last, and it seemed that Arpie Noss had been trying to fit as much as possible into whatever time he had.

Like buying Erner, for a start.

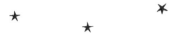

Erner was an apprentice in the Custodian Elite. Held in the highest esteem, the Custodians only accepted the best Pipers into their ranks.

The magical Songs that Pipers played could achieve wondrous things: there were Songs to conjure winds to sweep snow from blocked roads; Songs to make seeds sprout in barren fields; Songs that helped wounds to heal. There were even Songs that could defend against *armies*.

Pipers usually specialized in one kind of Song, but Custodians excelled at them all, using their skills with the Pipe to help wherever they could.

To the poor and downtrodden of the world, the Custodian Elite represented justice and hope, and for Erner there was no greater honor than being part of their ranks. For many, the greatest honor of all would be to become a member of the Pipers' Council, as they were the highest authority among Pipers, and decided the laws of Piping. But it was the

Custodian Elite who *upheld* those laws, and much more besides.

Erner had gone with Patch Brightwater to visit the castle of Underath the Sorcerer, hoping that the Sorcerer would help their friend Wren—a girl cursed into the shape of a rat.

When they'd reached the castle, however, they had found Underath seriously wounded and in hiding, his castle occupied by violent mercenaries. When the mercenaries had discovered them, the Sorcerer had hidden again; Erner and the others had fled on the back of Barver the dracogriff, as the mercenaries gave chase.

Just as they seemed to be out of danger, Patch had suddenly pushed Erner off Barver's back, into the lake below.

Erner had managed to swim to the side of the lake; exhausted, he'd expected the mercenaries to kill him. The moment they saw Erner's robes, however, they realized he was in the Custodian Elite. Killing him wasn't worth the kind of trouble it could bring down on their heads.

Instead, the mercenaries did what they always did: they tried to think of a way to make some money out of the situation. They'd already plundered everything of value from Underath's castle, and the time had come for them to move on; extra money would be welcome.

They considered holding him ransom, but the Custodian Elite was far too powerful a foe, with far too long a memory.

Such a course of action would end disastrously, they decided.

But there were, they knew, criminals in the world who were reckless enough, or foolish enough, to actually *enjoy* the thought of angering the Custodians.

Pirates.

So a letter was sent to the Pirate Kings and Queens of the territories of the Islands of the Eastern Sea, all two hundred and twelve of them. *We have come into the possession of a young apprentice in the Custodian Elite,* said the letter. *For a simple payment of one hundred gold muttles, you may have him as your prisoner, and show how little you fear the Custodians! Although none shall pay, for none would dare!*

The Custodian Elite tended to leave the Islands of the Eastern Sea alone, but it would take a particularly foolish and reckless pirate to think that a captive Custodian wouldn't be a huge risk. Luckily for the mercenaries, one of the Pirate Kings and Queens *was* particularly foolish and reckless.

Arpie Noss, newly crowned King of Pengersick, looking to make his mark in the pirate world. *What better way,* thought King Arpie, *than to do something nobody had ever done before?*

He wanted everyone to see how *fearless* he was!

He wanted everyone to see how *wealthy* he was!

And so Erner was sold. He spent a week blindfolded and chained in the stinking hull of a ship, his stomach heaving with every swell of the sea, and then he was brought before the King.

"Is this what I paid for?" said King Arpie. "Not exactly formidable..." The King prodded Erner with his staff. "Put him in a little cage hanging by my throne!" he said to a tall, skinny man standing beside him. The skinny man looked anxious. "Snap to it, Skreep! I gave you an order!"

"Yes, Your Majesty," said Skreep. "But surely the Custodians will be angry when they find out?"

"Of course they will!" said the King. "That's the whole *point*! Every pirate will know that I, King Arpie, fear nobody! You worry too much, Skreep. Worry less!" Skreep nodded and seemed to relax ever so slightly. "That's an order, by the way," added the King. "Worry less, or I will have you *killed*."

Skreep looked much less relaxed.

And so, they had built Erner a cage. It wasn't quite high enough for him to sit upright, or long enough for him to lie down, and in the weeks he'd been here he had yet to discover a way to sleep without some part of him being numb when he woke. He'd learned that as long as he was quiet, he was forgotten. Sometimes, one of King Arpie's pirates would amuse themselves by throwing insults to see if Erner responded. But Erner did not respond, and interest was soon lost.

He was given the bare minimum to eat and drink. Once a day, he was taken from the cage, manacled, and led outside;

there, he would do what needed to be done, and they would douse him with buckets of cold water when he was finished.

Yet Erner considered himself lucky. While King Arpie was eager to show how badly he treated his captive, Erner was a prized possession: no real harm was allowed to befall him.

Eventually, he knew, the Pipers' Council would do all in their power to find him, and they would make an example of King Arpie Noss. It would not be pleasant.

Then, once free, Erner could find Patch Brightwater.

He could finally ask him *why*.

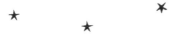

Once Erner had shifted his legs—without making the rope creak—the pins and needles subsided, and he dozed. After a while, the entrance to the throne room swung open; a nervous pirate came inside and woke Skreep, the King's advisor. A few whispers later, Skreep looked very worried indeed. He came over to the throne, and gave a little cough, but the King kept snoring. "Your Majesty . . . ," said Skreep, and then he just threw caution to the wind. "Arpie, wake up!"

King Arpie's eyes opened wide and he drew his sword, putting it to Skreep's throat. "Assassin!" he cried, then saw who it was and put his sword away. "Oh. What is it? Lunchtime already?"

"No, Your Majesty," said Skreep. "A couple of trouble-makers have been chained up and brought for your judgment, sire. They were asking questions about *him*." He threw a narrow-eyed glare at Erner, then looked back at the King, probably hoping for some sign of concern.

Instead, the King grinned. "Ah ha! They've got wind of it at last! Sent some spies to check! This is good news, Skreep!"

Skreep gave a huge sigh. "This is *bad* news, Your Majesty. It was only a matter of time, and I'd hoped to talk you 'round before the Custodians found out, but . . ."

King Arpie looked at him in horror. "*Talk me 'round?* I'm King Arpie Noss! I make the decisions! I fear nobody! What's the point of trying to make the Custodians look like fools if they don't know I'm doing it?" He reached to the floor and picked up a tankard, half-full of stale ale. He drank it down and started to bang the tankard against the metalwork that arched over his throne. It was the alarm call everyone in the palace knew well—the King has awoken, and when the King wakes up, all his subjects have to *damn well wake up, too.*

"Rise and shine, you lot!" shouted the King. There was a lot of wincing and blinking from the waking revelers, but absolutely no complaining—the heads on spikes were a constant reminder that an unbuttoned mouth was bad for your health. "Seems the Custodians have learned about my little *pet,*" he said, smiling at Erner. "And the idiots have sent some spies, who've been so kind as to be captured! I want you all to be on your best form, understand? Lots of sneering and glaring! *Bring in the spies!*"

Everyone in the throne room looked eagerly to the doorway, where, with a burly pirate at the front and another guarding the rear, in came a wretched pair of manacled prisoners, with sackcloth bags over their heads.

Erner felt sorry for them. In all likelihood, they were just two people who'd happened to ask about the King's new trophy because it was *interesting*. The King himself had wanted people *everywhere* to talk about it. To suddenly call someone a spy because they'd done what the King had been desperate for people to do . . . Well, that made Erner's sense of injustice burn deep inside him.

The two prisoners were led to the only clear area of the throne room floor, right in front of King Arpie and the spiked heads. There was a *reason* that area was left clear—a reason closely related to a certain *lever* by one arm of the King's throne.

A lever that, when pulled, opened up a large trapdoor right where the prisoners now stood.

"Let's have a look at them," said the King. One of the pirate guards stepped forward and pulled the cloth bag off the first prisoner's head.

A woman. Erner had seen her before, but for a moment he couldn't place where. She gave King Arpie a look of absolute contempt.

Then Erner remembered where he'd seen her, and his stomach lurched in a way it hadn't lurched since his horrible sea journey.

Alia, thought Erner. That was her name. She'd accompanied Patch and Wren back to Marwheel Abbey, after their trip to see the Witch of Gemspar Mountain. The trip had been a success—Wren, who had been cursed into the form of a rat, had been granted the ability to change back into her human shape, albeit just for short periods. He'd met Alia only briefly then—she had introduced herself as some kind of expert in magic and had seemed very friendly with Patch and Wren.

He turned his eyes to the second prisoner, who was quite a bit shorter than Alia, and a terrible feeling washed over him.

No, he thought. *It can't be.*

The guard gripped the cloth bag covering the second prisoner's head, and yanked.

There, only ten feet from Erner's cage, stood the whole reason that Erner was here at all.

Patch Brightwater. Looking terrified. And Erner could just make out a small shifting bulge in the chest pocket of Patch's coat, which he strongly suspected was a certain rat-shaped friend.

Erner had had plenty of time to wonder how he would feel when he saw Patch again—anger, perhaps, or even hatred. Now that the moment had arrived, he felt no animosity at all. What he felt was *apprehension*.

If they had come to rescue him, they had made a terrible, terrible mistake.

King Arpie cleared his throat. "Pitiful prisoners! You're accused of being spies for the Custodian Elite, on account of you asking questions about my pet Piper." He thwacked Erner's cage with his staff. "Do you confess?" He grinned, and at that moment Erner knew that the King didn't *care* if they were spies, not really. All he cared about was that *other people* would think it.

Alia's eyes narrowed as she spoke. "We don't represent the Custodian Elite, Your Majesty," she said. "We're here to ask you to show mercy and release a friend." She nodded to Erner. "He is a—"

But the King interrupted. "Yes, yes, blah, blah, yakkity yak! You're a spy, admit it! You admit he's a friend, so admit you're a spy and be done with it! We don't have all day."

Erner saw the King's hand move toward the lever. "No!" he cried, and the King gave him a sharp look and another *thwack*.

Alia was also looking at the King's hand, and at the lever it was now touching. "Don't do anything you might regret, sire," she said. Her voice was laced with the direst of warnings, a sound of deep foreboding woven into every word she uttered.

There was sorcery at work here, Erner realized. The woman's voice would make anyone with sense pause for a moment and wonder why it felt like the very stones of the throne room walls were shaking as she spoke. She was obviously powerful; ignoring her would be a very foolish thing indeed.

Unfortunately, King Arpie Noss was a very foolish man.

"This is how King Arpie deals with spies!" said the King. He pulled his lever. The floor under the prisoners swung down, and Erner watched them fall, their cries disappearing into the dark below. Everyone in the room listened, until at last the cries ceased and the trapdoor swung closed again.

Erner was in so much shock he could hardly breathe. He didn't know what awaited his would-be rescuers, but he did know *this*: the trapdoor led to a winding shaft, down which prisoners would tumble until they reached the bottom and found themselves in a place of absolute horror.

A place the pirates called "The Pit of Screaming Death."

King Arpie clapped his hands together in excitement and jumped out of his throne. "Come on, then," he said. "Everyone to the viewing gallery!" He nodded toward Erner. "Bring him along, Skreep. Let him watch. It'll be fun!"

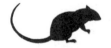

ACKNOWLEDGMENTS

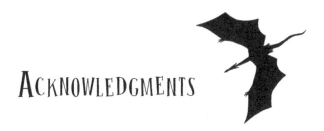

Patch, Wren, and Barver have been waiting a very long time for me to tell their story. I thank them for their patience.

Thanks also to my agent, Luigi Bonomi, who encouraged me to follow my heart when I was dithering about what to work on next.

I'm indebted to Anne Finnis, Rebecca Hill, and Sarah Stewart at Usborne for all their help and support in turning my early efforts into the finished work you have in your hands.

My final thanks, of course, go to my wife and children. Without you, there would be no music at all.

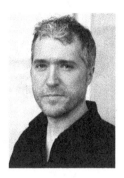

About the Author

S. A. Patrick was born in Belfast. When he was a child, he wanted to write video games, become an author, and have magical powers. The first two came true. If he does ever get magical powers, he hopes people like dragons and griffins because there'll suddenly be a lot of them around.

He has had four previous books published as Seth Patrick. *Songs of Magic: A Darkening of Dragons* is his first book for children.

Follow S. A. Patrick online

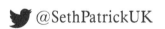 @SethPatrickUK

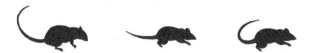